Running Group Visits in Your Practice

Edward B. Noffsinger, Ph.D.

Running Group Visits in Your Practice

Foreword by Zeev E. Neuwirth, MD

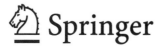 Springer

Edward B. Noffsinger, Ph.D.
Harvard Vanguard Medical Associates
275 Grove Street, Suite 300-3
Newton, MA 02466
USA

ISBN 978-1-4419-1413-2   (hardcover)
ISBN 978-0-387-33683-1   (softcover)   e-ISBN 978-0-387-68680-6
DOI 10.1007/b106441
Springer New York Dordrecht Heidelberg London

Library of Congress Control Number: 2009933983

Printed on acid-free paper

Springer is part of Springer Science+Business Media (www.springer.com)

First of all, I dedicate this book to my loving wife, Janet, who shared these experiences with me from the start, and whose warm love and gentle kindness nourished and sustained me throughout. Also to my dear children—Michael, Angie, and Kenny—whom I love dearly and are always in my heart. And finally to the many DIGMA and PSMA physicians and patients who had the courage to participate in this new healthcare innovation during its early stages, as they provided me with the multitude of practical experiences that were so necessary to my learning the many lessons that are presented in this book for the benefit of others.

Foreword

A Fateful Meeting

A year and a half ago, I was sitting at a conference listening to Ed Noffsinger speak, and suddenly had the most profound "Aha" moment of my professional career. Here was someone presenting a practical and tested solution to some of the most challenging problems currently plaguing the US healthcare system, problems such as poor access to primary and specialty care; the uncontainable and rising costs of healthcare; our nation's relatively poor quality outcomes; and finally, the sense of frustration, disempowerment, loneliness, and disenfranchisement that patients and their families too often experience.

Dr. Noffsinger's solution seemed deceptively simple—shared medical appointments (SMAs) that afford the highest quality healthcare to be delivered in the highest quality care experience—a group setting. Experience collected over a decade and involving more than 100,000 patient visits throughout the United States, Canada, and parts of Europe has demonstrated that SMAs, when used in primary care as well as in the medical and surgical subspecialties, lead to increased access to care, enhanced quality of care, and improved patient satisfaction. For physicians, the efficiency gains and team support from their participation in SMAs translate into much needed relief and improved career satisfaction.

Dr. Noffsinger's lecture was so inspiring that I waited in line over an hour after his presentation for the opportunity to speak to him. Our conversation that afternoon ended up lasting nearly 4 hours, at the conclusion of which I hesitantly asked if he and his lovely wife, Jan, would consider leaving their home in California and set up residence in Boston to join us at Harvard Vanguard Medical Associates, an affiliate of Atrius Health. Atrius Health is a multispecialty, ambulatory care practice of approximately 700 clinicians and 4000 non-clinical staff providing medical care to approximately 700,000 patients across eastern Massachusetts. By the end of our conversation that day, I was convinced that Ed's unconventional and creative approach to the delivery of ambulatory care had the potential to transform not only our practice, but quite possibly the delivery of medical care in the United States.

A Bold Vision

What I proposed to Ed and Jan that day had two elements—the first part was somewhat enterprising, but the second was audacious. First, I wanted Ed to join us at Atrius Health, as the Director of Shared Medical Appointments, and lead an organization-wide initiative in implementing his two SMA models—the Drop-In Group Medical Appointment (DIGMA) for follow-up visits and the Physical Shared Medical Appointment (PSMA) for physical examination visits. Second, Ed would create a world-class center of excellence for SMAs at Atrius Health and establish an institute for the study, training, and dissemination of SMAs to healthcare organizations across the country and around the world.

The vision we crafted that afternoon was bold. It was apparent to me that the DIGMA and PSMA models had profound implications for medical practice and patient care. While listening to Dr. Noffsinger speak that day, the fundamental question in my mind had quickly shifted from "Why should we offer SMAs to our patients?" to "How could we not offer SMAs, not only for our patients, but also for our providers of care?" This rapid shift may sound premature or even outlandish. But I can safely say that now, after a year of working closely with Dr. Noffsinger to implement SMAs throughout our practice, I've become even more convinced that the widespread implementation of SMAs in medical practice has the power to significantly improve the delivery of healthcare in the United States and across the globe.

The Physician's Job Is No Longer Doable and the Situation Is Getting Worse

We, in the United States, are facing a *perfect storm* in healthcare delivery today. Physicians, particularly in primary care and geriatrics medicine, are retiring and are not being sufficiently replaced by a new generation of doctors. Simultaneously, the baby boomers are about to enter their Medicare years and will be requiring increasing medical attention. In fact, the aging baby boomer population, due to their increased prevalence of obesity, will require more medical care than previous generations of similar age. And finally, to complete this perfect storm, the most obese and morbid pediatric population in our history will be entering adulthood and will also be requiring more medical attention than their young adult predecessors. Completing this perfect storm are the tens of millions of uninsured Americans to whom healthcare benefits are likely to be extended in the not too distant future. The question is "Who will take care of these people, and who will provide them with high quality, low cost, personalized, preventive primary care?"

Related to the critical issues of access and quality of care is the realization, based on a growing body of evidence, that the daily clinical responsibilities and demands placed on physicians are quite literally impossible to accomplish. A 2005 article in the *Annals of Family Medicine* estimated that it would require primary care physicians 18 hours a day to adequately and responsibly deliver evidence-based preventive and chronic disease management care to their patients (1). These 18 hours do not even include the diagnosis and treatment of acute medical problems. A reasonable solution might be to increase the number of primary care clinicians. However, in fact, the number of new entrants into primary care medicine has precipitously declined over the past decade. At this point in time—due in large part to the physician *job doability* issue mentioned previously—only 2% of medical students are entering general internal medicine (2).

A recent report by Sg2 (a health-care think tank located in Chicago) predicts that by 2020, given the rapidly declining supply of primary care physicians and the increasing primary care needs of our population, the typical primary care provider will be required to manage a panel size of 10,000 patients— nearly a five-fold increase above the current average panel size (3). Another recent report—this one from the Institute of Medicine— cites a current ratio of one geriatrician for every 2500 Americans who are 75 or older. They predict that this ratio is expected to worsen to one geriatrician per 4300 elderly Americans by 2030 (4). These scenarios are not vague predictions for some remote future. The impact on patient access is already being experienced by patients as evidenced by recent data from the Massachusetts Medical Society 2008 Physician Workforce study, which reveals that nearly half (48%) of Internal Medicine physicians are *not* accepting new patients (this is up from 31% only 2 years ago) and that the average wait time for an Internal Medicine appointment is 50 days. This study also lists 12 medical specialties in severe short supply, with nearly 75% of physician groups and hospitals reporting difficulty in filling their physician vacancies (5).

What Is Needed Is a Completely New Way of Thinking About Healthcare Delivery

So, what are we to do about this critical and escalating situation? I would argue that what is needed is not incremental change but radical and disruptive innovation—a substantial departure from the current way of delivering healthcare services. The DIGMA and PSMA models represent such a change. Albert Einstein noted that the solution to a problem cannot be derived from the same thinking or approach that led to the problem in the first place. Henry Ford reflected that if he had listened to the experts of his day, he would simply have built a better horse and buggy instead of developing the automobile. My concern with many of the current attempts to solve our healthcare system's problems is that, instead of moving us in a new direction of building the next paradigm, they continue to advance the *horse and buggy* of healthcare delivery. Professor Clayton Christensen of the Harvard Business School defines a *disruptive innovation* as one that allows for greater access and convenience to the public users of a product or service, at lower cost, and with quality outcomes that are deemed relatively sufficient for the purposes at hand as perceived by the consumers of that service or product (6). What I expect will become apparent over the next few pages and throughout the chapters of this book is that the DIGMA and PSMA models meet the criteria of a disruptive innovation and provide us with a new paradigm, a new approach to healthcare delivery—one that is more efficient, effective, and humane.

After Only 10 Months' Experience, Numerous Benefits Are Already Becoming Clear

It was with this hope for creating a better future that we at Harvard Vanguard Medical Associates and the other medical groups of Atrius Health asked Dr. Noffsinger to join our organization as Director of Shared Medical Appointments in December 2007. Fortunately, our own early (10-month) experience in implementing SMAs at Harvard Vanguard Medical Associates corroborates Dr. Noffsinger's 12-year track record of achievement. It is a testament to his success here that, within 1 year, he's been promoted to Vice President of Shared Medical Appointments and Group-Based Disease Management.

We are actively collecting data on numerous metrics and hope to have substantial and rigorous quantitative evidence of our success with SMAs. Our preliminary data and experience—based on the implementation of over 15 different DIGMAs and PSMAs to date—suggests that SMAs enhance: (1) the patient care experience and patient satisfaction with the care they receive; (2) clinician efficiency and job doability; (3) the morale and job satisfaction of the clinical and nonclinical support staff; (4) access to care for patients; (5) physicians' ability to increase their panel size and re-open their closed practices to new patients; (6) the cost-effectiveness of care; and (7) most importantly, the quality and safety of medical care that we are able to deliver to our patients.

The SMA Model Offers a Quantum Leap Forward in the Patient Care Experience

We are currently conducting patient satisfaction surveys (using a standardized and widely deployed assessment tool) and expect to have benchmarked data within a few months. In the meantime, our internally developed SMA patient satisfaction survey (which we've now had 120 patients complete) reveals that 96% of patients who have participated in a

DIGMA or PSMA would schedule another one and 98% would recommend it to their family and friends. One hundred percent of patients surveyed reported that the overall visit experience was the same as or better than their prior individual visits, with nearly 70% indicating that the SMA was actually better. These are impressive data given that many of these SMA visits were early experiences for the physicians and their teams, who were still on a steep learning curve. This is also a completely new offering and experience for our patients—a radical departure from the way they're used to receiving care, which makes the highly positive reception even more remarkable.

One major benefit to our patients, which we had not truly appreciated until recently, stems from the group dynamic itself; having patients in a room together, listening to and supporting one another. We are discovering that the social, psychological, and self-management benefits of the SMA experience are particularly significant. The effect is similar to a high performing sports team in which everyone's energy is intensely focused, with a strong feeling of intangible personal connection among the participants. This unique group dynamic is qualitatively different from the individual visit experience. Patients as well as the clinical team often come away from these SMA visits feeling refreshed, renewed, and energized. Our group visit implementation team constantly hears patients reporting on this specific aspect of SMAs. Comments gleaned from our in-house patient survey include: "I had felt so alone before, but in that room I felt like I was with family"; "It helped me to hear the answers to other patients' questions that I had not thought to ask, but which are important to me"; and "It's nice to know that other people are in the same boat and doing well." From our perspective, this experiential component is just as important as the more concrete and quantifiable benefits such as improved access.

The *healthful social benefits* of group visits should come as no surprise. Recent research in the treatment of obesity and diabetes has already demonstrated that group-based interventions have tremendous efficacy in producing positive health outcomes (7). Emerging understandings and concrete measurable results from such diverse fields as behavioral neuroscience, business management, and the social sciences are revealing that group-based interactions not only enhance an individual's experience but also lead to more efficient and effective outcomes. New terms such as *social intelligence, wisdom of the crowd, group genius, open sourcing, crowd sourcing, distributed leadership,* and *wikinomics* are being coined to describe the power of social networks and social networking within our personal and professional endeavors. The rapid increase, over the past decade, in the number of adults who are now using the Internet for healthcare-related purposes—the so-called Health 2.0 movement—underscores patients' desire to network and be in community with one another. In fact, the Harris Poll reported that in 2008, 66% of all US adults (or 81% of those who use the Internet) participated in online healthcare list services, web-based health-related social networking, and online patient communities (8).

We are so intrigued and excited by the interpersonal dynamics of group patient visits that we are planning to engage social scientists to help us better understand these phenomena and how they might translate not only into an enhanced patient experience, but also improved health. Again, this should come as no surprise as there is already a rich body of medical research that supports our observations and provides us with a theoretical framework. Dr. Arthur Kleinman, the noted Harvard medical anthropologist, has written about the *illness experience* and described it as a sociocultural phenomenon—not a technical or physiologic one (9). Our perception of illness is a social construct—formed by our family, our friends, our culture, *and* our healthcare providers. These perceptions, assumptions, and beliefs—all social phenomena—play a profound role in our motivations and behaviors around illness and health—behaviors that include medication taking, treatment follow-up, appropriate nutrition and physical activity, smoking cessation, and reducing alcohol consumption.

Over the past few years, there has been much emphasis in the medical literature on *patient activation* and *self-management*. This emphasis is based on our growing understanding that the behaviors of the patient are just as important in determining health outcomes—if not more so—than the activities or input of medical professionals (10). And despite this growing awareness, we still continue to practice medicine and deliver healthcare in ways that fundamentally underappreciate, underestimate, and underuse the power of social interaction and groups to create profound learning, action, and positive change in patients' health and well-being. It is in this space that group patient visits offer us a quantum leap forward in healthcare delivery.

Another significant benefit of the SMA approach has to do with the very simple act of a patient being listened to and being heard. Dr. Eric Cassell, a physician and noted medical bioethicist, distinguishes physical pain from human suffering and reminds us that a patient is a person, not a symptom, syndrome, disease, or list of medical problems. He defines suffering as any perceived threat to the integrity of one's person—that is, to the identification with and relationship to one's self, family, social group, work, and play (as well as to the transcendent meaning of one's life). From years of observation and study of the patient experience, he has discovered and eloquently described the critical importance of listening as a powerful therapeutic tool in the alleviation of suffering in illness (11).

Empathic listening, he explains, is how one person can lend strength to another and allow for the creation of meaning. Viewing medical encounters from this perspective, the individual medical visit affords a patient the opportunity to be heard by one person— the physician. We all recognize this to be a critical component of medical care. However, the present day reality is that the amount of time a physician can actually listen is quite limited—typically no more than a few brief minutes. More often than not, this time and listening are diluted and disrupted by the physician needing to document the visit and/or deal with any number of other concurrent clinic distractions. In contrast, the group patient visit provides the patient with the opportunity to be heard by the physician, who—in being assisted by a documenter (scribe) and multidisciplinary team—is able to devote more of his/her attention and time to the patient. Furthermore, in the SMA visit, a patient is also being listened to by a group of other patients, some of whom share his or her specific illness experience. If what Eric Cassell has described is correct, the group patient visit might actually be a much more powerful alleviator of patients' suffering than the individual one-on-one visit.

Numerous scholars have studied and described the experience of the patient, often from a first-hand account, and have documented the vital need of the patient to be listened to and heard. But, even more specifically, these scholar patients consistently report on the powerful healing effect of having others hear their stories (12–16). The opportunity to tell one's story of illness (and recovery), and to hear others' stories, may be one of the key reasons that patients experience the group patient visit to be so comforting, renewing, and meaningful.

In addition to being better listened to and heard, patients in the group visit also have the opportunity to teach. Being a patient can largely be a passive experience, as patients are acted upon. What we're finding in the group visit is that patients are becoming proactive participants in their healthcare experience as they begin to inform and teach one another. After all, chronically ill patients live their daily lives with their health problems and have, along the way, developed numerous strategies, skills, and resources for better coping with their situation. More than any other intervention, this very simple shift in dynamics—from passive recipient patient to proactive participant teacher—may lead to profound transformations in motivation and behavior change for patients. Here are two vignettes from recent SMAs at Harvard Vanguard Medical Associates that demonstrate this point. The specific details have been slightly modified to protect the anonymity of the patients.

Two Vignettes: Engaging Patients as Teachers

In the first case, a woman in her early thirties was recently diagnosed with a chronic life-long illness—an illness that will progressively impact her social interactions, particularly interactions with her spouse and her ability to function at work. When she was given this diagnosis (during the group patient visit), she immediately began to cry and talk about how her "life was over." The physician, as well as some of the other patients in the room, began to comfort her and assure her that she would be able to overcome this adversity. The response from the group was helpful, but one comment in particular was of tremendous benefit. One of the other women in the group, a woman in her fifties, turned to the younger patient and remarked that she should consider herself "lucky and actually quite fortunate to be diagnosed with this problem."

This comment caught everyone's attention. The younger woman asked why she should consider herself lucky. The older woman stated that she had herself lived with this problem for decades, but that it had gone undiagnosed for years. As a result, in addition to the direct pain and suffering that this illness engendered, her experience was overlaid with years of wondering if she was crazy; of her family and friends not understanding; of other physicians and clinicians not being able to help her; of doubt, depression and solitude. The older patient went on to point out to the young woman that she would be able to avoid all of this now that she had been properly diagnosed, particularly because she was diagnosed in the context of a group patient visit, where she could receive the understanding and social support of other patients and the clinical team. The younger patient was noticeably relieved by these comments and thanked the older woman for helping her.

In the second case, I received a phone call from a physician who had just emerged from one of his first DIGMA sessions. He was extremely excited and told me that he had already experienced a breakthrough patient interaction during the visit. He had been caring for a patient who was suffering from a chronic illness for many years. From the doctor's perspective, the illness was deeply compounded by his patients' recurring bouts of depression. Despite years of advice and urging on the part of the physician, the patient had refused to either recognize his depression or accept any medical treatment for it. Upsetting to this particular physician was the knowledge that depression in chronic illness not only is a common comorbidity but that it also, if left untreated, frequently leads to worse health outcomes.

During the course of this patient's first DIGMA visit, the patient courageously—albeit rather sheepishly and reluctantly—raised the issue of being depressed. The behaviorist in the room immediately picked up on it and began a brief dialogue with all the patients present, the majority of whom shared that they had also struggled with depression. A number of the patients described how their depression had held them back from getting better. The breakthrough came when this depressed patient shared that he had been struggling with depression for many years and had never realized it, but that he was now ready to do something about it.

As one might imagine, the physician almost fell off his chair—over 10 years of individual visits and even referrals to mental health colleagues, and he had not been able help this patient reach this understanding. And literally, within the first few minutes of a DIGMA session, the patient was able to arrive at this clear realization. Immediately after the session was over, this patient smiled and leaned over to the behaviorist stating: "I helped all these other patients, didn't I?" At a follow-up DIGMA visit 3 months later, the patient reported that he had, in fact, followed up with the treatment plan for his depression.

SMAs Improve Patients' Access to Care and Physicians' Capacity to Do Their Jobs

It is clear that SMAs offer patients and their families, as well as providers, the possibility of a much more empathetic, respectful, supportive, informative, and empowering environment. However, at the time of this writing and for the foreseeable future, the most critical drivers for SMAs as a mainstream modality of healthcare delivery are patients' access to healthcare, and the related issue of clinicians' ability to do their jobs, that is, their ability—given the demands, stressors, and clinical responsibilities upon them—to provide the type of care that is required.

As mentioned previously, fewer and fewer physicians are entering the field of primary care medicine. A disturbing statistic from the Massachusetts Medical Society 2008 Physician Workforce Study highlights this problem by pointing out that 42% of physicians are currently contemplating a career change because of the insurmountable challenges and lack of support they are experiencing from the practice of medicine in a highly bureaucratic and technocratic environment (17).

No doubt, what is required to solve these problems is a multipronged approach. Many of these solutions, such as creating the incentive for more physicians to select primary care as a career choice or creating the practice structures and supports to make the work more doable, will require a long time to implement. One immediate and practical solution would be the widespread implementation of DIGMAs and PSMAs. As an example of the immediate improvement in access to care that these SMA models can provide, we found that one of our highly respected and backlogged senior internal medicine physicians was able to reduce the wait time for his "third available" return appointment from 160 days down to 42 days after only 3 weeks of implementing his DIGMA visits.

This increased access was a direct result of increasing his net capacity by ten additional appointments each week. Each weekly DIGMA session created 13 follow-up visits with a net effect of adding 10 visits to his weekly capacity (13 visits in the DIGMA minus the 3 visits the physician would have seen in those 90 minutes had he not been doing a SMA). This increase of 10 visits (from the 29 follow-up visits he was currently offering to 39 follow-up visits per week) represented a remarkable 35% increase in this physician's capacity for follow-up visits. It was this dramatically increased capacity each week that so rapidly improved patient access to his practice. Once this internist's access was reduced to 42 days, he realized that for the first time in years he was now able to follow his out-of-control diabetic patients every 2 or 3 months, rather than every 5 months or longer due to the previous constraints on his schedule. The improvement in this physician's access led to an almost immediate improvement in his ability to care for his patients.

What we've discovered is that one SMA per week increases a physician's weekly capacity by approximately 3 hours, literally creating an extra 3 hours of time for a physician. How a physician uses this capacity is a function of the specific practice as well as the physician's specific needs. For example, this time can be used to see one's patients more frequently (as this doctor did), or the time can be used to see new patients who have been unable to get into the practice (as some of our other clinicians have done), or else it can be used to provide the physician with additional time each week to focus on preventive care or other clinical duties such as checking labs, responding to emails, and returning patients' phone calls.

Given this remarkable gain in capacity, we are currently engaging some of our physicians in the possibility of conducting five SMAs per week, one each day. This would create 15 hours of extra time per week for a physician. Imagine that! Although I've focused on examples from primary care internal medicine, we're implemented SMAs in various medical and surgical specialties (as well as in pediatrics and obstetrics and gynecology), and our early experience and data demonstrate an increase in access and capacity in these other specialties as well. As one example of this, one of our specialty gynecology centers was experiencing a waiting list of approximately 400 patients—women who literally were unable to get an appointment. Because of the highly specialized expertise involved in their care, these women, for the most part, were unable to obtain care at all. Within 3 or 4 months of implementing a PSMA program within this subspecialty service, the waiting list was rapidly decreased and is expected to soon be completely eliminated.

Related to access and capacity is the issue of *encounter volume*. From this perspective, the DIGMA and PSMA models offer a tremendous advantage to healthcare organizations, as well as to the physicians who are the primary generators of revenue for those entities. In our experience to date, we have discovered that, in a 90-minute SMA, a physician will experience anywhere between a 200 and 350% increase in encounter volume, with the average being approximately 250%. How can that be? In an average 90-minute period of clinic time, our primary care physicians are seeing approximately 3.5–4 patients, a number that includes follow-up visits as well as annual exams. They're typically scheduled to see more than that (i.e., during their 15–20 minute appointments for return visits and 30–40 minute appointments for private physical examinations), but once you remove no-shows, cancellations, and some physician down-time, the actual figure is pretty close to 3.5–4 on an average. In an average 90-minute SMA, the same physicians are now capable of seeing 10–13 patients in a DIGMA (for follow-up visits) and 7–10 patients in a PSMA (for private physical exams), which represents an approximate overall 200–350% increase in their encounter volume.

We have found that the impact of having just one well-attended DIGMA or PSMA per week on a full-time physician's schedule typically translates into a total encounter volume gain of approximately 10%. What's remarkable is that this increase is accompanied *not* by physicians spending less time with their patients, but by their actually spending *more* time, including a greater amount of quality time. The underlying reasons for this dramatic increase in efficiencies are due to: (1) physicians being able to delegate much of what they normally do, including most of their documenting, onto a multidisciplinary care team, which translates into the physician needing to do only that which he or she alone can uniquely do; (2) the ability to overbook sessions so as to eliminate the otherwise deleterious impact that no-shows and late cancellations can result in—not dissimilar from what the airlines do; and (3) the group setting itself, which leverages the physicians time and effort through a reduced repetition of information, since all patients in attendance can be addressed at once. As discussed in detail in this book, the DIGMA and PSMA teams include a documenter (transcriptionist); a behaviorist (group facilitator); and a usually both a medical assistant and a nurse or LPN.

This last efficiency gain is no small thing. Some of our surgical specialists have predicted that they could save anywhere between 60 and 90 minutes per day from this benefit alone. Physicians repeat instructions and health education mini-lectures numerous times throughout the course of a typical day. The SMA allows a physician to speak once and reach a dozen or more patients simultaneously. This is not only an efficiency gain, but because of the group dynamic and active patient participation, these mini-lectures and instructions are typically more effective and robust than in a one-on-one encounter.

SMAs Translate Directly into Efficiency Gains and Cost-Effective Care

These efficiency and capacity gains can also be translated into bottom line financial figures. Our finance department at Harvard Vanguard Medical Associates has constructed a pro-forma for the SMA program and conducted a number of sensitivity analyses that reveal that DIGMAs and PSMAs have the potential to deliver a significant financial return on investment.

Let me be clear that, as a non-profit healthcare organization, our primary goal is not profitability. However, it is also clear that the efficiency and capacity gains from SMAs can be readily applied to remedying some of the major problems facing our healthcare delivery system today. Implementation of the group patient visit model will allow physicians and other clinicians to: (1) appropriately see their patients more frequently for follow-up chronic disease management visits; (2) see new patients and, for the many physicians with closed practices, to open up their panels and accept new patients (thus providing access to care to those many patients who are unable to find a physician); (3) devote more time to the very serious responsibilities of checking patient test results and consultation reports; (4) be more available to return patients' phone calls and emails; (5) spend more time-practicing proactive preventive medicine instead of rushed reactive care; (6) have time to manage and lead their clinical teams (what our Chief Medical Officer has termed, "putting collaboration on the clock") and; (7) to also spend more time coordinating their patients' care across the very complex spectrum of our delivery system.

There is a growing opinion among some healthcare leaders, economists, and policy experts that provider payment should not be primarily a function of the volume of encounters or procedural activities (18), but should instead be coupled to what matters most—actual health outcomes, appropriate cost-effective medical care, and patients' experience of care (service excellence) (19). My personal conviction is aligned with these proposed reforms. What's interesting and quite remarkable to note about the SMA models is that they add value in any payment structure–i.e., the current fee-for-service and capitated models that we presently function within, as well as in the proposed primary care payment reform models such as the *patient centered medical home* (20) and *episode based payment systems* (18). In fact, group patient visits are included as an integral component of many of the innovative care models that are currently being piloted across the country (21,22).

Enhanced Quality of Care

Regarding the fundamentally critical issue of quality, we are currently putting into place longitudinal analyses of the healthcare quality outcomes of SMAs in comparison with those experienced by patients in individual visits. This analysis is somewhat flawed as we have already begun to notice a halo effect. That is, that the enhanced quality of care being provided in our SMA sessions is already spilling over into the care being provided to patients in individual visits. This is not surprising as our clinicians and staff are intent on providing the highest quality of care possible, and any intervention that appears to enhance quality would, and should, be adopted quickly throughout the practice.

One example of how quality is being improved is that of preventive care. Almost from the start, we've built quality in to the SMA visits. All of the preventive screenings (such as mammography, colonoscopies, immunizations, and cholesterol screening) have been programmed into the workflow of the SMA encounters; and therefore are not dependent on the individual physician remembering or being prompted (as with an electronic medical record) to complete these essential preventive functions. We're also building a number of back-up safeguards into the SMA workflow to make sure that every patient we see is assured the highest quality preventive care possible.

SMAs Can Create a More Transparent and Team-Oriented Medical Delivery System

It is apparent that the SMA group visit model offers many advantages to patients as well as to clinicians. However, there is another benefit that we have not discussed. Over the past few decades, the medical encounter between doctor and patient (in the outpatient setting) has been hidden, for the most part, behind the opaque closed door of the exam room. I'd like to suggest that this concealment has not been good for either the physician or the patient, nor is it good for the delivery system in general. Behind the closed door, the physician is alone and isolated, unable to be observed and thus less able to learn from feedback. Behind the closed door, there is no shared learning with colleagues, thus limiting clinicians' professional growth and development. Also, behind the closed door, it's difficult for a physician to teach others and share the wisdom of their experience.

Within healthcare, from the patients' perspective, there's a swelling public demand for, as well as a growing movement toward, greater transparency. I believe this transparency should also include the encounter between patient and doctor. Conducting the patient visit in a transparent group visit format affords physicians real-time feedback about their performance and their collective teams' performance. It also enhances the efficiency and effectiveness of the care team and fosters camaraderie that, as we know from the literature, leads to improved quality and safety of medical care. Our own experience indicates that physicians and their teams are highly enthusiastic and energized by the group visit format. We have a waiting list of nurses, medical assistants, psychologists, social workers, and administrators who are desirous of being a part of a SMA care team.

Here are a couple of quotes from SMA team members that illustrate the point: "We feel more connected and involved with the patients. The team venture is very different and promotes a camaraderie among different levels of staff that flattens the hierarchy." "These meetings function like a well-oiled machine. We can each pick up where the other leaves off during a session and support each other." From my perspective, the SMA approach is the most coordinated, team-oriented medical care I've ever encountered, outside of the surgical operating suite.

SMAs as a Forum for Teaching

Another related advantage of the SMA model of medical care is that it also allows other clinicians to attend the visit and learn. As one application of this, we're planning to have medical students and residents in training participate in the SMAs that their physician teachers (attending physicians) are holding. From the perspective of the physician teacher, it's challenging to teach effectively and efficiently in the ambulatory care setting. This is because it requires either that the attending physician be present during the entire time that the student or resident is speaking with and examining the patient or else that the attending physician review what the student or resident has done by listening to their report—a sort of second-hand method of teaching. Given the time and cost pressures of current day ambulatory care practice, it is very difficult for attending physicians to fully observe their students and provide real-time feedback as well as demonstration of appropriate care.

The SMA, however, represents a highly efficient and effective opportunity for teaching ambulatory care medicine. Imagine a physician teacher conducting a SMA with a couple of residents, fellows, and/or students in the room. The attending physician could begin the SMA and see the first two or three patients to get the group visit going, and then allow the residents, fellows, and students, in turn, to each see two or three patients while the physician is in the room. This approach would allow the attending physician full and direct observation of the student or resident in training, as well as the ability to demonstrate and teach their own approach and skills.

Another potential teaching application of SMAs, which we are planning, is to offer to our general internists to sit in on and participate in subspecialty SMA visits, such as geriatrics, nephrology, dermatology, otolaryngology, and orthopedics, to learn skills that they can apply in their own practice. This type of learning not only is a highly efficient and cost-effective way to foster clinicians' professional career development, it also can improve the quality and cost-effectiveness of medical care by expanding the services that primary care physicians can competently deliver.

How much more interesting and exciting would medical practice be if we opened our individual visit sessions to a group format? And, isn't this the way that we learned to be physicians in the first place—not in isolation, but in a group (i.e., during morning and afternoon hospital rounds) as part of a collective and multidisciplinary team? I, for one, would much prefer this mode of continuous learning over the more traditional continuing medical education (CME) training programs conducted in dark auditoriums with slide presentations.

Given our experience to date, it is my belief that most physicians would experience the open, transparent, and team-based group visit model as stimulating and liberating. It would allow highly competent and caring clinicians to showcase and share their knowledge, skill, and experience in an unprecedented way. In my own experience observing these groups, I find myself repeatedly touched and impressed by the trusting relationships and highly personal bonds that our physicians have formed with their patients and the profound gratitude and respect that our patients feel for their doctors, many of whom have cared for them and their families for decades. This is a lesson, something to be shared and celebrated, that is just as important as the more concrete technical skills and knowledge of our highly competent physicians.

Planning and Predictions

It is our hope, at Atrius Health, that our experiences and the lessons we've learned will assist others in implementing and sustaining their own successful SMA programs. Our experience is that the SMA represents a more organized, efficient, team-based, participatory, personalized, informative, and accessible way to deliver high-quality ambulatory medical care. It is for this reason that we, at Atrius Health, are planning to launch The Noffsinger Institute for Shared Medical Appointments. Through this institute, we will offer interested providers and medical groups all of the necessary training and support materials that are required to successfully design, launch, support, and sustain their own SMA programs. Our goals are to assist other organizations in avoiding the many beginners' mistakes that can so easily be made; to attend to the many predictable operational hurdles that will likely be encountered; and to create a community and network of learning and sharing among the many provider groups who will be deploying SMAs.

Predictions are always risky, but I believe that, given the current trends in healthcare, SMAs will become the predominant and preferred mode of face-to-face visit encounters in the ambulatory medicine setting and that the individual face-to-face visit will become the exception. As more and more clinicians and healthcare organizations begin to offer SMAs, we will begin to see medical schools and academic medical centers teaching SMAs as a core part of their training curriculum. As mentioned previously, I believe SMAs to be a tremendous opportunity for reinvigorating the practice of ambulatory medicine, particularly for primary care medicine. And, as SMAs gain traction around the country and around the world, we will begin to see collaboratives forming to share best practices and innovations in the implementation and delivery of SMAs.

Finally, with outpatient healthcare delivery increasingly shifting toward and leveraging web-based applications and electronic modes of communication, I can imagine *virtual SMAs* being offered to patients; that is, groups of patients being seen together online, perhaps on their cell phones. The social networking design of the web links very well with the group-based SMA format. For example, even at the present moment, we are contemplating the idea of the SMA behaviorist being online during the SMA to utilize, in real-time, web-based e-health applications such as the checking of medication interactions or looking up the answers to patients' questions that the physician does not immediately have at hand. From my perspective, the SMA is a real manifestation of the burgeoning virtual, web-based e-health solutions movement. Time will tell; however, my belief is that we will begin to see these predictions materialize within the next 5 years.

Why Read This Book

In this book, Dr. Ed Noffsinger presents the rationale behind SMAs and, most importantly, offers a practical, step-by-step approach to implementing DIGMAs, PSMAs, and CHCCs (Cooperative HealthCare Clinics) for clinicians, staffs, and entire organizations. In addition to presenting the accumulating body of outcomes data, common mistakes are emphasized and the systemic operational changes that must be implemented are discussed in detail. This book has been 8 years in the writing and over a dozen years in the making. It contains innumerable pearls of wisdom from Ed, the most experienced and pre-eminent expert in the area of group patient visits.

These pearls emanate not only from his 12 years of experience implementing literally hundreds of DIGMA and PSMA programs but also from his 35-year experience as a health psychologist conducting up to 15 group sessions each week, his intense analytic and systems training as a professional physicist, and his life-altering experience as a patient suffering with a serious illness. It is Ed Noffsinger's unusual amalgam of intelligence and experience, wit and wisdom, and perhaps most importantly, the dignity, respect, and generosity that he affords his family, friends, colleagues, and patients that make this book something akin to its author—unparalleled and one of a kind.

If I had to distill the ultimate value and meaning of Ed's mission, as well as that of group patient visits, I would have to say that it is to create a *community of caring* within each patient visit and to *change the story of the patient*—from one of isolation, frustration, and fear to one of hope, dignity, community, and empowerment. This is Ed's unique contribution to medicine and his gift to us all—patients, families, clinicians, and healthcare workers.

Healthcare executives, clinician leaders, and administrators who want to see a DIGMA and/or PSMA program implemented within their own healthcare system, as well as the physicians and allied healthcare providers who are interested in launching a SMA program within their own practices, will find this book to be indispensable. In addition, front-line administrators and operations personnel (as well as anyone interested in learning how to become a SMA behaviorist, nurse, LPN, MA, or documenter) will find this book to be an invaluable asset to them in designing, implementing, and running a successful group patient visit program. I have no doubt that this book will serve both as the definitive text and as the operational manual on group patient visits for many years to come.

Newton, MA   Zeev E. Neuwirth, MD
November 2008   Chief of Clinical Effectiveness & Innovation
                                     Harvard Vanguard Medical Associates/Atrius Health

References

1. Østbye T, Yarnall KS, Krause KM, et al. Is there time for management of patients with chronic diseases in primary care? *Annals of Family Medicine* 2005;3(3):209–214.
2. Brotherton SE, Etzel SI. Graduate medical education, 2007-2008. *Journal of the American Medical Association* 2008;300(10):1228–1243.

3. http://www.sg2.com/default.aspx
4. http://www.iom.edu/CMS/3809/40113/53452.aspx
5. Massachusetts Medical Society: 2008 Physician Workforce Study http://www.mass med.org/Content/NavigationMenu/NewsandPublications/ResearchReportsStudies/ PhysicianWorkforceStudy/MMS_Physician_Workf.htm
6. Clayton CM, Bohmer RMJ, Kenagy J. Will disruptive innovations cure healthcare? *Harvard Business Review* Sep–Oct 2000:102–117.
7. The Diabetes Prevention Program. Within-trial cost-effectiveness of lifestyle intervention or metformin for the primary prevention of Type 2 diabetes. *Diabetes Care* 2003;26:2518–2523.
8. www.harrisinteractive.com/news/newsletters/healthnews/HI_HealthCareNews2008 Vol8_Iss8.pdf
9. Kleinman A. The illness narratives – suffering, healing & the human condition. Basic Books, 1988.
10. Schroeder S. We can do better—improving the health of the American people. *New England Journal of Medicine* 2007;357:1221–1228.
11. Cassel EJ. The nature of suffering and the goals of medicine. *New England Journal of Medicine* 1982;306(11):639–645.
12. Cousin N. Anatomy of an illness. New York: Bantam Books, 1979.
13. Broyard A. Intoxicated by my illness. New York: Ballantine Books, 1992.
14. Frank AW. The wounded storyteller – body, illness, and ethics. Chicago and London: The University of Chicago Press, 1995.
15. Sacks O. A leg to stand on. New York: Harper Collins, 1987.
16. Brody H. Stories of sickness. New Haven and London: Yale University Press, 1987.
17. Massachusetts Medical Society: 2008 Physician Workforce Study, http://www.mass med.org/Content/NavigationMenu/NewsandPublications/ResearchReportsStudies/ PhysicianWorkforceStudy/MMS_Physician_Workf.htm
18. Rosenthal MB. Beyond pay for performance – emerging models of provider-payment reform. *New England Journal of Medicine* 2008;359:1198–1200.
19. Berwick DM, Nolan TW, Whittington J. The triple aim: care, health, and cost. Health Affairs 2008;27(3):759–769.
20. Goroll AH, Berenson RA, Schoenbaum SC, et al. Fundamental reform of payment for adult primary care: comprehensive payment for comprehensive care. Journal of General Internal Medicine 2007;22:410–415.
21. http://www.transformed.com/transformed.cfm
22. The Medical Home - Disruptive Innovation for a New Primary Care Model. Deloitte Center for Health Solutions. www.deloitte.com/us/healthsolutions

Preface

How It All Began

"The good news is that you scored higher on your exercise tolerance tests than anybody we've tested except for our young residents," I recall my renowned pulmonologist telling me as I apprehensively sat across from his desk to hear about my test results on that fateful day in late 1991. "Unfortunately, your tests are abnormal and we believe that you have primary pulmonary hypertension due to pulmonary vascular disease with a patent foramen ovale. Your tests showed considerable dead air space in your lungs due to destruction of the capillary bed, elevated pulmonary pressures, mild asthma, and what appears to be a cardiac shunt. However, in order to confirm your diagnosis we will have to redo the bubble study, as we thought we saw air bubbles on the wrong side of your heart in your recent exercise tolerance test—but the results were somewhat equivocal. If the follow-up test reveals a cardiac shunt that opens under exertion, then our diagnosis will be confirmed."

"What on earth is that?" I asked with concern as my wife sat silently by my side, "I never heard of such a condition."

"It's a rare condition that is uniformly fatal," he said. As I recall, he added something to the effect that "Seventy percent die within two years of onset of symptoms, and nobody has lived seven."

I could not believe what I was hearing. I was devastated, but clung to the remote hope that the definitive follow-up study would prove this diagnosis to be wrong. He ended the office visit by again stating: "If, in repeating the study, they find bubbles passing across your heart under exertion that will confirm our diagnosis."

At that time, I had been sick for over 3 years with some sort of serious cardiopulmonary condition that involved hypoxia, tachycardia, cardiac arrhythmias, profuse sweating, shortness of breath, and hospitalizations. Previous diagnoses variously ranged from bronchiolitis obliterans and pneumococcal pneumonia to suspicions that I had contracted some sort of exotic, destructive pulmonary condition from the truckloads of mushroom compost and various soil amendments that I had worked with over the years during extensive gardening activities in my yard. Prior to this devastating 1988–1992 illness episode, I had been a remarkably active, healthy, and fit 45-year-old man in excellent shape, capable of jogging 4 miles in less than 25 minutes and taking 100 + mile bike rides in the coastal mountains of Northern California. My illness, arrhythmias, tachycardia, and severe hypoxia had caused an all-too-rapid decline from being very healthy to extremely ill, ultimately resulting in structural changes to my heart and lungs, and eventually even a cerebellar stroke.

At my worst during these years, my highly variable blood oxygen level would drop as low as 43% while my irregular pulse rose to over 160, which would leave me sweating profusely, utterly fatigued, and panting endlessly while laboring to somehow catch my next breath. Throughout these years, I had undergone every imaginable pulmonary and cardiac diagnostic and imaging test. And finally, this multitude of test results were being drawn together by some of the best doctors in the country—especially my pulmonologist and cardiologist—to capture my definitive diagnosis, which now appeared to be very grim. However, I still clung to the hope that my upcoming *definitive* retest would prove this initial diagnosis to be incorrect.

While at my worst during these anoxic episodes, my energy was completely drained, and what little was left was spent in the sheer effort of breathing. Not infrequently, I was bedridden, except for when I could muster the energy to go over and sit in my recliner for an hour or so each day. Sometimes I lay listlessly in bed for days, with an irregular resting pulse of 140–160 beats per minute, sweating so profusely that it seemed like I had just run a marathon, and requiring my wife to change my soaking wet pajamas and bedding linen as much a eight times a night. Along with my closest physician friends, I felt that I was at death's door and feared for the welfare of my beloved wife and children, who, at that time, were only 5, 6, and 7 years old.

The Definitive Test

On the day of the fateful follow-up supine bicycle exercise bubble study, I lay down on the cold gurney in that sterile surgical room, dressed only in my exercise shorts, socks, and shoes—with IVs in and EKG leads all over. With my cardiologist, a nurse, an ultrasound tech, and a cardiology fellow present, the definitive diagnostic test—on the results of which my life presumably depended—now began. Lying there strapped to the gurney, I followed instructions and began pedaling at low resistance while watching my fragile-appearing heart beating on the small television monitor to my left side. "Go…go…go!" I kept thinking as I watched the delicate image of my heart pumping, for it looked as if it could stop beating at any time.

With regularity each time the pedaling resistance increased, my cardiologist told the nurse to inject another froth of air bubbles into the IV line, which she did immediately while lifting and massaging my affected extremity, with all in the room intently watching the TV screen in eager anticipation to determine if there was any evidence of bubbles crossing over from the right atrium to the left. In the midst of this study, when I was asked to do a Valsalva maneuver, all were witnesses to my heart's immediate response: the shunt opened up and the turbulent froth of bubbles unfortunately burst across the atrial septal defect from the right to left side of my heart.

The Stark Contrast Between My Feelings and the General Excitement Over a New Technology

Recognizing what this meant to me and my family in terms of confirming the dreaded diagnosis, I lay there distraught and unable to speak. However, the room became a hub of enthusiastic excitement. I remember somebody saying something to me like, "Do you realize how fortunate you are—that before we had developed this new technique for indirectly assessing pulmonary pressures, we would have had to intervene surgically in order to directly assess your elevated pressures?" It's not that I wasn't appreciative of this new technology, however, I was absolutely overwhelmed by the negative implications of this study. In their excitement over this cutting edge medical technology, the cardiologist and team asked if—because this was a teaching hospital—I wouldn't mind repeating the study so that their colleagues and residents could observe this remarkable new technology in action. Group after group witnessed the amazing results of the test, nodding with pleasure at its capabilities. In my numbed state, I wondered if I could die from someone injecting air bubbles into my bloodstream, although none of the excited witnesses to this new technology seemed concerned about that. Although I agreed to keep repeating the study, I was struck by how diametrically opposed my rapidly declining and disheartened mood was to the professional elation and fervor that permeated the room.

The Worst Moment

As quickly as the excitement had begun, it suddenly ended. I heard my cardiologist say that the test was over, and the entire team then promptly left the room, leaving me struck by the contrast between the dead stillness filled with my melancholy mood and the noisy hubbub of activity that had just occurred. As I lay there alone in that chilly room, I reflected on what the results of this study meant to me and my family. How long would I live? How would I die? Would I linger through a tortuous death of slow, progressive suffocation—gasping to catch my breath? Would I ever experience any semblance of energy again? What would I tell my wife, who was now patiently waiting in the adjacent lobby area? And what would become of my 7- and 5-year-old sons and my 6-year-old daughter? Devastated, I was overwhelmed and not thinking very clearly. It didn't seem fair. I suddenly felt cheated by God and I asked, "Why me?" I felt absolutely and totally alone and in despair.

"Well, they said the test was over," I thought to myself, "so I guess that I should get up, get dressed, and go home." I began to sit up and pull the various EKG patches from my chest, wiping the goop off from underneath them with my hand as best I could as I did this and looked toward my pile of clothes I had previously placed on the chair against the far wall when I came in for this study. As I got off the gurney to walk toward my clothing, my foot slipped. I had just stepped into a small puddle of my own blood that had dripped onto floor by the side of the gurney from my IV site. After slowly walking to the far wall, I sat down and put my face into my hands, despondent about what I could possibly tell my wife.

Just when I thought that things couldn't get worse, I looked up and could not believe what I was seeing. There was nothing warm, soothing, or comforting in this silent and dehumanized room, despite the excitement that had filled it just a few moments earlier. Instead, I saw a Salvador Dali-like picture of a cold, sterile room, with pure white walls and ceiling, a pewter-colored gurney in the middle, and a bloody, bright red footprint walking right toward me.

Be Careful Not to Neglect the Human Experience

My head whirled. I thought about how things might have come to this, and how modern medicine and technology could be so out of step with the human experience, so devoid of feeling and compassion, despite the best intentions of so many who cared deeply. What had gone wrong with the system?

I felt that I had the very best of doctors, especially my cardiologist and pulmonologist, both kind and gentle men, who always tried to spend as much time as they could with me, despite being overworked and somewhat harried. I had just undergone some of the newest and most sophisticated tests that contemporary medicine had to offer, yet now found myself feeling absolutely alone and in the depths of despair—right down to my soul. Despite the presence of so many dedicated healthcare professionals, where was the attention to the human spirit in all this and some basic empathy and emotional support for the patient undergoing such an ordeal?

Even with my dedicated and caring doctors, it took months to get appointments with them and their clinics frequently ran an hour or two late. To me, it seemed as if they were as tired out, pushed, and victimized by the system as I was. They tried to do the best they could for me; yet it seemed that the healthcare system itself was somehow broken, so that it was serving neither my physicians nor myself very well.

From Despair to the Earliest Beginnings of the Drop-In Group Medical Appointments Model

Some months later, while at home acutely ill from another severe illness episode, I was once again lying in bed one night and unable to sleep. Like so many times before, I was dripping wet with perspiration, panting, short of breath, utterly fatigued, and exhausted. I was also feeling more than a little anxious and depressed over my uncertain future. At that moment I felt desperately alone and yearned for some human understanding and companionship. Although it was still fairly early in the evening, I absolutely did not want to awaken my wife, as she had just gotten to sleep for some much needed rest after another hectically busy day of tending to our children and to her father, who was dying at that time from metastatic prostate cancer and advanced heart disease.

I got out of bed and struggled along into my boys' bedroom, where I promptly plopped down on the rocking chair next to their bed—the one that I had bought for my wife on that wonderful day when we initially found out that she was pregnant with our first child. As I gazed at my sleeping sons (my daughter was sound asleep next to my wife in the adjoining bedroom), I felt an unbelievably deep and foreboding sorrow. It simply wasn't fair that my children would be left to grow up without a father and that I wouldn't be there to enjoy playing with them through their childhood years, to watch them graduate from high school and college, to participate in their weddings, and to eventually relish my grandchildren.

Deep into despair, I telephoned my brothers, and then some old friends, hoping that they would cheer me up. They each offered advice, but I didn't find it helpful and just didn't feel that they understood. I wondered why these calls missed the mark and left me feeling so let down. It occurred to me that my friends and family, who really had my best interests at heart, did not seem to be supportive in the way I needed them to be because they were used to seeing me as a strong and capable caregiver, not as a sick person in need of caregiving. Seeing me so ill must have really scared and worried them.

I immediately began to reflect on the thousands of chronically ill patients that I had been privileged to work with during the past couple of decades as Director of Oncology Counseling and Chronic Illness Services in the Psychiatry Department at the Kaiser Permanente Santa Clara Medical Center, which served more than 300,000 patient members. I can't count the number of times my patients told me that, while they did not want to burden their friends and family with their health problems and worries, whenever they did in fact share their concerns they were often surprised at how unhelpful and unsupportive their friends often turned out to be, sometimes saying things such as, "Oh, you have breast cancer? My friend Mary had that also. Sadly, she died from it. I really miss her now." Many times these patients told me how much they wished that they could speak with other patients in the same boat because they felt that other patients could really understand.

Sitting there alone in my children's room that night, I felt myself spiraling downward emotionally and feeling evermore despondent. I told myself to stop complaining, buck up, and try to focus on more positive thoughts. I began to ask myself: "What do you really want?" In terms of my healthcare, what came through to me was very clear. First and foremost, I wanted prompt and barrier-free access to high-quality care, and, most importantly, more time with my own doctors (plus a more relaxed and less pressured pace of care). Despite having the best doctors I could have hoped for, I found that the system was somehow broken—traditional individual office visits were simply too inaccessible and too rushed. In addition, I wanted to be with other patients as I felt that they could truly understand.

Despite Having the Best of Doctors, Access and Service Were Poor

Although I was receiving my medical care in two major medical settings (a large HMO and a prestigious academic medical center), I was tired of calling for an appointment and hearing a recording say how important my phone call was, while at the same time forcing me to listen to elevator music for 20–40 minutes as I waited for a scheduler to pick up the line, and all this just to get a short appointment that was often several weeks away. Then, on the day of the scheduled appointment, I would often wait in the lobby for 1–2 hours or more for the nurse to call my name. I once waited more than 4 hours for a short office visit and had to wait more than 3 hours on a couple of other occasions. And then, even after I had been called in and roomed with vital signs taken, I would wait yet another 15–30 minutes in the exam room for the doctor to arrive. Finally, when the doctor did eventually come in (often appearing exhausted from a busy day that had been crammed full of too many patients), the visit frequently seemed all too pressured and rushed—with one of the physician's hands seemingly on the doorknob, while the other was busily writing notes in my medical chart.

Then, immediately after the doctor had left, I would often find myself thinking: "Oh no, I forgot to ask about this or that!" or "Did the doctor just tell me to take two pills or three?" Afterward, when I got home and telephoned the doctor's office to get an answer to my question, I would again listen to a recording about how important my telephone call was, waiting another 20–40 minutes for a live human to answer, only to have the entire vicious cycle repeat itself. In other words, after one appointment, I would often have to make yet another one just to get an answer to the question that would have been answered if only there had been just a little more time available during the original visit, i.e., if only the appointment had been just a little less rushed.

There Has Got to Be a Better Way

The entire system and appointment-making process seemed to not be patient oriented (and full of waste), and ultimately appeared to be very hard on patients and physicians alike. Indeed, the whole system supporting the individual office visit model of care seemed to be inefficient, flawed, and obsolete rather than patient centered and service oriented. "What other business," I wondered, "could survive with such pervasive waste and inefficiency built into it and with such poor service to its customers?" I thought that if you called a Toyota dealership about purchasing a car and (1) waited 20–40 minutes listening to music on the telephone; (2) then had to wait an additional several weeks to be able to come into the showroom; (3) still had to wait an additional hour or two in the lobby; (4) found that the waiting was still not over as this was followed by yet another half-hour spent in a separate room waiting for the sales person to arrive; and then (5) found out that you only had 7–10 minutes of the sales person's time—I wonder just how many people would end up buying a Toyota, or would they instead simply go down the street and purchase a Honda, assuming that their service was better.

The Drop-In Group Medical Appointments Model Begins to Take Shape

What I wanted most was prompt access and more time with my own doctors. When I asked myself how much time I wanted, what immediately came to mind (even though I still chuckle at the thought) was, "Ninety minutes seems just about right!" When I asked myself how quickly I wanted to get in, I felt that a week would be about as long as I would be willing to wait, giving birth to the idea of weekly 90-minute medical visits. Furthermore, I was so fed up with the entire inefficient appointment making process that I never wanted to go through it again. I was willing to call a day in advance to say that I was coming, but that was about it. Hence, the "drop-in" component of the DIGMA model was born.

Finally, I was feeling isolated and alone and yearned to be with other patients dealing with medical issues whom I felt could really understand. They did not have to be experiencing the exact medical condition that I had, which would have been impossible anyway due the rarity and swift lethality of my diagnosed condition. I felt like simply having any sort of medical condition would be sufficient for there to be an adequate degree of understanding and compassion. I was tired of waking up in the middle of the night, unable to sleep because I was feeling cheated, alone, isolated, worried, and depressed, yet not wanting to burden my family and friends with my problems (particularly since they might not turn out to be as supportive as I would like anyway).

I Was Feeling Just Like My Chronically Ill Patients Told Me They Had Felt

Interestingly, when I was at Kaiser, I had been working with many thousands of chronically ill medical patients over the years who had told me they were having the same types of thoughts and feelings as I was now experiencing personally. I was convinced that other patients could provide me with the warmth, support, and understanding that I craved and that this could occur in a group setting where my dignity and privacy would still be respected. Regarding how many other patients I would like to have present during my medical visits, I felt that 10–15 other patients would be just about right—thus, the idea of the group component of the DIGMA model was born.

In such a warm, compassionate, and supportive group setting, I would be able to have my unique medical needs addressed individually—but in front of others, who would be able to listen, learn, interact, and share their ideas while the doctor was working with me. I would similarly be able to learn as my doctor sequentially addressed the medical needs of each of the other patients in turn. In such a setting, I would be able to freely ask questions, receive emotional support, and exchange helpful information. It would be run very much like a series of individual office visits, but with other patients and their support persons acting as observers. Furthermore, I would get answers to important medical questions that I might not know to ask because others would ask. As time went on, the Drop-In Group Medical Appointment model was rapidly becoming progressively clearer to me.

I wanted this to be an additional healthcare choice (one that integrated the help and support of other patients into each patient's healthcare experience) that would always be voluntary to patients and physicians alike. I reasoned that a recipe for a disastrous group visit would be to force a physician who does not want to do one to have to run such a program. In addition, I always believed that patients should have freedom of choice when it comes to their healthcare options and that—for many—group visits would offer a refreshing option to the traditional individual office visit. I also felt that having a behaviorist—a mental health professional, such as a health psychologist or medical social worker—to manage the group and help patients with the emotional concomitants of their illness, would be an added benefit.

Since these original conceptualizations of the DIGMA model, I have subsequently found that having someone present to document the majority of patients' chart notes offers many efficiency benefits while also freeing the physician up to look at, enjoy, and interact in a more meaningful way with patients. I have also found that expanding the nursing and behaviorist roles to their full potential adds quality to the visit, as does having a nurse call patients a couple of days beforehand to confirm their appointment, conduct a med reconciliation, go through the HEDIS checklist, and ensure that all pre-visit labs have been completed. From the very beginning, my goals were to max-pack visits, to create a *one-stop healthcare shopping experience* for patients, to integrate the help and support of other patients into each patient's healthcare experience, and to better serve our patients by making their medical visit everything that it could be.

Why Would the Same Model of Care Be Best for Both Acute and Chronic Care?

I began to think about how the traditional individual visit model of care had evolved over centuries of acute care—prior to the development of antibiotics, when people suffered from a wide variety of deadly acute infectious illnesses—an era when patients were well yesterday, sick today, and dead tomorrow. But now we are living in an era of chronic care—with chronic illnesses absorbing the vast majority of our healthcare dollars—where patients were ill yesterday, are sick today, and will likely be coping with their illnesses for decades and possibly even for the rest of their lives. Such patients are trying to eke out the best possible quality of life that they can, despite struggling with the disastrous impact that chronic illness can have on them, their jobs, and their families.

So why would we think that the same model of care would be optimal for both types of circumstances—acute and chronic care? Although I have found DIGMAs to be appropriate for many types of acute care issues, they truly excel in the treatment of chronic illnesses, geriatric patients, and patients with psychosocial issues—areas where my professional experience (plus my personal story as a discouraged, chronically ill patient) has taught me that traditional care often falls short.

The DIGMA Model Crystallizes into Its Final Form

Thus it was that, in the muddled confusion of a frustrating 4-year illness episode from which I only very gradually improved (the medical impact of which has lingered throughout the subsequent decade and a half), I experienced first hand many of the frustrations, inefficiencies, and problems inherent in our modern healthcare system. It was out of these difficult personal medical challenges—combined with my professional experiences—that the basic elements of the Drop-In Group Medical Appointment (DIGMA) model gradually evolved and became clearer to me: That is, a highly accessible, weekly, 90-minute group medical appointment with the patient's own doctor that offered drop-in convenience (and had an ideal group size of between 10 and 16 patients)—run with the assistance of a behaviorist to better attend to group dynamics and psychosocial issues.

In DIGMAs, the focus from start to finish would be upon the delivery of medical care that sequentially addressed the unique medical needs of each person individually in a supportive group setting where all present could listen, interact, ask questions, and learn. Although the drop-in feature would be highly recommended due to its convenience in better servicing patients, I never considered this to be an essential feature of the model—so that physicians who preferred to have all patients pre-scheduled could do so if they so desired.

DIGMAs were always meant to be nothing more than an additional healthcare choice—and an added tool in the physician's *black bag* to better manage chronic illnesses and large, busy, and backlogged practices—a tool that would be voluntary to patients and physicians alike. One substantive change that has happened to the DIGMA model during the intervening years has been the strongly recommended addition of a documenter, especially in systems that are using electronic medical records—but only for those physicians who agree to consistently see an additional patient or two in their DIGMAs in order to cover the added cost of having a documenter.

Other changes have included expanding the nursing and behaviorist roles to achieve their full potential—such as having a nurse call patients a couple of days beforehand to confirm appointments, conduct med reconciliations, go through the HEDIS checklist, and ensure that all pre-visit labs were completed. Also, for nurses to update all routine health maintenance and injections during every visit, and for patients to get all appointments and referrals recommended by their doctor actually scheduled during the DIGMA visit—plus receive an *after visit summary* to take home with them which contains important parts of the chart note that the physician wants them to have, such as the treatment plan. My goal for the DIGMA model has always been to max-pack visits and better serve our patients by making their medical visit everything that it can be during each and every session.

My Recovery Begins

My slow path to recovery began one day in 1992 after I tried—for the first time in years—to take a walk outside with my children. On that morning, I awoke to find myself for some reason feeling surprisingly well and much like my good old pre-illness self. First thing that morning, I asked my kids (who were 6, 7, and 8 at the time) if they would like to go for a walk with daddy, thinking that I would take them on a mile or so long hike along the roads by my house in the coastal mountains of Santa Cruz, CA. What I had in mind was taking part of a 4-mile course on local coastal mountain roads that I used to jog on an almost daily basis prior to the beginning of this illness episode in 1988. My kids greeted this offer with glee and immediately got dressed with anticipatory excitement over the promised hike.

So off we went, on a hike that I expected would take approximately a half-hour to complete, but a hike that I felt confident I could do because I was feeling so good after so many consecutive days of feeling bad. However, what I discovered that day both shocked and frightened me. After walking down my driveway and perhaps the equivalent of a relatively level city block, I quickly became so profoundly fatigued that words fail, even now, to fully convey how utterly worn out and done in I felt. I was seeing flickering white and black spots all over the place, felt like I was about to black out, and had an extremely rapid and erratic pulse. My heart was fluttering with all sorts of missed beats and unusual feeling arrhythmias that seemed to be radiating strange sensations into my carotids (and with a peculiar pressure behind my eyes that made me feel as if they were about to explode right out of their sockets). Because of all the spots and visual disturbances I was experiencing, I couldn't even get my vision focused enough on my wristwatch to be able to take my pulse. Utterly exhausted and unable to go even one step further, I plopped down at the edge of the road and put my head in my hands for what seemed like an hour and a half, simply dreading the thought of somehow having to get enough energy to walk all the way back home. I no longer had any energy left to take even one more step. I sat there completely fatigued, despondent, feeling faint, and unable to catch my breath. My racing heart was absolutely pounding in my chest—racing erratically in excess of 180 beats per minute and I was clearly in A-fib.

When I finally did manage to get back home with my concerned children some time later, after making several rest stops along the short return journey, I could barely make it back to my bed, after which I immediately fell asleep for over 3 hours. Later that afternoon, my heart still raced and pounded irregularly, and I was still soaking wet with perspiration from the exhausting ordeal that I had just been through. I called both my pulmonologist and cardiologist to tell them about what had just happened and to relate a plan that had been hatching in my mind. I asked if it would be OK with them if I was to start an exercise program by trying to walk a little each day, hopefully going a little further and perhaps even a bit faster each day. After they each called me back and we had discussed my situation, I told them that—if I was going to die—I would prefer to have it happen out on the road while I was trying to do something to help myself, rather than passively giving up and just waiting around in my bed or in the hospital. They both agreed to my plan saying, as I recall, something like, "Why not give it a try? What do you have to lose?"

Now, as I look back at it, that is the day to which I attribute the beginning of my recovery. Yes, I was taking several inhalants and high doses of prednisone and many other medications that undoubtedly helped, but now I had a plan and better yet, it was a plan that I was prepared to start just as soon as I felt able. It is hard to put into words what a wonderful feeling it was to actually have a plan, one that gave me hope, could improve the quality of my life, and might possibly even offer the chance that I could eventually begin to feel better (and possibly even have some slight chance at recovery).

Then, I actually began my walking program. I started with the same single city block walk that I had just completed with my children, but took just a few extra steps each time. Every day that it was possible, I took this walk, going just a little further each day despite the myriad of serious cardiopulmonary symptoms that I continued to experience throughout—but trying to do it in the same amount of time as the previous day, so that I would be going just a little bit faster. I can still clearly remember how I would feel during those walks, especially during the early days of late 1992 and early 1993. I chronically felt exhausted and extremely short of breath. I frequently felt light headed, and feared that I was going to faint. I experienced strange sensations in my throat and carotids, extreme pressure behind my eyes, and often felt like I would pass out or throw up. My heart would pound in my chest and beat very rapidly, but irregularly. I had missed beats, strange feeling runs and arrhythmias, and occasional episodes of atrial fibrillation that lasted for many hours or days.

During these years, as I continued to carry out my walking recovery program, I continued to have recurrent episodes where I became seriously ill and bedridden with severe cardiopulmonary symptoms. Still, my lovely wife remained concerned, attentive, and supportive throughout, and I grew to love and appreciate her most profoundly. It was at this time that we even took what I told my children was to be a family vacation to North Carolina and Tennessee—the true purpose of which was to find an inexpensive home where we could relocate to a mild climate, a move that would financially enable my wife to stay home with the kids during their growing up years in the event that I did pass away. Fortunately, as it turned out, this move was to eventually prove unnecessary. Ever so gradually, I began to feel better. I was slowly beginning to succeed in my exercising efforts until finally, some 2 years later (in 1994), I was even able to combine some light jogging with my walking through what had by this time become a 7-mile course in the coastal mountains.

So despite my poor prognosis, I slowly began to improve and to gradually feel better. My pulmonary pressures slowly remitted over these years and my energy level began to incrementally increase, although never fully back to baseline. My bouts with anoxia, arrhythmias, tachycardia, fatigue, night sweats, and shortness of breath gradually became fewer and of shorter duration. Ever so slowly, my pulmonary and cardiac functioning began to improve, and various objective tests show that this increased functioning still continues. My physicians seemed to be as surprised as I was and had no explanation for why I recovered.

Although I still struggle with some negative reminders of this devastating illness episode (such as decreased energy, edema in my ankles, various cardiac arrhythmias, atrial fibrillation, occasional night sweats, the impact of a cerebral stroke, and profuse sweating with any exertion), my pulmonary pressures are now within the normal range, my right and left atria are no longer enlarged, and the thickness of my left ventricle has now returned to normal. All in all, I can only thank God for every added healthy day of life that I am able to experience. I am exceptionally pleased with this unanticipated (but most fortunate) outcome. Although my exercise program and the medical care that I received undoubtedly helped, to this day I am struck by the fact that out of the worst period of my entire life, something as good as the DIGMA model ultimately emerged, which is something that I can only thank God for. Other than this, I have no adequate explanation as to why I recovered, but am most grateful that I could somehow use this terrible personal experience in a helpful way to the benefit of others. The way that I look at it, I have already been blessed by having these 17 years of additional days—days that have allowed me to enjoy and raise my children, to see them all graduate from high school and college, to thoroughly enjoy and fully appreciate my cherished wife of 36 years, and to fully develop, implement, and test the DIGMA model.

By 1996, My Health Eventually Improved Enough to Implement 12 Weekly DIGMAs

Finally, by 1996, my job situation had changed. I had moved from the Kaiser Permanente Medical Center in Santa Clara to their medical center in San Jose, CA, and I was feeling well enough to put the DIGMA model that I had conceptualized to the test. Within the next 2 years, I successfully launched 12 different weekly DIGMAs (in oncology, nephrology, endocrinology, neurology, rheumatology, and family practice), in which I continued to act as the behaviorist until I took an early retirement package from Kaiser Permanente in 1999. Both during that time and ever since, I have tried out countless different iterations of the DIGMA model through efforts of continuous process improvement—some of which have been successful while others have not, as I explain in this book.

I went on to launch 18 different DIGMAs and Physicals Shared Medical Appointments (PSMA) per year during my 3 years of working half-time as SMA Champion and Director of Clinical Access Improvement between 2000 and 2003 at the Palo Alto Medical Foundation, which is where I developed the PSMA model. I am now enjoying my new job responsibilities as Vice President of Shared Medical Appointments and Group-Based Disease Management at Harvard Vanguard Medical Associates/Atrius Health, where I am also President of the Noffsinger Institute for Group Visits. I plan to have approximately 50 different DIGMAs and PSMAs in both primary and specialty care up and running throughout the various medical centers of our organization by the end of 2009.

These experiences, when coupled with the numerous DIGMAs and PSMAs that I have been privileged to help launch as a consultant working with medical groups nationally and internationally, have enabled me to participate in the launching of DIGMAs and PSMAs with more than 400 providers to date and to have personal experience with more than 20,000 patient visits in these two group visit models that I originated.

I can safely say that there is hardly any beginner's mistake that I have not already made at one time or another, yet every one of these experiences has provided a learning opportunity and some hard-earned pearls of wisdom that I am now able to pass along to the readers of this book. However, what is most important in understanding my passion for group visits—and the wonderful quality as well as service benefits that these SMA models can offer to our patients when they are properly designed, supported, and run—is to understand their humble beginnings as one frustrated patient's attempt to try to deliver healthcare in a way that could be better for patients, physicians, organizations, insurers, and purchasers alike.

I Thought that I Understood What My Patients Were Going Through, But Now Realize I Did Not

Looking back on this turbulent period of my life, I must admit that I am surprised at how much I have learned about health, illness, doctors, healthcare innovations, the medical system, and being a patient. When I originally experienced this 4-year illness episode, I had not only studied chronic illness, but had actually been working with chronically ill patients for more than a decade. I had received my first Ph.D. in psychology with a certificate in psychoanalysis and my second Ph.D. in counseling psychology at UC, Berkeley with my dissertation being on stress and illness.

As Director of Oncology Counseling and Chronic Illness Services at Kaiser Permanente, I had probably counseled more than 10,000 chronically ill patients with advanced disease (and their families), set up countless treatment programs for the medically ill, and felt that I truly understood my patients. I consider myself an empathetic person, and my wife and friends do as well. Given the unique perspective and understanding that my background and professional experience provided, if anyone should have recognized and truly appreciated the magnitude of such a life-altering experience as receiving a devastating medical diagnosis (and the emotional significance of then having to live with this horrible, life-threatening disease), I certainly should have, and I sincerely believed that I did.

Yet, looking back at it now in the light of my subsequent illness experiences, I realize that, in fact, I did not fully appreciate what my patients were experiencing. I know that there are doctors throughout the country (and undoubtedly around the world as well) who probably feel every day of their professional lives very much like I did and truly believe that they understand the illnesses they are dealing with and know what their patients are actually experiencing. While they might understand the diseases and organ systems they are treating, I doubt that they truly understand what's really going on inside of the patients they are caring for any more than I did, i.e., their innermost thoughts and feelings; worries about children, spouse, and family; wondering "Why me?"; feeling alone and cheated; experiencing the devastation to self-esteem that accompanies lingering illness and no longer being able to carry out one's normal roles and functions; and the anxiety, depression, and deathlike exhausting fatigue that so often grips the seriously ill. I believe now that to truly understand what our patients are experiencing, we must ourselves have faced serious illness.

DIGMAs Continue to Be a Work in Progress

It took many years for me to fully develop the DIGMA model (a work that is still in progress) and to feel well enough and have the opportunity to actually begin designing, implementing, and evaluating the very first DIGMAs in 1996. The basic elements of this model, as well as the reason that I am such an avid proponent of group visits, have been a direct result of my personal experience as a frustrated, gravely ill patient facing the shortcomings and limitations of individual office visits and traditional medical care in our broken healthcare system. The DIGMA was not originated, as some might believe (especially because I first implemented the DIGMA model in a large, staff model HMO setting), as a way to make doctors work harder by seeing even more patients or as a means for managed-care organizations to make more money by leveraging existing resources, containing costs, and improving their bottom line.

Providing patients with improved service and a better, higher quality healthcare experience has always been my first priority and ultimate personal objective. The remarkable efficiency and cost savings benefits of the DIGMA model were simply serendipitous side effects of this model. Only now am I able to look back to fully appreciate and marvel at how God was able to help me turn such a devastating personal tragedy into something as positive and beneficial to patients as properly run DIGMAs (and later, PSMAs).

Someday, when I am lying on my deathbed and reflecting back on my life's work, it is the fact that these shared medical appointment models—as they were originally conceived—provide patients with a better, more comprehensive, and more accessible healthcare experience (one that can increase both patient and physician professional satisfaction) that will make me the most proud. It will not be the fact that they happen to provide a means for physicians to be more productive or for a stronger bottom line to be realized. The enhanced productivity and cost savings provided by DIGMAs and PSMAs are serendipitous and nice and might even be a necessary prerequisite to economic viability and for continued growth and expansion. However, of primary importance are the improved service, care, and healing benefits which these group visit models can offer to our patients, i.e., rather than their direct efficiency and economic benefits.

Interest in Group Visits Continues to Grow

When I initially wrote the first article on DIGMAs and submitted it for publication in the *Journal of the American Medical Association* in 1998, they sent it out to two reviewers who came back with a split decision as a result of having diametrically opposing views on group visits in general and DIGMAs in particular. As I recall, one reviewer was rich in praise and thought that DIGMAs represented a remarkable healthcare innovation that had the potential to change healthcare for the better by offering benefits to doctors and patients alike and thought that the article definitely should be published. The other reviewer thought it was a terrible idea, was scathing in his criticism of group visits, and concluded in the strongest of terms that the article should not be published. I immediately recognized what a controversial issue group visits might become, and how divisive an issue they could prove to be in the medical community at large. After all, they involve a major paradigm shift and a great deal of change—and how many of us can truly claim that we are quick to embrace change, especially radical and disruptive change?

Furthermore, group visits can be perceived as threatening by many because, at first glance, they appear to chisel away at today's gold standard of traditional medical care and the very foundation bedrock of modern medicine, i.e., the individual office visit. I say "at first glance" because I see group visits as being very compatible with the judicious use of individual office visits, as DIGMAs, Cooperative HealthCare Clinics (CHCCs) and PSMAs were always meant to complement, and never to completely replace, individual office visits.

There is something that can be very healing about groups, where people are able to reach out and touch one another–and connect and support each other in a positive way. When properly designed and conducted, group visits can bring these healing properties into the medical appointment and into each patient's healthcare experience. That is why I sometimes say that DIGMAs and PSMAs are individual office visits *plus*, with the *plus* being the help and support provided by other patients and a multidisciplinary care delivery team—as well as the improved access, additional time with one's own doctor, greater patient education, and more relaxed pace of care delivery that these models offer.

Immediately after this rejection by the *Journal of the American Medical Association*, I submitted the original article on DIGMAs to the American Medical Group Association (AMGA) for consideration in their publication—which, upon thinking about it, I felt was a better venue anyway because *Group Practice Journal* tended to reach the high-level executive leadership of many (if not most) of the larger medical groups in the country. After the article was accepted for publication and the brown envelope containing the author's copies finally arrived at my home at the very beginning of 1999, I had my wife and children gather around it and say a prayer to the effect that it was well done and not filled with typos, inaccuracies, and errors that might prove embarrassing and result in irretrievable damage to the DIGMA concept.

What I found, to my absolute astonishment, was that AMGA felt so highly about this new healthcare innovation and its potential benefits to patients, physicians, and healthcare organizations alike that—for the first time in their history—they published an issue of *Group Practice Journal* with an author's face, rather than a graphic design, on the front cover—along with the words: "Dr. Ed Noffsinger Explains How To Take Care of Your Patients & Your Bottom Line" (Fig. 1).

The rest, as they say, is history. Immediately after this initial article was published, I got the following phone message from Dr. John Scott, the originator of the Cooperative HealthCare Clinic group model: "Noffsinger, this is John Scott out at Kaiser in Colorado. I've been reading your article, and this is great stuff! I do have one question, though: How the heck do you do it? Give me a call sometime and let's talk." This was the beginning of a lengthy and enduring professional friendship.

Interest in group visits has continued to grow steadily over the subsequent decade, during which time they have been the subject of numerous presentations and articles in medical journals. In 2002, while acting as Director of Clinical Access Improvement as well as the head of the Shared Medical Appointment Department at the Palo Alto Medical Foundation, I developed a group visit model for the efficient delivery of private physical examinations, which I called the Physicals Shared Medical Appointment

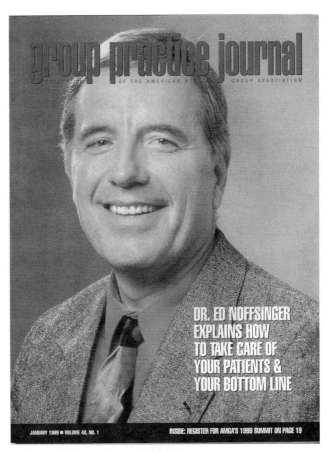

Fig. 1 For the first time in its history, *Group Practice Journal* put an author's photograph on the cover when they published Dr. Noffsinger's first article on DIGMAs because they believed so strongly in the concept of group medical appointments
(Courtesy of *Group Practice Journal*, American Medical Group Association, Alexandria, VA)

(PSMA) model. Like the DIGMA model before it, the PSMA model is also a multidisciplinary, team-based approach to care that offers several key benefits to patients and physicians alike, and it also garnered considerable attention in the press and medical community. Group visits have also received a great deal of positive press from the mass media, i.e., from television, radio, magazines, and newspapers. In addition, AMGA has continued to publish 19 of my articles during the past 9 years and recently told me that they were the most successful series of articles that they have ever published—as they have continued to receive requests for reprints of the entire series throughout the past several years.

As Dr. John Scott and I have continued to give numerous presentations over the years (both together and separately) to local, regional, national, and international audiences, we have noticed a tremendous growth in the number of attendees at our talks. Where there used to be 15–20 in the audience, it is no longer uncommon to have 100, 200, or more in attendance. While there has been an amazing growth of interest in shared medical appointments over the past few years, there is still much room for group visits to grow in the future. Gone is the not infrequent hostility that Dr. Scott and I used to receive from medical audiences during our presentations in those early years, which has been largely supplanted over time by "We know that we need to change by doing group visits, so please just show us how to do them correctly."

This book and accompanying DVD are designed to do just that—as they are not only intended to be a definitive treatise on group visits, but also a comprehensive *how-to* toolkit for doing them correctly. Group visits now appear to be on firm footing and should continue to grow rapidly throughout the coming years because of the multiple benefits they offer to patients, physicians, healthcare organizations, insurers, and corporate purchasers alike—that is, assuming that they are properly designed, supported, and run (and barring some unforeseen future negative turn of events regarding the issue of reimbursement, which is currently not completely resolved).

Boston, MA   Edward Noffsinger, Ph.D.
                            Vice President of Shared Medical Appointments
                                    and Group-Based Disease Management
                              President, Noffsinger Institute for Group Visits
                       Harvard Vanguard Medical Associates/Atrius Health

Acknowledgments

There are so many people I would like to acknowledge for their contributions to this book and attached DVD that there simply is not sufficient time or space to do so adequately here. I am both grateful for, and humbled by, the fact that so many have given as generously as they have of their time, talent, and energy in their contributions to this book and accompanying DVD. Nonetheless, I will attempt to do the best that I can within the limitations of space—apologizing in advance to the many others that I may have inadvertently omitted.

A Special Thanks to Kaiser Permanente, Palo Alto Medical Foundation, and Harvard Vanguard Medical Associates/Atrius Health

First of all, I would especially like to thank Kaiser Permanente, the Palo Alto Medical Foundation, and Harvard Vanguard Medical Associates/Atrius Health—their administrators, physicians, and patients—for the opportunities that they provided me to develop and implement my group visit models at their facilities. Without them, my pioneering work in originating these shared medical appointment models would never have been possible. Through their support and encouragement, I was able to create the innovative Drop-In Group Medical Appointment (DIGMA) model in 1996 at the Kaiser Permanente San Jose Medical Center and to develop the counterintuitive—but extremely efficient and satisfying—Physicals Shared Medical Appointment model in 2001 at the Palo Alto Medical Foundation. The Noffsinger Institute for Group Visits that we are currently developing at Harvard Vanguard Medical Associates/Atrius Health will be of lasting benefit to all those who want to learn how to design, implement, and evaluate successful group visit programs within their own medical groups, now and in the future.

In addition to the 12 initial physicians at Kaiser Permanente who were early adopters of the DIGMA model and with whom I developed such close relationships by acting as their behaviorist from 1996 to 1999, my thanks goes out to The Medical Editing Department of the Kaiser Foundation Research Institute for the editorial assistance that they provided for the early articles that I published.

A special thank you also needs to go out to my wife, Janet, and my children (Michael, Angie, and Kenny), who spent countless hours in word processing and proofreading these early articles. I would also like to thank Kaiser Permanente, as well as the American Medical Group Association (AMGA), for use of the DIGMA photographs that were originally taken to be utilized in my group visit articles published by AMGA's Group Practice Journal.

I would like to express my gratitude to the Palo Alto Medical Foundation (PAMF) for the generous contribution of all of their forms that are included on the DVD attached to this book, as well as for many photographs that have been used in this book.

Thanks to All the Medical Groups and Healthcare Organizations that Invited Me to Consult

I would also like to thank the numerous healthcare organizations that have invited me as an independent consultant to present in the area of group visits, quality, access, enhanced practice management, chronic disease management, and improved patient and physician satisfaction—such as Cleveland Clinic, Dartmouth–Hitchcock, Sutter Health, University of Virginia, Geisinger Health System, Woodland Healthcare, Advocate Health, Bristol Park Medical Group, Luther Midelfort-Mayo, St. Jude Heritage, Yale University Health Services, Austin Regional Clinic, Arnette Clinic, Northern Health in British Columbia, Everett Clinic, ProMed Healthcare, Mercy Clinic, Dutch Institute for Healthcare Improvement, Henry Ford Medical Center, Scripps Health, Texas Tech University, Scott and White, Sentara Healthcare, Fallon Clinic, WellSpan Health, Dreyer Medical Clinic, Rush-Presbyterian-St. Luke Medical Center, UC Davis Medical Center, and numerous DoD (Army, Air Force, and Navy), VHA medical centers, and public health facilities, to name just a few. In combination, these experiences provided me with a tremendous amount of experience in actually setting up and running group visit programs successfully in primary and specialty care in a wide variety of healthcare settings—practical experiences that I have drawn heavily from throughout the pages of this book.

Thanks to the Many Medical Organizations that Have Invited Me to Present at Their Conferences

In addition, I would also like to thank the various medical organizations in the private, public, and governmental sectors that have invited me to give innumerable presentations at their regional, national, and international medical conferences over the years—such as IHI, AMGA, AAFP, ACP-ACIM, ACC, HAP, NAPH, AANP, British Columbia Medical Association, Harvard Medical School's International Conference on Obesity, assorted regional medical societies, AMA, various DoD, VA, and Tri-Care Regional Conferences, etc. These presentations have enabled me not only to *spread the gospel* of group visits but also to learn about what others are doing with SMAs around the nation and world—which has added immeasurably to the contents of this book.

Acknowledgements for Contributions to the Body of this Book

There are so many people and organizations to thank for their positive contributions to this book that I fear that I may inadvertently forget to mention some of them; however, I will try to do my best.

A Special Thanks to American Medical Group Association

I would also like to thank my many friends at the American Medical Group Association (www.AMGA.org)—and most especially Tom Flatt, Senior Editor of *Group Practice Journal,* for all of his encouragement and editorial assistance over the years—for helping me to launch my DIGMA and PSMA models through the series of 19 articles on group visits that they published over the years in *Group Practice Journal*. In addition, I am most appreciative of their granting me permission to not only draw extensively from these articles in this book but also for use of photographs in which I was the behaviorist that were originally taken for use in some of my early DIGMA articles that they published in

Group Practice Journal. I would also like to thank AMGA for their permission to use the front cover of their January 1999 issue. I am extremely indebted to AMGA for all that they have done to further group visits over the years.

My Thanks to All Medical Journals, Trade Publications, and the Mass Media for Their Articles on Group Visits

A special thanks goes out to the numerous medical journals and trade publications that have published articles on group visits (and the writers of these articles), from which I have quoted extensively throughout this book. I also thank the numerous persons in the mass media that have carried write-ups and stories on group visits: (1) newspapers around the country such as The Wall Street Journal, The Boston Globe, The Orange County Register, The Washington Times, South Florida Sun-Sentinel, and San Jose Mercury News; (2) consumer-oriented magazines like Time, Good Housekeeping, AARP's Modern Maturity, and U.S. News & World Report; (3) electronic media such as WebMD; (4) radio stations (including national public radio and many local and regional stations); and (5) many local and national television stations, including CNN, CNN Headline News, PBS Healthweek, Northern California's Channel 3, etc. I have quoted many of these sources on numerous occasions throughout this book.

Thanks Also to the Many Specific Individuals Who Have Made Particularly Important Contributions to This Book and DVD

Nobody deserves a greater thanks for getting this book into final form than Margaret Burns, whom Springer assigned to this book, as she has spend countless hours during the past 2 years editing and re-editing both the manuscript for this book and the materials for its attached DVD. I greatly value and appreciate her professionalism, consummate skill, organizational abilities, and tireless efforts—all of which have proved to be critical to the final product. For that, I remain greatly in her debt. I would like to thank Rob Albano of Springer for his vision in seeing that this book could be a part of the dialogue on healthcare in this country and thanks as well to Kathy Cacace of Springer for seeing the book through to publication.

A special thank you goes to Zeev E. Neuwirth, MD, Chief of Clinical Effectiveness & Innovation, Harvard Vanguard Medical Associates/Atrius Health (HVMA/AH) in Newton, MA, for the remarkable and thought provoking foreword to this book. Dr. Neuwirth has an encyclopedic grasp of healthcare innovations, process improvement, and clinical effectiveness—as well as of the multifarious challenges facing our broken healthcare system today. A thoughtful innovator and valued friend and colleague, he has an in-depth appreciation of group visits and the multiple benefits they can provide to patients, physicians, and healthcare organizations alike—but possesses a deep and abiding respect for the positive impact that, when properly designed and implemented, shared medical appointments can have on our patients' healing experience. He (along with my SMA Program Coordinator, Deb Prescott, and SMA/IT Project Manager, Nancy Curtin) has stood shoulder-to-shoulder with me during the past year, sharing excitement and frustrations alike, initially in setting up our shared medical appointment program, then in fine-tuning and perfecting it, and finally in launching it organization-wide at HVMA/AH. Thank you to Roanne Weisman for editing and rewriting on the preface to the book and to Ann Marie Frakes, Vice President, Development in Administration at Harvard Vanguard Medical Associates/Atrius Health for providing the budget for this to be done.

I would also like to extend my appreciation to all the physicians who allowed their group visit programs to be photographed for use as illustrations in this book—many of whose photos, unfortunately, could not be included due to limited space and the large number of contributing physicians and healthcare organizations. Most especially, I would like to thank those physicians whose DIGMA and PSMA photos were used as illustrations in this book: Drs. Tom Morledge, Holly Thacker, and Patricio Aycinena at Cleveland Clinic; Dr. Jan Millermaier at ProMed Family Practice; Dr. Lynn Dowdell at Kaiser Permanente Medical Center in San Jose; Dr. Keith Novak at Memphis Tennessee VA Medical Center; and Drs. John Lu, Mary Ann Sarda-Maduro, Margaret Forsyth, Barry Eisenberg, Richard Greene, and Melvin Britton at the Palo Alto Medical Foundation.

I would also like to thank Dr. Richard A. Maxwell and Dr. David L. Bronson at Cleveland Clinic; Dr. Ed Millermaier at ProMed Family Practice; Alice Domes at Northern Health; the Regional Multimedia Department at Kaiser Permanente; and Dr. David Hooper, Gina Earle, and Joan Colvin at the Palo Alto Medical Foundation for being instrumental in obtaining these photos and submitting them for use in this book. Thank you to Margie Namie, RN, MPH, CPHQ, Vice President of Chronic Care Management, Mercy Health Partners in Cincinnati, OH, for the examples of their coordinated invitation letter, flier, and poster. Thanks to Marci Sindell, Vice President of Marketing, Harvard Vanguard Medical Associates for their sample poster and flier seen in the book and on the DVD.

In addition, I would also like to acknowledge Dr. John C. Scott, a fellow pioneer in group visits and the originator of the Cooperative HealthCare Clinic model, for his friendship, encouragement, and advice over the years. I find him to be a generous person, a constant source of inspiration, and a fountain of knowledge in the area of group visits—and count myself fortunate to have known and associated with him. As it turns out, our independently conceived group visit models are mutually supportive and enhancing rather than mutually exclusive. In addition to numerous copresentations that we have given to international, national, and local audiences over the years, we have coauthored several articles regarding understanding today's major group visit models, practical tips for establishing successful group visit programs, and preventing potential abuses of group visits that were published in *Group Practice Journal* and *The Permanente Journal*—articles that I have drawn from in this book. I would also like to thank Dr. Scott for having reviewed and edited Chapter 4 of this book, which is on his CHCC model. I have learned much from John over the years that has helped to shape my own thinking and which has undoubtedly contributed to this book in numerous ways.

Finally, I would like to let the medical folks in the Army, Navy, Air Force, and VA know that they hold a warm place in my heart and that it makes me especially proud when my DIGMA and PSMA models are of help to them in the special work that they do every day. This sentiment is expressed in the following brief vignette, which is meant as a tribute to both my uncle, Ernest Sterka, and to those who care for our fighting men and women—whose sacrifices, patriotism, and courage preserve the freedoms that we all enjoy every day of our lives. Born in 1943, my first memory in life was of my uncle in the Army Air Corps coming home in his tan uniform on leave from the European theater and joyfully tossing me up in the air while my mother and father hugged and greeted him with tender love. It was an especially warm and loving moment that touched me and became indelibly etched into my heart throughout life. Sadly, he was killed the following month in the Battle of the Bulge—something which neither the family nor I could ever fully accept. As a result, I never forget the price paid by our fighting men and women for the freedoms that we all enjoy and am particularly pleased when my work helps those medical caregivers who care for them in the Veterans Health Administration and Department of Defense (Air Force, Army, Navy, Marine Corps, and Coast Guard). Thanks for your service.

Contributors to the Outcomes Chapter

I am particularly grateful to all of the contributors to the Outcomes chapter of this book. I thank Stacey Lutz-McCain, a Certified Registered Nurse Practitioner (CRNP), for sharing her personal story as a provider who went from initial outright refusal, to a willingness to try, to great anxiety during the initial launch, and ultimately to clinical success with her group visit—and who eventually came to enjoy her DIGMA so much that she soon wanted to do DIGMAs full time. I wish to also extend my thanks to Karen E. Jones, MD, FACP (and Meagan Renninger VanScyoc, PA-C, MBA, who assisted her), both because of their specialized application of the PSMA model (i.e., for preoperative gastric bypass pulmonary consultations and sleep apnea consultations) and because it clearly demonstrates the robustness of this group visit model. They found that even though their PSMA group census was substantially below the recommended target of tripling provider productivity whenever possible (which is something that I never recommend, since reduced census translates into increased likely of failure for the entire SMA program), the PSMA model was nonetheless so efficient and productive that it was still capable of solving access problems and of doing so with high levels of patient and provider satisfaction.

I also want to thank Dr. Thomas N. Atkins, Chief Medical Officer at the Sutter Medical Foundation in Sacramento, California, for his contribution to the outcomes chapter, which was based on the series of three articles we coauthored that were published in the March, April, and May 2001 issues of AMGA's *Group Practice Journal*. These articles were based upon a 6-session pilot project (which involved four physicians at two different Sutter sites) that was conducted under his leadership while I was a consultant at Sutter Medical Foundation. The results are important because they are fairly typical of DIGMA pilot studies conducted with multiple physicians in primary and specialty care over time and because they contain several important teaching points.

I would also like to recognize Dr. Keith W. Novak, the Associate Chief of Staff for Ambulatory Care at the Memphis Tennessee VA Medical Center (VAMC), who discusses some of the experiences that he has had over the years in using the DIGMA and PSMA models. Dr. Novak (who now also runs a DIGMA for homeless veterans) has been instrumental not only in moving group visits forward within the Memphis VAMC but also in establishing the highly recognized Combat Veterans Physicals SMA. In addition to working with Dr. Novak in implementing DIGMAs and PSMAs in his own practice, it was also an honor to help him launch the first ever Physicals SMA for Combat Veterans returning from Iraq and Afghanistan.

I would similarly like to thank Dr. Kenneth Meehan (who published an article entitled "Group Medical Appointments: Organization and Implementation in the Bone Marrow Transplantation Clinic" in the January 2006 issue of *Supportive Cancer Therapy*) who presents another specialized application of the PSMA. Dr. Kenneth Meehan et al. report that using the PSMA model in their bone marrow transplantation unit resulted in Transplant PSMAs that were surprisingly satisfying to patients, providers, and caregivers alike.

I also appreciate Dr. Richard A. Maxwell's contribution, in which he writes about the DIGMA and PSMA program at Cleveland Clinic, i.e., the background and current status of Cleveland Clinic's SMA program, why they selected the DIGMA and PSMA models, how they bill for these visits, how their program is evolving, and the access and patient satisfaction benefits that they are experiencing through this program. A pediatrician at the Cleveland Clinic Wooster Family Health Center, Dr. Maxwell has been the shared medical appointment champion for Cleveland Clinic since its inception and is in a unique position to discuss lessons learned, hurdles that needed to be overcome, how Cleveland Clinic's SMA program is currently evolving, and specific recommendations to other medical groups interested in launching a SMA program of their own. Dr. Maxwell is a personal friend with whom I have stayed in contact and have enjoyed giving many presentations over the years. I am also indebted to both Dr. Maxwell and Dr. David L. Bronson for their assistance in obtaining—and to the many physicians and SMA teams at Cleveland Clinic for their willingness to provide—numerous photographs of their DIGMA and PSMA sessions for use as illustrations in this book.

My thanks go out to Louis A. Kazal, Jr., M.D. (Associate Professor and Chief Clinical Officer, Department of Community and Family Medicine, Dartmouth Medical School, Hanover, New Hampshire and Chief, Section of Family Medicine, Dartmouth–Hitchcock Medical Center, Lebanon, New Hampshire) and to Gillian C. Jackson (Quality Improvement Coordinator, Dartmouth–Hitchcock Community Health Center, Lebanon, New Hampshire) who assisted him in this project and write-up regarding their diabetes program, which is largely based on the CHCC model. Their contribution to the Outcomes chapter is of interest because they demonstrate that group medical visits—when applied to patients with diabetes in a setting where access was not a problem—not only increased the frequency of obtaining recommended diabetes tests and preventive medicine measures but also resulted in very high levels of patient satisfaction.

My appreciation likewise goes out to Carolyn L. Kerrigan, MD, Professor of Surgery at Dartmouth, who has been championing SMAs at Dartmouth–Hitchcock since 2003. In the Outcomes chapter, she discusses her use of the PSMA model for surgical intake visits for women seeking consultation for breast reduction surgery (which she terms the "BRITE" visit). This has so dramatically increased the efficiency and quality of her surgical intake process that Dr. Kerrigan has been able to retool her master schedule to dedicate more time to surgery—and less time to individual intakes—during her work-week. Because of the remarkable success that she was able to achieve through this application of the PSMA model to breast reduction surgery intakes, Dr. Kerrigan has concluded that she cannot compete with herself in the quality of care that she is able to offer her patients in group versus individual office visits and has therefore shifted to doing group visits almost entirely for these patients. In addition, she has expanded this work to carpal tunnel surgical intake visits as well.

I also thank Janet M. Carroll, RD, LD, CDE, DIGMA Coordinator at the Kansas City VA Medical Center (KCVA) and Wayne L. Fowler, Jr., M.D., Ph.D., FACP, Endocrinologist at the KCVA for their contribution to the Outcomes chapter. They discuss their experience with using DIGMAs in a chronic illness treatment paradigm for diabetes—a write-up that is important because, to my knowledge, they were the first healthcare system in the country to use the chronic disease population management paradigm I developed for fully using group visits in the treatment of chronic illness. I first published on this chronic disease population management paradigm that makes full use of shared medical appointments in the February 2008 issue of Group Practice Journal (volume 57, number 2), a paradigm that is discussed in great detail in Chapter 7 of this book. Estimating that the KCVA serves approximately 20,000 veterans with diabetes, their large Diabetes DIGMA program is of particular interest because their preliminary clinical outcomes data indicates that, even at this early point of operations, patients seen in their Diabetes DIGMA program are able to achieve better control over their diabetic symptoms.

I would also like to acknowledge Brian E. Logue, Maj, USAF, BSC, Chief Clinical Pharmacy 1st Medical Group, 1st Fighter Wing, Air Combat Command, Langley Air Force Base (who is a Clinical Assistant Professor at the Medical College of Virginia) for his contribution in which he addresses pharmacist managed group medical appointments at the 1st Medical Group, Langley AFB. This contribution regarding the successful SAR, URI, and Lipid DIGMAs run at Langley AFB is of interest because of their implications for applying DIGMAs to urgent care, cold and flu, allergy, and primary care settings—especially when there is a need to treat and triage facility-overwhelming acute infections in order to relieve workload from overcrowded and inundated ER, urgent care, and primary care clinics.

I would also like to thank Andrew H. Lin, M.D., Jeffrey J. Cavendish, M.D., and Daniel F. Seidensticker, M.D. from the Department of Internal Medicine and Division of Cardiology at the Naval Medical Center San Diego in San Diego, California for their study, which demonstrates how the PSMA model can be used in a heart failure clinic to reduce hospitalizations among this costly high-risk patient population. Furthermore, they report that this reduction in hospitalizations was accomplished while simultaneously achieving high levels of patient satisfaction and enhancing other outcomes as well—such as improved medication utilization, increased use of cardiac rehabilitation services, improved compliance with lifestyle recommendations, decreased depression, and enhanced quality of life.

I similarly appreciate the contribution by James B. Sutton, RPA-C (Director of Clinton Family Health Center in Rochester, New York, a large outpatient Medicare and Medicaid provider in the Rochester area), who also serves as Adjunct Clinical Faculty for the Rochester Institute of Technology (RIT) Physician Assistant Program and precepts PA students in Family Medicine. His write-up demonstrates the remarkable benefit that even severely backlogged and overloaded healthcare systems can realize when they simultaneously launch Open Access (or Advance Clinic Access, ACA) and well-designed shared medical appointments (SMAs) in their system—work for which their facility has been recognized both locally and nationally for the changes being undertaken and the resulting outcomes being achieved.

I would like to express my personal appreciation to my friend Dr. Ed Millermaier, MD, MBA (Chief Medical Officer, Ambulatory Care, Borgess Health and Medical Director of ProMed Healthcare in Kalamazoo, Michigan) for the two previously unpublished outcomes studies that he provided. These studies underscore how DIGMAs and PSMAs can be successfully employed to (1) significantly enhance the likelihood of consistently updating screening tests, performance measures, and routine health maintenance for chronically ill patients in attendance (in this case, diabetic patients); and (2) improve clinical outcomes for diabetic patients attending DIGMAs and PSMAs. For virtually all clinical outcomes that were measured, the trend was for SMA patients to outperform those receiving usual one-on-one office care—even when the results were not statistically significant. I also appreciated the many DIGMA and PSMA photographs that Dr. Millermaier and his staff (particularly Dr. Jan Millermaier) contributed for use in this book.

Finally, although international applications are just beginning and still in their earliest stages, DIGMAs and PSMAs are now beginning to find their way onto the international scene—especially when there are workload and access problems, or when there is a mismatch between supply and demand (which is often the case for capitated systems and socialized medicine). In this regard, I would like to thank Alice Domes, RN, BScN, Regional CDPM Coordinator for Northern Health, and Judy Huska, Executive Director, Health Services Integration, Northern Health in Canada for their contribution to the Outcomes chapter. Here, they discuss the early work with shared medical appointments that Northern Health is now undertaking in their Health Service Delivery Area in British Columbia, Canada, which encompasses approximately two-thirds of the upper portion of the province and delivers healthcare to a population of over 300,000, many of whom live in northern and rural settings. I also thank Ms. Domes—as well as the physicians, staffs, and patients at their facilities—for the photographs they contributed to this book. Similarly, I would like to acknowledge Stan Janssen RN, MS, Senior Advisor Radboud University, Nijmegen, the Netherlands, and Femke Seesing, MSC, Advisor, Dutch Institute for Healthcare Improvement (CBO) for their contribution to the Outcomes chapter with regard to how DIGMAs are beginning to be introduced into the Netherlands.

Acknowledgments for Contributions to the DVD Attached to this Book

There are many individuals to whom I am indebted for their contributions to the DVD attached to this book. This DVD certainly adds value to the book and its readers by providing extensive edited video segments of medical grand rounds, behaviorist training, and mock DIGMA presentations that I personally made at Northern Health in British Columbia. It also includes templates and examples of all of the forms and promotional materials that readers will need in order to launch their own successful DIGMA and/or PSMA program.

I would like to extend a very special *thank you* to my many friends at Northern Health in British Columbia for their generous contributions to this book and its attached DVD. I am particularly appreciative of their willingness to have me include (i.e., in the DVD attached to this book) the behaviorist training and *mock DIGMA* sessions that I conducted with them while spending a week there in February 2005. I am especially indebted to Marvin Barg of the Care North Resource Team for the great job that he did in spending countless hours pulling together and editing the massive amount of videotaped material that was taken during the week that I spent with them and in reformatting this material for use in the DVD attached to this book. I would also like to thank Dr. Paul Murray for use of the *behaviorist training* and *mock DIGMA* training presentations contained in the attached DVD, which were centered on preparation for his upcoming DIGMA.

Templates of All Forms and Promotional Materials Needed for a Successful SMA Program

One of the great benefits of this book is that it has a DVD attached that contains templates and examples of all the forms and promotional materials that providers and healthcare systems will need in order to launch a successful group visit program in their own system. It is important to note that these forms are meant as examples and templates to be used for illustrative purposes only and are not meant to be used *carte blanche* exactly as presented. Ultimately, each healthcare organization will need to develop the appropriate forms and promotional materials for its own system. In addition, certain forms (such as the confidentiality agreement/release form) will be subject to various local, regional, and national guidelines and regulations—and will therefore need to be specifically developed by each medical group in consultation with their own medical risk management department and/ or corporate attorney for their own specific needs, regulations, and requirements.

I would especially like to acknowledge the Palo Alto Medical Foundation for allowing me to use all of their SMA forms, many of which were developed while I was SMA Champion and headed their DIGMA and PSMA program. In addition, I would also like to thank Alice Domes and Marvin Barg at Northern Health in British Columbia for use of their SMA forms; Dr. Richard Maxwell of Cleveland Clinic for use of their SMA materials; Karen Jones at WellSpan in York PA (for their "Frequently Asked Questions" and Diabetes Paper Chart Note Template forms); Dr. Wayne Fowler and Janet Carroll at the Kansas City VAMC (for the many forms included in their VA Toolkit and the tri-fold program description flier used in Dr. Fowler's Diabetes DIGMA); Annie Tuttle at the Loma Linda VA Healthcare System (for use of their CHF flier); Dr. Mark Schafer at Bristol Park Medical; and Dr. Thom Atkins at Sutter Medical Group (for use of their SMA Wall Poster).

Disclaimer

The views expressed by Dr. Edward Noffsinger are based on his best available knowledge, both as the originator of two of today's three major group visit models and as a result of approximately 20,000 patient visits in DIGMAs and PSMAs with over 400 different providers that he has been involved with in developing their group visit programs during the past 12 years. Nonetheless, one must keep in mind that group visits are still an evolving and comparatively new phenomenon and that much about them is still unknown or changing. Based on his extensive experience in the field, the author is expressing his personal knowledge and viewpoint to the best of his ability in this book; however, no guarantees or warrantees exist or are implied. Therefore, it is not only prudent but also incumbent upon readers to do their own independent research and due diligence—i.e., in addition to reading this book and studying the attached DVD—before proceeding with any group visit program.

Although it contains a remarkable amount of information, the attached DVD is not meant to stand-alone, but rather to be utilized in conjunction with the much more detailed information contained in this book. The reader must keep in mind that the medical grand rounds presentation—as well as the behaviorist and mock DIGMA training sessions—depicted in the DVD was, in the interest of time and available storage space, heavily edited from its original format by Northern Health. Also, whereas the author spent 8 years in the writing of this book, the events depicted in the videos on the attached DVD transpired over just 1 week's time.

The reader should find all of the forms and promotional materials included in the DVD to be very helpful; however, they are meant as templates and examples for illustrative purposes only. It is imperative that each system not only develop its own specific look for their SMA program but also develop—and have their medical-legal team review—all of its own SMA forms to best meet their own particular organizational needs, regulatory demands, billing requirements, confidentiality requirements, etc.

Contents

Contents of the DVD

Part I
Group Visits: The Next Step in Medical Care

Chapter 1
Introduction to Group Visits

It's called a group visit, and it's the latest twist on the most fundamental encounter in medicine: the doctor–patient relationship. Health clinics across the country, from a Mayo Clinic affiliate in Wisconsin to Stanford University School of Medicine in California, have recently introduced programs. . .Some doctors set up their group visits around patients with specific chronic ailments—such as diabetes, arthritis or hypertension, or for routine pediatric or geriatric complains. Fallon Clinic Inc., Worcester, Mass., has such visits, and its medical director, Jonathan Harding, praises their efficiency. Rather than saying the same thing 20 different times to 20 different patients, he says, the doctor only has to say it once. Though it seems paradoxical, both doctors and patients maintain the arrangement reclaims the closeness of the doctor–patient relationship that many argue has been eroded in the era of managed care.

Martinez B. Now it's mass medicine—doctors start seeing groups of patients to save time; one-on-one vs. one-on-12. *Wall Street Journal* Monday, August 21, 2000; p. B1.

Would you be interested in a care delivery model that could simultaneously: (1) increase productivity, access, and efficiency; (2) improve patient education, prevention, and chronic disease management; (3) enhance quality, clinical outcomes, and the patient's healing experience; (4) more closely attend to mind as well as body needs—psychosocial needs that are known to drive a large percentage of all medical visits; (5) control costs while max-packing visits and providing patients with a one-stop healthcare shopping experience; (6) deliver consistently high levels of patient and physician professional satisfaction, and bring some joy back into the practice of medicine; (7) increase job performance by optimally off-loading as many provider responsibilities as possible onto less costly members of a multidisciplinary care team; (8) provide a value-added service that offered more time with the provider and a more relaxed pace of care; and (9) make use of the greatest untapped resource in every healthcare system (i.e., the patients themselves, not only in their own disease self-management, but also in the more altruistic sense of helping, encouraging, and supporting each other)? If so, then read on.

First and foremost, *group visits* are medical appointments in which multiple patients are seen simultaneously by the physician in a supportive group setting—i.e., the focus is upon the actual delivery of medical care. However, they also bring a great deal of patient education and emotional support into the appointment by integrating the help and support of other patients as well as an entire multidisciplinary care delivery team into each patient's healthcare experience. Confronted by today's quality mandates and multiple healthcare challenges, the potential of group visits (also referred to as *shared medical appointments* [SMAs], shared visits, shared medical visits, group medical appointments, group appointments, etc.) to both redesign the physician office practice and enhance care for the chronically ill is just beginning to emerge. Managed care demands for increased productivity, when coupled with reduced reimbursements and dwindling bottom lines, have sliced the time pie into ever smaller pieces and led to shorter, more pressured appointments. The economic imperatives of today's managed care environment and the fast-paced treadmill of outpatient care has impacted physicians' practices in that it has increased their roles as gatekeepers, diagnosticians, documenters, and technicians fighting disease—and has decreased the amount of time they have to comfort, console, educate, emotionally support, and get to know their patients.

By off-loading as many duties as possible onto the multidisciplinary team, group visits provide an innovative alternative to the trend of putting evermore responsibilities onto the shoulders of the physicians so that they are able to look at, and have more direct contact time with, their patients. Group visits are particularly helpful in better managing busy, backlogged practices and in

E.B. Noffsinger, *Running Group Visits in Your Practice*, DOI 10.1007/b106441_1,
© Springer Science+Business Media, LLC 2009

meeting the complex needs of the chronically ill, patients with mind as well as body needs, and elderly patients and their families.

Three Major Group Visit Models

Three major group visit models are currently in widespread use: the *drop-in group medical appointment* (DIGMA) and *physicals shared medical appointment* (PSMA) models originated by the author, and the *cooperative healthcare clinic* (CHCC) model developed by Dr. John C. Scott. DIGMAs and CHCCs focus primarily on follow-up visits, but PSMAs (as the name implies) are specifically designed for increasing the efficiency of delivering complete private physical examinations in primary care as well as in the various medical and surgical subspecialties. Table 1.1 summarizes the unique and differentiating features of today's three major SMA models.

In a 2004 article on SMAs, *Private Practice Success* presents the case for group visits as follows: "Imagine

Table 1.1 Unique features of the three major group visit models

	Drop-in group medical appointment	Cooperative healthcare clinic	Physicals shared medical appointment
Primary focus	Follow-up visits (sometimes intakes)	Follow-up visits only	Physical examinations (new and established patients)
Target patients	Most patients in provider's practice or chronic illness program needing a follow-up visit (or sometimes an intake)	Same 15–20 high-utilizing, multi-morbid geriatric patients for monthly follow-ups	Most patients in provider's practice or chronic illness program needing a private physical examination
Same or different patients	Different	Same	Different
Formal educational presentation	No	Yes	No
Is run like a series of individual office visits?	Yes	No	Yes
Medical care from start to finish?	Yes	No	Yes
Patients come on a regular basis (or just when they need to be seen)	Only when medically necessary	Regular (typically monthly)	Only when medically necessary
Ideal group size	10–16 patients	15–20 patients	*Primary care*: 7–9 males; 6–8 females *Medical and surgical subspecialties*: 10–13 patients
SMA team members	MD, 1–2 nurses, documenter, behaviorist, dedicated scheduler	MD, RN/MA, guest speakers as needed	MD, 2 MAs or nurses, documenter, behaviorist, dedicated scheduler
Other personnel (in larger systems)	Champion and program coordinator	Program coordinator	Champion and program coordinator
Frequency of sessions	Weekly (or twice weekly, daily, etc.)	Monthly (or per best practice guidelines for Specialty CHCC)	Weekly (sometimes twice a week)
Typical length of sessions	90 minutes	2½ hours (1½ hour group followed by 1 hour of individual care to about one-third of patients)	90 minutes
Unique benefits	⇧ Productivity ⇧ Access ⇧ Practice & disease management FFS billing	Reduced nursing home, emergency room, and hospitalization costs; intense patient bonding	⇧ Productivity ⇧ Access ⇧ Practice management FFS billing
Drop-in convenience	Yes	No	No
Subtypes of model	Heterogeneous, homogeneous, and mixed	Specialty CHCC (same format, but for medical subspecialties and meets irregularly)	Heterogeneous, homogeneous, and mixed

Table 1.1 (continued)

	Drop-in group medical appointment	Cooperative healthcare clinic	Physicals shared medical appointment
Much medical care conducted in group (in front of others)	Yes (almost all, except private discussions and examinations)	No (most care is provided individually and in private)	Yes (during interactive group segment only)
Greatest weaknesses	Maintaining census	Not being seen as a class; FFS billing	Maintaining census
Common patient benefits of all 3 SMA models	⇧ Quality; ⇧ patient education; ⇧ attention to psychosocial needs; reduced repetition; ⇧ compliance; ⇧ lifestyle medicine; ⇧ self-efficacy; ⇧ disease self-management skills; help and support of peers; multidisciplinary, team-based care; enhanced continuity; closer follow-up care; improved outcomes; immunity to no-shows by overbooking sessions; cost containment; ⇧ patient and physician satisfaction; better management of elderly and chronically ill patients; extra treatment choice		

FFS, fee-for-service; SMA, shared medical appointment

providing 20 of your hypertension patients the care they need, but only having to offer advice about behavior modification once. Physicians who use shared medical appointments swear these appointments help them provide better care, see more patients, and rekindle the joy of practicing medicine…'Doctors who have backlogs to physical exams will want the physical shared medical appointment (PSMA),' says consultant Edward B. Noffsinger, PhD. 'Doctors with access problems to return visits will want drop in group medical appointments (DIGMAs). And if their primary problem is that they have a small group of very costly patients, they'd want to start with the cooperative healthcare clinic (CHCC)'" (1).

Group Visits for Better Managing Busy Practices and Chronic Illnesses

Group visits or SMAs—terms that are used interchangeably throughout this book—can address many of the critically important economic challenges facing healthcare delivery systems today. They can be used as practice management tools for better and more efficiently managing large, busy, and backlogged practices as well as tools for better managing both chronic illnesses and geriatric patients. Group visits can offer remarkable benefits in today's integrated healthcare delivery systems by addressing many of the most important healthcare challenges of our time: double digit annual increases in the cost of care; ongoing access problems; inadequate attention to performance measures and health maintenance updates; the lack of job doability; increasing demands from today's informed patients; the growing medical needs of an aging patient population; decreasing reimbursements and stressed bottom lines; and the rising dissatisfaction of patients and physicians alike.

In addition, because so many healthcare dollars go toward the treatment of chronic illnesses, highly productive and efficient group visits can enhance quality and help to contain the rapidly rising cost of providing care to the chronically ill. These high-risk medical patients have the potential for both poor outcomes and high cost to the system and often have extensive mind as well as body needs, complex needs that are difficult or impossible to meet in the brief amount of time available during traditional individual office visits. Group visits offer the additional benefits of not only a multidisciplinary healthcare delivery team, but also of the help and support that is provided by other patients, which represents one of the greatest untapped resources in healthcare today.

See Chapter 7 for an in-depth discussion of a high quality, cost-effective chronic disease management paradigm developed by the author that makes full use of group visits—one which is not just theoretical, but has already been successfully utilized in actual practice. This paradigm can be used with equal benefit for virtually any chronic disease (diabetes, CHF, depression, asthma, MS, hypertension, etc.), and excels when there are large volumes of patients whose illness needs to be successfully and cost-effectively managed—such as ten or more thousands of diabetic patients. Group visits can benefit all of our patients (i.e., those with acute as well as chronic needs); however, by providing accessible, high-quality, and high-value medical care to some of our most challenging and costly patients, SMAs offer a creative new approach to the effective management of high-risk, high-cost patients with chronic conditions and the potential for reduced medical costs in both fee-for-service and capitated healthcare delivery systems (as well as in the Veterans Administration, Department of Defense, and public health sectors). Also, because (when properly run) they have the ability to increase capacity and reduce demand, SMAs can be used to treat underserved populations, i.e., the uninsured, disenfranchised, underserved minorities, urban poor, patients currently falling between the cracks, and so forth.

Efficiency is enhanced because sessions can be over-booked to compensate for patient no-shows and late cancellations, because physicians can delegate much to a multidisciplinary team, and because repetition can be avoided. Meant to be voluntary to patients and physicians alike, group visits are also designed to provide individual one-on-one time with the physician on an *as-needed* basis to all patients.

Although the term *physician* is used throughout this book, all *providers* of medical care are included (i.e., providers of follow-up visits and physical examinations), such as nurse practitioners, podiatrists, pharmacists, Pharm.Ds, and physician assistants, who would set up their group visits in exactly the same manner, using the same types of staffing, facilities, and promotional materials.

The Many Benefits of Shared Medical Appointments

Representing a biopsychosocial and multidisciplinary team-based approach to medical care, SMAs are meant to enhance quality and outcomes, improve patient–physician relationships, increase productivity and access to care, and enhance both patient and physician professional satisfaction. Carefully designed and properly run group visit programs can offer a multitude of benefits to doctors, patients, healthcare organizations, third-party payors, and corporate purchasers alike. They can also be an integral component to new healthcare innovations such as the patient-centered medical home—in which group visits could not only be an access, quality, and satisfaction enhancers, but also an economic driver help-ing to improve the bottom line. It is because of these multifarious benefits that so many articles have been published on group visits and that such an extensive body of literature has already been generated (e.g., see Suggested Readings at the back of this book).

The DIGMA model for return visits and the PSMA model for private physical examinations have emerged as revolutionary access solutions in both primary and speci-alty care. Unlike the CHCC model, which is not designed to improve either physician productivity or access to care, increased physician productivity and improved access are hallmarks of the DIGMA and PSMA models. DIGMAs and PSMAs efficiently provide extended medical appointments with the patient's own physician, which can not only improve access but also increase both con-tinuity of care and time spent with one's own physician.

First and foremost, SMAs are medical appointments; therefore, they are not support groups, health education classes, behavioral medicine programs, or psychotherapy groups (although they are inclusive rather than exclusive, and can work well together with any such group programs as well as with individual office visits). DIGMAs have been demonstrated to be extremely effective in solving access problems at both the individual physician and departmental levels (2,3).

DIGMAs and PSMAs reverse the trend that has been occurring in medicine during recent years in that, rather than adding evermore responsibilities, they reduce physi-cian responsibilities to an absolute minimum and place these duties instead on the shoulders of a less costly and specifically trained, multidisciplinary care delivery team. Even a documenter can be provided to assist the physician in documenting chart notes. This leverages the physician's time by enabling the physician to focus on patients and doing that which the physician alone can do—i.e., deliver high-quality, high-value, and individualized medical care to each and every patient in the room.

DIGMAs and PSMAs Resemble a Series of Individual Office Visits with Observers

Among all group visit models, DIGMAs and PSMAs stand alone in that they so closely resemble traditional office visits, i.e., by delivering medical care from start to finish, and by being run just like a series of individual office visits with observers. DIGMAs and PSMAs are similar to individual office visits in that: (1) the physician sequentially attends to the unique medical needs of each patient individually (i.e., without any preplanned class-type presentation); (2) the same medical services, and often more, are provided (history, examination, risk-assessment and reduction, medical decision-making, counseling, treatment, etc.); (3) the physician is present throughout the entire session; (4) a comprehensive and individualized chart note is documented on each patient; and (5) the focus from start to finish is on the delivery of medical care through a series of one doctor–one patient encounters (but in the supportive group setting where all can listen, learn, interact, and benefit). In fact, these two unique group visit models are best envisioned as a sequence of individual office visits with other patients as observers and in which as much medical care as appropriate and possible is provided in the supportive group setting (Fig. 1.1). For these reasons, patients never confuse a properly run DIGMA or PSMA with a class, support group, behavioral medicine program, or psychotherapy group.

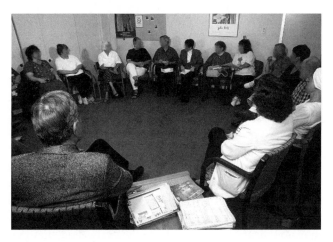

Fig. 1.1 DIGMAs and PSMAs are run as a series of individual office visits with other patients as observers, where all present can listen and learn. The author is shown (left, back to camera), serving as behaviorist in a large DIGMA (courtesy of American Medical Group Association and Dr. Lynn Dowdell, the Kaiser Permanente Medical Center, San Jose, CA)

Much about group visits is counterintuitive. Because of this, their many frustrating beginner's mistakes can easily be made (which are more fully discussed later in this book) and initial development faced many challenges. While many physicians initially viewed group medical appointments as just another unwanted change in their routine, most now recognize their multifarious benefits and just want to know how to implement them (4).

Cooperative Healthcare Clinics Follow the Same 15–20 Patients Over Time

Whereas the DIGMA and PSMA models represent two of today's three major group visit models currently in widespread use, the third model—the CHCC model—is used to follow the same group of high utilizing, often multi-morbid geriatric patients over time through structured group sessions containing a formal educational presentation with some care delivered followed immediately afterward by individual care for those patients who need it. This model, which differs dramatically from (but works well together with) the DIGMA and PSMA models, is discussed in greater detail in Chapter 4. Unlike DIGMAs and PSMAs, which focus on most if not all patients in the physician's practice or the chronic illness management program (and closely resemble individual office visits), CHCCs focus on the same group of 15–20 patients over time and have a different structure from traditional office visits. CHCCs—as well as the related Specialty CHCC subtype of the CHCC model—do not necessarily increase physician productivity or improve

access to care in physicians' practices. However, CHCCs and Specialty CHCCs represent great care for those patients fortunate enough to receive it, and they have been shown to reduce hospitalization, emergency department, and nursing home costs for these costly, high-risk patients (5–10).

Other Applications for Shared Medical Appointments

In addition to being ideally suited to the treatment of geriatric patients and the chronically ill, SMAs can play equally important roles in

- Improved physician management of busy, backlogged practices
- Better meeting the medical needs of most patients— those with routine, acute issues as well as patients with chronic conditions
- Providing improved access benefits to both follow-up visits (DIGMAs) and physical examinations (PSMAs)— and therefore in helping to achieve the goals of advanced access
- Reducing patient phone call volume
- Effectively managing difficult patients (such as psychologically needy patients; extreme information seekers; angry, high-using, or noncompliant patients; and those with diagnoses often seen as difficult to treat in the traditional office visit setting, such as chronic pain, headache, fibromyalgia, and irritable bowel)

The wide-ranging applications for group visits are much broader than one might at first envision. Personally, I believe that the majority of the medical care that we currently provide in ambulatory outpatient settings could be as well (or better) provided in the group visit paradigm. When most people think about group visits, they think about them in the more limited sense of just treating the chronically ill, the elderly, or high utilizers—all applications for which SMAs are admirably suited. However, what most do not realize is that SMAs can play an equally important role in managing busy and backlogged practices, in outpatient ambulatory care settings for virtually all medical subspecialties in both primary and specialty care, in training residents and fellows in academic settings, and in some inpatient, urgent care, and nursing home settings as well. When carefully designed, adequately supported, and properly run, SMAs have the potential to offer many advantages, which can include benefits to patients, physicians, healthcare organizations, insurers, and corporate purchasers of medical care alike.

Positive results have been achieved in both primary and specialty care in a wide variety of healthcare delivery systems in the commercial (fee-for-service, capitated, profit, not-for-profit, PPO, HMO, IPA, etc.), public, and governmental (Department of Defense and Veterans Health Administration) sectors. Despite the multiple potential economic and productivity benefits that properly run SMAs are able to offer, it is the service, quality of care, patient education, and disease self-management benefits that they can offer to our patients that is of greatest importance to the medical community and is the source of greatest satisfaction to me, personally.

Today's major group visit models work well not only with each other and other types of group programs, but also in combination with traditional individual office visits, which they are meant to complement and not to completely replace. It is anticipated that both group and individual visits will play an important role in the future of healthcare delivery. The challenge facing us now is how to optimize the use of both types of appointments so that we can best match the type of service offered to the actual needs of the patient.

Use in Medical and Surgical Subspecialties

Although group visits are still relatively new, it is worth noting that they have already been successfully employed not only in virtually every medical and surgical subspecialty, but also in many ways within each subspecialty. For example, in cardiology DIGMAs and PSMAs have been used in numerous ways: general cardiology, CHF, arrhythmias, atrial fibrillation, post-MI follow-ups, cardiovascular disease, pacemaker interrogations, etc. In dermatology, these group visit models have been used for general dermatology, acne, skin cancer, cosmetic dermatology, eczema, psoriasis, sun damage, etc. In oncology and hematology, they have been used for all types of cancer, autologous bone marrow transplants, breast cancer, prostate cancer, etc. In nephrology, DIGMAs and PSMAs have been designed for all of the nephrologist's kidney patients, dialysis patients, pre-dialysis patients, kidney stones, end-stage kidney disease, hypertension, etc.

In internal medicine and family practice, DIGMAs and PSMAs have been used in countless ways: for most or all of the primary care provider's patients; diabetes; endocrine syndrome; cardiopulmonary patients; women's health; GI patients; stress, anxiety, and depression; high utilizers; geriatric patients; morbid obesity; cardiovascular disease; etc.—to name but a few. Do keep in mind, however, that you must always design your group visit programs in such a way that all sessions can be

consistently kept full—which means designing DIGMAs and PSMAs around patient demand rather than simply around physician interest.

Why Group Visits?

Many physicians view the individual office visit model in which they have been trained and practicing as the *gold standard* of care, i.e., the best possible form of care that they can offer to their patients. Although many physicians might like to maintain the status quo, this option may no longer be viable—due to the decreasing numbers of primary care physicians, closed practices, increasing costs, declining reimbursements, large practice sizes, increasingly large backlogs, dwindling patient as well as physician professional satisfaction, the brief and rushed nature of care, and the inability of patients to secure the timely appointments that are commensurate with good care. In addition, there are many benefits inherent in the group visit that simply cannot be matched by individual office visits—such as a multidisciplinary team. More time, and the help and support of other patients being built into each patient's healthcare experience. It is clear that our healthcare system is increasingly stressed (some would even say that it's broken) and in need of positive innovations that can offer the multiple benefits that group visits do.

In a June 2000 *Modern Healthcare* article, the case is stated this way: "Advocates for group medical appointments claim that the quality of care is improved while both patient and doctor are more satisfied" (11).

Improved Access to Care

Maintaining excellent access to both follow-up appointments and physical examinations through use of existing resources represents a major contemporary healthcare challenge because many care delivery systems have a marked mismatch between capacity and demand. All too often, when efforts are made to improve access to follow-up care, physical examinations get pushed out even further and vice versa. Group practices and healthcare organizations recognize that there simply is not enough money in the system (nor the number of physicians and professional staff available) to hire the required numbers of physicians and support staff to solve existing access, service, economic, and quality of care problems through traditional office visits alone, i.e., by throwing still more doctors at the problem. For both return appointments and physical examinations, a tool is needed that will dramatically increase productivity and efficiency, improve access and quality of care, and contain costs while strengthening the bottom line.

Despite being a more expensive form of medical care to deliver (due to their additional personnel, promotional, and facilities requirements)—costs that can be more than offset by the remarkable productivity gains that these models offer—DIGMAs and PSMAs are the right thing to do for our patients because of the multiple benefits they offer. SMAs offer patients an additional healthcare choice, one that not only enhances quality and performance measures but also integrates the help and support of other patients and a multidisciplinary care delivery team into each patient's healthcare experience.

Patient Benefits

From the patient's point of view, DIGMAs, CHCCs, and PSMAs offer patients what they most want (Table 1.2). DIGMAs are successful because they offer effective medical treatment at a reasonable cost, while also addressing (with the assistance of the behaviorist and the group itself) the problematic psychosocial and lifestyle issues that impact the patient's health and use of healthcare services, often better than can be accomplished in the brief time span of an individual appointment. This is especially important because a large percentage of all medical visits are driven by behavioral health and psychosocial issues, rather than true medical need. Because of the extensive amount of time that the patient is able to spend with

the physician and care delivery team, patients receive a great deal more information about healthy lifestyles and disease self-management strategies during each and every DIGMA, CHCC, and PSMA session than could possibly be worked into a relatively brief individual office visit (Fig. 1.2).

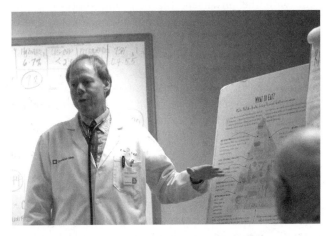

Fig. 1.2 Because of the additional time available, there is an opportunity for the physician and multidisciplinary SMA team members to deliver a great deal of patient education about healthy lifestyles and disease self-management skills during every SMA session (courtesy of Dr. Thomas Morledge, Men's Primary Care PSMA, Cleveland Clinic, Cleveland, OH)

DIGMAs, CHCCs, and PSMAs offer their own unique quality of care benefits, as they can offer better care, not just more efficient care. The presence of a specially trained behaviorist (typically a psychologist or social worker, but occasionally a nurse, diabetes nurse educator, Pharm.D., nurse practitioner, or other specially trained professional) is one of the hallmarks of the

Table 1.2 Benefits to patients of drop-in group medical appointments and physicals shared medical appointments

- Prompt access to care
- Extra time with their own physician and a more relaxed pace of care
- Answers to questions they might not have thought to ask (because others ask)
- Like CHCCs, they provide greater patient education and attention to psychosocial issues
- Max-packed visits, a one-stop shopping healthcare experience, and multiple quality of care benefits
- Mind as well as body needs are met
- Professional skills of a behaviorist to better address psychosocial needs
- Like CHCCs, they integrate the help and support of other patients into each patient's healthcare experience
- Personalized care (as each patient's unique medical needs are addressed individually)
- Appropriate privacy is maintained at all times—private time with physician is available as needed
- A means of reaching out to the underserved and patients who might be falling through the cracks
- Enhanced physician–patient relationships
- Helpful information for family members and caregivers
- Like CHCCs, high levels of patient satisfaction
- Closer follow-up care
- Like CHCCs, an additional healthcare choice
- DIGMAs offer patients drop-in convenience
- Like CHCCs, they are meant to be fun for patients, physicians, and medical staff

CHCC, cooperative healthcare clinic

DIGMA and PSMA models. The behaviorist can be most helpful in addressing patients' behavioral health and psychological issues, which often go under-diagnosed and under-treated in the primary care setting, because behaviorists are often better able to address these mind needs than physicians. These group visit models provide more time with the physician, the help and support of the behaviorist and group itself, and a means for addressing many of the lifestyle and psychosocial issues that are affecting patients' quality of life and utilization of healthcare services. This benefit is especially important given the substantial under-diagnosis of depression, anxiety, and substance abuse that is known to occur in the primary care setting (12,13).

Patient Satisfaction

Time and time again, the level of patient satisfaction with DIGMAs has been demonstrated to be very high. The author reported high levels of patient satisfaction in a 6-week pilot study at Sutter Medical Group in Sacramento (14), in a 1-year study involving all three neurologists in the Neurology Department at the Kaiser Permanente Medical Center in San Jose (plus improved patient–physician relationships) (3), and in the first 12 DIGMAs that the author ran between 1996 and 1999 (15,16). I have also found the level of patient satisfaction to be consistently high in the more than 50 DIGMAs and PSMAs that I launched as SMA champion and Director of Clinical Access Improvement at the Palo Alto Medical Foundation (and in the more than 50 DIGMAs and PSMAs that I have launched as SMA champion and Vice President of Shared Medical Appointments and Group-Based Disease management at Harvard Vanguard Medical Associates/ Atrius Health), and in the more that 300 DIGMAs and PSMAs that I have helped launch between 1999 and 2007 as a healthcare consultant specializing in group visits to healthcare systems both nationally and internationally.

Dr. John Scott (the originator of the CHCC group visit model) has also found patient satisfaction with DIGMAs to be very high. He relates that when Kaiser Permanente conducted a 1-year pilot study on DIGMAs in their Colorado region, they found that (1) over 90% of the patients who attended reported being satisfied with the DIGMA visit and (2) more than 60% of patients stated that they would *not* have preferred an individual office visit (John Scott, personal communication, 2005). This latter finding is especially remarkable when one considers that the majority of these patients were attending a DIGMA for the first time and that they previously had a lifetime of expecting a traditional individual office visit when they went to see their doctor.

Many other healthcare organizations have reported similar findings regarding the high level of patient satisfaction with SMAs. For example, as reported in Chapter 9 on outcomes, Cleveland Clinic found that (1) 85% of patients attending a DIGMA rescheduled their next visit into a future DIGMA and (2) that the percentage of patients rating their overall satisfaction with the visit as excellent was much higher for DIGMAs and PSMAs (74.67%) than for either individual office visits with the same providers (59.17%) or for Cleveland Clinic Regional Medical Practice providers on average (63.00%).

Shared Medical Appointment Reception in the Popular Press

Because of the many patient benefits that properly run and supported group visit programs can offer, they have created quite a stir in the popular press—from *Time Magazine, U.S. News & World Report, WebMD, The Minneapolis Star Tribune,* and *The Wall Street Journal to Good Housekeeping, AARP's Modern Maturity, The Washington Times,* and *The Boston Globe.* In addition, they have been featured both locally and nationally on CNN, PBS, National Public Radio, and numerous local radio and television stations. Because of the pushback that one would normally anticipate with any new innovation requiring so much change, I have been surprised at the overall positive tone of the mass media coverage. I believe that it is because, at least to date, of the consistent emphasis on group visits always being for the benefit of our patients. There are many reasons that group visits are so patient centered, especially because of the enhanced quality, time, access, education, support, and follow-up care benefits that they offer to patients.

Also, it is important to always remember that I originally developed my two group visit models as a result of being seriously ill in order to give patients *more* rather than *less*—i.e., out of personal frustration with traditional medical care as it was being delivered—and this despite having the best doctors that one could hope to have. It is extremely important that the focus of SMAs always remain on our patients and that extreme caution be taken to ensure that group visits are never perceived (or used) as a means for physicians and healthcare organizations to extract more money out of their patients in order to spend less time at work and more on the golf course, which is how one newspaper editor put it to me. This is but one of many reasons why it is imperative that our patients always come first and that group visits never be abused, which is a subject to which our attention will return later in this book (see Chapter 8).

An article in *Good Housekeeping* magazine points out that sessions are voluntary: "Imagine a doctor who never keeps you waiting. Your appointment lasts at least an hour, with time to get in all your questions. The catch? You're one of a dozen or more patients vying for the physician's attention. Welcome to the group visit, a trend that's spreading at healthcare centers across the country" (17). AARP's *Modern Maturity* has reported on DIGMAs as well (18). In a front page article, *The Boston Globe* reported that thousands of groups have been started, including at institutions such as the Department of Veterans Affairs and Dartmouth-Hitchcock Medical Center in New Hampshire, and Harvard Vanguard Medical Associates and Boston Medical Center in Massachusetts (19).

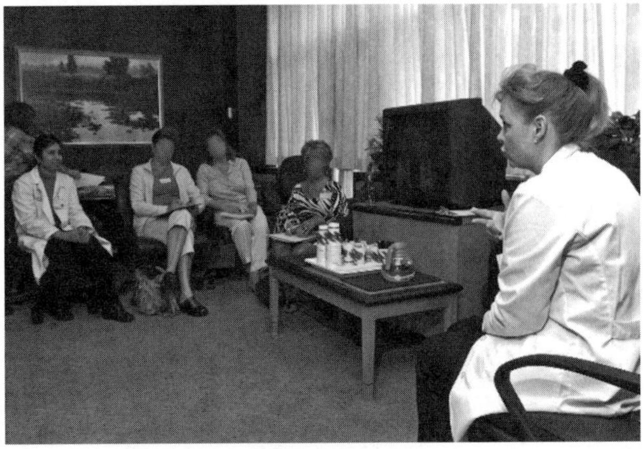

Fig. 1.3 SMAs and PSMAs offer a more informative and relaxed pace of care, a benefit to both patients and physicians (courtesy of Dr. Holly Thacker, Women's Health Physicals SMA, Cleveland Clinic, Cleveland, OH)

Physician Benefits

In addition to the benefits they offer patients, DIGMAs, CHCCs, and PSMAs also offer significant benefits to the physicians running them—benefits that physicians must clearly understand if they are expected to embrace these group visit models. Many physicians may at first be reluctant to initiate SMAs for their practices due to a variety of concerns with these innovative new models as well as a certain comfort level with the status quo and perhaps even a deep-seated belief that the individual treatment model in which they were trained and have been practicing is simply the best form of providing medical care. Naturally, such concerns must be balanced against the many real benefits that properly run DIGMAs, CHCCs, and PSMAs can offer to patients and physicians alike.

Unlike individual office visits, where physicians must do almost everything themselves, SMAs offer physicians real and meaningful help—both from the treatment team (nurse, behaviorist, documenter, dedicated scheduler, champion, program coordinator, and support staff) and from other patients. Due to the greater amount of time available and their inherent efficiencies (because group visits provide a multidisciplinary team-based approach to care, because the same information does not need to be repeated to different patients individually, and due to the ability to overbook these SMA sessions to nullify potential physician downtime from no-shows and late-cancels), SMAs offer a more informative and relaxed pace of care, unlike comparatively rushed and brief individual visits (Fig. 1.3).

Because they are less intuitively obvious than the CHCC model (in which the same group of high-using, multi-morbid geriatric patients is followed over time), physician acceptance is critical to the ultimate success of any DIGMA and PSMA program, which requires that all physician questions and concerns be addressed and that the many real physician benefits that they offer be made clear (see Chapter 6). When establishing a new group visit program, great attention must be directed toward extracting every possible benefit from the group visit, especially those most important to the individual physician for whom the DIGMA or PSMA is being customized. By so doing, the physician will become aware of the multiple physician benefits that the customized DIGMA or PSMA will offer—which can range from better managing busy and backlogged practices and the opportunity of doing something interesting and different, to seeing dramatically more patients in the same amount of time and experiencing greater professional satisfaction (Table 1.3).

Organization Benefits

DIGMAs, CHCCs, and PSMAs can also provide a multitude of benefits to healthcare organizations (Table 1.4). Through SMAs, the organization can achieve the benefits of increased productivity, improved access, reopened practices, enhanced job doability, the leveraging of existing resources, more satisfied patients and providers, and a stronger bottom line. Furthermore, happier patients and providers should ultimately translate into retained patients and providers. The increased productivity and efficiency provided by DIGMAs and PSMAs can be used to solve access problems, to enable physicians to better manage their large practices, to better address the needs of the elderly and

Table 1.3 Benefits to physicians of drop-in group medical appointments and physicals shared medical appointments

- An effective tool for working smarter, not harder
- An important tool for better managing both physicians' practices and chronic illnesses
- An opportunity for physicians to do something different, interesting, and fun
- They can enhance quality, outcomes, and the patient's healing experience
- They can contain costs and increase physician income
- They are able to leverage existing resources to increase physician productivity by 200–300% or more
- They can solve access problems to physician's practices and chronic illness treatment programs
- Physicians enjoy more time with patients, a more relaxed pace of care, and a temporary reprieve from ongoing clinic demands and distractions
- SMAs offer backlogged physicians the opportunity to provide closer follow-up care
- A chance to get to know their patients better
- Consistently high levels of patient and physician professional satisfaction
- An opportunity to get off the fast-paced treadmill of individual office visits
- Reduced patient phone call volume and patient complaints about poor access
- Decreased need to work-in or double book patients
- Documentation support can be provided
- Real help from the multidisciplinary team (nurse, behaviorist, documenter, dedicated scheduler)
- Additional help from the patients themselves
- Enjoyment of collegiality with the entire SMA team (especially the behaviorist)
- The SMA program is customized to the physician's particular needs and practice
- Reduced repetition of information
- Increased opportunity for providing patient education and addressing psychosocial needs
- A helpful tool for managing difficult, time-consuming, and psychosocially needy patients
- SMAs help physicians to optimize their master schedule and appointment mix

SMA, shared medical appointments

chronically ill, and to improve the customer focus of the organization. In addition to the competitive advantage of offering a positive new service, SMAs can also improve the quality of care offered by the organization through max-packed visits, expanded nursing and behaviorist roles, and greater attention to performance measures, disease self-management skills, and prevention.

Properly run DIGMAs, CHCCs, and PSMAs are highly productive and efficient, which certainly represents a benefit to healthcare organizations. They provide a team-based paradigm of care that leverages physician time by enabling many physician responsibilities to be appropriately delegated to less costly care providers. In DIGMAs and PSMAs, the nursing role is greatly expanded beyond normal clinic duties, and a behaviorist is introduced into the care delivery process to better address the behavioral health and psychosocial needs of patients (needs known to drive a large percentage of all office visits).

The MA or nurse can also do some previsit work a couple of days prior to the SMA session by doing the medication reconciliation, checking for injections and health maintenance due, and updating the HEDIS measures on each patient when the confirmation phone call is made for the upcoming SMA visit. In addition, once the MA's duties have been completed during the DIGMA or PSMA (i.e. on all patients at the front end of the DIGMA or PSMA session), the MA can then act as a "Care

Table 1.4 Benefits to organizations of drop-in group medical appointments, cooperative healthcare clinic, and physicals shared medical appointments

- Improved quality of care (max-packed visits, improved health maintenance, etc.)
- Improved access at both the individual physician and departmental levels (DIGMAs and PSMAs only)
- Increased efficiency and the leveraging of existing resources
- Dramatically increased physician productivity of 200–300%, or more (DIGMAs and PSMAs only)
- Better physician management of busy, backlogged practices
- An important tool in chronic illness population management programs
- High levels of patient and physician professional satisfaction
- The competitive advantage of a new service and an additional healthcare choice
- Improved customer focus for the organization
- Potential for increasing revenues and RVUs, leveraging existing resources, containing costs, and improving the bottom line

DIGMA, drop-in group medical appointments; PMSA, physicals shared medical appointments

Coordinator" for the group (as they do at Harvard Vanguard Medical Associates/Atrius Health)—i.e. by calling each patient out of the group room in turn once the physician has finished working with them and their SMA chart note has been completed. The care coordinator then schedules all of the patient's upcoming appointments, tests, referrals, and procedures that the physician has ordered during the SMA—and then gives each patient a copy of their "after-visit summary" (which is that portion of the patient's chart note preselected by the physician to give to the patient towards the end of the session to take home with them). DIGMAs and PSMAs often also introduce a documenter to handle the majority of documentation responsibilities for the session, with the documenter being trained by the physician, using the physician's own chart note template so that a superior chart note is generated that is both contemporaneous and comprehensive. The documenter is also trained by the organization's billing and compliance officer so that all elements impacting billing are certainly entered into each patient's chart note—which should optimize the billing process. Also, these models often use a dedicated scheduler to *top-off* census and ensure that all group sessions are consistently kept full. However, because, of all the group visit models, DIGMAs and PSMAs most closely resemble traditional office visits, be certain to run these from start to finish like a series of one doctor–one patient encounters with observers—while giving other patients the opportunity to listen, learn, and interact as you sequentially address the medical needs of each patient individually (Fig. 1.4).

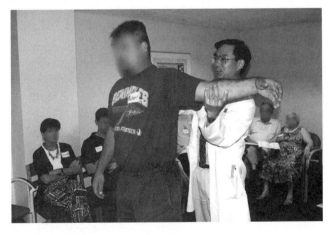

Fig. 1.4 With DIGMAs and PSMAs, there are efficiency and patient education benefits to running the entire session as a series of one doctor–one patient encounters, but with as much medical care as possible and appropriate being conducted in the group setting where all can ask questions, share experiences, and learn (courtesy of Dr. John Lu, Physiatry DIGMA, Palo Alto Medical Foundation, Palo Alto, CA)

Organizations also benefit from the multitude of patient benefits that well-run SMAs can offer. DIGMAs and PSMAs are designed to enhance the patient's care experience by providing patients with the benefits of prompt access, more time, *max-packed* visits, and a *one-stop shopping* healthcare experience. Here, the various healthcare needs of each patient are addressed, injections and routine health maintenance are brought current, greater patient education and attention to psychosocial issues is provided, and the help and support of other patients is built into the care experience—and all this is accomplished with a minimum outlay of physician time. In addition, DIGMAs and PSMAs are efficient because the physician gets real help from the entire SMA team—nurse(s), behaviorist, documenter, and dedicated scheduler—as well as from other patients in the group.

Interestingly, patients do not abuse the improved access that DIGMAs and PSMAs provide. In a study at the Kaiser Permanente San Jose Medical Center in which all three neurologists in the Neurology Department simultaneously started a DIGMA for their practice in order to solve their serious access problems both individually and departmentally, it was found that despite the remarkable accessibility that these patients now had to care with their neurologists (patients with headache, stroke, multiple sclerosis, Parkinson's disease, dementia, etc., who were often quite needy both medically and psychologically), they did not abuse this privilege. In fact, those neurology patients who attended the DIGMA program only came to the Neurology DIGMA an average of 2.0 sessions during the entire year of the study (i.e., despite high levels of patient satisfaction with the program) (15).

Are There Applications in Which DIGMAs and PSMAs Will Not Work?

Because these models have proven to be so robust and have worked well in such a wide variety of different medical subspecialties and settings (provided that they are designed in such a manner that sessions can be consistently filled), I began to wonder what the limits of these models might actually be. I began to ask: "Are there applications where DIGMAs and PSMAs simply will not work?" In an effort to determine what these limits might be, I set up and ran a DIGMA and a PSMA that I felt would have a very high likelihood of failure and, when they were in fact launched, watched very carefully to see if they would fail.

Homeless Patients

One DIGMA that I felt would test the limits of the model and have a high likelihood of failure was designed for homeless veterans on the east coast. Because much of the previous social interaction that these patients would have had would have been distinctly negative (i.e., with people often looking down on them and humiliating them), I believed that this DIGMA would likely not prove to be successful. Furthermore, it was felt that many of these patients would have mental health, substance abuse, and hepatitis C issues—and that they would have limited personal resources and interpersonal skills. For all of these reasons as well as others, I felt that these patients would not be very favorably disposed toward receiving their medical care in a group visit format. Therefore, I went to the east coast and assisted in setting up such a DIGMA for the homeless. One hour before the session was to start, the group room was empty and we sent the vans out to the streets, soup kitchens, flop houses, and the emergency department to find if any such patients were in the lobby waiting for care. Our hope was to find enough homeless patients willing to participate to promptly fill the group session at the last minute.

What I found was that, far from being the failure that I had anticipated, this homeless patients' DIGMA was not only a success, but also an absolutely touching and heartwarming experience for all. These patients were extremely appreciative of the care we were offering to them. They simply could not believe that anyone would care enough about them to reach out and provide them with such a high-quality healthcare experience. Not only was this DIGMA no failure, but was one of the most successful DIGMAs that I have ever been privileged to witness. The heartfelt warmth and support that these patients shared (both with each other and with the medical staff), the deep appreciation that was shown for everything that was provided, the amount of acute care needs that we were able to meet, and the upbeat atmosphere in which much healing laughter was shared by all left me both humbled and with a deep sense of satisfaction—and with more than one tear in my eyes. Furthermore, this finding was recently replicated when I helped to set up a DIGMA for impoverished, street involved aboriginal people in Canada, which, again, turned out to be a successful and heartwarming experience. As a result of such experiences, I am a firm believer that group visits are a wonderful way to reach out and provide care to the medically underserved.

However, there is one important word of caution to anyone considering setting up DIGMAs or PSMAs that reach out to such needy and underserved populations: Be certain to be organized and have everything possible done during the session, which includes getting lab test results back before the session is over, as you would not want to find out that the patient has a HbA1C of 12 after they are back out on the street and cannot be located. Similarly, diabetic foot lesions will need to be cleaned and dressed before patients leave the session and disappear back into the streets. Nonetheless, for those who feel such a calling, I cannot encourage you enough to apply the increased capacity and multiple benefits that properly run SMAs can offer to such underserved and needy patient populations, and then see if you are not also as moved as I was through this satisfying experience.

Digital Rectal Examinations for Elderly Hermits Living in the Bush of Alaska

As a result of the high-risk Homeless DIGMA actually turning out to be such a success, I was even more resolute about making yet another attempt to determine the limits of applicability of these models. How about digital rectal examinations for elderly hermits living in the bush of Alaska, especially one provided by a young female urologist? Would you feel that such a PSMA could ever succeed? Here we have elderly patients, most of whom are living alone in remote areas of Alaska with an absolute minimum of social contact, and we are going to give them a group medical appointment focused upon digital rectal exams, prostate problems, erectile problems, and male incontinence—I don't think so! Certainly this could not succeed. So off I went to Alaska to assist in setting up a Urology PSMA program that would largely include just such patients.

There were 10 patients originally scheduled to attend the initial session of this PSMA, all of whom came. In addition, there was one support person in attendance, as the wife of one of these patients insisted on staying despite my diplomatic attempts to dissuade her—i.e., out of concern that she would further dampen the likelihood of discussing personal matters during the session. In addition to all 10 of the originally scheduled patients actually attending (surprisingly, there were no late-cancels or no-shows), another elderly patient (who had driven over 300 miles from his remote cabin in the bush) dropped in unannounced. This patient had arrived a couple of hours early for his individual medical appointment with the urologist and decided to simply drop-in at the last minute on hearing about the group when he registered. Now we had 11 male patients (plus a female support person) in attendance for the first session of this Urology Prostate PSMA. My initial feelings regarding the high likelihood of failure for this PSMA were now even stronger.

However, far from not working, what we found was that this group was actually quite successful in practice. The urologist came in wearing an "Ask me about ED" button to encourage discussion about such personal topics as erectile dysfunction. There was a great deal of warmth, camaraderie, and shared emotional support, plus much laughter throughout the session. This included many humorous comments from these elderly patients, such as, "As I've always said, there's no Niagara without Viagra." To my surprise, even the presence of the assertive wife worked out quite successfully as the various male patients seemed to make an extra effort to make her feel welcome. Everyone received their digital rectal exam in the privacy of the examination room; however, as is typical of PSMAs, almost all of the discussion was deferred to the subsequent interactive group room setting—where we discussed such serious medical issues as prostate cancer, benign prostatic hyperplasia, erectile dysfunction, male incontinence, and so forth (but in the context of the urologist working with each patient individually in the supportive group setting, rather than as a class-type presentation). Others have similarly found that DIGMAs and PSMAs can be successfully implemented in urologic practices, and with high levels of patient satisfaction, despite the sensitive nature of many of the issues discussed (20).

In the end, the success of these programs still leaves me looking around for a type of DIGMA or PSMA application that would simply not work in actual practice. To date, I have not found one. Virtually all DIGMA and PSMA failures to date have been because they were either poorly designed or inadequately promoted to patients, with the end result being that sessions could not be consistently kept filled to targeted census levels over time and were therefore not economically viable. Out of all the hundreds of DIGMAs and PSMAs that I have helped to design and launch to date, inadequate group census has been the only reason for failure—never has it been because either patients or physicians did not like them. In short, despite having specifically designed some DIGMAs and PSMAs to have a high likelihood of failure in order to test their limits of applicability, those limits are as yet undetermined.

The Ultimate Goal: Precisely Match the Type of Care Offered to the Needs of Patients

As long as they are designed and promoted to patients in such a way that predetermined census requirements can be consistently met, the DIGMA, CHCC, and PSMA models can continue to be successfully used in an extremely wide variety of settings and applications. As time goes by, and as more and more SMAs are implemented, we will undoubtedly find occasions where they will not work. Although I have already had considerable personal experience with these models (i.e., over 20,000 patient visits in DIGMAs and PSMAs to date, with more than 400 different physicians and other providers in a wide variety of healthcare settings), there will undoubtedly come a time when these SMA models will have been used much more extensively—eventually for millions of patient visits and thousands of providers in a wide variety of medical subspecialties and healthcare settings. Once we more fully understand where SMAs work and don't work—and where they do and don't offer substantial benefits over traditional individual office visits—we will be better able to more precisely match the specific type of care that we offer (i.e., particular types of group visits vs. individual office visits) to the specific needs of our patients.

Shared Medical Appointments Must Be Carefully Planned, Adequately Supported, and Properly Run

It is important to note that the full benefits of a DIGMA, CHCC, or PSMA program will only be achieved with optimal success when it is carefully designed, adequately supported, appropriately promoted, and properly run. This is because SMAs represent a major paradigm shift from traditional office visits, are something that patients and physicians are as yet largely unfamiliar with, and it is very easy to make many beginners' mistakes when setting them up. When DIGMAs and PSMAs do fail, inadequate census is almost always at fault; therefore, take particular care when designing and promoting your SMA to ensure that you will be able to consistently fill sessions over time (see Part II for specifics on planning for new SMAs and filling sessions).

Successful DIGMAs and PSMAs pose a multitude of operational challenges, tend to stress the system and exacerbate any pre-existing problems, and have many support requirements (personnel, facilities, promotional, and budgetary) that must be met for success—issues that are fully explored throughout this book (see Part II for detailed discussions). Although they provide a rare combination of benefits that can be extremely beneficial to patients, physicians, and organizations alike, as with all other recent healthcare innovations, these SMA models clearly cannot solve all of the challenges facing medical groups today.

Create a Culture of Excellence Around Your Group Visit Program

It has never been my intention to convince others to do group visits, especially those who do not have any desire to run them in their practice. Rather, my intent has always been to convince those who have chosen to start a group visit program to do so correctly. It is my strong conviction that there is so much benefit to be derived from a properly run group visit program that there is simply no good reason for not creating a culture of excellence around SMA programs. Because so much good can come out of a well-run DIGMA, CHCC, and PSMA program, be certain that your group visits are carefully designed, adequately supported, appropriately promoted, properly run, and thoroughly evaluated on an ongoing basis. Do not cut corners, fail to provide the necessary personnel and facilities, launch prematurely without proper training for all involved, or fail to take the necessary precautions to prevent any potential for abuse. Use the best and most appropriate SMA team members, not just the cheapest and most readily available. In addition, build all possible quality into the program—e.g., by updating injections, routine health maintenance, and HEDIS measures on all patients; by inviting patients to bring a support person; by distributing high quality Patient Packets to all attendees; by providing patients with max-packed visits and a comprehensive healthcare experience; etc. It is for this reason that I want to discuss, right at the beginning of this book and at the conclusion of the first chapter, how to create a culture of excellence surrounding whatever group visit program you might choose to initiate.

I personally feel that sometime in the future, when used to the greatest possible extent, group visits could eventually account for as much as 60–80% of all outpatient ambulatory care, plus make significant contributions to other forms of medical care as well (urgent care, residential care, skilled nursing facilities, inpatient care, etc.).

Build Excellent Quality and Service into Your Shared Medical Appointment Program

Be certain at all times to maximize the quality and service that you build into all of your group visit programs. Max-pack visits, optimize the nursing and behaviorist functions, use quality promotional materials, serve snacks, employ a documenter, ensure that everybody involved receives appropriate training, and provide the best—rather than the cheapest—SMA team members. In his thought-provoking book, *The Ice Cream Maker,* Subir Chowdhury underscores the importance of quality—and

makes several points that hold as true for group visits as they do for corporate cultures (21). Never cut corners or settle for less than what is optimal and constantly evaluate what you are doing so that you can strive to improve the product that you are delivering, i.e., through continuous process improvement.

Focus on Maximizing Long-Term Benefit

In this country, we too often seem obsessed with profits and the need to show quick results. The net result is a tendency to focus on immediate benefit and the *bottom line*—i.e., rather than upon quality, service, and process improvement over the long run. I am very concerned that the same thing could happen to the way we set up, support, and run our group visit programs. The old adage about "Quality in, quality out" vs. "Garbage in, garbage out" holds equally true for group visits. My hope is that physicians and healthcare organizations will accurately recognize the numerous benefits that SMAs can realistically offer to patients, providers, and healthcare organizations alike, so that they cherish and protect these benefits by maintaining a focus on quality and service to our patients that is long term in nature. Strive to build the quality into your SMA program, to avoid the pitfalls of potential abuses, to improve processes, to measure results on an ongoing basis, and to maintain a constant focus upon better servicing our patient–customers.

Some Concluding Comments

Although the traditional one-on-one office visit has been the bedrock of medical practice for over a 100 years, it is now being eroded and threatened by rapidly expanding new forms of medical care that are more efficient, less costly, and better aligned to the specific needs of patients. Increasingly, patients are being offered a menu of options from which they can choose the particular form of medical care they desire. Patients are increasingly able to receive prompt medical advice through 24/7 telephone and e-mail availability of their care providers, which offers many advantages: immediate access; avoiding the scheduling of appointments; no drive time and no need to come into the office; not waiting in either the lobby or the examination room; and not being exposed the germs of many other sick people. The convenience of the highly accessible "doc-in-a-box" at your local drugstore or superstore is increasingly becoming an available option for many patients. Internet-based medicine is also progressing on many fronts and is increasingly becoming the preferred source of information and medical care for many patients and conditions.

Team-based medicine (which includes SMAs) continues to emerge and expand and is transferring evermore components of direct medical care from the physician to less costly members of the multidisciplinary healthcare team (Fig. 1.5). Group visits are continuing to proliferate and to offer a viable, highly beneficial treatment choice that is preferred by many. This list of choices will continue to grow rapidly as we move toward a future that increasingly includes telehealth, automated triage, Web-based care, and SMAs. Although traditional office visits will always have a role to play in medical care, that role is certainly changing and its predominance is decreasing.

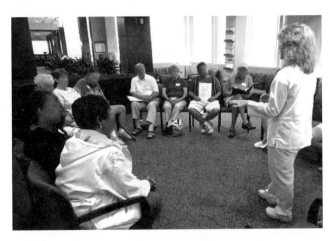

Fig. 1.5 In DIGMAs and PSMAs, the physician delegates as many duties as appropriate and possible, such as having the behaviorist temporarily take over the group (focusing on behavioral health and psychosocial issues) while the physician is documenting a chart note or conducting a brief private examination (courtesy of Dr. Patricio Aycinena, Diabetes DIGMA, Cleveland Clinic, Cleveland, OH)

Because many physicians view the traditional individual office visit model of care in which they have been trained and practicing for years as being the best form of care (i.e., and thus the *gold standard* of care), they would simply like to maintain the status quo. Unfortunately, the all-too-common consequence of this sole focus on the individual office visit and the current physician–patient dyad has been increasingly large panel sizes, visits that often feel rushed, backlogged practices with lengthy wait-lists, high costs, and a level of accessibility that is not commensurate with good care—problems that cannot simply be solved by throwing more physicians and support staff at them. Group visits provide a refreshing alternative that can leverage physician time, improve access, increase productivity, max-pack visits, enhance care, improve outcomes, strengthen the patient–physician relationship, and increase both patient and physician professional satisfaction.

Fostering group interaction and integrating the help and support of other patients into each patient's SMA healthcare experience enables patients to help patients, which also reduces the sense of isolation that patients often feel. Medical patients leave the group visit session recognizing that they are not alone, that their situation could be worse, that there is still much that they can do which others cannot, and that they can build on their strengths rather than perseverating on the limitations imposed by their illnesses. In SMAs, patients teach each other by exchanging helpful information, sharing personal experiences, discussing successful coping strategies, and providing one another with beneficial emotional support. In addition, patients appreciate the opportunity to meet and talk with others dealing with similar issues, frequently comment upon how they no longer feel alone, and often refer to their group visit experience as being like "Dr. Welby care." Because of the greater amount of time available, the pace of care in a SMA often feels quite relaxed—especially relative to comparatively rushed individual office visits.

Unlike traditional office visits, in which physicians need to do almost everything themselves, in SMAs other patients and an entire multidisciplinary care delivery team provide help. In fact, one of the important overarching goals of any successful DIGMA or PSMA program is to remove everything possible and appropriate from the shoulders of the physician and to place it instead on less costly members of the SMA team. In this manner, physicians are left with much less to do; however, that "much less" is what the physician alone can do—i.e., what the physician has gone to medical school to learn and typically most enjoys doing. However, because they delegate so much and need to do less in the DIGMA and PSMA settings, providers can efficiently see many more patients in the same amount of time—yet emerge after the group feeling energized rather than depleted, which is how they would likely feel after another hour and a half on the same old fast-paced treadmill of individual office visits.

In addition, the fact that medical care is delivered in a group setting also offers certain efficiency advantages. For example, SMAs also eliminate the need to keep repeating the same information over and over all week long to different patients individually—instead, the physician can say it once to the benefit of the entire group, often going into greater detail. In addition, the fact that it is a group allows the physician to do like the airlines do by overbooking sessions according to the expected number of no-shows and late-cancels—thus eliminating expensive physician downtime due to these problems, which can prove to be so vexing and costly in the traditional individual office visit setting.

Why Not Consider Group Visits as Your Primary Means of Delivering Care?

As you read this book, I would encourage you to think about how you might use group visits, at least in certain circumstances, as your primary care delivery modality. I have often thought about, and sometimes advocated, running group visits as a primary means of delivering medical care, i.e., rather than as some sort of add-on or extra service that is secondary to individual office visits. All too often, healthcare organizations approach group visits in a very limited way, with a singular focus on access, productivity, patient satisfaction, patient education, emotional support, practice management, or chronic disease management. In so doing, they miss just how broad the application of group visits could be throughout all areas of the organization, as well as the many benefits that SMAs, when fully utilized, could provide to patients, physicians, and the healthcare organization.

Whereas the individual office visit model of care was developed long ago, during an era when acute medical care needs were predominant (and prior to the introduction of antibiotics and most of today's modern therapeutic interventions), we are now in an era of chronic care—i.e., in which the majority of patient demands upon our medical services, as well as healthcare dollars spent, are in the area of chronic disease management. It is with chronic illnesses that group visits truly excel. During this historic focus on acute care, patients were well yesterday, sick today, and dead tomorrow. Yet, in today's era of chronic care, patients were often sick yesterday, sick today, and will be sick for the rest of their lives, so the question often becomes how to live life as fully as possible despite having a chronic illness. So why would we think that the same model of healthcare delivery would be best in both situations?

While the individual office visit model has heretofore been the gold standard in acute care settings, my experience has been that properly run DIGMAs and PSMAs are equally capable of addressing many acute care needs—and that they are often much better at addressing the multifarious, complex medical needs of our burgeoning geriatric and chronically ill patient populations. As will be seen in this book, group visits—especially properly run DIGMAs, CHCCs, and PSMAs (as well as other SMA models yet to come)—offer a practical and refreshing solution to many of today's healthcare woes.

In 1996, I had the privilege of being involved with Kaiser Permanente's Regional Planning Committee for Adult Primary Care Redesign. Although it was still too early in the development of today's major group visit models for this suggestion to be taken seriously at that time, as we examined how to optimally redesign adult primary care, I often thought about a radically different approach to delivering medical care—one that did not just offer group visits, but put them into a salient position of predominance. If we were going to go to a concept of *modules* for a specific number of covered patients (sometimes referred to as *teams, units,* or *pods* by various healthcare systems) that involved not only a particular number of providers, but also specific auxiliary personnel—such as a certain number of nursing personnel, a behavioral medicine specialist, and a part time physical therapist—then why not take a couple of these modules and measure the impact of a completely different paradigm of care delivery?

Specifically, why not take one or two such modules (i.e., in which all providers are in agreement with this concept, as group visits are meant to always be voluntary to patients and providers alike) and have them focus on DIGMAs and PSMAs as their primary, frontline modality of delivering medical care, i.e., rather than relegating these SMA models to secondary, add-on status? It would then be a comparatively simple matter to measure their efficiencies, costs, satisfaction levels, and outcomes vs. those of the other modules delivering standard individual office visit care alone. While such thoughts were only a personal dream back in 1996, group visits have subsequently advanced to a point where this approach could certainly be implemented and tested in larger integrated delivery systems today. If you decide to try any type of related approach within your own healthcare system, and you take care to incorporate the suggestions in this book to ensure that your DIGMA and PSMA programs are properly designed, supported, and run, then be sure to contact me at TheDIGMAmodel@aol.com as I would be most interested in hearing from you about your findings and results.

References

1. McLeod L. (ed.). Multitask in the exam room—three shared-appointment models help physicians see more patients. Private Practice Success, July 2004;6–8.
2. Noffsinger EB. Enhance satisfaction with drop-in group visits. *Hippocrates* 2001;15(2):30–36.
3. Noffsinger EB. Solving departmental access problems with DIGMAs. *Group Practice Journal* 2001;50(10):26–36.
4. Belfiglio G. Crowd control—group office visits provide efficiencies, patient support. *Modern Physician*, June 2001;34–36.
5. Scott JC, Conner DA, et al. Effectiveness of a group outpatient visit model for chronically ill older health maintenance organization members: a 2 year randomized trial of the Cooperative Health Care Clinic. *Journal of the American Geriatrics Society* 2004;52(9):1463—1470.
6. Coleman EA, Eilertsen TB, et al. Reducing emergency visits in older adults with chronic illness—a randomized, controlled trial of group visits. *Effective Clinical Practice* 2001;4(2):49–57.

7. Scott J, Gade, G, et al. Cooperative health care clinics: a group approach to individualized care. *Geriatrics* 1996;53(5): 69–81.

8. Beck A, Scott JC, et al. A randomized trial of group outpatient visits for chronically ill older HMO members: the Cooperative Health Care Clinic. *Journal of the American Geriatric Society* 1997;45(5):543–549.

9. Scott JC, Robertson BJ. Kaiser Colorado's Cooperative Health Care Clinic: a group approach to patient care. *Managed Care Quarterly* 1996;4(3):41–45.

10. Martinez B. Now it's mass medicine—doctors start seeing groups of patients to save time; one-on-one vs. one-on-12. *Wall Street Journal*, Monday, August 21 2000; p. B1.

11. Thompson E. The power of group visits: improved quality of care, increased productivity entice physicians to see up to 15 patients at a time. *Modern Healthcare*, June 5, 2000;30(23):54, 56, 62.

12. Cummings NA. Behavioral health in primary care: dollars and sense. In: Cummings NA, Cummings JL, Johnson JN, editors. Behavioral health in primary care: a guide for clinical integration. Madison, CT: Psychosocial Press; 1997. p. 3–21.

13. Mechanic D. Response factors in illness: the study of illness behavior. *Social Psychiatry and Psychiatric Epidemiology* 1966;1:52–73.

14. Noffsinger EB, Atkins TN. assessing a group medical appointment program: A case study at Sutter Medical Foundation. *Group Practice Journal* 2001;50(4):47–48.

15. Noffsinger EB. Benefits of Drop-In Group Medical Appointments (DIGMAs) to physicians and patients. *Group Practice Journal* 1999;48(3):26–28.

16. Noffsinger EB. Establishing successful primary care and subspecialty Drop-In Group Medical Appointments (DIGMAs) in your group practice. *Group Practice Journal* 1999;48(4):20–21.

17. Goff L. Checkup club: The doctor is ready to see all 15 of you now. *Good Housekeeping*, July 2001; p. 187.

18. Nelson R. Club Medical—the new way to get more quality time with your doc: join a group. *AARP's Modern Maturity*, November–December 2002; pp. 17–18.

19. Dembner A. Patients, doctors turn to care in groups—shared settings bring quicker access. *The Boston Globe*, Tuesday, June 22 2004; pp. A1, A9.

20. Fletcher SG, Clark SJ, Overstreet DL, et al. An improved approach to follow-up care for the urological patient: Drop-In Group Medical Appointments. *Journal of Urology* 2006;176:1122–1126.

21. Chowdhury S. The ice cream maker: an inspiring tale about making quality the key ingredient in everything you do. New York, Currency, 2005.

Chapter 2
The Drop-In Group Medical Appointment Model: A Revolutionary Access Solution for Follow-Up Visits

The group appointment may seem like a tall order: See twice as many patients per hour while raising the quality of care, boosting patient satisfaction, and improving physician job satisfaction. But at several large group practices that have launched group appointments in recent years, many physicians have become firm believers in the efficiency of this unusual format....The physician saves time by not having to repeat basic medical information or shuttle between exam rooms....But physicians report that thousands of patients are participating because they appreciate the extended appointment time and the opportunity to exchange ideas with other patient. Moreover, patients often can be scheduled sooner for a group appointment than for an individual appointment....Reimbursement has not been a problem, despite the unconventional format of group visits....Further, there are no separate CPT codes for group visits, so insurers are obligated to pay for them at the same level as individual patient visits....Although group visits are voluntary for physicians as well as for patients, officials report that many doctors are enthusiastic about the new approach.

Internal Medicine News, October 15, 2001, p. 39, Practice Trends, Leigh Page, "Group Visit Format Raises Efficiency and Eyebrows."

Today's rapidly changing managed healthcare environment has had a dramatic, and often negative, impact on the practices and professional satisfaction of physicians in both primary care and the medical and surgical subspecialties. While working as hard and efficiently as possible, many find themselves barely able to keep up and struggling with diminishing bottom lines. Physicians feel ill-equipped to handle any further increases in their already jam-packed caseloads, yet many feel that this is inevitable and just a matter of time. Capacity is decreasing just as patient demand is increasing—i.e., with the number of geriatric and primary care physicians declining dramatically just as the baby boomers are retiring and the most obese pediatric population in history is reaching adulthood. What is needed is a completely new paradigm for delivering medical care—a tool for working smarter, not harder—which is something for which the DIGMA model is particularly well equipped. DIGMAs enable providers to see dramatically more patients in the same amount of time (often three times as many), but accomplish this while simultaneously providing improved accessibility, max-packed visits, greater attention to patient education and psychosocial issues, and higher levels of patient and physician professional satisfaction. All three of today's major group visit models (i.e., the DIGMA, CHCC, and PSMA models) provide new, innovative medical care delivery systems that are intended to be voluntary, efficient, holistic, interactive, cost-effective, and highly satisfying to patients and physicians alike.

Overview of the Drop-In Group Medical Appointment Model

Throughout the entire DIGMA session, the physician attends sequentially to each patient's unique medical needs individually in a supportive group setting. In DIGMAs, physicians manage, advise, and treat each patient individually, but in front of others (except for brief private discussions and examinations that require disrobing, which occur with the physician in the privacy of a nearby examination room). This avoids repetition and increases patient education, plus allows others who are present to listen, learn, ask questions, and actively participate (by sharing personal experiences, information, their thoughts and feelings, etc.).

DIGMAs, which provide a multidisciplinary team-based approach to care, typically include one to two

E.B. Noffsinger, *Running Group Visits in Your Practice*, DOI 10.1007/b106441_2,
© Springer Science+Business Media, LLC 2009

nursing personnel (often a MA and a RN or LVN), a behaviorist, a dedicated scheduler, and a documenter. There are homogeneous, heterogeneous, and mixed subtypes of the model. Visits are often max-packed with vital signs, injections, and routine health maintenance brought current. Patients typically wear name tags bearing their first names, healthy refreshments are often served to encourage a relaxed atmosphere, and patients (as well as any support persons accompanying them) sign a confidentiality release in which they consent to having their medical information discussed in front of others and agree not to discuss the personal information of others once the group is over.

While DIGMAs do offer drop-in convenience, the vast majority of patients are typically prescheduled just like traditional office visits. While the drop-in component of DIGMAs offers an added convenience to patients, it is not an essential feature of the DIGMA model, and physicians can have all attendees preschedule their group appointments if the physicians prefer. Most commonly held weekly for 90 minutes, DIGMAs provide patients with the benefits of more time, improved access, greater patient education, and attention to mind as well as body needs, and physicians with the benefit of dramatically increased productivity and better practice management without extra hours being spent in the clinic. Although DIGMAs are occasionally used for intake visits and new patient appointments, they primarily focus on return or follow-up appointments in most cases (where they are open to most established patients in the provider's practice).

Drop-In Group Medical Appointments Provide Four Major Benefits

DIGMAs that are carefully designed, properly supported, well promoted, and correctly run have consistently been demonstrated to work in actual practice in primary care and almost all medical and surgical subspecialties—and to simultaneously meet the following four major objectives that this group visit model has been designed to achieve:

1. To enhance the patient's healing experience by max-packing visits; offering more time with the patient's own doctor; delivering barrier-free access to medical care; increasing the amount of patient education; more closely attending to psychosocial issues; integrating the help and support of other patients, plus a behaviorist, into each patient's healthcare experience; providing continuity of care with the patient's own physician;

improving patient–physician relationships; and enabling closer follow-up care to be provided;
2. To dramatically increase physician productivity (and, as a result, patient accessibility to quality care) by leveraging existing resources and enabling physicians to see two, three, or more times as many patients in the same amount of time;
3. To provide a useful tool that will enable physicians to better manage both busy, backlogged practices and chronic illnesses (i.e., through carefully designed chronic illness population management programs that make full use of SMAs, such as that discussed in Chapter 7);
4. To deliver high levels of both patient satisfaction and physician professional satisfaction.

Basic Parameters of a Drop-In Group Medical Appointment

As shown in Table 2.1, a combination of features makes the DIGMA model unique. DIGMAs are typically designed for follow-up visits with established visits; however, they are usually open only to the provider's own patients, or to patients in a chronic illness population management program that the physician is attached to (although they are occasionally designed to also be open to other patients from the module or pod that the physician works in). They can include most or all of the patients in the physician's practice (or all patients in the physician's practice with particular diagnoses or conditions) or in the chronic illness treatment program.

DIGMAs provide medically necessary visits. Because patients only attend when they have a medical need, different patients typically attend each DIGMA session (sessions which are often held weekly or even more frequently), which differs in a major way from CHCCs, where the same 15–20 patients typically attend all monthly sessions, often for years—regardless of whether or not they happen to have a medical need at that time. Therefore, effective promotion of the DIGMA program and ongoing vigilance regarding consistently meeting pre-established census targets are critical to successfully achieving full benefit from a DIGMA. See Part II of this book for specific information about setting up and managing DIGMAs and PSMAs. Another substantial difference between CHCCs and DIGMAs is that, in DIGMAs, the agenda of the group is totally open to (and driven by) the needs of those present at any given session (i.e., as the physician sequentially addresses the medical needs of each patient individually while others listen and learn) and not by a topic determined during a

Table 2.1 Features that make drop-in group medical appointments unique

- Although DIGMAs are sometimes used to take in new patients (or for the first part of two-part physicals), they are typically designed for follow-up visits with established patients
- DIGMAs are typically open to most or all patients in the physician's practice (or the chronic disease management program) and are typically only attended by the physician's own patients (and their support persons)
- DIGMAs are specifically designed to increase the physician's productivity by 200–300% or more, with 300% being most common
- There are heterogeneous, homogeneous, and mixed subtypes of the DIGMA model (as discussed in greater detail later in this chapter)
- DIGMAs can be customized to the needs, goals, practice style, and patient panel constituency of the individual physician
- In DIGMAs, different patients typically attend each DIGMA session (because DIGMAs are open to most or all patients in the physician's panel and because patients only attend when they have an actual medical need and want to be seen)
- DIGMAs are meant to be voluntary to patients and providers alike
- DIGMAs typically offer drop-in convenience, although the vast majority of patients are usually pre-booked into DIGMA sessions in lieu of an individual office visit (although the drop-in feature is not an essential component of the DIGMA model)
- An important defining characteristic of DIGMAs is that, throughout the session, properly run DIGMAs provide a series of one physician–one patient encounters with observers (and are best viewed as being a series of individual office visits with observers that occurs in a supportive group setting with the added benefits of the behaviorist and group interaction)
- From start to finish, the focus in DIGMAs is on delivery of medical care, addressing the unique medical needs of each patient individually
- To the maximum extent possible, well-designed DIGMA visits are meant to be max-packed and to provide a one-stop shopping healthcare experience for patients (in which all of their healthcare needs are addressed during each visit, including not only the medical issues that are bringing them in but also the updating of injections and routine health maintenance)
- An important defining characteristic of DIGMAs is that almost all medical care is delivered in the group setting, where all can listen and learn and where information does not need to be repeated (only truly private exams and discussions are typically conducted outside of the group room and in the nearby exam room)
- Private time with the physician is made available as needed to all patients for brief private exams and discussions—typically toward the end of the session
- Because of the greater amount of time available (plus the help and support of a behaviorist and other patients), the DIGMA model better addresses the mind needs of patients, which is important as a large percentage of all medical visits are driven by lifestyle issues and psychosocial needs
- Although DIGMAs provide a great deal of medical information, all patient education occurs in the context of the physician working with one patient at a time while others are able to listen, and not in a preplanned, formal class-type educational presentation like CHCCs
- The presence of a behaviorist (health psychologist, social worker, nurse, diabetes nurse educator, etc.) is characteristic of the DIGMA and PSMA models
- The physician receives real and meaningful help from the entire DIGMA team: a behaviorist (typically a psychologist or social worker); one to two nursing personnel; a documenter (whenever possible); a dedicated scheduler; and a champion and program coordinator (in larger systems only)
- The DIGMA typically consists of 10–16 patients, 2–6 family members or caregivers, the physician, the behaviorist, and possibly a documenter—and usually includes a nurse and/or medical assistant (MA), who could either return to normal clinic duties or join the group after their DIGMA nursing duties are completed (or else act as a *care coordinator* to schedule all referrals and follow-up appointments made by the provider, plus give patients their after visit summary, or AVS, consisting of those parts of their DIGMA chart note that the provider wants them to have and take home with them)
- DIGMAs work equally well for low-, medium-, and high-utilizing patients and can even be used to reach out to underserved patients
  - For example, the physician can ask the scheduler to call a number of inappropriately under-utilizing patients who have not been in for more than a couple of years to attend the next DIGMA session for a *let's get to know each other and bring your health maintenance current* session
  - Similarly, the physician could ask the scheduler to call several high-risk patients who have fallen through the cracks and invite them to attend an upcoming DIGMA session, such as diabetic patients who have not been seen for more than 6 months, or patients started on psychotropic medications more than a year ago that have not been back since
- Because DIGMAs are run like a series of individual office visits with observers, they are being billed by many fee-for-service healthcare organizations much like individual office visits, i.e., according to the level of care delivered and documented using existing E&M codes, except for the following:
  - The behaviorist's time is typically not billed and is instead considered an overhead expense to the program (in order to keep patients from receiving two bills and co-payments for a single visit)
  - Providers bill for history, exam, and medical decision-making but not for counseling time (as many patients might benefit at once and it would be egregious, and likely fraudulent, to bill several times for the same block of counseling time)
  - Because the documenter used in DIGMAs is specifically trained and produces a comprehensive and contemporaneous chart note (as opposed to the individual office visit, where the physician often completes the chart note at lunch, after work, or on Saturday mornings, by which time some of that which has actually been provided is often forgotten), billing for DIGMAs is anticipated to be optimized.
  - These healthcare organizations stand ready to adapt to any future changes in coding and billing policies that might occur—e.g., should specific billing codes be developed for the different types of group visit models

previous session while planning for the next session, as is the case for CHCCs. Yet another difference is that, whenever possible and appropriate, medical care is delivered in the group setting where all present can listen and benefit, so that repetition can be avoided and efficiency gained.

Scheduling

The single most important part of a DIGMA is the scheduling of patients, because a full group virtually always translates into a successful one. With DIGMAs (and PSMAs), the key to success lies in consistently meeting pre-established census targets during all sessions. DIGMA sessions typically range between 60 and 120 minutes in length and can be held daily, twice weekly, weekly, biweekly, monthly, or even quarterly; however, weekly 90-minute DIGMAs are by far the most common and are generally most highly recommended (especially when they are held on the day of the week that the physician experiences the greatest patient demand), at least to start with. Later, if the weekly DIGMA is consistently kept full to targeted census levels, then the physician can expand to two DIGMAs per week, and so forth.

Although patients can drop in on an as-needed basis (a convenience that is most appreciated by patients), the vast majority of patients are typically prescheduled into the DIGMA for their follow-up visits, i.e., in exactly the same manner as patients are prescheduled into individual visits. Typically, there are no drop-ins at all during the initial sessions, as patients do not yet know enough about the program and its many benefits to do so. However, even for DIGMAs that are well established and have been running for years, it is typical that only 10–25% or so of the patients who attend sessions will drop in.

However, when patients do drop in, they are asked, if at all possible, to telephone the physician's office at least a business day in advance to let staff know they are coming, so that charts can be ordered (i.e., for systems still using paper charts), census can be monitored (so that the group does not become too large), and patients can check to see if the DIGMA will be meeting that week—as the physician will occasionally be absent due to vacations, meetings, or illnesses. Furthermore, should the session need to be canceled at the last minute, patients who have let the office know that they will be dropping in can be telephoned and save a drive to the clinic. Nonetheless, in the unlikely event that the patient happens to experience a last-minute medical need that does not allow sufficient time to call the office (and if the patient is willing to take the chance of coming to the office without first checking to ensure that the DIGMA

will in fact be meeting), they are still encouraged to drop in to the cost-effective and highly efficient DIGMA rather than scheduling a more costly and less accessible individual office visit.

Patients Enter Drop-In Group Medical Appointments in Six Different Ways

Patients can enter the DIGMA in any of six different ways:

1. By invitation from the physician and support staff during routine office visits to have their next visit be a DIGMA visit;
2. By patients being encouraged by scheduling staff to make a DIGMA appointment rather than an individual office visit appointment when they telephone the office to make a follow-up appointment with their doctor;
3. By a dedicated scheduler attached to the DIGMA program telephoning a list of patients selected by the physician (usually patients from the physician's practice who have particular diagnoses or are on a waiting list) and inviting them via a scripted message to attend an upcoming DIGMA session;
4. By patients scheduling their follow-up visit during a DIGMA back into a future DIGMA session;
5. By self-referral from the program's promotional materials (program announcement, invitation letter, wall poster, program flier, patient newsletter article, etc.);
6. By patients, sometimes accompanied by a support person (such as a spouse, adult child, friend, or caregiver) simply dropping in any week that they have a medical need and want to be seen.

The Drop-In Group Medical Appointment Team

The physician receives real and meaningful help from the entire DIGMA team, i.e., the behaviorist, nurse/MA(s), documenter, dedicated scheduler, champion, and program coordinator. The physician also receives support from administration and from the physician's own front and back office staff (especially the physician's receptionists, nurses, and schedulers), who need to be specifically trained to invite and schedule patients into the DIGMA. Because the DIGMA and PSMA models represent a multidisciplinary, team-based approach to care, they work best with a dedicated and cohesive team of motivated, skilled, and well-trained people with complementary skill sets. Each team member needs to be professionally competent, courteous to patients, and a firm believer in the group visit program.

Real and meaningful help from the entire SMA team is help that physicians are not used to receiving during traditional, individual office visits. This help greatly increases their efficiency in (as well as their enjoyment of) the DIGMA/PSMA program—and therefore it is most appreciated. Along with the increased efficiencies offered by the group setting itself (where things only need to be said once, so that repetition can be avoided, and where sessions can be overbooked to make oneself immune to the downtime of no-shows and late-cancels), it is this ability to delegate as many duties as appropriate and possible to an entire SMA team that makes DIGMAs and PSMAs so efficient. This leaves the physician with much less to do; however, that *much less* is that which the physician alone can do, i.e., nobody else is qualified to do it.

The Behaviorist

The physician leads the DIGMA with the assistance of a behavioral health professional (although this is sometimes a nurse or diabetes nurse educator), which I refer to as a *behaviorist* (such as a health psychologist, social worker). Both the physician and the behaviorist are typically present throughout the entire session. In addition to arriving early to warm the group up and write down patients' concerns, giving the introduction at the start of each session, and helping to keep the group running smoothly and on time, the behaviorist performs myriad other duties in the DIGMA setting. For example, the behaviorist manages the group dynamics (drawing out the quiet patient, containing the talkative or dominating patient, intervening when two patients start distracting side-conversations with each other, etc.); paces the group so that it finishes on time with all patients' medical needs addressed; addresses patients' psychosocial and behavioral health needs (including conditions that are known to go under-diagnosed and under-treated in the primary care setting, such as depression, anxiety, and substance abuse); takes over running the group (focusing on behavioral health and psychosocial issues) while the physician is drafting the chart note or out of the group room for brief private examinations or discussions; and stays afterward to address any last-minute patient issues and to straighten up the group room.

The behaviorist is typically a psychologist or social worker, but occasionally a nurse, nurse practitioner, diabetic nurse educator, Pharm.D., etc. Ideally, this person must have group management skills, be adept at fostering group interaction, have the professional skills to tactfully address the psychosocial issues of medical patients and their families, and be able to work closely with the provider. The behaviorist's experience and skill set needs to complement (rather than be identical to) that of the physician, which helps to relieve physician anxieties about managing the group, including worries about having it spiral negatively out of control.

Because the role of the behaviorist is a much more active and structured one in a DIGMA than in a traditional mental health group, this can lead to problems in how behaviorists fulfill their role in a DIGMA—especially if they have not had specific training for these new DIGMA responsibilities. For this reason, I caution would-be DIGMA behaviorists to read about (and to fully understand) the role of the behaviorist in the DIGMA model before taking on this responsibility—despite the possible initial feelings that he or she knows how to run groups and can probably just wing it with current professional skills and experience (see Part II for more information about the behaviorist's role).

In an article entitled "Drop-In Visits Help to Improve Service," family physician Dr. Mark Attermeier (whose group is part of the Mayo Health System) underscores the critically important role that the behaviorist plays in his DIGMA: "The physician provides the medical expertise, while the behaviorist gives behavioral guidance and leads the patients to provide affirmation for one another, to feel empowered, and to become more active in their own care and more responsible for their own health....This method is so much better than if I simply referred my patients to a behaviorist. This way, if the behaviorist and I choose to debate treatment options in front of the group, the patients can chime in, and everyone gains understanding....We have finally hit on something that can cause behavioral change more rapidly than anything we have used before" (1). Another article emphasizes the importance of the behaviorist, who can sometimes identify issues that aren't recognized in a short visit with a physician (2).

The Nursing Personnel

One or two nursing personnel (RN, LVN, MA, Nursing Tech., etc.), which typically includes the physician's own nurse or medical assistant, are also attached to the DIGMA. Whenever possible, I recommend the use of a nurse and a medical assistant (MA) because it is twice as efficient (as the nursing duties can then be completed in half the time) and because the nurse and MA can have more fun and enjoy each other. Also, if the two nursing personnel have different levels of training and skill sets, then they can divide the DIGMA duties up accordingly, such as the RN or LVN giving injections, updating routine health maintenance, and providing diabetic foot exams, while the MA or nursing tech takes routine vital signs.

In general, the nursing role is typically expanded in the DIGMA setting to be all that it can be, beyond what it normally encompasses during traditional individual office visits. The nurse/MA(s) can take all applicable vital signs; update injections; help to bring performance measures and routine health maintenance current (and then pull the appropriate paper or electronic medical records referral forms, and fill out the patient identifying information on each form); perform other special nursing duties, such as taking blood glucose levels and examining the feet of diabetic patients (and indicating which patients' feet the physician needs to personally examine), checking the peak flow and PO_2 levels of asthmatic patients, etc.; and document the results of these nursing duties on each patient's chart note (Fig. 2.1).

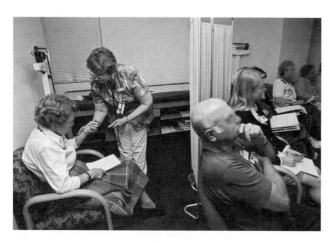

Fig. 2.1 The nurse takes all applicable vital signs and documents the results on each patient's chart note while the group is in process. Whenever possible, this should occur in a nearby examination room, rather than behind a curtain in a corner of the examination room, as is being done here. (Courtesy of Dr. Melvin Britton, Rheumatology DIGMA, Palo Alto Medical Foundation, Palo Alto, CA)

There are two additional duties that nursing personnel can fulfill, both of which we routinely conduct at Harvard Vanguard Medical Associates/Atrius Health. First, a couple of days prior to the session, nursing personnel can dispatch previsit duties by conducting medication reconciliations, reviewing health maintenance due, ensuring that all previsit labs have been completed, and reviewing HEDIS checklists during the confirmation calls made to all patients scheduled for the upcoming SMA session—and then entering this data into the patients' DIGMA chart notes. Also, once all nursing duties have been completed on all patients during the DIGMA (that is, after each patient has been called out of the group room to the

nearby exam room for vitals, injections, special nursing duties, etc.), the nurse or MA can then become the Care Coordinator for the DIGMA during the remainder of the session. Here, the MA calls each patient out of the group room, one at a time (i.e. after the physician has completed reviewing and modifying each patient's chart note in turn), and schedules all referrals, procedures, follow-up visits, etc., that the physician has recommended for that patient during the DIGMA. The Care Coordinator also provides patients with their "after visit summary," or AVS. The AVS consists of those parts of the chart note that the physician wishes for the patient to have and take home with them after the DIGMA is over. Amongst other things, the AVS always includes the "treatment plan" and "medication list" for each patient. In the event that no appointments need to be scheduled on any particular patient, the Care Coordinator simply takes the AVS into the group room and gives it to that patient—thus avoiding disrupting the group unnecessarily by calling such patients out during group time.

The Documenter

Especially in systems using electronic medical records, it is highly recommended that a specially trained *documenter*, sitting at the computer throughout the DIGMA session, assist the provider in the documentation process by drafting a comprehensive and contemporaneous chart note on each and every patient in turn (using the physician's own instructions and chart note template) as that care is being delivered to that patient in the DIGMA setting. The result should be a superior chart note that accurately documents everything that occurs in the DIGMA setting while it is actually happening and one that is therefore optimal for billing purposes. It is the physician, however, who determines the level of care delivered. The physician would typically review, modify, update, and sign off on these chart notes immediately after working with each patient in turn in the group setting, while everything about that patient is still fresh in the physician's mind before moving on to the next patient.

Afterward, the organization's billing and compliance officer should also review these DIGMA chart notes periodically (perhaps checking all chart notes documented during the first 2 months that the DIGMA is run, and then randomly spot-checking them thereafter) to ensure that they are in compliance with all applicable policies, regulations, and guidelines. In fact, physicians should include their organization's billing and compliance as well as documentation officers in the initial design, training, and planning phases of their DIGMA (including when they develop their chart note template for the program and when their documenter is trained), as they often have valuable suggestions and recommendations with regard to optimizing the documentation and billing process.

The documenter used in DIGMAs has often been a nurse, MA, resident, fellow, medical transcriptionist, or motivated member of the physician's staff with good typing and computer skills who is familiar with medical terminology, capable of deftly navigating the EMR system, and able to work closely with the physician. Even other providers, such as nurse practitioners and Pharm.Ds, have occasionally been used as documenters with great success as they can add an important extra dimension to the group—plus the additional benefit of acting in a consultation capacity to the DIGMA with their unique skill set. However, before selecting another provider as your documenter, make certain that the overhead expense assessed to the program is the provider's hourly wage and not the revenues that the provider could have generated for the system if they would instead have spent the group time seeing other patients themselves, which could drive the overhead expense up to the point where the DIGMA program is no longer seen as economically viable. This problem can often be circumvented by using other providers only when they are clearly providing extra hours to the clinic at their hourly wage (and preferably not at overtime pay, in order to keep overhead expenses for the program down).

The Champion and Program Coordinator

In larger systems (say of 20 or more providers), a *champion* is typically charged with the overall responsibility of moving the DIGMA program forward throughout the organization. In extremely large systems with multiple large facilities or medical centers, there may even need to be a site champion at each facility. The DIGMA champion attends departmental meetings, gives staff presentations, recruits physicians, develops forms and promotional materials (in template form whenever possible), custom designs each provider's DIGMA, and interacts with high-level administration.

When I was the SMA champion at the Palo Alto Medical Foundation (as well as now at HVMA/AH), my duties included developing a DIGMA and PSMA implementation plan to become a part of the organization's long-range business plan; assisting in designing and developing templates of all forms, marketing, and training materials to be used in the SMA program; selecting and training a program coordinator for the program; attending and making presentations at numerous primary care and medical subspecialty departmental meetings;

recruiting primary and specialty care physicians on an ongoing basis to run SMAs for their practices; custom designing and implementing 18 DIGMAs and PSMAs per year throughout the entire system; assisting in hiring and training behaviorists and dedicated schedulers as needed; helping to train the support personnel associated with all DIGMAs and PSMAs implemented (such as office staff, nurses, medical assistants, PSRs, advice nurses, scheduling personnel, documenters); developing the evaluative measures and periodic reports necessary for analyzing the SMA program on an ongoing basis; and sometimes co-leading each newly launched DIGMA and PSMA with the physician during its initial stages while simultaneously training a behaviorist well matched to both the physician and the patients (to later take over the responsibilities of the new SMA once it was running smoothly and any system problems were solved). In addition, as the SMA champion, I would both sit in on approximately three of the initial sessions to observe and critique the DIGMA/PSMA session, plus help out as appropriate. I would also debrief with the physician and SMA team 2–4 times for approximately 15 minutes after these initial sessions were over (i.e., during the first month or two). My dual focuses during these early debriefing sessions were twofold: first, how to make the program even better during the next session; and second, how to make the next session even more efficient and on time.

Larger systems also need to have a *program coordinator,* whose primary responsibility is to assist the champion in every way possible, while also handling many of the DIGMA program's administrative, management, and operational details. For example, the program coordinator supervises the schedulers, documenters, nurses, and behaviorists used in the SMA program; assists with the forms, implementation details, and training necessary for launching each new DIGMA; and takes primary responsibility for producing the periodic productivity, quality, outcomes, and patient/provider satisfaction reports that are necessary for overall evaluation of the program. See Chapter 11 for detailed information on the roles of the champion and program coordinator.

The Dedicated Schedulers

In addition, larger systems often hire *dedicated schedulers* for the SMA program, perhaps one full-time scheduler for every 15–25 DIGMAs and PSMAs that are up and running. These DIGMA schedulers must have good interpersonal, telephone, and telemarketing skills, as they must be able to inform patients about the program and persuade them to attend in a relatively short amount of telephone time. They are specifically trained to monitor the census of all DIGMA and PSMA sessions that they are responsible for and to take immediate corrective action when an upcoming session is not filled to targeted levels by telephoning and inviting additional patients as requested by the provider. The job of the dedicated SMA scheduler is not to take primary responsibility for filling sessions (which must remain the responsibility of the provider, the provider's support staff, and the healthcare system's regular scheduling staff) but rather to top off and fill to capacity any upcoming DIGMA or PSMA sessions that might fail to meet target or minimum census requirements. Ultimately, the primary responsibility for filling DIGMAs and Physicals SMAs must always remain with the provider, as nothing is more likely to succeed in getting a patient to attend a future DIGMA session for their next follow-up appointment than a carefully worded personal invitation from their own doctor.

The dedicated schedulers for the SMA program (i.e., for those systems fortunate enough to have them) have the more limited but extremely important role of spending a couple of hours per week on average per DIGMA or PSMA ensuring that all of the upcoming sessions meet their target census requirements. If upcoming sessions fail to meet desired census levels, then the dedicated scheduler attached to the DIGMA or PSMA takes immediate action by promptly alerting the physician and the physician's scheduling staff, and by personally inviting more appropriate patients (i.e., from lists of patients that have already been preapproved by the physician).

Physician Satisfaction Is High

In actual practice, physician professional satisfaction with DIGMAs and Physicals SMAs has been demonstrated to be uniformly high. Experience to date reveals that even physicians who are initially reluctant to start a SMA, but who are willing to try one for their practice and give it their best shot, rapidly become comfortable with this new venue of care and grow to like it. As a result, DIGMAs and PSMAs can gradually but steadily win over all but the most resistant physicians at the grassroots level, i.e., on the basis of provider self-interest. Interestingly, even in the case of the relatively small percentage of DIGMAs and PSMAs that ultimately fail in actual practice (almost invariably due to insufficient ongoing census), the physicians involved have almost universally expressed that they enjoyed running them and wished

that they could continue. Nonetheless, there will undoubtedly always be some physicians and patients who will choose not to participate in a group visit program and will prefer to continue with the status quo of traditional office visits alone.

Physicians appreciate the fact that DIGMAs and PSMAs can provide extremely helpful tools for better managing a large, busy, and backlogged practice—as well as for better managing chronic illnesses. They also value the remarkable increase in productivity and access (and possibly even income) that these group visit models can help them to achieve by improving operational efficiencies, leveraging existing resources, and improving value in the healthcare services rendered. Physicians like the fact that they no longer need to repeat the same information over and over in the exam room to different patients individually and enjoy the positive feedback that they so often receive from patients in the SMA setting— e.g., when was the last time you had a standing ovation from your patients? Providers report that they enjoy the group dynamic, the greater time available, the sheltering from outside clinic distractions, and the amount of patient education that they are able to provide in the SMA setting. Physicians also appreciate the fact that their DIGMA and/or PSMA has been custom designed to their specific needs and practice and that they are now able to better optimize the appointment mix on their master schedule— i.e., by opening up more new patient appointment slots or by having more time for doing procedures and surgeries (i.e., because so many individual follow-up appointments or physical examinations can be off-loaded onto their highly efficient DIGMAs or PSMAs). Physicians also appreciate the positive team building that DIGMAs provide, as well as the beneficial venue in which patients often open up and share difficult and personal issues with each other— thus providing a healing experience for all in attendance.

In one case, a neurologist from Kaiser Permanente's San Jose Medical Center reported that a patient indicated that she wanted to come to her neurologist's DIGMA, but that she would be embarrassed if it was mentioned in front of the group that she had been seeing a psychiatrist to deal with the extreme pain she had been experiencing. However, when she attended the group, she brought up on her own that she had been seeing a psychiatrist and gave his name. Several other members of the group said they were seeing the same psychiatrist and liked him too. The neurologist running the group was surprised, but pleased, at how "empowering" the group was for this patient (3).

Physicians value getting meaningful help from the entire DIGMA team and enjoy the collegiality they share with all members of the team. Nowhere is this truer than with the behaviorist, whose complementary skill set they soon grow to appreciate and with whom they spend so many hours working closely together within the group setting (and, as a result, often develop a close professional relationship). In addition, physicians often report that their SMAs provide an oasis during their otherwise hectic workweek—an opportunity to learn something new, to do something interesting and different, to get off the fast-paced treadmill of individual office visit care, to develop better relationships with their patients, to have some fun, and to deliver a more satisfying level of medical care.

in the medical center, as often happens in other types of group programs or classes. There are, however, two relatively common exceptions to this. First, if the DIGMA is designed for a chronic illness treatment program, then patients with that diagnosis who happen to be from other physicians' practices could also be included. Second, several physicians working closely together in a module, pod, or small department might mutually decide to open their DIGMAs to not only their own patients but those from their colleagues' practices as well in order to improve access to all of their practices. As depicted in the table, DIGMAs can be customized by adjusting any of a number of parameters to the specific needs of the provider.

Drop-In Group Medical Appointments Are Customized to Each Provider

In each and every case, DIGMAs are customized to the particular needs, goals, practice style, and patient panel constituency of the individual physician (Table 2.2). DIGMAs are typically open only to the physician's own patients (and their support persons); however, they can be designed to encompass the majority (or even the entirety) of the physician's patient panel. Patients are not generally drawn from other physicians' practices or from elsewhere

Drop-In Group Medical Appointments Can Increase Productivity 200–300% or More

The DIGMA model was originated to enhance the patients' healing experience, i.e., to improve quality and access to follow-up appointments. However, DIGMAs have also been shown to increase physician productivity, enable physicians to better manage their large practices, enhance treatment of the chronically ill, and provide high levels of patient and physician satisfaction. Both the inherent efficiencies of the group, such as lack of repetition and ability to overbook sessions to compensate for

Table 2.2 Drop-in group medical appointment variables that can be customized to the provider

- The target, minimum, and maximum census requirements set for each DIGMA
- The DIGMA subtype used (homogeneous, heterogeneous, or mixed)
- The types of patients, conditions, and diagnoses that will be included and excluded
- Will it involve only the physician's own patients, or other provider's patients as well (as in a chronic disease population management program or from other referring providers in the physician's own module, team, or pod)
- What types of medical care will be provided (and how much) during each session
- The length of sessions and the frequency with which they will be held
- The weekday and time of day that the DIGMA is to be held
- The particular behaviorist, nurse/MA(s), and dedicated scheduler to be utilized
- Whether or not to use the drop-in component of the DIGMA
- The expanded duties that the behaviorist and nurse(s) will provide
- The specific responsibilities of the dedicated scheduler and the amount of time allocated to the DIGMA each week
- Whether a documenter will be employed and what their specific duties will be
- What charting template will be used and what the final chart note will look like
- Which group and exam rooms will be used
- How is the behaviorist to prompt the physician to hurry up and move along when time is running short and too much time is seemingly being spent on a particular patient
- What marketing materials will be used and how the DIGMA will be promoted
- What help the SMA champion and program coordinator will provide, both initially and on an ongoing basis
- Whether or not to use the drop-in component of the DIGMA model (which I generally recommend, but some providers refuse to use)
- What types of training will be provided for the physician, DIGMA team, and the physician's support staff
- How will the DIGMA be evaluated on an ongoing basis and what reports will be generated (and how often)
- Specifically, what corrective actions are to be promptly taken whenever the census for an upcoming session is low

no-shows, and the multidisciplinary team-based nature of care (in which as many physician responsibilities as appropriate and possible are delegated to less costly members of the SMA team) contribute to the DIGMA's remarkable efficiency.

DIGMAs have repeatedly been demonstrated to enable physicians to see dramatically more patients in the same amount of time, generally 200–300% or more, with 300% being the most common goal. Furthermore, experience shows that this dramatically increased efficiency can often be accomplished while simultaneously enhancing patient and physician professional satisfaction, improving service and quality of care, and providing brief private examinations and discussions (as well as minor procedures) as needed toward the end of each session. Experience has shown that the ideal census for a DIGMA is typically between 10 and 16 patients, plus 2–6 family members and support persons, for an optimal group size of between 12 and 22 members. However, sessions are usually overbooked by one to three patients, like the airlines do, in order to compensate for the expected number of no-shows and late cancelations. For many primary care DIGMAs, the "sweet spot" for actual attendance appears to be around 13 patients.

Design the Drop-In Group Medical Appointment to Triple Productivity

Although in some circumstances DIGMAs can only double productivity (typically for providers who are already extremely productive during individual office visits, such as pediatricians in delivering well baby checks and school, camp, and sports physicals, obstetricians in providing prenatal examinations, dermatologists providing full-body skin exams, and primary care physicians offering only 10-minute return appointments), DIGMAs are typically designed to triple the provider's actual productivity with respect to similar types of individual office visits. However, in order to achieve this, the physician needs to receive the supports discussed in this book: an appropriate SMA team, the assistance of a dedicated scheduler, the help of a champion and program coordinator, help from the physician's scheduling staff, etc. Here, we are referring to tripling the provider's actual productivity over the number of individual return visits provided during the same amount of clinic time as the DIGMA session lasts (i.e., not with respect to the number of individual return visits scheduled, but rather to the number actually seen on average during 90 minutes of clinic time). Notice that the actual number of patients seen is typically less than the number scheduled, as there are usually some no-shows and late cancelations (plus some unfilled appointments and provider downtime on the schedule) that reduce the provider's

actual productivity for traditional office visits from the number of patients scheduled.

While it may not seem like much to triple a provider's productivity during 1½ hours of clinic time each week (i.e., for 90-minute DIGMAs held on a weekly basis), this actually translates into a substantial net gain in productivity for the entire week. For example, for a full-time physician whose workweek contains 36 hours of direct patient contact time in the clinic, running one 90-minute DIGMA per week that increases actual productivity during the group visit by 300% would result in an approximate 8.3% increase in the physician's overall productivity for the entire week. Running two such DIGMAs per week would correspondingly increase the full-time physician's weekly productivity by approximately 16.6%. Furthermore, running such DIGMAs five times a week (i.e., daily) could increase this physician's productivity for the entire week by 41.5%—and without extra hours being spent in the clinic. On the other hand, the corresponding numbers for half-time physicians would be 16.6, 33.2, and 83.0%—i.e., for one, two, and five DIGMAs per week, respectively. Similarly, the actual percentage increase in weekly productivity would be correspondingly greater for physicians in systems requiring 34 hours of direct patient contact time rather than 36 or 38—and still greater for systems requiring that only 32 hours be scheduled with patients.

Increased Productivity Can Improve Access

This increased productivity and capacity that comes from the DIGMA model (and the consequent leveraging of existing resources) can be used to work down backlogs and wait-lists and to improve access to the physician's practice without extra time being spent in the clinic. In addition, DIGMAs often turn out to be a positive, motivating, and enjoyable experience for those physicians who choose to run them. Furthermore, physicians running DIGMAs in their practice often report that they leave the group feeling energized rather than depleted or exhausted. For physicians who choose to run a DIGMA for their practices primarily because of the program's productivity and efficiency benefits, this can be a most pleasant and enjoyable surprise.

Specialists Can Often Increase Productivity Even More Than 300%

Even more dramatic increases in weekly productivity can sometimes be achieved when the individual appointments that are being replaced by the DIGMA are longer than 15 or 20 minutes, for example, when the physician's individual appointments are 30, 45, or even 60 minutes (which is sometimes the case for intake visits and certain types of follow-up appointments with specialists who provide procedures and surgeries). In addition, certain specialists (such as gastroenterologists, urologists, general surgeons, plastic surgeons, orthopedic surgeons) are able to efficiently off-load lower compensated pre-procedure intake visits and post-procedure follow-up visits onto their DIGMAs or PSMAs. As a result, they are often able to restructure their master schedules so as to offer more procedures and surgeries each week, which are typically more highly compensated and of greater interest to many such specialists.

In addition, some other medical and surgical subspecialists (plus a few primary care providers, especially those dealing with complex, multi-morbid geriatric patients) still have some longer return appointments, such as 30-minute slots. Generally speaking, the longer that the underlying individual office visit is (i.e., that the DIGMA is replacing or leveraging), the greater the productivity gain that the DIGMA will provide. To understand why this is true, consider a physician with 15-minute return appointments in the clinic who happens to increase productivity by 300% through the DIGMA. Then, this physician would actually increase productivity by 600% through the DIGMA by seeing the same number of patients in the group, i.e., provided the physician's return appointments in the clinic were 30 minutes in duration rather than 15 minutes.

Subtypes of Drop-In Group Medical Appointments and Physicals Shared Medical Appointments

There are three subtypes of the DIGMA and PSMA models: heterogeneous; homogeneous; and mixed, which is in between the heterogeneous and homogeneous subtypes. These three designs offer great flexibility when customizing DIGMAs and PSMAs to the physician. The relative frequency with which these three designs are actually being used in practice (as well as the different types of applications for which they are being used) is quite surprising—and not at all intuitively obvious. In all three subtypes, patients can be invited to bring a support person along, usually the patient's spouse, although it is occasionally an adult child, a friend, or a caregiver. However, I caution that it be made clear that the patient is invited to bring a support person along, as I once had a patient enter the DIGMA accompanied by 13 family members—which was a group unto itself!

The Heterogeneous Subtype

In the heterogeneous subtype, most if not all patients from the physician's practice are invited to attend the DIGMA any week they want, regardless of their condition, diagnosis, or utilization behavior. Heterogeneous DIGMAs and PSMAs are broadly inclusive, encompassing most or all of the types of patients in the physician's practice. For example, almost all of an oncologist's cancer patients could be included in every heterogeneous oncology DIGMA session, regardless of type and site of cancer, stage of disease, prognosis, presence or absence of metastases, etc. Similarly, a nephrologist's heterogeneous DIGMA could be open to all patients with kidney disease in the nephrologist's practice, including diabetic and hypertensive patients with advanced kidney disease, patients in the early stages of kidney disease, patients experiencing end-stage renal disease, pre-dialysis patients, patients currently receiving dialysis treatments, and patients who are recipients of a kidney transplant.

That Heterogeneous DIGMAs Work at All Is Counterintuitive

Many things about group visits are surprising and not at all intuitively obvious—which is a major reason that contributes to why, with group visits, frustrating beginner's mistakes can so easily be made. The fact that confidentiality has not proven to be more of an impediment to group visits is one such example (a problem that is often addressed by handling the issue of confidentiality conservatively, which includes having all attendees sign a confidentiality agreement prior to the start of each and every DIGMA or PSMA session). It is also counterintuitive that patients often speak more openly and frankly in the group setting than they do one-on-one with their physician during traditional individual office visits—a problem which I believe is a reflection of the power mismatch that exists between the physician and patient in the normal office visit, a disparity that is largely ameliorated by the presence of numerous other patients in the group setting (especially when other patients bring up an embarrassing issue first).

Perhaps one of the greatest surprises is that the heterogeneous subtype works exceptionally well in actual practice, especially as a practice management tool and in improving access to care. In such medical disciplines as family practice, internal medicine, women's health, neurology, rheumatology, and endocrinology—subspecialties that encompass some very diverse patient populations and health conditions—it is by no means obvious that the heterogeneous model would be so much more popular in

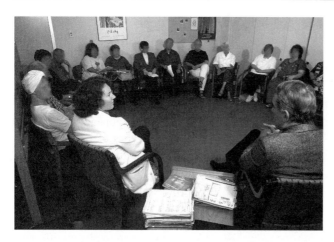

Fig. 2.2 Heterogeneous DIGMAs work well in actual practice, especially as a practice management tool and in improving access to care in medical disciplines such as family practice, internal medicine, women's health, neurology, rheumatology, oncology, and endocrinology. (Courtesy of American Medical Group Association and Dr. Lynn Dowdell, Kaiser Permanante Medical Center, San Jose, CA)

actual practice for managing a physician's practice than the homogeneous and mixed DIGMA models (Fig. 2.2). In fact, when the homogeneous and mixed subtypes of the DIGMA model are initially used in many of these medical subspecialties, they are frequently observed to either fail due to lack of adequate census or to gradually evolve into the heterogeneous subtype over time.

The reason that the heterogeneous DIGMA works so well in primary care is that the patients who attend simply represent a cross-section of the physician's practice as a whole. For example, if 13 patients attend a heterogeneous primary care DIGMA, it is likely that 7 or 8 will have hyperlipidemia, 6 or 7 hypertension, 3 or 4 diabetes, and 2 or 3 headache—so that even in the heterogeneous subtype, there is still a great deal of commonality between patients in attendance.

In Heterogeneous DIGMAs, Patients Still Share Many Common Issues

Perhaps one reason that heterogeneous DIGMAs are so successful is that, in a heterogeneous DIGMA, all of the patients not only share that particular physician but also have many common concerns, even though the specifics of their illnesses happen to differ. Especially for the chronically ill, such common concerns include: the adjustments that must be made to having a chronic illness; the frustration of facing new limitations and not being able to do what one used to do; the erosion of self-esteem that comes from not being able to fulfill one's normal roles and responsibilities, and the anxiety created by facing a

worrisome and uncertain future. Despite having different diagnoses, chronically ill patients nonetheless share many common threads—as they all have some type of chronic illness that will require frequent, routine medical visits together with emotional support and the need to see a physician for a lifetime. Patients with severe chronic illness know what it is like: to wake up with a jolt in the middle of the night worrying about what tomorrow will bring; to feel sick, fatigued, overwhelmed, and unable to cope; to worry about the impact that their illness is having upon their job, family, and friends; and to feel isolated, alone, cheated, and ask "Why me?" Regardless of the specifics of their particular illness, the chronically ill in general know what it is like to face these issues—as well as having the desire to not burden their family and friends with their difficulties.

As can be seen, even though the DIGMA happens to be heterogeneous in terms of diagnoses, there are still many psychosocial issues and feelings shared between patients. Because patients have so much in common, they provide each other with a great deal of compassion and emotional support in the group setting, and sometimes patients even form friendships and provide off-site unofficial support for each other. This is something that tends to happen more with serious chronic illnesses that can have a substantial psychosocial overlay, such as cancer, end-stage kidney disease, AIDS, bone marrow transplants, congestive heart failure, multiple sclerosis, and Parkinson's disease. When relationships outside of the clinic are likely to happen, or have in fact happened, it is important to clarify the confidentiality issues with these patients.

Patients Listen When Others with Different Conditions Are Treated

Many find it difficult to envision how such a heterogeneous mix of patients could possibly work in their practice. They even find it more astonishing that because of its operational simplicity and the ease of filling sessions, the heterogeneous design is turning out to be the most common DIGMA subtype in actual practice, at least when it comes to improving access and better managing a busy, backlogged practice. It is important to note, however, that this is not true for chronic illness population management programs, in which the homogeneous subtype tends to predominate (because there are typically so many patients having a particular diagnosis that there is no difficulty in consistently filling homogeneous DIGMA sessions). In fact, when I first started DIGMAs in primary and specialty care at Kaiser Permanente in 1996, I wondered whether other patients would be interested in listening when the physician was working with a patient who had a completely different set of health problems. At that time, I believed this issue was the lynchpin as to whether the heterogeneous DIGMA subtype would or would not succeed in actual practice.

For over 2 years, I stopped DIGMA groups time and time again in order to ask patients questions such as the following: "Mary, you look interested in what the doctor is saying; however, you have multiple sclerosis, while John, who is three times older than you, has Parkinson's disease. Are you really interested and, if so, why?" "Oh yes, I am very interested," was the answer I almost always received, although occasionally patients were disinterested because they were preoccupied only with their own issues. When I asked patients such as Mary why they were interested in issues that did not directly pertain to them, there were four types of answers: (1) "Because I might get it myself some-day"; (2) "Because my mother [brother, neighbor] has it"; (3) "Because this is like a mini-medical school class taught by my own doctor"; or (4) "This is better than watching ER!"

Heterogeneous Model in Primary Care and Medical Subspecialties

Many primary care physicians feel that the heterogeneous DIGMA model would not work for them, pointing out that their practice is much more heterogeneous than that of most medical specialists for whom they could see it work-ing. My counterargument would be that the most hetero-geneous DIGMAs I have ever witnessed were not in pri-mary care, but rather in neurology—but even here, the heterogeneous subtype was quite successful. I say this because these heterogeneous neurology DIGMAs would have young neurology patients diagnosed with headache, multiple sclerosis, and seizure disorder frequently mixed in with elderly men and women experiencing stroke, demen-tia, and Parkinson's disease. What I discovered with this diverse mix of patients was that, despite the fact that their ages and conditions varied substantially, many of the issues that these patients were dealing with were common issues.

Many of these neurology patients shared the fact that they were discouraged, anxious, or depressed about their illness and uncertain future. Another common factor for many of them was that they knew what it was like to wake up in a panic in the middle of the night feeling isolated and alone, worrying about burdening their family with their illness and uncertain future, and asking, "Why me, God?" It turned out that, even though the medical diagnoses and conditions of these neurology patients varied consider-ably, they still shared a wide range of common medical, lifestyle, and psychosocial issues, which enabled them to be interested in one another because they could identify with, and relate to, each other. In addition, because each

of these patients had already made some adjustments to their own particular illness, they all tended to see certain others in the group as being worse off than they were—which they often found to be uplifting as they now saw that there was still much that they could do which others cannot.

Mixed and Homogeneous Groups Often Evolve into Heterogeneous Groups

At one large staff model HMO, I started three different weekly 90-minute neurology DIGMAs (one with each of the three different neurologists in the neurology depart-ment) back to back on the same weekday; however, only one of these neurologists chose to have a heterogeneous design. The other two neurology DIGMAs started out with a mixed design because those neurologists wanted to have more of a condition-specific focus during their ses-sions. For these two mixed neurology DIGMAs, head-ache patients were the focus on the first week of the month; multiple sclerosis, seizure disorder, and younger neurology patients the second week; Parkinson's disease, stroke, dementia, and older neurology patients were the focus the fourth week; and the third (and the occasional fifth session) each month was heterogeneous and open to all of the neurologist's patients, so that no patient had to wait more than a couple of weeks to be seen in the next appropriate group session. What we found was that the two mixed models gradually evolved into a straight het-erogeneous design by the end of 1 year of operations, by which time all three of these neurology DIGMAs were of the heterogeneous subtype.

Here is what would sometimes happen in the hetero-geneous neurology DIGMAs. The neurologist would sequentially work with each of the patients in attendance, i.e., patients with multiple sclerosis, stroke, dementia, Parkinson's disease, etc., either by going around the room in a counterclockwise or clockwise fashion or by clustering patients by diagnoses and treating them sequentially, one condition after another. One patient might be a young woman in a wheelchair accompanied by her parents, who are despondent about their daugh-ter's rapid decline. Others could be patients who have recently had serious strokes, one of whom might be pro-foundly depressed and while another has lost impulse control. Often, there would also be several patients with Parkinson's disease. Then, there would be other patients with migraines or cluster headaches, who just wanted the lights to be turned down and for everyone to be quiet. Finally, in the middle of it all, another patient in the group with seizure disorder might suddenly and unexpectedly drop onto the floor and have a seizure. One might very well ask what good could possibly come out of such a seemingly disorganized hodgepodge and heterogeneous mix of patients. Yet, I found that a great deal of good almost always came out of this diverse mix.

What we found was that patients encouraged and supported each other, even in these heterogeneous groupings. They no longer felt as alone and isolated, and everyone left these sessions with a more balanced perspective on life, realizing that, despite their own particular affliction, there was often still much which they could do that others were no longer able to accomplish. In addition, patients often met others with similar conditions, occasionally for the first time and even exchanged telephone numbers. Sometimes, these neurology patients could be found in the lobby or parking lot 1 or 2 hours after the DIGMA was over, still talking with each other.

It appears that one of the reasons that such heterogeneous DIGMAs work so well in actual practice is that what is most important is that patients have some sort of illness or health problem and therefore can identify and empathize with one another (especially when that illness is impacting their daily life and emotional well-being, and when it is creating an uncertain future), and not necessarily that they have the same illness. Often, patients do not want to burden their families and closest loved ones with their worries, health concerns, and problems. However, they also indicate that they would still like some type of social support—someone they could talk to who could understand, such as another patient who is also dealing with an illness. Patients point out that what they want is to feel that others can truly appreciate the difficulties that they are going through with their health problems—and that they are able to provide compassion, helpful information, and emotional support.

Patients Benefit from Seeing Others Perceived as Being Worse Off

During the heterogeneous neurology DIGMA session previously discussed, just as everyone was looking at the patient on the floor who had just suffered a seizure, one of the patients looked up and said, "God, I'm glad I have brain cancer and not *that*!" I wondered at that moment what this patient with brain cancer would have said earlier that morning if someone had told him beforehand that, before the day was out, he would actually state that he was glad that he had brain cancer—under any circumstances. Others agreed that they were also glad that they had what they did, rather than the seizure disorder that this patient was suffering from.

Interestingly, the seizure patient was seen by all other patients in the room as being the most unfortunate of all. Of course, medically speaking, this was certainly not the case. This had the immediate salutary effect of causing everyone else in the group room to instantly feel better about their own conditions. Whether they realize it or not, almost all patients have already made some adjustments toward accommodating their own illnesses. This makes it more likely that they will be able to see others as being worse off than they are, so that everyone is likely to leave the group feeling a little better. This is especially true when patients witness something as dramatic as a seizure in the group setting.

However, as it turned out, even the seizure patient benefited greatly from this session. Once this patient came around and regained consciousness, her first words to the group were, "Well, I guess that I don't need to tell you why I see the doctor." This lightened up the moment and caused everyone to laugh in a warm and accepting manner. At the end of the session, this patient said that even though she frequently had seizures, the worst part of the illness for her was the agoraphobic symptoms she had subsequently developed, i.e., out of fear that she would go out, have a seizure, and embarrass herself. However, she added, "Because you folks have been so kind to me, I'll tell you what I'm going to do. If my friends call me this afternoon and invite me out to dinner, I'm going to go."

At that moment, I could not help but appreciate the emotional support benefits—the healing properties—that properly run DIGMA groups are able to offer, as everyone present in the group that day benefited a great deal from this remarkable interchange. Furthermore, I have witnessed countless similar incidences in DIGMAs over the years, so this is by no means an uncommon benefit of the group dynamic.

The Heterogeneous Subtype Can Be Less Threatening to Other Patients

A heterogeneous mix of patients often makes it less threatening for other patients in the group, because patients in a truly homogeneous group might tend to look at each other as being somewhere on a linear progression of that disease. For example, when one woman in a group that is specific to breast cancer (or, worse yet, a particular type and stage of breast cancer) happens to have a metastasis, then this could be quite threatening to other patients in the group who happen to have the same type of disease and fear that the exact same thing could happen to them next.

However, if the group included a heterogeneous mix of patients with all types of cancers (colon, lung, breast, prostate, cervical, ovarian, brain, head and neck, leukemias, lymphomas, melanomas, etc.), then this event would likely not be nearly as disquieting and threatening to other patients, many of whom would probably have different cancers and stages of disease. Furthermore, because there would then be far more patients to draw from for the heterogeneous group, it would also have the additional benefit of being easier to consistently fill sessions, which is the key to a successful group visit.

Heterogeneous Drop-In Group Medical Appointments Are Best for Half-Time Physicians

The heterogeneous subtype of the DIGMA model is the design of choice for most part-time physicians. For example, in the case of a half-time physician, the panel size would typically only be approximately half as large as the panel size of a full-time physician, and consequently there would only be half as many patients to draw from in order to fill the half-time physician's DIGMA sessions. As a result, experience demonstrates that half-time physicians often have great difficulty consistently meeting pre-established census requirements when they employ either the homogeneous or mixed DIGMA designs. However, by changing to the heterogeneous subtype of the DIGMA model, where virtually every patient in the physician's practice qualifies to attend sessions whenever they have a medical need, these half-time physicians are typically much better able to meet the census requirements of their DIGMA (4).

Operational Advantages of Heterogeneous Drop-In Group Medical Appointments

It is worth noting that, as a practice management tool, the heterogeneous subtype of the DIGMA model is often the easiest to run and keep full. First of all, the sessions are easy for patients and staff to keep track of because all of the physician's patients wanting or needing a follow-up visit qualify to attend any of the heterogeneous DIGMA's sessions—and because all sessions are therefore open to exactly the same large group of patients. Second, the physician's scheduling staff is more willing to schedule heterogeneous DIGMAs because they are not worried about being reprimanded for scheduling the wrong type of patient into any given session. Third, it is easier to keep all sessions full which, as we have repeatedly discussed, is the key to a successful DIGMA program.

As an example of the heterogeneous subtype of the DIGMA model being operationally easier to run and keep full, consider two young and energetic dermatologists with large practices at one mid-sized integrated healthcare delivery system. One of these dermatologists specialized in skin cancer and cosmetic dermatology, whereas the other had a special interest in acne. However, both also had an on-call day each week in which they were responsible for covering all patients needing to be seen in the dermatology department at the last minute that day, regardless of their diagnosis. Therefore, the first dermatologist decided to run a homogeneous dermatology DIGMA each week for skin cancer and another for cosmetic dermatology, whereas the other decided to run a homogeneous dermatology DIGMA for acne. However, both dermatologists decided to also run a heterogeneous dermatology DIGMA on their on-call day—which they humorously referred to as their "garbage can DIGMA" because all of the leftovers of the day were spilled into it, regardless of diagnosis (skin cancer, rosacea, warts, sun damage, acne, keratoses, cosmetic issues, etc.).

So which of these DIGMAs would you guess to be the most successful? The correct answer, as you might have guessed by now, was the two heterogeneous DIGMAs, because, whereas it was often difficult to find even eight patients with skin cancer, cosmetic issues, or acne who were willing to attend the group and happened to need to be seen on the days that these weekly homogeneous dermatology DIGMAs were held, it was relatively easy to fill the heterogeneous DIGMAs on their on-call days with 12–15 patients. Remember, a full DIGMA is almost always a lively, interesting, interactive, and successful DIGMA, i.e., both psychodynamically and economically.

The Homogeneous Subtype

There are two basic forms of the intuitively appealing homogeneous DIGMA design. The first basic form, which is frequently used in chronic illness population management programs, is one in which all of the homogeneous DIGMA sessions are dedicated to the same disease or condition, such as diabetes, congestive heart failure, hypertension, hyperlipidemia, peri-menopausal issues, morbid obesity, or dialysis. The second basic form, which is sometimes used by physicians employing the DIGMA as a practice management tool, is one in which the physician's patient panel is partitioned into a series of relatively homogeneous subpopulations, with each patient grouping being the focus of a different DIGMA session. For example, a primary care physician might divide her practice up and use the homogeneous DIGMA design to see the following sequence of homogeneous patient groupings on successive weeks: diabetes and obesity, hypertension and hyperlipidemia, chronic pain, peri-menopausal issues, geriatric patients, asthma, irritable bowel syndrome, GERD, etc. Each diagnostic group of patients would attend the DIGMA session that focused on their particular condition, and the entire sequence of sessions would then be repeated over and over on an ongoing basis.

Homogeneous Subtype Has Limitations

While intuitively appealing, the homogeneous DIGMA suffers from several important shortcomings, the result of which is that the homogeneous design tends to be the least frequently used of the three DIGMA subtypes in actual practice, at least when it comes to managing a busy, backlogged practice (which is where the heterogeneous subtype predominates). The exception to this would be in diagnostic-specific applications, such as chronic illness treatment programs or surgical intakes or follow-ups for specific conditions (such as intakes for breast reduction or carpal tunnel surgeries), where enough patients of a particular type can often be found to ensure that all homogeneous DIGMA sessions are consistently filled, thus making the homogeneous design a viable option.

Physicians all too often make this common beginners' mistake: They design their DIGMA homogeneously around a specific patient population that happens to be of particular interest to them (i.e., even if there does not happen to be much patient demand for such a service) rather than designing it for the majority of their practice, which is where their greatest patient demand exists. As a result, these homogeneous DIGMAs often end up failing due to patient attendance being insufficient, i.e., both for a lively and interactive group session and for an economically viable program.

One shortcoming of the second homogeneous approach discussed in the previous section is that, if there are too many different diagnostic-specific sessions in the sequence being offered, individual office visits might be available to patients before the next appropriate homogeneous DIGMA session is held—even for backlogged physicians with access problems. This goes against the entire intent of the DIGMA program, which is to improve access and offload, whenever appropriate and possible, costly individual follow-up visits onto highly efficient DIGMA sessions.

In addition, although it would not be a problem if the entire homogeneous DIGMA program were for a single disease or condition (such as diabetes), in the second situation discussed previously (i.e., where there is a series of different homogeneous sessions, each focusing upon a different illness or condition), it can be difficult for staff and patients to keep track of the sequence of sessions so that they know what session will be meeting on which week. This is especially true whenever there is a holiday break, or when the sequence is interrupted by the physician being absent due to illness, vacation, or meetings. When this does happen, does the physician skip the particular patient grouping in the sequence that the canceled session was to focus upon (and thus continue with the remainder of the sequence of sessions as previously scheduled)—or does the physician simply postpone that grouping of patients until the next session that is held, with the result being that all future sessions would also be correspondingly postponed (so that any patients prescheduled for these sessions would then need to be called and rescheduled)? As can be seen, any interruption to the established sequence of sessions throws the schedule off and makes it that much more difficult for patients and staff (especially the physician's scheduling staff) to keep track of. It is for this reason that I seldom recommend this approach.

Patient with Different Condition Attending a Homogeneous Group

An additional complication of the homogeneous subtype is the problem of what to do with the patient with a different condition who happens to attend, or the patient who mistakenly attends the wrong session (i.e., a session that focuses on a different type of health problem than the one the patient has). Or the patient might have the correct condition—for example diabetes, when the homogeneous DIGMA session is focusing on diabetes—but the patient is not interested in diabetes that week and instead wants to discuss an unrelated symptom or problem (such as an earache, headache, acne, or sprained ankle). When this happens, would you treat the patient anyway for such issues that are unrelated to diabetes and thereby make the homogeneous DIGMA session more heterogeneous? Or would you refuse to see the patient and thereby risk alienating the patient or having the patient instead schedule a more costly individual office visit, both of which are undesirable options and antithetical to the goals of a well-run DIGMA program? Almost always, the physician will go ahead and see the patient in the group and find out that it all works out just fine (and that other patients are often interested in what is being discussed), which is why homogeneous and mixed DIGMAs so often gradually evolve into heterogeneous DIGMAs over time.

Handling Patients Who Bring Lengthy Lists of Health Concerns to a Homogeneous Group

However, the most problematic difficulty of all for the homogeneous DIGMA subtype is the long list of other medical issues that each patient frequently brings to the visit and wants to have addressed, i.e., their laundry list of medical concerns. This is especially problematic for physicians having access problems, as patients then tend to store up a list of health complaints for their next visit, rather than coming in promptly for a focused single issue visit. For example, a hypertensive patient might be scheduled into a homogeneous DIGMA session focusing on hypertension; however, at the time the session is held, high blood pressure might be the least of the patient's concerns, as the patient might instead be preoccupied by a host of other medical issues. If these other concerns are not dealt with during the DIGMA session (an approach that I do not recommend taking), several consequences will result.

First of all, convenience to the patient will be reduced, which can be upsetting to some patients and is counter to the one-stop shopping healthcare philosophy of the DIGMA model. Second, extra visits will likely be created, because the patient will probably then want to return for a subsequent individual visit in order to have these other issues addressed, which, again, goes counter to the entire underlying philosophy of group visits regarding replacing (not adding) visits. On the other hand, if the physician does address these diverse medical issues, which might be unrelated to the central theme of the homogeneous DIGMA session, then the group will automatically become more heterogeneous in nature. In fact, this is precisely what very often does happen in practice. This is the central reason that the homogeneous and mixed DIGMA subtypes are so often observed to gradually evolve into the heterogeneous subtype over time.

Homogeneous Drop-In Group Medical Appointments Are Best for Chronic Illness Treatment Programs

After a great deal of experience as a consultant in healthcare organizations nationwide participating in hundreds of primary and specialty care DIGMAs of various types, my observation has been that the homogeneous subtype of the DIGMA model is generally best used in chronic illness population management programs, rather than for better managing a large, backlogged practice (unless, of course, it happens to be a physician whose practice almost entirely consists of a particular diagnosis or condition). This is because it is a relatively easy matter to consistently fill homogeneous DIGMA sessions when there are a large pool of patients available that happen to have a particular illness, which is the case for chronic illness population management programs (but is typically not the case when it comes to an individual physician's own particular practice).

For example, there can be thousands or even tens of thousands of patients in the hypertension, hyperlipidemia, or diabetes chronic illness treatment programs of larger healthcare systems, which makes it relatively easy to consistently fill all homogeneous DIGMA sessions

within these treatment programs. On the other hand, an individual physician might have a very difficult time filling a homogeneous Diabetes DIGMA designed just for his/her own patient panel as there might only be 300 diabetic patients in his/her practice to draw from–and they must have both diabetes and a medical need to be seen that week in order to attend a DIGMA session.

In addition to larger chronic illness treatment programs, the homogeneous DIGMA model can be successfully used in a couple of other circumstances. For example, homogeneous DIGMAs can sometimes be successfully employed in certain medical subspecialties where one medical condition tends to dominate their practice, such as an endocrinologist who has a homogeneous DIGMA for diabetes in general (or for type 2 diabetes, in particular) or a rheumatologist specializing in patients with arthritis.

The homogeneous DIGMA model can also be used by certain specialists (such as plastic surgeons, general surgeons, orthopedic surgeons, urologists, gastroenterologists) who are able to design a homogeneous DIGMA or PSMA for intakes and/or follow-up visits for the types of surgeries and procedures that they frequently perform—breast reductions, hip replacements, knee replacements, carpal tunnel surgeries, bariatric surgery, etc.—provided that they do enough of them to ensure that their homogeneous SMA sessions will be consistently filled. Homogeneous DIGMAs have similarly been successfully employed in travel medicine for short-term and long-term travelers.

The Mixed Subtype

The mixed DIGMA design, which is almost as frequently used in practice as the heterogeneous design (at least initially, when physicians first start their DIGMAs), represents a compromise between the heterogeneous and homogeneous subtypes—and combines some elements of both of these. Also, the mixed subtype is frequently used for PSMAs, because patients requiring physical examinations can often readily be divided into four major subgroupings, e.g., according to sex and age groupings, with one of these being the focus during each of the four weekly sessions held each month (such as men under 50 being the focus of the PSMA on the first week of the month, men over 50 on the second, women under 40 or 45 on the third week, and women over that age being the focus on the fourth week each month).

The mixed design typically divides the provider's entire patient panel into four large groupings, with one of these groupings being the focus for each week of the month. The same sequence is then repeated every month, so that patients and staff alike can easily keep track of which session is being held on any given week of the month (except for those couple of months each year that happen to have five weekly sessions). In one mixed primary care DIGMA, the first week of the month focused on all of the physician's cardiopulmonary patients; the second week on diabetes and obesity; the third week on all gastrointestinal patients; and the fourth on woman's health issues. In the couple of months each year having five SMA sessions, the fifth week of a mixed DIGMA is often a heterogeneous session open to all of the physician's patients, although it can also focus on the largest grouping (or whichever patient grouping the physician wants). On the other hand, if the physician prefers, these fifth weekly sessions that happen to occur just a couple of times during the year could simply not be held.

The mixed DIGMA resembles the heterogeneous subtype in several respects, because (1) each of the four weekly sessions can be broadly inclusive of several diagnoses; (2) the fifth weekly session is often heterogeneous; and (3) patients are welcome to attend any session that better fits their schedule in the event that they cannot attend the most appropriate one. On the other hand, each of the weekly sessions has a different diagnostic-specific focus, which is reminiscent of the homogeneous subtype. The mixed subtype is therefore best viewed as a design that lies in between the heterogeneous and homogeneous subtypes, and which contains some of the attributes of each.

Patients Unable to Attend the Most Appropriate Session Can Attend Another

One important provision of the mixed design is worth noting: If, for reasons of personal convenience (or because of a scheduling conflict), the patient is not able to attend the most appropriate session that month for his or her particular health problem, then—in the mixed subtype—the patient is typically invited to attend any other *appropriate* session that better fits the patient's schedule. I say *appropriate* because, for example, men would not be invited to attend a women's health issues session. In addition to providing better, more convenient service to our patients, the reason for this provision is in line with an important goal that we always have for DIGMAs and Physicals SMAs, i.e., whenever possible, of off-loading as many costly individual appointments as appropriate and possible onto highly efficient SMA sessions.

Example 1: Mixed Endocrinology Drop-In Group Medical Appointments

For example, the two endocrinologists at one facility of a larger healthcare organization started off using a mixed

design for their DIGMAs—one in which virtually all of their endocrine patients were invited to attend one or another of their DIGMA sessions during the month, but with each weekly session during the month dedicated to its own specific focus. In these mixed endocrinology DIGMAs type I diabetes was the focus of the first week of the month; type II diabetes was the focus of the second and fourth weeks; thyroid, parathyroid, adrenal, pituitary, and other endocrine disorders were the focus of the third week; and, for the couple of month's each year having five sessions, all of the endocrinologist's patients were invited to attend the fifth session of the month, regardless of diagnosis.

Evolution of Mixed to Heterogeneous Drop-In Group Medical Appointments

Even though they might initially be more intuitively appealing to the physicians who choose to start them (i.e., because the mixed DIGMA subtype still retains at least some focus upon specific diseases and conditions), mixed DIGMAs (like homogeneous DIGMAs) are often found in practice to gradually evolve over time into the counterintuitive heterogeneous DIGMA model. For example, in the cases of the previously mentioned endocrinology DIGMAs of mixed design that I personally participated in implementing and running (as both champion and behaviorist), they gradually evolved into a heterogeneous design during the first year of operations and then stayed heterogeneous thereafter.

This evolution happened because some patients entered either in the wrong session for their condition or with a lengthy *laundry list* of diverse medical concerns, some of which were inevitably outside of the focus of that week's session. Perhaps the single most important reason that heterogeneous DIGMAs work so well in practice is that patients seldom bring a single issue (such as headache or diabetes) to their office visit. It is much more common for patients to bring to their visit a fairly lengthy list of diverse issues which they want attended to. However, as soon as the physician addresses this laundry list of diverse issues, mixed DIGMA sessions (like homogeneous DIGMAs) quickly begin to evolve into a more heterogeneous design. The other patients in attendance often find these seemingly unrelated health issues to be interesting in their own right, and sometimes potentially helpful to themselves as well. Therefore, the physician soon realizes that he is perfectly able to address these seemingly unrelated issues in the mixed DIGMA setting and in such a way that it holds everyone's interest.

Once this evolution to a heterogeneous DIGMA occurs, physicians quickly discover that the heterogeneous design offers certain advantages—both in terms of operational simplicity and in terms of filling all sessions with relative ease (as all of the physician's patients are welcome to attend any given heterogeneous DIGMA session, regardless of diagnosis). Also, patients and staff alike have no problem in keeping track of heterogeneous DIGMA sessions, because all of the physician's appropriate patients qualify to attend any and all heterogeneous DIGMA sessions for their follow-up care. Schedulers are therefore less hesitant to schedule heterogeneous DIGMA sessions, because they do not need to worry about being chastised for scheduling a patient into the wrong session.

Preparing Chart Notes in Drop-In Group Medical Appointments

Well-executed DIGMAs that are properly run by the physician and behaviorist consistently provide a highly interactive group experience, with everyone present being attentive and playing a more or less active role in the session. The physician spends most of the time in the DIGMA group setting delivering the same medical services as the physician would normally provide during traditional office visits for follow-up appointments. However, in order to accomplish the goal of seeing 10–16 patients in the DIGMA session, the physician will have to learn to be highly efficient in completing the chart notes on all patients in attendance in order to finish documenting these chart notes during the allotted amount of group time, i.e., without occupying too much of the physician's time during DIGMA sessions.

The Goal: Finish on Time with All Chart Notes Completed

The goal of each and every DIGMA and PSMA session is to have full groups and to start and end on time with all of the physician's duties completed, including drafting an individualized chart note on each and every patient in attendance, before the session is over. In other words, when the DIGMA is over, all of the work should be done. During a typical DIGMA session, it is normally best for the physician to complete the chart note on each patient immediately after finishing working with that patient in the group setting before moving on to the next patient. By doing so, each chart note will be completed while all medical services provided to that patient are still fresh in the physician's mind—and therefore mistakes and omissions are less likely to occur. Although, for a variety of reasons, some physicians might prefer to document the

chart note after the DIGMA session is over, my strong recommendation is to strive to complete all chart notes during the group time (i.e., immediately after completing the work with each patient) whenever possible.

Use a Documenter Whenever Possible

Completing the chart note on each patient immediately after finishing working with that patient is a process that requires pacing, time management skills, and coordinated teamwork between the physician and both the behaviorist and documenter, i.e., if the physician is fortunate enough to have a documenter. The last thing that a provider will want to do is to leave the DIGMA session without having completed all chart notes, so that the physician still needs to complete the chart notes on these 10–16 patients in attendance after the session is over. The physician would then have not only an overwhelming task facing him or her after the DIGMA is over, but also a very difficult time recalling exactly what medical services were provided to each of the many patients in attendance—i.e., without confusing what was done to whom, or without forgetting (and omitting from the chart note) much of the care that was actually delivered. It is important for the physician to use a documenter in the DIGMA whenever possible, especially in systems using electronic medical records, in order to optimize both productivity and the ability to finish the group on time with all documentation done.

Efficiency in the charting process—a chart note that meets all applicable regulatory, ethical, documentation, billing, and compliance requirements—can be gained in several different ways, although the best way, whenever possible, is through use of a documenter throughout the DIGMA session (especially for systems using electronic medical records).

Physicians Using Paper Charts

Physicians who are still using paper charts can sometimes efficiently document chart notes in the DIGMA without a documenter by using a chart note template that is largely preprinted and in check-off form. The confidentiality release form that patients and support persons sign can be printed onto the back of this chart note template in order to save paper and make clear that the release applies to this DIGMA session. It is important to note that even when such largely preprinted chart note templates are used, it is nonetheless important to generate a unique and individualized chart note on each patient in the DIGMA to accurately document and bill for the care that each patient has actually received during today's session.

Physicians who dictate chart notes by telephone or microcassette will often use a paper chart note template during the DIGMA that later serves as a *crib sheet* after the session is over from which to dictate. Or better yet, because it enables chart notes to be efficiently dictated during the SMA session, physicians can use the dictation process as a teaching point for the entire group immediately after working with each patient in turn by saying something such as, "OK, I'm going to dictate the chart note on John. So, listen up everybody and let me know if I leave anything out." Patients love hearing their case summarized by their doctor, and others in the group appreciate the learning opportunity that this provides for them as well.

I first experienced this process when my own cardiologist told me that he was going to dictate my chart note toward the end of a traditional office visit. I found it so helpful to have my case summarized in front of me by my own doctor that I subsequently carried this efficient, useful approach forward into the DIGMA setting. Nonetheless, there are two serious problems that I do not like about dictating chart notes as a teaching point during the DIGMA setting: (1) it eliminates the behaviorist's opportunity to foster some group interaction and to focus on relevant psychosocial (or, in the case of a nurse behaviorist, nursing) issues while the physician is completing the chart note; and (2) it means that the physician will still have to review, modify, and sign off on all chart notes when they eventually come back to his or her office sometime after the DIGMA session is over. Personally, I always recommend strongly that all of the work for the group be completed during the DIGMA session, which is a goal that having a documenter can be most helpful in achieving.

Physicians Using Electronic Medical Records

Physicians using electronic medical records who do not have a documenter can turn to the computer located toward the side of them in the group setting to complete the chart note after working with each patient in turn, using keystroke shortcuts and the physician's own chart note template. In this case, try not to place the desktop computer between you and the patient, as it can create an inhibiting psychological barrier. Physicians who are touch typists might prefer to simply place the keyboard on their lap (or to use a laptop computer) and type while interacting with the patient. However, I strongly recommend using a documenter because it will likely take something like 5 minutes on average with electronic medical records to complete a good chart note on each patient in the DIGMA. In other words, if there are 15 patients present in the group that day, it will likely take you approximately 1 hour and 15 minutes on the computer

to do the required documenting for the 90-minute session. That is a sure way to get the same proverbial complaint that providers using electronic medical records already get all too often during traditional office visits: "The doctor looked at the computer the whole time and never looked at me!"

Another way to gain efficiency in the DIGMA or PSMA chart note process (although this is not neraly as helpful as using a documenter) is for the physician to think of ways to include others in the documentation process, although the help requested from others must always be appropriate, commensurate with their skill set, and within their scope of practice. For example, consider having the nurse/MA enter the reason for today's visit and the results of all nursing functions performed (i.e., vital signs, routine health maintenance, injections provided, performance measures, current medications, drug allergies, etc.) into each patient's chart note at the beginning of the SMA session. Also, in the event that the nurse joins the DIGMA after vital signs and all nursing duties have been completed, he or she could be asked to provide documentation support while sitting in on the group.

Also consider ways that the behaviorist might be of assistance in the documentation process. For example, consider having the behaviorist double as the documenter. Or else, consider having the behaviorist write the physician's treatment recommendations for each patient on a duplicate form that is to be reviewed and signed by the physician, with one copy then given to the patient and the other used for charting purposes by the physician. Neither of these approaches is ideal in that the behaviorist already has a full plate of responsibilities to fulfill in the DIGMA setting, and adding further to these duties will likely dilute their ability to perform their normal behaviorist responsibilities. Therefore, keep in mind that none of these approaches for increasing the efficiency of the documentation process in the DIGMA is nearly as efficient as using a documenter whenever possible.

A Documenter Saves Time and Money and Adds Quality

Having a documenter can enable the physician to gain enough efficiency to see additional patients during each group session, typically not just one or two additional patients, but several. It also makes the DIGMA much more enjoyable to the physician as few enjoy the tedium of the documentation process and most would prefer to spend their time focusing on the patients and addressing their various medical needs (Fig. 2.3).

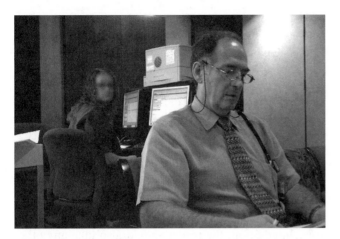

Fig. 2.3 Comprehensive, contemporaneous chart notes are created on the computer by the documenter (who typically sits behind the physician) while the physician leads the group. (Courtesy of Dr. Patricio Aycinena's Diabetes DIGMA, Cleveland Clinic, Cleveland, OH)

Remember that if it takes 3–5 minutes on average to draft a chart note on each patient, this translates into 30–80 minutes time being spent by somebody (the physician, nurse, behaviorist, or documenter) in the documentation process during the DIGMA session—i.e., this is the amount of somebody's time that will be taken up during the session just to complete all of the chart notes on the 10–16 patients attending the DIGMA. One would certainly not want to have the physician spend more than approximately 20 minutes time during a 90-minute DIGMA on documenting chart notes; however, this would require that the physician be able to finish chart notes on patients during the group session in just 1–2 minutes on average, which is unrealistic without some type of documenter.

However, having a documenter will certainly help a great deal in accomplishing this goal, while also helping to eliminate the common patient complaint during individual office visits about the doctor looking at the computer the whole time. The documenter's training can take the form of (1) reviewing many of the physician's chart notes beforehand to become familiar with the physician's way of drafting chart notes; (2) shadowing the physician during individual office visits for a couple of days prior to the launch and drafting the chart notes (which are then immediately reviewed, corrected, and approved by the physician); and (3) working with the physician beforehand to develop a basic chart note template of the physician's choosing for use during DIGMA sessions. The main point here is that you want the documenter to be fairly well trained prior to the first DIGMA session, so that the documenter knows what the physician wants—and how to accomplish it—prior to the first group session. Although the documenter will continue to learn in the DIGMA

setting as the physician continuously reviews and modifies each patient's chart note in turn, what you absolutely do not want is to have a documenter enter the DIGMA without knowing what to do and hoping to learn through "on the job training" alone. If the documenter has been trained by the physician to use the physician's own chart note template and to generate the type of chart note that the physician is satisfied with (as well as by the billing and compliance officer as to what elements are most critical to include in the chart note), then that documenter can eventually assume perhaps 80–90% of the documentation responsibilities for the DIGMA session. Once this level of accuracy is achieved by the documenter, the physician will then only need to take a minute or so reviewing, modifying, and completing the chart note immediately after working with each patient in the group setting. It is during this time (i.e., when the physician is quickly reviewing, modifying, updating, and signing off on the documenter's chart note before moving on to the next patient) that the behaviorist can temporarily take over running the DIGMA, i.e., fostering some interaction and focusing on psychosocial issues of relevance to the group. This intervention by the behaviorist, in small doses, can enhance the value of the SMA to patients, i.e., by providing them with important information and by keeping everyone attentive and actively involved in the process.

While Having One Documenter Is Recommended, Having Two Is Not

Although having a documenter is good, having two documenters is not better. This is just one of the many things about group visits that are counterintuitive. It is true that there are many benefits to having a documenter, including: increased physician efficiency and productivity; a better chart note (i.e., one that is both comprehensive and contemporaneous in nature); and the ability for the physician to focus upon patients and give them his or her undivided attention.

By having two documenters, with each one efficiently drafting the chart note on every other patient, you lose this interactive group benefit provided by the behaviorist and risk turning your DIGMA into a *mass medicine* experience in which one patient is treated immediately after the other. A sure sign that this is happening is when each patient gets up and leaves immediately after the physician has finished working with them—i.e., because without any group interaction, there is nothing left for them to stay for. This is something that I personally witnessed when I observed one physician turn a previously well-run, warm, highly interactive, and successful DIGMA into an efficient mass medicine machine employing 2 documenters in which more patients were treated, but in which most of the interaction and education benefits were lost, as revealed by the fact that each patient got up and left as soon as the physician had finished working with them.

The Chart Note Must Support the Bill and Comply with Billing Standards

It is important that the chart note documented on each patient supports the bill on that patient and that all bills generated through DIGMAs or PSMAs be in full compliance with all applicable billing standards and regulations. To accomplish this in fee-for-service systems, it is recommended that the initial bills going out from every newly launched DIGMA and PSMA be carefully reviewed by the organization's billing and compliance officer to ensure that they meet all applicable standards—perhaps by checking every bill generated during the first couple of months of operations and by randomly spot-checking bills thereafter. In addition, the organization's documentation as well as billing and compliance officers can even be involved during the early planning, training, and design stages of the DIGMA. The reader should note that the issue of billing for group visits is covered in Chapter 10.

Confidentiality in Drop-In Group Medical Appointments

A guiding principle of DIGMAs and PSMAs is that everything that can appropriately be conducted in the highly efficient group setting is provided there. However, because so much medical care is delivered in the group setting, physicians invariably wonder about the issue of confidentiality and how this can be successfully handled in a group visit setting. In fact, confidentiality is so important that it has been brought up by the audience in virtually every speaking engagement I have made covering DIGMAs and PSMAs during the past decade with medical groups both nationally and internationally. (The next most commonly asked question is, "What about billing?" which is discussed in Chapter 10.)

In the more than 400 DIGMAs and PSMAs (and more than 20,000 patient visits) that I have personally been associated with to date as champion, behaviorist, and consultant, to my knowledge the issue of confidentiality has never been brought up by patients or healthcare organizations as being a problem. Undoubtedly, this is due in part to patients' surprising willingness to discuss almost anything in the group setting, but also in part due to the conservative manner in which I recommend that the issue of confidentiality be handled in shared appointment settings. In general, patients feel safe and comfortable in a well-run DIGMA and are surprisingly open and candid—often discussing the most intimate and personal of issues. Those patients who do not want their medical issues discussed in front of others will generally opt not to attend a SMA in the first place, which is fine because group visits are always meant to be voluntary to patients and providers alike.

The following six steps toward successfully addressing confidentiality in a DIGMA and PSMA program are highly recommended in order to avoid problems in this area. In addition, the reader should also take any other steps that might prove to be appropriate and necessary.

Step 1: Address Confidentiality in All Promotional Materials

Make certain that all promotional materials for the DIGMA and Physicals SMA program (framed wall posters, program description fliers, announcements, invitations, follow-up letters, Patient Packets, etc.) clearly indicate that this is a shared medical appointment, where patients' medical care will be delivered in front of others in a supportive group setting, and that all who attend will need to sign a confidentiality release at the beginning of the session.

Step 2: The Physician and Staff Must Be Properly Trained in How to Refer Patients

Ensure that the physician and all staff involved with inviting and scheduling patients into the DIGMA and PSMA programs (schedulers, receptionists, call center personnel, nurses, medical assistants, etc.) are properly trained in how to word their referrals. In particular, it is imperative that they make clear to all invited patients that this is a shared medical appointment that will be conducted with many of the physician's other patients and that everyone's medical issues will be discussed in front of each other in the group setting. The physician must also be appropriately trained in how to successfully invite patients while making it clear to all who are referred that this will be a group visit.

One thing that will really anger patients is to come in with the understanding that they have a 90-minute one-on-one appointment with their physician, only to see that there are 9–15 other patients in the group room also waiting to be seen by the doctor. There is nothing that will anger patients more than feeling that they have been subjected to some sort of "bait and switch" exercise because they were led to believe that they were scheduled to have a 90-min individual appointment with their own provider, but arrive to find out that many other patients are also present to share this healthcare experience. When this does happens, it is often due to all of the scheduling personnel (including the replacement personnel used when the primary schedulers are out ill)

each healthcare organization draft all of its own DIGMA and PSMA forms, including their own confidentiality release form (which needs to be specific to all of the particular needs, statutes, rules, and regulations that they are subject to). However, the confidentiality release form developed by the organization must adequately cover all of the important points regarding confidentiality, including the points shown in Table 2.3.

Table 2.3 Some points to cover in the confidentiality agreement/release form[a]

- Medical care will be delivered in a group setting
- Patients understand that their medical issues will be discussed in front of others in the group setting and agree that this is OK with them
- Patients can request brief private time with the doctor for discussing personal matters, which will typically be made available toward the end of the session
- After the group is over, patients agree to not identify or discuss the medical concerns of others in attendance (either directly or indirectly)
- Participation is completely voluntary, and patients are free to leave at any point; however, if they do choose to leave early, they will miss out on some of the program's educational and support benefits
- There will be no reprisals whatsoever to patients who leave early or choose not to attend a DIGMA or PSMA, and patients will still have individual appointments available to them just like before
- Patients are welcome to take home and share with others anything that they learn in the DIGMA or PSMA that is helpful to them in managing their own health and illness, as long as they do not identify others or discuss the health problems of others outside of the group

[a]It is imperative that each healthcare organization draft its own confidentiality release form that is specific to the particular needs, statutes, rules, and regulations to which it is subject

not being properly trained regarding how to appropriately schedule patients into a DIGMA—so take great care to ensure that this never happens at your organization.

Step 3: Have Your Corporate Attorney or Medical Risk Department Draft a Confidentiality Release

A comprehensive confidentiality agreement and release form should be drafted by the healthcare organization's own corporate attorney or risk management personnel. However, it will likely need to be subsequently reviewed and simplified by administration and the champion in order to ensure that it is relatively brief (perhaps only half a page in length) and written in such a manner that it is both understandable and patient friendly.

For systems still using paper charts, consider printing the confidentiality release on the backside of the paper chart note template for the DIGMA session (perhaps with a little space immediately above it for the patient to write down the reason for today's visit, as well as any medical issues they might want to have addressed during today's session), so that paper is saved and the signed release is permanently affixed to the chart note to which it refers.

Sample confidentiality release forms are included in the DVD attached to this book; however, it is critical to note that these forms are for illustrative purposes only and are not meant to be used as is. It is imperative that

Step 4: All Attendees Must Sign the Confidentiality Release

Being conservative by nature, I always have each patient sign his or her own copy of the confidentiality release at the beginning of every session, preferably prior to entering the group room. In addition, I also have any support persons that patients happen to bring with them to the DIGMA setting also sign the same release, usually underneath or above the patient's signature. It must be made clear that signing the release is a necessary condition for attendance in the DIGMA session. However, it should also be pointed out that anyone not comfortable with signing the release would not have to—in which case, even though they would not be able to attend today's group session, they would still be able to have individual appointments just like before.

As a psychologist, I am held to a high standard regarding confidentiality; however, I strongly recommend that others also have all patients (along with their support persons) sign the confidentiality release before each session begins, i.e., until this is eventually proven to be unnecessary. Corporate attorneys have told me that they actually prefer to have patients sign the confidentiality release before they even enter the group room in order to minimize any possible risk, as patients could theoretically come into the group room and recognize some of the patients (or hear some of their health concerns), but then decide not to sign the release, leave, and later talk about others in attendance outside of the group.

However, there are a couple of healthcare systems that are looking into the possibility of just having the patients and their support persons sign a confidentiality release periodically, such as every 6 months. Then, when patients and support persons later return to the DIGMA or PSMA, they can sign either the original release (if there are several lines for the signatures and dates at the bottom of the confidentiality release form) or a separate release each time they attend, which is, by far, the most common approach. The latter approach is usually preferable, because it is typically easier and less time consuming to sign a new release form than it is to try and locate an old confidentiality release form for re-signature—especially as patients might bring different support persons to various sessions.

Occasionally, systems instead choose to use a single confidentiality release for each group session, which all attendees (patients and support persons) must sign and date, with this release then being stored as a separate medical–legal document for each SMA session (an approach that should only be used if it is compliant with the Health Insurance Portability and Accountability Act [HIPAA]). One system is even using a purely verbal release that the behaviorist simply reads off during the introduction at the beginning of the session, to which all attendees must respond in the affirmative before the session can start, an approach that I must admit to personally not being comfortable with, even though this is a major, respected healthcare organization and this approach was supposedly cleared by their medical–legal staff.

Step 5: The Behaviorist Must Discuss Confidentiality in the Introduction

At the beginning of every DIGMA and PSMA session, the behaviorist needs to thoroughly address all aspects of confidentiality during the introduction given to patients. The behaviorist points out that, while patients are welcome to take home and share with their loved ones whatever they learn during today's session regarding disease self-management and better managing their own health, patients must agree not to identify other patients in attendance (either directly or indirectly) and not to discuss the medical issues of others once the session is over. The behaviorist also points out that everyone's medical issues will be discussed in front of others in the group and asks if this is OK with everybody to ensure that this is acceptable and that nobody who is uncomfortable with this stays and attends the session. However, the behaviorist also points out in the introduction that private time with the physician for brief private discussions or examinations will be

made available to any patients requesting it, although it will typically be toward the end of the session so as to not interrupt the flow of the group. The behaviorist then asks if everybody (patients and their support persons) has already signed the confidentiality agreement and release for today's session and, if not, promptly gives them one to sign—at least until such time as this is proven unnecessary, or a better process is developed.

Step 6: Place the Signed Confidentiality Release in Each Patient's Medical Chart

For systems still using paper charts, the signed confidentiality releases should be placed into the patients' medical charts. For systems using electronic medical records, the signed confidentiality release could be scanned into the patient's electronic medical record or kept in a safe place as a separate medical–legal document. As mentioned earlier, patients should sign the confidentiality release each time they attend the DIGMA or PSMA, as should any support persons who accompany them.

Drop-In Group Medical Appointments Are Not Appropriate for All Physicians and Patients

Although DIGMAs are appropriate for *most* physicians (especially busy and backlogged, full-time physicians) and patients, it is important to note that they will not work well for *all* physicians and patients.

Physicians for Whom Drop-In Group Medical Appointments Might Not Work

While DIGMAs and PSMAs have been shown to work for most physicians (and to be largely independent of physician personality), there are some types of physicians for whom running a DIGMA or PSMA program will prove to be difficult.

Physicians with New or Unfilled Practices or with No Access Problems

For example, physicians who have new practices that are not yet filled, small practices with many open appointment slots, or no access problems will likely have difficulty consistently maintaining targeted census requirements in their DIGMA or PSMA sessions. This is because DIGMAs and PSMAs dramatically increase capacity, which is something that these physicians already have enough of. I say this because each DIGMA and PSMA that is run per week will further increase the full-time physician's capacity by approximately 8–10%, and there is already insufficient patient demand in the aforementioned practices to ensure full groups. However, such physicians might still choose to institute a DIGMA and/or PSMA because of the improvements in patient care and the patient–physician relationships that they can provide, in which case particular emphasis must be placed on how these SMA sessions will be consistently kept filled.

Physicians with new or small practices, as well as physicians without access problems, could use a DIGMA or PSMA to intake new patients if they wanted to increase the size of their practices while continuing to maintain good access. Which model to use would depend on whether a private physical examination is needed as part of the intake process. Similarly, if such physicians desire to change their master schedule to include fewer follow-up visits by either working a shorter workweek or by opening up more appointment slots of other types (such as intakes, consults, procedures, surgeries, physical examinations, desktop medicine, teaching, or administrative time), this could theoretically be achieved by placing many return patients into a DIGMA instead of individual follow-up appointments (or into PSMAs instead of traditional individual physical examinations).

Physicians Who Do Not Follow Their Patients over Time

Similarly, some physicians who do not follow their patients over time, perhaps because they primarily provide one-time consults, might not benefit as much from a DIGMA—although, when the DIGMA is properly designed, it could still work. For example, a cardiologist who primarily reads EKGs and provides one-time consultations will likely have limited benefit from group visits, except perhaps for certain types of intake appointments. However, a SMA might work under specific circumstances, for example, the PSMA model has been used in ophthalmology to provide the physical examination that is, by protocol, a prerequisite to cataract surgery at one integrated healthcare delivery system and in another for breast reduction and carpal tunnel surgery intakes.

Physicians Unwilling to Put Time or Energy into Their Shared Medical Appointments

Some physicians might expect a DIGMA or PSMA to succeed due solely to the efforts of others. In larger systems, the SMA champion and program coordinator will make every reasonable effort to minimize the outlay of physician time during clinic hours in launching a new DIGMA or PSMA program. Nonetheless, some time and energy investment will always be required of physicians wanting to run a successful DIGMA or PSMA in their practices. For example, there will be initial planning and training sessions that will need to include the physician, some of which will only include the physician and champion, but others of which will include the SMA team as well as the physician's support staff. Also, the physician will need to take the time to customize the promotional materials and chart note template for their DIGMA (i.e., from templates already developed for the SMA program)—and to develop the handouts that will ultimately be used in the Patient Packet distributed to patients during the DIGMA or PSMA session.

Physicians Not Willing to Invite All Appropriate Patients During Regular Office Visits

Finally, it is extremely important to the success of any DIGMA or PSMA that the physician be willing to take 30–60 seconds during every regular office visit to invite all appropriate patients to have their next visit be a DIGMA or PSMA visit—i.e., in a succinct but carefully and positive-worded manner that accurately describes the program and its benefits to patients. Physicians who are not willing or able to promote their own DIGMA or PSMA program to patients will make poor candidates for running a group visit in their practice, as they will likely fail to consistently meet census requirements.

Part-Time Physicians

DIGMAs might not always be appropriate for the part-time or half-time physician, especially with the homogeneous and mixed subtypes, in which only a fraction of the physician's already reduced patient panel size would qualify to attend any particular session. This is because the half-time physician typically has only half the practice size of full-time physicians and consequently half the number of patients with whom to fill their DIGMA sessions. In order to have a successful group visit that consistently meets pre-established census requirements, it is therefore recommended that half-time physicians interested in running a successful DIGMA for their practice seriously consider using the heterogeneous subtype, so that most or all patients in the physician's practice would qualify to attend any given session, thus giving the part-time physician the greatest possible opportunity to fill sessions and meet census targets.

Are There Certain Physician Personalities That Are Unsuitable to Group Visits?

When I began my first DIGMAs in 1996, I used to think that, for the DIGMA to be fully successful, the physician would need to be either an Albert Einstein or a Jay Leno, i.e., either a brilliant physician or one who is very outgoing, engaging, and entertaining. What I subsequently observed during the past decade has been quite the opposite.

The Shy, Introverted Physician

On several occasions, I have observed providers who were so painfully shy and introverted that they actually shook during their first few sessions (or their voice kept cracking, or, as actually happened in one case, the provider even broke out in full body hives during the first DIGMA session), yet they were still able to run successful DIGMAs for their practices. In fact, such physicians have even grown to enjoy their SMAs tremendously, so long as they had the motivation and courage to actually try a DIGMA in the first place. In the case of the provider who broke out in full body hives during her first session, she grew to enjoy her DIGMA so much that a year later she wanted to alter her master schedule to do nothing but DIGMAs all day, every day (her story is more fully discussed in Chapter 9).

The Physician with Many Worries and Concerns about Starting a Drop-In Group Medical Appointment

I have also witnessed physicians who were initially resistant to starting a DIGMA for their practices due to their many worries and concerns end up running successful group visit programs, so long as they were willing to try one and give it their best shot. I have set up successful DIGMAs and PSMAs with providers who were fearful about: losing control of the group; saying something stupid in front of 15 patients at once; not knowing the answer to questions that patients might ask; or being embarrassed by the fact that the DIGMA model might not work for them. Although not true in every case, most of these initially reluctant

physicians have subsequently grown to enjoy their SMAs so much that some now run more than one DIGMA per week (i.e., despite all of their initial resistances and concerns). Simply put, their DIGMAs eventually won them over.

Physicians Perceived as Being Boring, Poor Communicators, or Difficult

In addition, I have run successful SMAs with physicians perceived by their colleagues as being boring—only to see their patients give the physician a standing ovation and a thank you for being so thoughtful and deliberate in their approach. I have even set up successful DIGMAs with physicians having very low patient satisfaction scores, as well as with physicians who were viewed by their colleagues as being extremely poor communicators and unlikely to succeed. In fact, the results were so positive that I now believe (because of the salutary effect that properly run DIGMAs can have on physician communication skills and the patient–physician relationship) that DIGMAs might even be used as an effective—albeit benign and not at all embarrassing—tool for increasing the patient satisfaction scores of low-scoring physicians. This is especially true when such a physician is paired with a behaviorist who demonstrates very good communication skills, which can then be picked up and learned by the physician.

Finally, I have even been able to set up successful DIGMAs with physicians perceived by administration and their colleagues alike as being *impossible*, i.e., as being the least likely physician in the entire department to be willing to try one for their practice and, even if they were to try one, the least likely to succeed. By pairing such a physician off with a behaviorist possessing exceptional communication skills, the physician can gradually learn—almost by osmosis, after months of working together with the behaviorist—to communicate with their patients in a much more positive and effective manner. In fact, I have found that, by winning over the physician perceived by colleagues as being impossible, the DIGMA could be advanced throughout the system faster than perhaps by any other means, as other physicians feel that if this physician can succeed, then they certainly should be able to as well.

To Be Successful, Physicians Only Need to Be Themselves

Extensive experience with many different DIGMAs and PSMAs during the past decade has caused me to come to the conclusion that success in a SMA is almost independent of physician personality—and that all physicians need to be in order to run a successful DIGMA or PSMA is to be themselves. Remember, your patients have selected you as their doctor for any of a variety of reasons. All they want from you in a DIGMA or PSMA is for you to be the same doctor that they have grown to like and trust during their individual office visits. Try not to be different because the medical care is being delivered in a group setting, e.g., by trying to be perfect, all-knowing, uncharacteristically entertaining, overly solicitous, humorous, or by putting on airs. Just be yourself and you will likely find that you will be quite successful in running your SMA!

Patients for Whom Drop-In Group Medical Appointments Are and Are Not Appropriate

Patients and Conditions Best Suited to Drop-In Group Medical Appointments

DIGMAs and PSMAs are meant to work in conjunction with other forms of group care as well as with the judicious use of individual office visits—and not to completely replace them. DIGMAs and PSMAs work exceptionally well for patients seeking: prompt access; routine follow-up care; chronic illness follow-ups; re-check appointments; peer support; or extra professional handholding. They also work well with time-consuming problematic patients; patients with extensive informational or psychosocial issues; and patients with extensive mind as well as body needs. Because of the professional skills of the behaviorist and the emotional support provided by other patients, DIGMAs provide an exceptional venue for drawing together the mind and body aspects of care. They can not only provide the medical care that is normally delivered during individual office visits (and often more), but also better address the full spectrum of issues that patients bring to their medical providers, so that considerable attention is paid to the behavioral health and psychosocial issues that are known to drive a large percentage of medical visits (5–9).

Of relevance here is the following quotation taken from an article in Medical Economics focusing on the benefits that a behavioral specialist can bring into a physician's practice, an article which naturally covers DIGMAs: " 'Since I started group appointments (DIGMAs) three months ago, I've discovered so many things about my patients that I never would have during individual office visits,' says FP Mark Attermeier of the Midelfort Clinic in Eau Claire, WI. 'I always thought of the one-on-one setting as the gold standard, but for some conditions, it's definitely not. Group appointments are an efficient way to educate large numbers of patients. But, more important, they bring together the psychosocial and medical models in one setting. They treat the whole person rather than just the disease' " (8). Table 2.4 presents guidelines regarding the types of patients, situations, and conditions to best refer to your DIGMA.

Drop-In Group Medical Appointments Are Not for All Types of Patients

Despite being appropriate for most patients and conditions, DIGMAs and PSMAs are not appropriate for all types. In this segment, we examine those types of patients for whom a DIGMA or PSMA might not be appropriate—noting that this is a relatively short list (Table 2.5).

Patients Who Do Not Speak the Language

Inappropriate patients would include monolingual patients who do not speak the language in which the SMA is being conducted. Again, one could offer a specialized DIGMA or PSMA in the patients' native language (i.e., if the physician happened to speak their language or if an interpreter was available), provided there were enough patients speaking that language to ensure consistently full sessions. Another possibility would be for the physician to conduct the first SMA session each month in that language. While one or two such patients could be accommodated in a regular DIGMA session, what you certainly would not want to happen is for several patients who do not speak the language to attend SMA sessions with their family members acting as interpreters. The resulting cacophony of ongoing background noise from so many different family members simultaneously acting as translators in the group room (especially if the monolingual patient happens to be hard of hearing) would likely prove to be a distraction to the group process.

Patients Too Hearing Impaired or Demented to Benefit

In addition, patients who are too hearing impaired or demented to comprehend or follow what is being discussed would also be inappropriate. However, one could run a specialized DIGMA or PSMA for the hearing impaired (assuming that there were enough such patients to meet the SMA's census requirements) by using microphones and loud speakers—with the physician, staff, and support

Table 2.4 Guidelines for types of patients and conditions to refer into your drop-in group medical appointment

- When it comes to the routine follow-up care of established patients, the physician and staff should first consider referral into the DIGMA and reserve costly individual office visits for patients that are clearly inappropriate for the DIGMA (although this always needs to be a voluntary choice on the part of the patient)
- Follow-up visits for relatively stable chronically ill patients are generally ideal for DIGMAs (diabetes, hypertension, arthritis, irritable bowel, asthma, chronic pain, congestive heart failure, etc.)
- When patients want to be seen promptly, the DIGMA is often an excellent choice as sessions are typically available that week, even if the physician's next available individual office visit happens to still be weeks away.
- All patients requiring re-check appointments (e.g., for medications, procedures, and lab tests) could be offered the DIGMA—except for inappropriate patients, such as those who are severely hearing impaired or only speak a foreign language
- Patients who are newly diagnosed, or are starting a new medication or treatment regimen, can often be appropriately referred to the DIGMA for routine monitoring and surveillance, education and support, closer follow-up care, etc.
- Although DIGMAs are not appropriate for serious and highly contagious illnesses (such as bird flu, tuberculosis, SARS), they are often used for minor infectious illnesses such as colds and flues—to which patients are often exposed in the lobby anyway, especially during the cold and flu season (plus, such preventative measures as masks and hand washing can easily be incorporated into such DIGMAs)
- DIGMAs work well with high, medium, and low utilizers alike, and can even be used to reach out to patients who inappropriately under-utilize healthcare services, are currently being underserved, or are somehow currently *falling between the cracks* of the system
- Inappropriate high utilizers (such as the *worried well* and patients who seem to need more professional handholding by their physician) also make excellent candidates for DIGMAs and Physicals SMAs
- Psychosocially needy patients who are anxious, highly information seeking, or telephoning the office frequently can often be appropriately seen in DIGMAs because it provides a venue wherein the help and support of a behaviorist and other patients is available, greater time and patient education is offered, injections and routine health maintenance can be updated, and patients can be personally evaluated, examined, and closely followed by their physician
- Many types of patients for whom the physician is constantly repeating the same information over and over throughout the workweek can often better be seen in a DIGMA or PSMA, where the physician only needs to say things once, but can often go into greater detail
- Noncompliant patients are often better managed in DIGMAs and PSMAs than in traditional office visits due to the help, encouragement, and gentle confrontation of the behaviorist and other patients
- Patients with extensive informational needs (long lists of questions, multiple articles downloaded from the Internet, questions about pharmaceutical ads, extensive concerns based on their reading of lay literature, etc.) that the physician does not have the time to address during the relatively brief time available during an individual office visit are often better served in DIGMAs due to the greater time and patient education that is available, as well as helpful tips shared by other patients
- Patients needing peer support (including those whose medical condition is affecting their ability to function at work, socially, or at home) often find DIGMAs to be a helpful and encouraging venue of care
- Patients perceived as being difficult, time consuming, demanding, distrustful, or angry are often better followed in the DIGMA—where there are the benefits of more time, group support, and the professional skills of the behaviorist
- Because they provide emotional support and better attend to psychosocial needs, well run DIGMAs are often a superior choice for conditions frequently perceived as difficult to treat in the individual office visit setting (e.g., fibromyalgia, irritable bowel, headache, chronic pain, etc.).
- Some physical exams and new patient intakes (especially when the exams do not require disrobing and can appropriately be done in the group room setting, such as is often the case in podiatry, endocrinology, rheumatology, etc.) can be appropriately handled in a DIGMA
- DIGMAs have also been used for the first part (where most of the discussion occurs) of *two-part physical exams*, with the second part being completed shortly thereafter in the form of a brief individual office visit—which is where the actual private exam is provided. Although less efficient than the PSMA model, this two-part approach to physical examinations in a DIGMA has the advantage of getting patients in promptly for their physical exam, even when the physician might otherwise have extensive backlogs and long waits for physical examination appointments (i.e., for physicians who run a DIGMA but do not run a PSMA). It also occupies a single short individual appointment slot on the physician's clinic office visit schedule rather than a long physical examination appointment
- Consider DIGMAs for all appropriate patients who are voluntary and willing to share their medical issues with other patients

Table 2.5 Types of patients and conditions for which DIGMAs and PSMAs are not suitable

- Monolingual patients not speaking the language in which the DIGMA is conducted (although one or two can sometimes be worked into DIGMA sessions)
- Patients too hearing impaired or demented to comprehend what is being said (although such specialized groups can sometimes be run, provided sessions can be kept full)
- Patients with severe, highly contagious illnesses (SARS, bird flu, tuberculosis)
- Medical emergencies
- Complex medical procedures
- Initial intakes that require a private physical examination (for which the PSMA model can be used)
- Physical examinations for established patients that require disrobing (although one or two such patients are OK as they can be examined in the privacy of the nearby examination room, typically toward the end of the session)
- Any patients who the physician prefers to see individually
- Patients who refuse to maintain confidentiality
- Patients who refuse to attend a group visit

persons possessing normal hearing using earplugs. Similarly, assuming that there were enough such patients, there could also be specialized DIGMAs for dementia, especially early in the disease process or when the patients are accompanied by a caregiver with whom the physician is able to communicate and provide benefit.

Patients with Serious Infectious Illnesses

Also, DIGMAs would not be appropriate for patients suffering from severe, infectious illnesses that are highly contagious, such as tuberculosis, bird flu, or severe acute respiratory syndrome. On the other hand, mild cold and flu symptoms are sometimes acceptable; in fact, some healthcare organizations have even set up cold and flu DIGMAs during the cold and flu season because these symptoms are so widespread, prevalent, and consuming of individual office visits. They do this because DIGMAs are highly productive, can eliminate the waste of no-shows (as they can be overbooked accordingly), and are able to get rid of repetition, as the physician does not need to repeat the same information over and over to different patients individually. In fact, whenever a physician is repeating the same information time and time again to different patients individually throughout the week, this is almost a sure sign to set up a DIGMA and say it once for everybody.

Keeping in mind that patients are exposed to colds and flu in the lobby anyway, in most DIGMAs, patients with mild cold and flu symptoms could simply be kept to one side of the group room where they would be somewhat isolated from others. They could be provided with masks and asked to wash their hands. Those with cold and flu symptoms could even be treated first in the DIGMA session by the physician and given the standard treatment for cold and flu symptoms. For example, the physician might listen to their heart and lungs, examine their throats, tell them to drink plenty of fluids, and recommend that they to go home and get plenty of rest, so as to not further expose others in the room. In addition, those patients requiring an antibiotic could be prescribed one; however, the physician would only need to give the antibiotic talk to everybody once (e.g., use only when there is a bacterial component, take the full course). However, patients with 105 degree temperatures who are coughing up blood are clearly inappropriate for DIGMAs.

It is worth mentioning that I used to be a purist about not allowing any patients with acute contagious illnesses to attend a DIGMA or PSMA, even those with minor cold and flu symptoms. However, one day a clearly sick patient (who was coughing, sneezing, and generally looking miserable) entered a DIGMA for which I was the behaviorist. When I met this patient at the group room

door and told him that this was not the appropriate venue of care, suggesting that he go to Urgent Care instead, he replied, "I'm sick and have a bad cough, so I'm coming here to get some help—that's my problem. If you don't like it, that's your problem." The patient then walked right past me, entered the group room, and took a seat. Somewhat taken aback, I realized immediately that I did not have as much power as I might have thought. However, it all worked out just fine as the physician simply treated him first and then told him that he was free to go so that others wouldn't get infected, which he was all too glad to do, as he felt miserable. From then on, I have not been nearly as scrupulous about not allowing patients with minor acute cold and flu infectious symptoms to come in—which has made running SMAs easier and has generally worked out well.

Patients Having Medical Emergencies

In addition, patients suffering from rapidly evolving medical conditions requiring urgent or emergency care would clearly be inappropriate for a DIGMA. Be certain that your scheduling staff does not tell the patient who happens to call in with severe acute chest pains and shortness of breath that the doctor has a DIGMA tomorrow at 3:00 p.m. Should this happen, an immediate 911 call and an ambulance ride to the emergency room are the appropriate actions to be taken. Although this should be self-evident, it does bear repeating because this did happen one time (fortunately without incident) due to a scheduler not being properly trained on what types of patients should and should not be referred into a DIGMA.

Patients Needing Complex Medical Procedures or Private Examinations

Although some simple procedures can be provided during the DIGMA (nitrogen freezes of skin tags, brief hearing tests, trigger point injections, flu shots, etc.), complex medical procedures are generally inappropriate in this setting. Some initial visits and one-time consultations are inappropriate (especially when they are too time consuming or require a private physical examination), although DIGMAs are sometimes used for new patient intakes when a private physical examination is not required. It would clearly be inappropriate for numerous patients to enter the DIGMA who require a private physical examination that involves disrobing—although they could be efficiently and successfully treated in a PSMA.

Nonetheless, if only one or two patients enter the DIGMA needing a simple procedure, a private exam, or a brief private discussion, then this can usually be accommodated—typically by the physician stepping out of the group room and taking the patient to a nearby exam room. This typically occurs toward the end of the session so as to not interrupt the flow of the group, i.e., while the behaviorist temporarily takes over running the group. This occasionally does happen, such as when a patient enters the DIGMA and mentions that she just this morning found a lump on her breast. Complex medical procedures, however, are best left to referrals or individual office visits rather than DIGMAs.

Patients Who Opt Not to Attend

Finally, patients refusing to attend a SMA would be inappropriate, as group visits are meant to be voluntary to patients and providers alike. However, when the DIGMA or PSMA program is properly promoted to patients, the population of patients refusing to attend the group setting is typically found to decrease over time. It is often the case that patients who have been refusing a group visit, even those who have steadfastly refused to attend for some time, are eventually persuaded to attend when they hear positive reports from a friend who did attend—or when they overhear other patients talking in the lobby about what a positive expreience attending the group had been for them. It has consistently been observed that once patients do in fact attend a SMA session—even for those who are initially quite resistant and reluctant—they almost always like it and are willing to return. Therefore, the key to success lies in getting patients to agree to attend a DIGMA or PSMA for the first time. This is accomplished primarily by: (1) effectively promoting the program to patients; (2) ensuring that the physician and staff consistently invite all appropriate patients seen during routine office visits to attend the DIGMA or PSMA for their next visit; (3) ascertaining that the physician's entire scheduling staff is taking the time necessary to consistently encourage patients to attend and, whenever appropriate and possible, to schedule a SMA for their next medical appointment; and (4) having the dedicated scheduler reach out by telephoning appropriate patients and inviting them to attend.

How to DIGMA: The Flow of a Typical Session

A typical DIGMA session is most commonly 90 minutes in duration, held weekly, and of a heterogeneous, homogeneous, or mixed design. Let us take a closer look at the various steps involved in the flow of a typical DIGMA session (Table 2.6).

Previsit Work

A couple of days prior to the session, it is often the case that a MA or nurse will call all patients scheduled to attend the DIGMA to (1) confirm the appointment; (2) do a medication reconciliation; (3) go through the HEDIS checklist; and (4) ensure that all previsit labs have been completed. Some physicians will want to review patients' chart notes prior to the DIGMA session—although most will not, instead preferring to review chart notes in the group room while working with each patient individually. Please note that it is imperative that all computers in the group and exam rooms, as well as the entire IT infrastructure, must be correctly installed prior to the initial DIGMA session.

Register Patients for the Session

Upon entering the clinic for the DIGMA session, patients must first register for the appointment. For patients who are new to the clinic, or when patients need to register in an area that is different from what they are used to, signs might need to be posted prior to each session in order to direct patients where to register. Patients typically register in either the physician's own office area or in the group room. The disadvantage of the physician's office is that it is often some distance from the group room and consequently inconvenient for patients. On the other hand, the disadvantage of having patients register in the group room can be even worse because some patients might arrive quite early (perhaps an hour or more early), resulting in their entering the group room when an earlier SMA is still occurring. Even though we usually allow a half-hour separation between DIGMAs and PSMAs in any given group room, the previous physician can run late, and patients can arrive sufficiently early to enter the wrong SMA, which can be quite disruptive.

In addition, if patients are to be registered in the group room, somebody needs to be there to register them, which introduces an additional logistical wrinkle (and an extra overhead cost) into the equation. Therefore, most healthcare organizations choose to have patients register for the DIGMA in the physician's own office area, which is something that they are used to doing anyway. Occasionally, if the DIGMA is large and the registration process fairly lengthy, the organization might also arrange to have some extra help at the front desk during the half-hour preceding the DIGMA to ensure that all patients are registered expeditiously.

Table 2.6 The flow of a typical DIGMA session

Pre-visit work
- A couple of days prior to the session, a MA or nurse can call all patients scheduled to attend the DIGMA to:
  - confirm the appointment
  - do a medication reconciliation
  - go through the HEDIS checklist
  - ensure that all pre-visit labs have been completed
- The physician sometimes chooses to review patients' medical records prior to the DIGMA session
- The computers and IT infrastructure need to be correctly installed in the group and exam rooms prior to starting the DIGMA

15–30 minutes prior to start of session
- Nurse writes down patients' pre-visit labs on whiteboard, circling abnormal findings in red
- Early-arriving patients register for session
  - Patients register for SMA
  - Patients given Patient Packet
  - Name tag filled out and put on (usually first name only)
  - Patients and support persons sign and return confidentiality release
  - Patients are directed by receptionist to sit down in lobby or go to group room
- As additional patients arrive and register, the same process occurs and they join group

15–30 minutes prior to session
- Early-arriving patients escorted or directed from lobby to group room
- Patients sit in circular or elliptical arrangement with no table or clutter in middle
- MA/Nurse starts calling patients out of group to exam room (one or two at a time)
- Each patient gets vital signs taken, injections and health maintenance updated, etc.
- Once all nursing duties are completed, each patient is taken back to the group room
- The next patient is then called out to the exam room by the nurse
- This process continues until nursing duties are finished on all patients
- This process often continues well into the actual DIGMA session
- Once nursing duties are finished on all patients, nurse returns to normal clinic duties (whereas MA rechecks high blood pressures and then becomes the care coordinator)

10–15 minutes prior to start of session
- Behaviorist arrives early to group room, introduces self, and welcomes patients
- Behaviorist begins to *warm up* group and get patients talking
- Behaviorist asks each patient what issues they want to discuss with the physician today
- Behaviorist writes issues down next to each patient's name on a flip chart or whiteboard

Behaviorist starts session on time with an introduction
- Behaviorist starts session on time with introduction, even if provider has not yet arrived
- Introduction should only take 3–5 minutes, by which time provider should be there
- The following points are covered in the behaviorist's introduction:
  - Introduction starts by welcoming all and introducing SMA team (as well as any observers)
  - Behaviorist explains why physician is running the DIGMA and patient benefits
  - Behaviorist then covers what to expect during the session and how to best use it
  - Behaviorist ensures that all attendees have signed the confidentiality agreement
  - All aspects of confidentiality are covered in detail (confirm acceptance by all)
  - Patients are told that private time with physician is available to all upon request
    - Private time will usually be toward end of session (to not interrupt flow)
  - Personal comfort items are also discussed (stretching, bathrooms, snacks, etc.)
  - Patients are encouraged to ask questions, share experiences, and participate
  - Although they can still have individual visits, patients are encouraged to return
    - Return to DIGMA the next time they have a medical need
    - Patients only come when they have a medical need, not every week
  - If physician wants it asked, behaviorist ends by asking if anyone must leave early

3–5 minutes after start until 5–10 minutes before end of session
- By the time introduction is over, physician enters group room, says "Hello," and welcomes patients
- Physician sequentially delivers medical care to each patient individually
  - Each patient's unique medical needs are addressed individually
  - Entire DIGMA session consists of delivery of medical care
  - History, exam, medical decision-making, counseling, etc. are done, as appropriate, on all

Table 2.6 (continued)

- ○ Physician tries to deliver some personal one-on-one care to each patient
  - ■ Walk over and examine patient's wrists, thyroid, tremors, etc.
  - ■ Can routinely listen to patients' heart and lungs
  - ■ Can give patient a refill, referral, etc.
- ○ All education occurs in context of provider caring for each patient individually
  - ■ There is no separate educational or class-type component to a DIGMA
  - ■ Truly private discussions or exams are done in privacy of the exam room
  - ■ When possible, private discussions/exams are done toward session's end
- ○ DIGMA starts by delivering medical care to a patient of physician's choosing
  - ■ Physician briefly gives group appropriate background information
  - ■ Start with any patients needing to leave early who have had nursing duties completed
  - ■ Physician then typically addresses any patients with cold and/or flu symptoms
  - ■ Then select mothers with children and others who are best treated first
  - ■ From then on, select others with vital signs and nursing duties completed
  - ■ Start with volunteers or patients the physician is comfortable with
  - ■ Sometimes (e.g., in medical subspecialties) physician starts by diagnosis
  - ■ Physician always maintains appropriate privacy in group room
  - ■ Documenter (if used) drafts comprehensive, contemporaneous chart note
  - ■ When finished with each patient in turn, physician completes chart note
- • Physicians reviews, modifies, and signs off on documenter's chart note
- • If no documenter, provider starts note while working with patient
- • Right after finishing with patient, provider completes chart note
- • While provider documents, behaviorist temporarily takes over group
  - ■ Typically focusing upon relevant psychosocial or lifestyle issues
  - ■ Addresses noncompliance, smoking cessation, exercise, diet, etc.
- • Behaviorist watches physician to see when chart note is finished
  - ■ As soon as chart note is completed, focus promptly shifts to next patient
  - ■ This process is repeated over and over until all patients receive their care
- • Provider often goes around room clockwise or counterclockwise
- • Provider sometimes addresses patients in order by diagnoses
- • A particularly challenging patient could be treated last
- • For rest of session, care is delivered to each patient individually
  - ○ The same medical care (and often more) is delivered as in regular office visits
  - ○ Whenever appropriate, care is delivered in group room (all can listen and learn)
  - ○ One at a time, the physician sequentially addresses each patient's medical needs
  - ○ From start to finish, run it like a series of individual office visits with observers

After all nursing duties are finished (usually 45 minutes into the session)
- • MA becomes Care Coordinator
  - ○ MA calls patients whose chart notes are completed out of group room, one at a time
  - ○ MA schedules all follow-up visits, referrals, procedures, etc. that physician has ordered on the patient
  - ○ MA gives patient the after visit summary (AVS)—i.e., parts of chart note physician wants patient to have, which always includes
treatment plan and recommendations
  - ○ For patients not needing to schedule any appointments, MA goes into the group room and hands AVS to them
- • MA continues acting as Care Coordinator with all patients until end of session

Final 5–10 minutes can be for brief private exams and discussions
- • This only occurs if there are patients needing private time (there's typically only one or two)
- • Physician steps out of group to take these patients individually to privacy of exam room
- • Behaviorist temporarily takes over group, focusing on relevant psychosocial or nursing issues
- • Physician formally ends session on time by thanking patients for attending
  - ○ If physician is in exam room, the behaviorist can wrap up and end the session
- • If provider finishes early, he or she can stop early or cover patient issues in greater depth
- • Patients can be given copy of DIGMA chart note, (i.e., AVS) including treatment recommendations

End of session
- • Always strive to finish on time with all chart notes finished
- • Physician must leave group room when finished, or else patients will continue to stay
- • Patients and any support persons complete a patient satisfaction form anonymously
  - ○ Some systems ask all attendees to complete patient satisfaction form after group
  - ○ Do this anonymously—put it in box without any patient identifying information
  - ○ Other systems prefer to later send patient satisfaction form by mail

10–15 minutes after session is over
- • Patients often stay to talk with each other, exchange information, and ask questions
- • Behaviorist stays with patients (answering logistical questions and clearing room)
- • Behaviorist then quickly straightens up the group room

Table 2.6 (continued)

For the first 2 months, provider and SMA team debrief for 15–20 minutes after sessions
- Debriefing sessions occur outside of group room, otherwise patients will linger
- The provider and team focus on how to make future sessions better and more efficient
- After the first 2 months, it is usually only necessary to debrief occasionally (as needed)
- Thereafter, physician and documenter only need to schedule 90 minutes for DIGMA
- However, because behaviorist starts early and stays late, 2 hours needs to be scheduled

The Patient Packet

When they register for the DIGMA visit, patients are often given a Patient Packet for the session by the receptionist (Fig. 2.4). From a patient's point of view, receiving a Patient Packet when registering for a DIGMA suggests a high-quality service. It also creates a favorable impression to the effect that a lot of people have worked very hard to make this a special healthcare experience for the patient, plus it gives the patient something to take home to read later on, after the session is over. In addition, it can dispel any initial bias the patient might have had regarding this being mass medicine and an attempt on the organization's part to save time and money at the patient's expense. The Patient Packet can include any of the items listed in Table 2.7, as well as any other materials that the physician might want included. For more detailed information, see the forms section of the DVD for sample forms and promotional materials that can be included in the Patient Packet. Patients will often use the blank sheet of paper included in

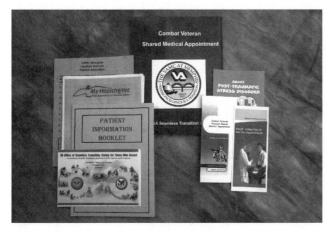

Fig. 2.4 Sample Patient Packet sent to patients when they make an appointment in a PSMA. (Combat Veterans Patient Packet courtesy of Dr. Keith Novak, Memphis Veterans Administration, Memphis, TN; photograph courtesy of Lorraine Burns)

the Patient Packet (i.e., that simply says "Notes" at the top) to take notes upon during the session.

If the receptionist gives a Patient Packet to patients as they register, the receptionist will usually quickly go over

its contents with the patient. I tend to place all materials that the patient will need for the DIGMA session (descriptive flier, name tag, confidentiality release, patient satisfaction form, blank sheet of paper saying "Notes" at the top, etc.) in the left inside flap of the Patient Packet, and any educational handouts and PR materials on the physician's medical group (i.e., that the patient is to take home and read later) in the right inside flap. The receptionist then typically asks patients (as well as any support person they might have brought with them) to sign the confidentiality agreement/release, and generally collects the signed releases immediately, before the patient goes into the group room. The receptionist then completes each patient's (and support person's) name tag using a fat felt marker in large, dark letters (perhaps black for patients and red for support persons) that can easily be read from across the room so that patients more easily get to know each other and the physician is not embarrassed by not knowing the patient's name. Usually, the patient's first name (or nickname that the patient likes to go by) is used, unless the physician wants to call patients by their last name. I strongly prefer to use first names because it is less revealing of patients' identities; however, in some systems, calling patients Mr. or Mrs. is the accepted norm. If there happen to be two patients named Jim or Mary in the session, then the receptionist will often also include the first letter of the patient's last name. Patients are then asked to have a seat in the lobby, unless they are directed or escorted directly to the group room, which usually happens 30 minutes or less prior to the start of the session.

The Nursing Functions

As soon as the patients who have arrived early have completed the registration process, the various nursing functions of the DIGMA are initiated. After rooming the physician's last individual patient prior to the DIGMA, one of the nurses or medical assistants attached to the DIGMA (typically the physician's own nurse or MA) goes to the physician's lobby approximately 30 minutes before the group is start and escorts those who have arrived early to the group room. These are the patients

Table 2.7 Contents of the DIGMA Patient Packet

- A cover letter from the physician welcoming patients and explaining the DIGMA
- A program description flier
- An assortment of appropriate patient education handouts (usually 4 or 5) selected by the physician (on smoking cessation, exercise, nutrition, diabetes, osteoporosis, PSA, hypertension, hyperlipidemia, colorectal cancer screening, breast self-examination, etc.)
- Any information about the physician's medical group and the various programs that it offers to patients that the physician might want to have included
- Possibly a list of internal and external community resources that are relevant to the patients in attendance
- A blank sheet of paper (one that simply says "Notes" at the top) for the patient to take notes on during the session, plus a pen or pencil to write with
- A name tag (on which the receptionist typically writes the patient's first name in large, dark letters with a thick felt marker so that it can easily be read from across the room)
- A confidentiality agreement and release form for the patient and accompanying support person to sign and return to the receptionist prior to going to the group room)
- A patient satisfaction form to be completed and returned anonymously after the session is over

who have already registered for the DIGMA, received their Patient Packet and name tags, and signed the confidentiality release. From this point forward (i.e., for patients who arrive later on to register for the session), the receptionists themselves will direct patients to the group room as soon as they have registered and signed the confidentiality agreement. Patients are usually directed to the group room either verbally or by signs; however, they can also be escorted by the receptionist or nurse/MA.

In DIGMAs and PSMAs, the nursing role is typically maximized—as this enables visits to be max-packed, consistency to be achieved, quality to be enhanced, performance measures to be optimized, routine health maintenance and injections to be updated, and the physician's productivity and efficiency to be maximized. One of the major goals of the DIGMA is to introduce consistency and efficiency by off-loading as many duties as appropriate and possible onto the nurse/MA—such as expanded vital signs, providing injections, completing forms, bringing routine health maintenance current, and assisting in documenting so that the physician is able to maximize productivity by focusing upon providing just those medical services that the physician alone can uniquely provide. When these duties are made a part of the nursing protocol for the DIGMA, consistency is introduced as these functions are then provided to all patients in attendance.

Each patient's pre-visit labs can be written by the nurse or MA prior to the SMA session (i.e., on a whiteboard with grid lines permanently imprinted on it so as to make drawing the chart much easier), perhaps with abnormal findings circled in red. The nurse and/or MA/ typically arrive 15–30 minutes prior to the start of the DIGMA and begin calling patients who have arrived early, one or two at a time, out of the group room and into the nearby examination room, where they take vital signs, update injections and health maintenance, and

perform any other special duties requested by the physician. One or two nursing personnel are typically used, although I prefer two (at least one of whom is usually the physician's own nurse or MA) because the nursing duties can then be logically divided up between them according to skill set and scope of practice and completed in half the time. In addition, two nursing personnel working together often have more fun than a single nurse working alone, and one of the goals of every DIGMA and PSMA session is for it to be an enjoyable experience for all, which includes the nurse/MA(s).

In addition, the physician might request that the nursing personnel do any or all of the following as long as it is in the nurse/MA's skill set and scope of practice under licensure: (1) assist in documenting chart notes (by entering the reason for today's visit, current medications, allergies, recent health changes, vitals, injections provided, etc.); (2) expand the number of vital signs taken to all that are important to the physician and relevant to the patients in attendance; (3) update injections (e.g., flu shots, tetanus, pneumovax), performance measures, and routine health maintenance on all patients; and (4) provide special duties such as taking blood glucose levels and doing preliminary diabetic foot examinations on diabetic patients (red flagging any feet of concern that the provider should look at), checking pulse oximetry readings and peak flows on asthmatic patients, etc.

Nursing personnel could pull and complete the patient information sections of lab slips and referral forms (regardless of whether they are paper or electronic) for tests, procedures, and additional medical services that might be needed. The nurse(s) could also search patients' medical charts for routine health maintenance that is due and then pull the appropriate referral forms that might be needed and complete the patient information sections. Work together with your

DIGMA nursing personnel to maximize their roles and responsibilities—especially during the design and planning stages of your DIGMA, but also on an ongoing basis later on.

Nurses/MAs Stop Calling Patients out When the Behaviorist Gives the Introduction

Typically, the nurse/MA(s) will only have completed vital signs and other duties on some (but not all) of the patients by the time the group is scheduled to start—at which time the behaviorist begins the session promptly on time with a brief 3- to 5-minute introduction, even if the physician has not yet arrived. The nurse/MA stops calling patients out of the group room when the behaviorist starts giving the introduction and then only resumes calling patients out for vital signs and other nursing duties after the introduction is completed. The nurse/MA(s) typically do not take vitals and perform other nursing duties during the behaviorist's introduction that all patients can hear it.

Nurse/MA(s) Resume by Next Calling out Any Patients Needing to Leave Early

After the completion of the behaviorist's introduction, the nurse/MA resumes taking vital signs on the remaining patients in attendance, one at a time, until all are inished—beginning with those patients who state they must leave the session early (i.e., when asked by the behaviorist during the introduction), but have not yet had their vitals taken.

Nursing Duties Continue Until All Patients Are Finished, at Which Time the Nurse Returns to Normal Clinic Duties and MA Becomes Care Coordinator

After completing vitals, injections, performance measures, health maintenance, and any other special nursing duties on all patients attending the DIGMA session (which normally takes two nursing personnel approximately 30–60 minutes for 10–16 patients), the nurse most frequently then returns to the clinic to resume normal clinic duties. By returning to regular nursing duties as soon as possible, any disruption to the nurses' normal working routine is minimized and the overhead expense of these nursing duties to the SMA program is also kept to a minimum. Because, like the physician, nursing personnel typically see far more patients in the DIGMA than in a comparable amount of time spent on individual office visits in the clinic, they actually represent a cost savings (rather than an expense) to the program.

However, it is sometimes the physician's preference (especially when it is the physician's own nurse) for the nurse to join the DIGMA to assist the physician in the group rather than returning to regular nursing duties—where they can then help with documentation, get any forms and handouts requested by the physician, provide nursing information to patients, find any medical equipment that the physician might need, be a *go-for*, etc. When this occurs, it is usually enjoyed by the physician's nurse or medical assistant—who comes to feel more a part of the DIGMA program. In addition, the nurse/MA is then able to observe their physician actually delivering medical care firsthand in the DIGMA setting—something much enjoyed by nurses, but often not possible during traditional office visits.

Also, by attending the remainder of the DIGMA session, the nurse/MA gets to personally observe what a warm, caring, and informative experience it is for patients. By so doing, the nurse/MA is subsequently better able to promote the program to patients when they come in for traditional individual office visits by encouraging appropriate patients to have their next follow-up visit in a future DIGMA session.

However, the most frequent arrangement is for the MA—when all nursing functions are completed on all patients in the SMA—to first recheck all blood pressures that were high (because the combination of the group plus white coat hypertension makes high blood pressure readings at the beginning of the session fairly common) and then become the care coordinator—calling patients out of the group room, one at a time, to schedule all recommended appointments and to give patients their after visit summary (AVS).

Approximately 45 Minutes Into the DIGMA Session, the MA Can Become the Care Coordinator

I am always learning new things about the DIGMA model and how to optimize it. One of the things that I have only recently started doing with DIGMAs at Harvard Vanguard Medical Associates/Atrius Health is to have the medical assistant become the Care Coordinator for the DIGMA approximately 45 minutes into the DIGMA session—or as soon as the MA has completed the MA duties on all patients attending the session. Typically, the MA will first recheck blood pressures in the group room on any patients whose blood pressures were initially found to be high when their vital signs were first taken, after which the MA will leave the group room and become the Care Coordinator.

As Care Coordinator, the MA begins to call patients out of the group room one at a time, beginning with those patients that the physician has already finished working with (and completed the chart notes on). At Harvard Vanguard, once the physician has finished working with a patient and completed reviewing their chart note, the documenter places a green dot by that patient's name—which lets the Care Coordinator know that they can now call that patient out of the group room. Once the Care Coordinator has later finished with that patient outside of the group room, the green dot is then changed to red.

As Care Coordinator, the MA schedules all follow-up visits, referrals, procedures, etc., that physician has ordered on the patient. The MA then gives the patient an After Visit Summary (AVS) that contains those parts of DIGMA chart note that the physician wants the patient to have and take home with them—which always includes the patient's medication list, treatment plan, and follow-up recommendations. When finished with that patient, the MA then escorts the patient back into the group room and calls another patient with a green dot next to their name out of the group room, and so forth—i.e. until the end of the DIGMA session, when the MA has finished working as Care Coordinator with all patients in attendance. One final nuance of this process is to have the Care Coordinator take the After Visit Summaries into the group room to give to those patients who do not need to have any referrals, procedures, or follow-up appointments scheduled—which minimizes any disruption to the flow of the group process and eliminates patient complaints about being called out of the group room unnecessarily.

The Behaviorist's Functions

Before the Session

The behaviorist, who—like the nurse/MA—has a fully expanded role in the DIGMA in order to optimize the quality and efficiency of the visit, typically arrives approximately 10–15 minutes early to greet patients, begin fostering some group interaction, and warm up the group. This is because, when the group does start, you want patients to already be comfortable, talking, and interacting with one another, not just sitting on their chairs and staring at the ceiling. One helpful technique for warming up the group is for the behaviorist to ask all patients what issues they want to discuss with the doctor today. The behaviorist then writes down each patient's

issues on an erasable whiteboard or a flip chart next to the patient's name, which the physician can then readily see on entering the group room.

This increases efficiency and saves the physician the considerable amount of time that it would otherwise take to find out each patient's reason for today's visit when later going around the room and working with each patient individually–and accomplishes this while also fostering some group interaction. It also enables the physician, should he or she choose to proceed in such a manner, to cluster the order in which the physician works with the various patients in the group according to commonalities in their reasons for today's visit, e.g., by first dealing with all patients having cold and flu symptoms, and then treating all patients with headaches, and so forth.

The Behaviorist Starts the Group on Time with an Introduction

The behaviorist can even point out, and encourage discussion between, those patients who share common issues. If the behaviorist has not yet completed writing each patient's medical issues down on the whiteboard, they should nonetheless start the DIGMA session on time with the introduction. Later, they can continue this process of writing down patient's issues by asking the late arriving patients what medical issues they want to cover with their doctor today—i.e., when they temporarily take over running the group while the physician is reviewing and modifying the chart notes on the first couple of patients. The behaviorist starts the group on time with a brief 3- to 5-minute introduction (see the behaviorists' training portion of the DVD). Even if the nursing duties are not completed on all patients by the designated start time for the session, the behaviorist starts the DIGMA on time, even when the physician is running late and has not yet entered the group room. Having the behaviorist give the introduction creates a brief buffer for the physician—as physicians are often running a few minutes late in the clinic. However, it is important that the physician arrive in the group room by the time the behaviorist's introduction is over. I would recommend that physicians who are notorious for running late in the clinic hold their DIGMAs either first thing in the morning or right after lunch, at which times they should temporarily be back to running on schedule.

Points Covered in the Behaviorist's Introduction

In the introduction, the behaviorist welcomes all attendees; introduces the SMA team; explains the DIGMA program and its multiple benefits to patients; covers what to expect during the session and how patients can make the best use of their time in the group today; points out that individual private time with the physician is available to anyone requesting it (typically toward the end of the session); discusses housekeeping and personal comfort issues; and thoroughly addresses the entire issue of confidentiality, including reviewing all points covered in the confidentiality release that they signed. The behaviorist also asks if everyone present—patients and support persons—has already signed the confidentiality release and then immediately gives a release for signature to anyone who has not already done so. The behaviorist also explains that patients are still entitled to regular office visits just like before and that they are welcome to return to the DIGMA setting any time in the future when they have a medical need and want to be seen, but that they are not expected to come regularly. Also, that the doctor will be providing the same types of medical services during today's DIGMA session that he or she normally delivers in regular office visits, but in the group setting, where all can listen, learn, and interact.

In addition, the behaviorist mentions in the introduction that, because of the additional time available and more relaxed pace of care, patients are encouraged to actively participate and interact with one another. Nonetheless, the physician and behaviorist will need at all times to stay focused and succinct, as there are many patients needing care during the next 90 minutes. Patients are asked to turn off their cell phones and to not enter into distracting side conversations with those sitting close to them during the session. Because the doctor will be sequentially focusing on one patient at a time in the group setting (running the DIGMA much like a series of individual office visits), patients are told that they are invited to briefly share any personal experiences that might prove helpful to the patient that the physician is working with. Also, the behaviorist points out to patients that, when the physician comes to them, they should immediately bring up the one or two most important issues that they especially want to have the physician address with them today, so that they are certain to have their most important medical needs addressed.

The behaviorist also explains during the introduction that the nurse/MA(s) will be continuing to call patients out, one at a time, for vital signs and other nursing duties until all are finished. In addition, the behaviorist addresses personal comfort issues and points out that the last 5–10 minutes of the session will be reserved for brief private examinations and discussions, that individual appointments will still be available to patients as before, and that—if patients like it—this is a new service that will continue to be available to them in the future on an ongoing basis.

The behaviorist also emphasizes to patients that it is important to finish on time because the physician has other patients to see in the clinic as soon as the group is over. Therefore, the behaviorist states that he or she will act as a timekeeper to ensure both that the DIGMA is able to finish on time and that everyone will have sufficient time to get their needs met today.

Patients Are Encouraged to Return to the DIGMA for Their Next Visit

In the introduction, the behaviorist also explains that patients are invited to return to the DIGMA setting the next time they have a medical need, preferably by pre-scheduling their appointment into a future DIGMA session, although drop-in convenience is also available to them if they prefer it. However, patients are told that if they ever do choose to drop in, they should telephone the office a business day or two prior to the session in order to let staff know that they are coming and to make certain that the DIGMA is going to be held that day because the physician will sometimes be away due to meetings, vacation, or illness.

The Introduction Ends by Asking If Anyone Needs to Leave Early

Finally, depending on whether or not the physician wants this question asked (most do want it asked), the behaviorist can end the introduction by asking whether anyone needs to leave early (so that they can be among the first treated during today's session). However, it should then also be pointed out by the behaviorist that by leaving early, patients will miss out on some of the important educational and support benefits that the DIGMA is designed to provide them with and that, whenever possible, patients should therefore try to stay for the entire session. Nonetheless, the behaviorist also points out that it is understandable that patients will sometimes have pressing job, sitting, or personal issues that need to be promptly addressed, and that we would rather have them attend the DIGMA for part of the time than not at all. Therefore, these patients are welcome to stay in the group as long as they are able. When the behaviorist's introduction does in fact conclude by asking if any patients need to leave early today, the behaviorist then asks the nurse/MA to next take those patients who must leave early but have not yet had their vitals taken—i.e., in order to have their vitals taken, injections and health maintenance updated, and other nursing duties performed as soon as possible.

Behaviorist Duties Throughout the Session

The behaviorist has many responsibilities throughout the entire DIGMA session, which include keeping the DIGMA running smoothly and on time. After the introduction, the behaviorist continues to play a major role throughout the remainder of the entire DIGMA session by managing the group dynamics, fostering some group interaction, addressing behavioral health and psychosocial needs, assisting the physician in every way possible, keeping the group running smoothly, and pacing the group to finish on time. In addition, the behaviorist temporarily takes over the group for a minute or two (typically focusing on behavioral health and psychosocial issues, or nursing issues in the case of a nurse behaviorist) whenever the physician completes documenting the chart note after working with each patient in turn or reviews and modifies the chart note created by the documenter on that patient. The behaviorist also temporarily takes over running the group whenever the physician steps out of the group room to conduct brief private examinations and discussions with patients individually (usually with no more than one or two patients, and typically toward the end of the session) or needs to step out of the group room to attend to a pressing clinic emergency.

Finish on Time, After Which the Behaviorist Stays Late for a Few Minutes

Although the physician must leave the group room as soon as the last patient is finished and the session is over (because patients will otherwise stay as long as the physician remains in the group room), the behaviorist needs to stay approximately 10–15 minutes to answer any last minute questions that patients might have, such as where to go for their colonoscopy or the smoking cessation program that was recommended. The fact that patients want to stay longer and have even more time is often surprising to physicians, who quite often undervalue their importance to patients and initially worry that they are burdening their patients by expecting them to stay through a 90-minute DIGMA, i.e., until they think about it and realize that the cycle time, from initially entering the clinic's door prior to an individual office visit until later departing through it after the visit, is often 90 minutes or longer. Once the patients have gone, the behaviorist then quickly straightens up the group room for the next SMA.

The Physician Delivers One Doctor–One Patient Medical Care to Each Patient

Immediately after the 3- to 5-minute introduction by the behaviorist has been completed, the physician (who should have arrived in the group room by this time) immediately begins delivering medical care to one patient at a time. Some physicians like to have patients briefly introduce themselves and state what their medical condition is—along with specifically what they would like to get from today's DIGMA visit. Actually, this is somewhat redundant (as the behaviorist has already written down patients' reasons for being here today) and a common beginner's mistake that physicians often make, as even if each patient only took 30 seconds, this would add up to 7 minutes of the session being used up. Worse yet, some patients might take several minutes in introducing themselves, which would dramatically reduce efficiency and ultimately the number of patients that could be seen during the DIGMA (plus divert from the medical care delivery nature of the visit).

Some physicians will start by taking patients in the order in which they arrived, while others simply look at a patient whom they are comfortable with and say something such as "Mary, tell us what's going on with you" or "Tell us what brings you in today, John." The most common strategy is for the physician to start with any patients who need to leave early, then treat any patients with head colds or flu symptoms, followed by any patients who are accompanied by young children (who could become restless and whiny), before sequentially treating the remaining patients in the room—possibly starting with any patients who might be suffering from headaches or chronic pain, who might not be able to stay for the entire session. Interestingly, even though the physician typically starts with those patients who have indicated that they need to leave early, many of these patients (often as many as half or more) will nonetheless stay for the entire session, because they become engaged in the process and find it to be an interesting learning opportunity.

The physician delivers the exact same medical services to patients in the DIGMA as during traditional individual office visits (history, examination, risk assessment and reduction, counseling, medical decision-making, documentation, etc.). Figure 2.5 depicts how examinations are often conducted in the DIGMA group setting (i.e., whenever appropriate and possible), where other patients are able to listen and learn. This reflects just how closely the one-on-one care that is delivered in a DIGMA can resemble that provided in traditional individual office visits, with the main differences simply being the setting in which the care is delivered (i.e., a group room vs. an examination room) and the number of observers present. Interestingly, these

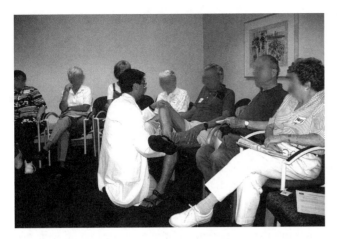

Fig. 2.5 In DIGMAs and PSMAs, whenever it is appropriate and possible, examinations are conducted in the group setting, where other patients are able to listen and learn. (Courtesy of Dr. John Lu, Physiatry DIGMA, Palo Alto Medical Foundation, Palo Alto, CA)

two issues do not seem to be addressed at present with regards to coding and billing. In addition, even more medical care is often provided during DIGMAs than in regular individual office visits, such as greater patient education, more attention to psychosocial issues, and consistent application of expanded nursing duties.

Difficult, Time-Consuming, and Problematic Patients Can Be Handled in Various Ways

Sometimes physicians go into the group room and spot one of their most demanding, time-consuming, and psychosocially needy patients sitting there. When this happens, they will often choose to start the DIGMA session with the patient on either side of this problematic patient, and then go around the group room in the opposite direction, so that this difficult patient ultimately only has whatever time is left toward the end of the session. This is especially important when the physician recognizes that starting with this patient could result in tying up much of the group time on this one patient. In the event that there is not enough time left toward the end of the session to finish working with this patient, then this patient could be invited to attend a future DIGMA session to address any remaining issues that are not covered adequately during today's session. By using this strategy, we have been able to contain some of the most challenging and difficult of patients in the DIGMA setting, and to do it with high levels of both patient and physician professional satisfaction.

The Physician Completes the Chart Note Immediately After Finishing with Each Patient

Documentation is completed on each patient immediately after the physician has finished working with that patient in the group setting (while the behaviorist temporarily takes over running the group), preferably by reviewing and modifying the chart note created by the documenter, but sometimes by finishing the chart note that the physician has personally started while working with that patient if there is no documenter. Some group interaction is fostered throughout the entire DIGMA session, usually in the direction of having other patients help the patient with whom the physician happens to be working at any given moment. However, when this happens, the behaviorist must be attentive and skillful in ensuring that the focus of the group does not then shift from the patient that the physician is working with to the other patients who are interacting (e.g., by providing information and advice or by sharing a personal experience). In addition, while the physician is completing the chart note (i.e., after finishing with each patient in turn), the behaviorist has a great opportunity to foster additional interaction and to address psychosocial issues. Do not lose control of the group by letting the focus of the group shift from patient to patient around the room; instead, try to keep the group interactions in the direction of helping that patient with whom the physician is currently working.

Foster Some Group Interaction, But Not Too Much

For maximum benefit, the physician and behaviorist need to foster some limited amount of group interaction throughout the session as this keeps all attendees involved and attentive. However, the physician and behaviorist must also remain cognizant of time—as well as focused and succinct in their interventions—because group interaction can take a lot of group time and must therefore be limited and used with care. Although DIGMAs can increase efficiency and provide patients more time with their physician, the behaviorist and physician must nonetheless pace the session so as to consistently finish on time—as there are many patients present and only 90 minutes in which to deliver care to all of them. If a patient has been cut off by another patient and has had his or her feelings hurt, the behaviorist can play a comforting role by being sympathetic and going back to quickly ask the patient what it was that they were about to say.

While it is important for the behaviorist to foster discussion and be attentive, empathic, accepting, and a good listener, it is equally important not to be critical, confrontational, argumentative, loquacious, or defensive. A useful time to foster some group interaction is when a patient is clearly being noncompliant with recommended treatment regimens. This is a time when other patients can often be most helpful in supporting the physician's recommendations and encouraging the patient to comply via specific helpful hints that they will often offer.

Always Strive to Finish on Time

With the help of the behaviorist in pacing the group (a function that is very important to some physicians, but is scarcely needed by others who happen to be good time managers), the goal of every DIGMA session is to finish on time, with everyone's medical needs adequately addressed and with chart notes on all patients completed—-and with all appropriate patients invited to have their next visit scheduled into a future DIGMA session. I recommend that physicians always try to finish working with all patients in the group a little early, so that 5–10 minutes still remain in the session. The leftover time can be used by the physician for providing brief private discussions or examinations (i.e., where disrobing is required) in the nearby examination room for the one or two patients who might need or request such one-on-one time. If no patients need to be seen privately, then further counseling, more patient education, or more in-depth discussions around medical or psychosocial issues of importance to the group can be provided during this time.

Recognizing that patients generally want more time with their doctor, whereas the physician has the opposite motivation and wants to finish the group on time, one endocrinologist developed an interesting strategy for aligning the motives of patients with his own in the DIGMA setting. He would start the group off by saying something such as "I just read the most fascinating article on the latest upcoming treatment for diabetes. If we finish a few minutes early today, I'd like to discuss those exciting findings with you." This of course held great interest to his diabetic patients, who were now motivated to keep things moving along so that the DIGMA did in fact finish a few minutes early.

Physicians Seldom Need to See More Than One or Two Patients Privately

The majority of physicians find that they do not need to see any patients privately toward the end of the DIGMA

session, or just one or two patients at most. However, a few physicians might find that they consistently need to see two or three patients for brief private examinations, personal discussions, or simple procedures toward the end of the session. For example, a rheumatologist might choose to provide some trigger point injections. Physician's practices and needs vary, so only time will tell how many patients will need to be seen in private, although it is most commonly none, followed by one and then two patients, in that order. This runs counter to the initial fears of many physicians, who are concerned that virtually all of their patients in attendance will request private one-on-one time with them.

There appear to be three major reasons why such a small number of patients request or need to be seen privately by the physician toward the end of the group session—another counterintuitive finding regarding group visits that many physicians find surprising. First, patients are generally surprisingly open and candid in the DIGMA so that almost all discussions can appropriately be conducted in the group setting; patients who are reluctant to speak in group will typically opt out and choose not to attend a DIGMA in the first place. Second, the physician is able to provide most examinations in the DIGMA group setting, as a relatively small percentage of the examinations provided during follow-up visits require disrobing. Third, patients often end up discussing issues that they might never have brought up because other patients bring them up first, and the patient then admits to having a similar problem.

There are some *quasi group visit* models that are being specifically developed around physician's concerns that each patient should have some private time with the physician outside of the group room (often this is motivated by billing considerations and a residual attachment to the same old individual office visit model)—i.e., instead of having all possible care that can be appropriately provided in the group milieu actually being delivered there. I view the latter as being the goal of true group visit models such as DIGMAs, because providing as much medical care as appropriate and possible in the group room optimizes both efficiency and patient education. It is not uncommon for physicians to make the beginner's mistake of spending some private one-on-one time in the exam room with each patient who attends the DIGMA. This appears to be a holdover from the individual office visit model of care that they have been trained in and are used to, where physicians feel that they are giving the best possible care because they are delivering it to patients individually and in the privacy of the exam room. Some may even be doing this because they feel that they can then more easily bill for the DIGMA. Because this approach not only is inefficient but also ultimately deprives all patients in attendance of much physician-provided education and helpful information, I generally consider it to be a mistake that is to be avoided whenever possible.

Once the DIGMA Is over, the Physician Needs to Leave the Group Room Promptly

The goal of every DIGMA is to end on time with all chart notes completed—after which the physician needs to promptly leave the group room to resume normal clinic duties. If the physician lingers, the patients will tend to stay also. Therefore, it is important for the physician to leave immediately after the group is over and the work is finished. This is something that the behaviorist can prepare the patients for during the introduction by emphasizing that it is important to finish on time because the physician has other appointments in the clinic right after the group is over.

Regardless of whether or not the physician was able to finish the session on time, it is courteous and a nice touch for the physician to, on finishing with the last patient, take a moment to formally conclude the session by telling patients that the session is now over, thanking them for actively participating and recognizing their contribution toward making this session all that it was. The behaviorist might also help to quickly conclude the DIGMA or PSMA session with a few warm and carefully chosen words to thank all patients and support persons for coming, for their openness and willingness to share, and for how they helped and supported one another. In the event that the physician had to step out for a brief private discussion or exam, it might only be the behaviorist who can formally conclude the session and thank patients for their participation and who can encourage them to return to the DIGMA the next time that they have a medical need and want to be seen. The behaviorist then lingers in the group room for approximately 10–15 minutes or so after the session is over, initially to answer any last-minute logistical questions from patients (e.g., "Where do I go for my colonoscopy?"), and then to clear the group room and quickly straighten it up for the next group visit session.

Financial Analysis

There are many financial benefits that a carefully designed, adequately supported, and well-run DIGMA and PSMA program can provide to the physician and organization. However, the analysis that follows primarily examines only one such potential economic benefit, i.e., that resulting from the increased productivity that comes from dramatically leveraging physician time in the DIGMA and PSMA models (but not the CHCC model, which does not increase physician productivity). This increased productivity can solve access problems to both follow-up visits and physical examinations by effectively creating additional physician full-time equivalents (FTEs) out of existing resources, thus creating extra capacity without the need to hire additional physicians and support staff, which saves money. All other sources of financial benefit simply add to and compound the gains derived from this increased physician productivity.

In addition to the financial benefits that result from the increased productivity of a well-run DIGMA and PSMA program, as depicted in Table 2.8, there are also many other (albeit more difficult to assess) economic advantages to physicians and the organization—many of which will only be realized downstream and over time.

The DIGMA and PSMA models can save money not only by increasing provider productivity and enhancing supply but also by decreasing utilization (and thus patient demand upon medical services) by enhancing patients' self-efficacy and disease self-management skills. Because they can enhance supply, reduce demand, and better match supply to demand, DIGMAs and PSMAs can play important roles in both achieving the goals of advanced access and containing the rapidly escalating costs of healthcare. Greater capacity coupled with decreased demand can translate into closed practices being re-opened, panel sizes being increased, new patients being brought into the system, and enhanced downstream profitability being the ultimate result. In addition to increasing revenues and containing costs, a well-run DIGMA and PSMA program can better meet informational and psychosocial needs—plus provide patients with an enhanced healing experience. Thus, properly run DIGMAs and PSMAs can provide a wide variety of economic benefits, in addition to the increased physician productivity, which they can certainly deliver.

Financial Benefits from One Source Alone—Increased Productivity

Because DIGMAs and PSMAs can frequently increase physician productivity by 200–300% or more (and most typically 300%), providers are able to see as many patients in a 90-minute weekly DIGMA or PSMA as it would normally take 4½ hours to see during traditional office visits. This results in a net weekly savings of 3 hours of physician time per weekly DIGMA/PSMA session that triples productivity on average, or 36 hours of physician time saved per week for every 12 such weekly DIGMAs and PSMAs that are run. In systems requiring 36 hours of clinic time for a full-time physician, this effectively represents an extra physician FTE being created by the SMA

Table 2.8 Potential sources of economic benefit of DIGMAs and PSMAs

- By dramatically increasing productivity and efficiency, and by leveraging physician time through use of existing resources, supply can be enhanced and access improved without the need of hiring additional physician staff—and improved access translates into many benefits, economic and otherwise
- The productivity and access benefits that DIGMAs and PSMAs offer can result in many sources of increased downstream revenue to the system–more RVUs, more open panels, increased panel sizes, additional new patients, financial benefits from additional labs and medications, etc.
- Because DIGMAs are readily accessible, patients will often pre-schedule or drop into a highly efficient DIGMA any week that they happen to have a medical need, rather than scheduling a more costly individual office visit, demanding an urgent work-in appointment, complaining about poor access, or telephoning the office
- This can save money by reducing the number of individual office visits, by creating fewer patient demands on services and support staff and by decreased phone call volume
- Also, by off-loading numerous individual return and physical examination appointments onto highly efficient, cost-effective DIGMA and PSMA visits, costly individual office visits are thereby freed up and eventually made more accessible to those patients needing or wanting them
- DIGMAs and PSMAs can play a major role in virtually all chronic illness population management programs by making efficient, accessible, consistent, multidisciplinary, and cost-effective medical care available to all—high quality and consistent care that can improved outcomes
- By overbooking sessions according to the expected number of no-shows and late-cancels, DIGMAs and PSMAs can be made immune to this vexing and costly source of physician downtime
- By utilizing a documenter, DIGMAs and PSMAs can generate superior chart notes that are comprehensive and contemporaneous in nature, which can thus optimize billing for medical services actually rendered (and reduce the likelihood of under-billing for these services by forgetting to include them in the chart note)
- By offering improved access and more time, costs can be contained by providing timely care that can help to keep chronic health conditions from turning into acute medical emergencies
- DIGMAs and PSMAs support advanced clinic access by providing a helpful tool for achieving and maintaining same-day accessibility, but without extra hours needing to be spent in the clinic—i.e., to work down backlogs or increase capacity
- DIGMAs and PSMAs offer high-quality care and max-packed visits in which injections, health maintenance, and performance measures are consistently updated—thus offering patients the benefits of a *one-stop* healthcare experience and helping to reduce long-term healthcare costs
- By better addressing the emotional and psychosocial issues that are known to drive a large percentage of all office visits, DIGMAs and PSMAs can end up reducing utilization and demand upon medical services
- The help and support of others is integrated into each patient's healthcare experience, social support that can reduce utilization by decreasing one's sense of isolation as patients realize that they are not alone, many others are worse off, and there is much they still can do which others cannot
- Group visits generally provide greater patient education, more opportunity to get questions answered, and increased teaching of disease self-management skills, which can decrease utilization and costs
- In SMAs, inappropriately high-utilizing patients can be taught by the physician, behaviorist, and other patients to more appropriately utilize urgent care, the emergency room, and other medical services
- Designed to handle many of the most problematic, difficult, time-consuming, and psychologically needy patients in the physician's practice, DIGMAs and PSMA can provide an effective format wherein these challenging patients can often be better treated at lower cost
- By providing the gentle confrontation of other patients, answers to questions they may not have thought to ask, and the professional skills of a behaviorist, SMAs can enhance compliance with recommended treatment regimens
- DIGMAs and PSMAs can be used to reach out to underserved patients (inappropriate under-utilizers, those with unhealthy lifestyles, noncompliant patients, those currently *falling between the cracks*, etc.)—*ticking time bombs* that can drive up long-term healthcare costs
- DIGMAs and PSMAs offer the competitive advantage of a new service
- By maintaining a strong customer focus, it is not uncommon for the DIGMA and PSMA program to receive valuable positive PR from local newspaper, radio, and TV coverage
- Although it has never been tested, I hypothesize that well-run group visit programs could potentially reduce malpractice risk (i.e., due to the improved access and enhanced amount of time available, the more relaxed pace of care, the greater attention to mind as well as body needs, the high levels of patient satisfaction, and the improved patient–physician relationships they can engender)—an intriguing, but untested, hypothesis
- Although DIGMAs have not yet been formally studied in this way, they could potentially be used to increase patient satisfaction scores of physicians with low scores by pairing them off with behaviorists possessing excellent communication skills
- Because DIGMAs and PSMAs provide high levels of patient and physician professional satisfaction, they have the potential of offering the financial benefit of reduced turnover—as happy patients and physicians translate into retained patients and physicians, and thus to reduced costs—such as not having the normal recruitment costs that would otherwise be involved for hiring the additional physicians that DIGMAs and PSMAs can effectively provide

program out of existing resources for every 12 such 90-minute weekly DIGMAs and PSMAs that are run. Because they are being created by the DIGMA and PSMA program through more efficient use of existing resources, these physician FTEs do not require the additional offices, examination rooms, capital equipment, nursing personnel, support staff, medical equipment, recruitment costs, etc., all of which would be required if you were

Table 2.9 The assumptions on which the financial analysis shown in Table 2.10 is based

- On average, DIGMAs and PSMAs increase physician productivity by 300% (it is absolutely critical that physicians take primary responsibility for maintaining the census of their SMAs, something which offering a documenter helps achieve by aligning the interests of physicians and administration)
- The champion and program coordinator establish 21 new DIGMAs and PSMAs per week at a uniform rate throughout each year
- Assume that of these 21 newly launched DIGMAs and PSMAs, 3 fail (i.e., 14.3%) due to lack of adequate census or physicians leaving the system; thus, a net 18 new weekly DIGMAs and PSMAs gets successfully launched each year
- To keep this analysis simple, all numbers (except marketing materials) are rounded off and based on the number of DIGMAs and PSMAs projected to be up and running at the middle of each year, e.g., since a net of 18 SMAs are launched uniformly throughout the first year, the average number up and running during the first year is therefore taken to be nine
- Patients attend the DIGMA or PSMA for their follow-up visit or physical examination in lieu of an individual office visit (i.e., visits are being replaced, not added)
- Assume that the same level of care is being delivered and documented and that reimbursement for a given level of medical care is the same for DIGMAs and PSMAs as it is for traditional office visits, which is an assumption as the entire matter of billing for group visits is still evolving and not yet completely resolved
- Physicians can run between one and five 90-minute DIGMAs and PSMAs per week, with physicians having busy and backlogged practices often running more than one DIGMA per week
- It is assumed that full-time primary and specialty care physicians work 36 hours per week in the clinic and receive an average salary (including benefits) of $230 K per year
- The cost of the SMA champion is assumed to be $125 K annually (i.e., salary plus benefits)
- The program coordinator's cost, including benefits, is $75 K per year
- Assume that behaviorists are hired as needed and only paid for DIGMA and PSMA sessions actually held—and that half-time behaviorists cost $40 K per year with benefits, and are responsible for nine 90-minute DIGMAs and/or PSMAs per week
- As is the case for physicians, the time of nursing personnel employed in the SMA program is also leveraged; however, because the exact gain is more difficult to assess, it is not included
- Assume that there is no net cost to the SMA program for the documenter as, in return for having a documenter, the physician must agree to see 300% more patients on average plus one extra patient in the SMA to cover this added cost
- Including benefits, the cost of full-time dedicated schedulers (hired as needed) is assumed to be $48 K per year (salary plus benefits)—with each scheduler being responsible for 24 DIGMAs and PSMAs each week
- For each SMA, healthy snacks cost an average of approximately $500 per year
- It is assumed that nonproductive DIGMAs and PSMAs (i.e., where physicians do not meet their census requirements) will be terminated and replaced relatively promptly
- The one-time cost of promotional materials (framed wall posters, flier holder, initial fliers and invitations, announcements mailed to 500 patients, etc.) is approximately $1 K per SMA—thus, $18 K needs to be budgeted for marketing materials for the 18 successful SMAs launched each year
- It is assumed that the necessary group and exam room space exists—and is available on an as-needed basis at no cost to the SMA program
- The actual savings from reduced future physician hires would be equal to 1.5 times the number of physician FTEs saved by the program, i.e., 1.5 times the average physician's salary plus benefits of $230 K per year. This is because these extra physician full-time equivalents are being generated from existing staffing so that there is no need for the additional recruitment costs, offices, exam rooms, medical equipment, nursing staff, and support staff that new physician hires would require
- The behaviorists and dedicated schedulers required for the SMA program are hired contractually on an as-needed basis so that their cost is only incurred by the SMA department for sessions actually held

to actually hire this number of additional physicians. Table 2.9 shows the assumptions on which the financial analysis is based. Although it is based on several fairly realistic assumptions in order to keep this financial analysis relatively simple, this analysis represents the estimated net profit that would be generated by the DIGMA program—i.e., as it takes into account the increased productivity and additional physician FTEs generated on the one hand, and subtracts the personnel and promotional costs of the program on the other.

As a result of not needing additional space or personnel (i.e., other than the behaviorist, dedicated scheduler, and documenter), these additional physician FTEs are being created out of existing resources. Therefore, the true savings of the DIGMA and PSMA program to the

system are approximately 1.5 times the average physician's salary (or approximately $1.5 \times \$230\ K = \$345\ K$) for every extra physician FTE created out of existing resources in systems wherein the average physician cost (salary plus benefits) is $230,000 per year. In addition to the economic benefits that come from leveraging the physicians' time, there is a similar financial benefit for nurses/MAs as their time is also leveraged a great deal on average. However, the additional savings that also comes from increasing the productivity of the nurse/MA(s) is not included in the financial analysis that follows—i.e., because the nurses are also asked to do far more in the DIGMA and PSMA settings, so that they might not end up actually seeing three times as many patients in the same amount of time. As a result, although the nurses

Table 2.10 Projected economic benefits from increased productivity

No. of DIGMAs and PSMAs at mid-year		1st yr 9 SMAs	2nd yr 27 SMAs	3rd yr 45 SMAs	4th yr 63 SMAs	5th yr 81 SMAs	6th yr 99 SMAs	7th yr 117 SMAs
Expenses (×$1000)	Champion	125 K	125 K	125 K	125 K	125 K	125 K	125 K
	Program coordinator	75 K	75 K	75 K	75 K	75 K	75 K	75 K
	Behaviorists	40 K	120 K	200 K	280 K	360 K	440 K	520 K
	Dedicated scheduler	18 K	54 K	90 K	126 K	162 K	198 K	234 K
	Marketing materials	18 K	18 K	18 K	18 K	18 K	18 K	18 K
	Snacks	4.5 K	13.5 K	22.5 K	31.5 K	40.5 K	49.5 K	58.5 K
	Total	280.5 K	405.5 K	530.5 K	655.5 K	780.5 K	905.5 K	1030.5 K
Savings (×$1000)	MD FTEs saved	0.75	2.25	3.75	5.25	6.75	8.25	9.75
	#FTE×MD salary	172.5 K	517.5 K	862.5 K	1207.5 K	1552.5 K	1897.5 K	2242.5 K
	Total (1.5×MD$)	258.75 K	776.25 K	1293.75 K	1811.25 K	2328.75 K	2846.25 K	3363.75 K
Total net savings		−21.75 K	370.75 K	763.25 K	1155.75 K	1548.25 K	1940.75 K	2333.25 K

Total net savings—first 7 years of SMA program = $8,090,250[a]

[a]This estimated $8,090,250 dollar savings during the first 7 years is just from leveraging physician time. Other potential sources of financial gain discussed in Table 2.8 will add to this benefit over time (enhanced care, more time, improved access, improved patient–physician relationships, better-informed and empowered patients, decreased utilization, improved healing experience, favorable publicity, reduced patient and physician turnover, increased panel sizes, opened practices, additional new patients, increased downstream revenues, etc.)

will also end up having their time leveraged to some degree, it is difficult to assess exactly actually how much, e.g., it might be 150–200% rather than 300% due to the extra nursing duties.

Million Dollar Savings from Increased Physician Productivity over Time

As is depicted in Table 2.10, we must then deduct from the economic gains that result from increased physician productivity the extra costs associated with the SMA program (e.g., the expenses of the champion, program coordinator, behaviorists, dedicated schedulers, promotional materials, and snacks). The documenter is not being shown as an expense in Table 2.10 because the physician will likely be asked to see an extra patient—i.e., beyond the number necessary to increase productivity by 300% on average—in order to cover the cost of having a documenter. While relatively small compared with the multiple benefits that a properly run DIGMA and PSMA program can provide financially and otherwise, these costs are nonetheless substantial and must be taken into account.

As seen in Table 2.10 (which is based on the assumptions depicted in Table 2.9), the savings can amount to millions of dollars annually in just a few years' time—savings that can then increase dramatically over subsequent years. However, readers will need to substitute the values that are accurate within their own system in order for this analysis to be of meaning in their own

particular cases. It is interesting to note that, while the financial officers within healthcare organizations will look at the economic side of their DIGMA program in different ways, it is not uncommon for their numbers to represent a reasonable approximation to those generated in the relatively simple financial analysis depicted here.

Economic Requirements and Ideal Group Size Coincide

There is a fortuitous finding that is central to the success of DIGMAs and PSMAs: consistently achieving optimal census targets in order to increase provider productivity by 200–400% (most typically 300%) also serendipitously results in an ideal group size from a psychodynamic perspective, i.e., between 10 and 16 patients for most DIGMAs, 6–9 patients for primary care PSMAs (6–8 female patients or 7–9 male patients), and 10–13 patients for most PSMAs in the medical and surgical subspecialties. Although not true in every case, the census targets generally required to increase physician productivity by 300% on average also turn out to be ideal group sizes from a psychodynamic perspective, i.e., from the standpoint of being manageable, lively, interactive, interesting, and helpful to patients. In addition to being optimal economically, these group sizes seem to be just about optimal in terms of quality, the patient's healing experience, and both patient and physician professional satisfaction.

Consistently Meeting Census Targets Requires Physicians and Support Staff to Personally Invite All Appropriate Patients

Despite all efforts by the champion and program coordinator to minimize the physician's time commitment to the program (especially during the early stages), there remains one responsibility that each and every DIGMA and PSMA provider must commit to fulfilling on an ongoing basis. During each and every office visit, the provider must commit to taking 30–60 seconds to briefly explain the SMA program in positive terms to all appropriate patients and then to personally inviting all appropriate patients to attend the DIGMA or PSMA the next time they need a follow-up visit or physical examination, respectively—and then promptly scheduling all who accept this invitation. In the long run, nothing is more important to a successful SMA than positively worded personal invitations from the physician to all appropriate patients in the physician's practice whenever they are seen for regular office visits. Nobody else—not the scheduling personnel, receptionists, nurses, behaviorist, champion, program coordinator, or dedicated scheduler—can be as successful at inviting patients to attend the DIGMA or PSMA as the physician can be. For example, I have found that for every ten patients that physicians invite via a carefully worded, positive personal invitation, roughly 7–9 patients will likely accept the offer; however, it could very well take as many as 50 to 80 or more cold phone calls by well trained dedicated schedulers to get the same number of patients to attend.

A Fully Used Shared Medical Appointment Group Room Can Create 2.5 Physician Full-Time Equivalents

Another way to look at the economics of group visits is that, because up to thirty 90-minute DIGMAs and PSMAs (i.e., separated by 30 minutes) could be run back to back in a single group room per week, a fully used group room could leverage existing resources to provide the equivalent of an additional 2½ physician FTEs. Recall that each weekly DIGMA or PSMA that increases physician productivity on average by 300% enables the physician to see as many patients in the 90-minute group as it would take 4½ hours to see individually during an equivalent amount of time spent in the clinic—which, on average, saves 3 hours of physician time per week. For every 12 such weekly DIGMAs and PSMAs, this amounts to 36 hours of physician time saved per week—or 1 FTE saved per 12 such weekly DIGMAs and PSMAs in systems that require full-time physicians to have 36 hours of

physician contact time (or 1.13 FTEs saved in systems requiring 32 hours of clinic time). Therefore, 30 weekly DIGMAs and PSMAs that increase productivity by 300% on average translate into a net savings of 2½ physician FTEs per week in systems requiring 36 hours of direct patient contact time each week. Along with the increased quality that a properly run SMA program can provide, it is this remarkable potential efficiency benefit that behooves us to alter the physical plant to create the group room and examination room space that is needed to accommodate DIGMAs and PSMAs.

Champion Trains Site Champions Throughout the System

By having the SMA champion also train site champions at each of the major sites within the system (i.e., those with more than 20–25 physicians) and then overseeing their work on an ongoing basis, even greater efficiencies and economies of scale could be achieved with the DIGMA and PSMA program. Once the SMA champion and program coordinator have established five or so well-functioning DIGMA and PSMA programs at a given facility or medical center within the organization, a less costly site champion could be trained within that facility to move the program forward from that point onwards at that particular facility. These site champions could use the five or so DIGMAs and PSMAs that have been established by the SMA champion and SMA program coordinator as *A-Teams* and training groups (i.e., for other interested physicians and SMA teams at that site to sit in on). Furthermore, all such site champions would receive ongoing training and support from the SMA champion and program coordinator over time—perhaps through monthly 2-3 hour meetings shared by all site champions, discussing challenges and sharing successes. Thus, the SMA champion would focus on setting up the initial DIGMAs and PSMAs at each site and then train a site champion to take over that responsibility at each facility, which would thus allow the SMA program to grow exponentially over time at a much more rapid rate than the SMA champion alone could accomplish. It is also a best use of the SMA champion's time in moving the SMA program forward throughout the entire organization with optimal speed.

Caution! Caution! Caution!

I would like to end this discussion of the DIGMA model on a strong cautionary note with regard to doing research studies that involve this relatively new and innovative group visit model—i.e., a caution regarding studies in which data from DIGMAs is combined with data from other types of group visit models.

Start Your Shared Medical Appointment Program with One of the Established Models

In addition, one needs to realize that the DIGMA, CHCC, and PSMA models discussed in this book have gradually evolved and been optimized over time through countless iterations and refinements as they have been used in hundreds of different applications. Therefore, rather than just jumping into group visits with some sort of new design that might hold intuitive appeal to you, a more successful strategy would be to first start with one of these established models and only later, after some success and experience has been gained, slowly depart from them should you feel that you need to do so, being ready to promptly retreat from any such deviation should it not work.

This book makes clear that there are different types of group visit models, with each having its own strengths and weaknesses as well as its own design, support, personnel, facilities, promotional, and census requirements. Some are more oriented toward the delivery of medical care, whereas others are more educational and/or supportive in nature (or designed to utilize mid-level providers rather than the patient's own physician)—although, by definition, all group visits have some degree of focus on the actual delivery of medical care. In the case of DIGMAs and PSMAs, this focus upon delivery of medical care is exceptionally strong, as they represent medical care from start to finish—and can best be envisioned as a series of individual office visits with observers (which is why they have proven to be so successful in the fee-for-service environment).

Drop-In Group Medical Appointments and Physical Shared Medical Appointments Differ Dramatically from Other Group Visit Models

As discussed in this book, DIGMAs and PSMAs differ dramatically from all other types of group visit models in a number of very important ways. For example, they are designed to dramatically increase physician productivity, max-pack visits, enhance quality and outcome, improve access to care, and provide patients with a one-stop healthcare *shopping* experience. In addition, DIGMAs and PSMAs: (1) are run throughout just like a series of individual office visits with observers; (2) deliver as much medical care as appropriate and possible in the group setting; (3) have definite facilities and personnel requirements (including a behaviorist, nursing personnel, a dedicated scheduler, and often a documenter); and (4) involve clear promotional and census mandates.

Unlike other types of group visits (such as CHCCs), DIGMAs and PSMAs do not include a separate, preplanned educational presentation—as all of the patient education in these models occurs in the context of the physician working with each patient individually while others are able to listen, learn, interact, and share experiences. This is not to say, however, that a separate educational program could not be *piggy-backed* on, either prior to the start or immediately after, the DIGMA or PSMA session (for example, a diabetes nurse educator could take advantage of there being a preformed group by presenting to patients in attendance for perhaps 20–30 minutes before or after the DIGMA). Rather, it means that this educational presentation would not be part of the session itself, as every minute spent on such an educational presentation during the DIGMA or PSMA session would directly translate into a minute's less time for the physician to deliver medical care—and hence ultimately to reduced census and efficiency.

Do Not Combine Data from Drop-In Group Medical Appointments and Physical Shared Medical Appointments with Other Types of Group Visit Models

When done properly, DIGMAs and PSMAs offer many unique benefits. These are distinct SMA models that are not equivalent to other types of group visits. Therefore, they should not be massed, lumped, combined, or compiled with other group visit models in any sort of overall data collection scheme for supposedly doing *research* on group visits in general—which is something that, unfortunately, is already beginning to occur (10). In fact, due to their similarity to traditional individual office visits, if one were to insist on batching data across models, it would probably be a better fit to batch DIGMAs and PSMAs with individual office visits rather than with other types of group visit models, especially when those traditional office visits have been max-packed.

References

1. Ann B. Gordon, Drop-in visits help to improve service. MDComplianceAlert.com, Dec 2001.

2. Thompson E. The power of group visits—improved quality of care, increased productivity entice physicians to see up to 15 patients at a time. *Modern Healthcare* June 5, 2000;54.

3. Heimoff S. Waiting room crowded? Put a few people in the examining room at once. *Managed Care* June 2000;9(6):34–37.

4. Noffsinger EB, Atkins TN. Assessing a group medical appointment program: a case study at Sutter Medical Foundation. *Group Practice Journal* 2001;50(4):44–45.

5. Noffsinger EB. Drop-In Group Medical Appointments (DIGMAs): history and development. Counseling for Health Newsletter, No. 23, Spring 1999;3–4.

6. Cummings NA. Behavioral health in primary care: dollars and sense. In: Cummings NA, Cummings JL, Johnson JN, editors. Behavioral health in primary care: a guide for clinical integration. Madison, CT: Psychosocial Press, 1997. pp. 3–21.

7. Mechanic D. Response factors in illness: the study of illness behavior. *Social Psychiatry* 1966;1:52–73.

8. Slomski AJ. What a behavioral specialist could add to your practice. *Medical Economics* June 5, 2000;77(11):149–171.

9. Noffsinger EB, Mason JE Jr., Culberson CG, et al. Physicians evaluate the impact of drop-in group medical appointments (DIGMAs) on their medical practices. *Group Practice Journal* 1999;48(6):29–30.

10. Jaber R, Braksmajer A, Trilling JS. Group visits: a qualitative review of current research. *Journal of the American Board of Family Medicine* 2006;19:276–290.

Chapter 3
DIGMAs: Strengths, Weaknesses, and Real-Life Examples

Other organizations using or exploring the role of shared appointments include Palo Alto Medical Foundation, Dartmouth Hitchcock Medical Center, University of Virginia, Christus Medical Group, University of Michigan, Massachusetts General Hospital, and the US Department of Defense....Some practitioners avoid the term "group visits," which may connote impersonal care and a lecture-style format. Instead these are truly shared medical visits, in which each patient has an individual appointment in which other patients are also present in the room as observers...We are presently using the model for such problems as cardiac risk factor follow-up, hypertension, diabetes, weight loss and lifestyle management, movement disorders, asthma, fibromyalgia and chronic pain management, hematology (leukemia, lymphoma, and chronic anemia), women's health care, and bariatric surgery patients....These visits should be viewed as enhanced care, not less care. Physicians need to remember that these are regular medical encounters with individual patients done in a group setting. Avoid the temptation to turn these into a "class."

From Bronson DL, Maxwell RA. Shared medical appointments: increasing patient access without increasing physician hours. *Cleveland Clinic Journal of Medicine* 2004;71(5):369–377. Reprinted with permission. Copyright © 2004 Cleveland Clinic Foundation. All rights reserved.

Major Strengths of the Drop-In Group Medical Appointment Model

Properly run DIGMAs are designed to efficiently deliver high-quality, high-value medical care to each and every patient in attendance and to provide patients with more patient education, greater attention to psychosocial issues, and better disease self-management skills. First and foremost, DIGMAs are meant to provide high-quality medical care with a warm, personal touch by enabling physicians to interact with their patients in ways that rushed, brief individual office visits simply do not permit. Because of their remarkable economic and efficiency benefits, it is easy to lose sight of the many quality and care benefits that DIGMAs were originally intended to offer to patients (Table 3.1). However, it was this desire to increase each patient's healing experience that originally motivated me to develop the DIGMA model, and it remains the aspect of the group visit models of which I am most proud.

Every possible effort should be made to design the maximum quality of care benefits into each and every DIGMA (and PSMA), especially prevention, health maintenance, and performance measures. This approach is a convenience to patients, as well as a sound business policy as it can improve outcomes, reduce utilization, and enhance patient satisfaction. Then, in addition to addressing the medical concerns that bring patients into their DIGMA visit that day, all recommended injections (flu shots, pneumovax, tetanus, etc.) can be updated, all routine health maintenance can be brought current (blood screening tests, colon cancer screening, mammograms, etc.), and all important performance measures and prevention issues can be addressed.

Because DIGMAs and PSMAs enable physicians to delegate as many responsibilities to the SMA team as appropriate and possible, the role of the nurse, behaviorist (e.g., in dealing with group dynamic as well as patients' psychosocial and behavioral health issues), and documenter attached to the program are all meant to be maximized and fully expanded. By off-loading as many responsibilities as possible onto the shoulders of the less expensive, multidisciplinary care deliver team, the physician's duties in the group setting are correspondingly reduced—ideally to doing only that which the physician alone can do, which is typically what physicians most enjoy doing.

E.B. Noffsinger, *Running Group Visits in Your Practice*, DOI 10.1007/b106441_3,
© Springer Science+Business Media, LLC 2009

Table 3.1 Some strengths of well-run DIGMAs

- Enhancement of the patient's healing experience
- Max-packed visits that bring injections and routine health maintenance current—offers a *one-stop* healthcare experience
- Greater focus on prevention and performance measures
- Dramatically increased productivity
- Improved patient access to care
- Access improves immediately for group visits, later for individual visits
- Medical care from start to finish, and run like a series of office visits
- Increased efficiency by reducing repetition and overbooking sessions
- Provides drop-in convenience
- Provides more time with physician and a more relaxed pace of care
- Increases continuity of care with one's own physician, as capacity is increased and patients do not need to be shunted off to mid-level providers
- Enhances the physician–patient relationship
- Addresses mind as well as body needs
- Delivers greater patient education and attention to psychosocial needs
- Provides the help and support of other patients
- Offers the professional skills of a behaviorist and a multidisciplinary team
- Excellent venue for treating difficult, problematic, and demanding patients
- Ideal milieu for information-seeking and psychosocially needy patients
- Can increase patient compliance and reduce one's sense of isolation
- Can reveal different types of medically important patient information or previously undisclosed patient symptoms
- Physicians get to know their patients better
- Patients can get answers to important questions they did not know to ask
- Can reach out to underserved or overlooked patients
- Offers patients the opportunity for closer follow-up care
- Gives patients an additional healthcare choice
- Also offers helpful information to family members and caregivers
- Provides an enjoyable healthcare experience as well as high levels of patient and physician professional satisfaction

DIGMAs Can Be Used Either Alone or in Conjunction with Advanced Clinic Access

DIGMAs can be used to improve access to care either as stand-alone programs or in conjunction with Mark Murray's *advanced clinic access* model (sometimes referred to as *advanced access, open access,* and *same-day access*) (Table 3.2) (1–5). The central tenant of advanced clinic access is the matching of supply and demand: (1) if demand exceeds supply, then backlogs and wait-lists will accumulate and lengthen (with the result being delays in the delivery of care); (2) if supply exceeds demand, then there will be unfilled appointments, and resources will be wasted, whereas (3) if supply matches demand, a balance is struck between the availability of appointments and patient

Table 3.2 DIGMAs support advanced access by demand reduction, supply enhancement, and backlog reduction

Demand reduction

- DIGMAs improve access to return visits, which can itself reduce demand—e.g., nursing staff no longer needs to be deployed to keep patients in a *holding pattern*
- Patients can drop into highly efficient DIGMAs rather than using individual visits
- Many patients prefer DIGMAs to individual visits, which reduces demand on them
- For the most part, properly run DIGMAs replace visits rather than adding them
- DIGMAs can improve access, so patients no longer need to make unnecessary "just in case I need it" future appointments
- Prompt, accessible care can help keep a chronic condition from evolving into an acute medical emergency
- Because patients see their own doctor, have more time, and enjoy better access, DIGMAs increase continuity of care, which can reduce demand
- Patients sometimes reveal different, medically important information in DIGMAs, which enables important prevention measures to be taken
- DIGMAs can enhance the patient–physician relationship—the *value stream* in healthcare—which can reduce *doctor shopping* and unneeded visits
- Well-run DIGMAs provide *one-stop shopping*, which reduces unnecessary visits
- Greater patient education enables patients to better manage chronic conditions
- More attention is paid to the psychosocial issues that drive many visits
- Added help and support from other patients is integrated into each patient's healthcare experience, which can increase self-efficacy and reduce demand
- DIGMAs can increase patient compliance with recommended medical regimens, which should reduce future demand
- Highly efficient DIGMAs can handle the follow-up care for many, if not most, established patients
- DIGMAs are an efficient venue for *physician-driven* returns, patients in the *holding tank,* and those wanting to schedule future visits
- Because of the remarkable access benefits they offer, DIGMAs can reduce the demand created by work-ins, patient phone calls, and complaints about poor access
- The *overflow* from each day can be referred to the physician's DIGMA
- DIGMAs provide high levels of patient, staff, and physician satisfaction

Supply enhancement

- Improved access and efficiency are hallmarks of the DIGMA model
- DIGMAs add capacity by increasing provider productivity by 200–300%, or more
- DIGMAs provide an efficient, additional healthcare choice that many patients prefer
- Physician efficiency increases by delegating to the behaviorist, nurse, and documenter
- Patients can attend highly efficient DIGMAs in lieu of more costly and time-consuming individual office visits
- 1 extra physician full-time equivalent (FTE) can be created by every 12 properly run DIGMAs that triple productivity

Table 3.2 (continued)

• DIGMAs help do today's work today, thereby reducing bottlenecks and constraints

• DIGMAs add flexibility, and a means of matching supply to demand (e.g., hold them on your highest demand day, such as on Monday afternoon)

• By appropriately over-booking DIGMAs, waste can be avoided and—unlike individual office visits—they can be made immune to late-cancels and no-shows

• DIGMAs offer physicians a tool for better managing both busy, backlogged practices and chronic illnesses

• DIGMAs provide a tool for optimizing the provider's schedule

• A weekly DIGMA can enhance a full-time physician's supply by 8–9%, and without extra hours being spent in the clinic

Backlog reduction

• DIGMAs provide a means of increasing productivity, reducing demand, containing costs, working down backlogs, and enhancing revenues—and accomplishing all this without the need of spending extra hours in the clinic. In addition, they can also help to maintain same-day access once it is achieved

• DIGMAs offer an effective and appropriate tool for reducing backlog with less pain (and then for maintaining same-day access once it is achieved), and an additional service for distinguishing oneself in a tight market

Matching Supply to Demand

• By leveraging existing resources, DIGMAs can increase supply to match demand

• DIGMAs add flexibility, and a means of matching supply to demand

• By offering DIGMAs at times of peak demand during the workweek (such as at the end of Monday mornings or Monday afternoons), they can help to better match supply and demand both within the clinic and in the individual provider's own schedule

demand on these appointments each day, so that a homeostasis is struck in which there is neither waste nor delays in the provision of care (i.e., once scheduling backlogs have first been worked down and eliminated). As depicted in Table 3.2, DIGMAs can help to achieve advanced clinic access goals by reducing patient demand, by increasing supply, by working down backlogs, and by matching supply to demand.

True patient demand reflects the total number of requests (for all types of medical services combined) that are received by the clinic each day from both internal and external resources, whereas actual supply reflects the total resources available to the clinic each day to provide these medical services. When there is a balance between supply and demand (and when the resources available to the clinic are well managed), the result is an openness in the scheduling of patients and an improvement in the availability of clinic appointments. When capacity (which reflects the total amount of clinician time dedicated to appointments) and patient demand are matched each day and when other steps are also taken such as reducing the number of appointment types, aligning providers' schedules so as to meet peak demand periods during each day of the week, equitable

patient empanelment in primary and specialty care practices, streamlining the referral process, and redesigning the system to optimize supply, there is a sufficient supply of available appointments to exactly meet patient demand each day, so that same-day access can be achieved.

The advanced access model involves accurately measuring both supply and demand, initially working down backlogs, doing today's work today, reducing demand (max-pack visits, increased patient involvement in care, extend appointment intervals, create one-on-one care delivery alternatives, etc.), finding and managing constraints, reducing the number of appointment types, using "huddles" and effective communication, planning for contingencies, optimizing the care team and facilities, etc.

While Dr. Mark Murray's advanced clinic access model (which is currently in widespread use) offers a scheduling optimization plan for improving access, it does not increase physician productivity, something that well-run DIGMAs and PSMAs can accomplish quite well (see Chapter 9 on outcomes). However, because DIGMAs can increase physician productivity and improve access in their own right, they can work well either as a stand-alone program or in conjunction with advanced access in improving access to care—where they can be used to achieve the goals of advanced access, but without needing to work extra hours in the clinic in order to immediately increase capacity and work down the backlog. By dramatically leveraging existing resources, increasing provider productivity, and rapidly reducing return appointment backlogs, well-run DIGMAs have been shown to solve access problems at both the individual physician (6) and departmental levels (7), as discussed in Chapter 9 on outcomes.

DIGMAs Offer an Efficient Venue for Handling Good Backlog

Furthermore, DIGMAs provide a highly efficient venue of care for handling *good backlog* and physician-driven follow-up visits, as many patients needing to be scheduled for appropriate follow-up appointments weeks or months ahead can be pre-booked into highly efficient DIGMA sessions in lieu of more costly and less efficient individual office visits.

Once Achieved, DIGMAs Can Help Maintain Same-Day Access

DIGMAs permit advanced access goals to be more easily maintained once the backlog has been worked down and same-day access has been achieved by enhancing supply, reducing demand, helping to match supply to demand, and scheduling appointments into highly efficient group visits that dramatically increase physician productivity rather than costly individual office visits whenever appropriate and possible.

DIGMAs Introduce Four Issues with Regard to Advanced Access

Although, because of the dramatic productivity benefits they offer, DIGMAs are the most effective healthcare innovation I am aware of for supporting and helping to achieve the goals of advanced access, there are none-theless four issues that need to be mentioned and discussed in this regard. Three of these issues could be considered negatives with regard to advanced access, whereas I view the fourth as being a definite positive (Table 3.3).

DIGMAs Introduce an Extra Appointment Type

First, whereas advanced access tries to reduce the number of appointment types on a physician's schedule to an absolute minimum, DIGMAs necessarily introduce an extra group visit appointment type. It is only by introducing a separate appointment type for SMAs that patients can be consistently made aware that they have a 90-minute group appointment and do not end up mistakenly believing that they have *hit the jackpot* and landed a 90-minute individual appointment with their physician. One thing that I have found will really anger patients about group visits is when they mistakenly enter the group room believing that they instead have a 90-minute individual office visit with their doctor (i.e., rather than a group visit) and end up feeling betrayed because they sense that some *bait and switch* type of tactic has been used on them.

Certainly, this would happen more often if there were not separate appointment types on the schedule for group and individual office visits—and possibly even for the different types of group visit models (e.g., DIGMA, CHCC, and PSMA). In the case of the homogeneous and mixed subtypes, you might even want a separate computer code for each patient grouping that occurs. This type of mistake is something that seems to most commonly happen when a scheduler who has been well trained on the group visit program is out ill and is replaced by a

Table 3.3 Disadvantages of DIGMAs for advanced access

- DIGMAs create an additional visit type
- Once backlog is reduced and same-day access is achieved, keeping DIGMAs full poses an ongoing challenge
- Advanced access would have you spread your visits out, but this is not so for DIGMAs (where follow-ups can be scheduled as the physician ideally wants them)
- DIGMAs represent a major paradigm shift and pose many operational challenges
- Therefore, you must be seriously committed to making DIGMAs work

temporary who has not yet been adequately trained. Although the behaviorist and physician can usually deal with this matter adequately by tactfully explaining the situation to the patient, why not save yourself the aggravation and take the necessary safeguards to ensure that this does not happen to you in the first place?

How Will DIGMAs Be Kept Full Once Open Access Is Achieved?

Second, while DIGMAs can be extremely helpful in increasing supply and reducing backlogs without physicians spending extra hours in the clinic, one must ask how a DIGMA (i.e., that has previously been filled to capacity and quite successful while the backlog was being worked down) will be able to continue being successful once same-day access has in fact been achieved. In other words, why would a patient calling the office for an appointment go to a DIGMA that is not being held until tomorrow when they can have an individual appointment with the doctor today?

To keep DIGMAs full once same-day access has been achieved, the provider and support staff will need to be especially effective in promoting the DIGMA. Keeping DIGMA sessions full even after advanced access goals are achieved will depend in large part upon how effectively and persuasively the provider (as well as the physician's entire scheduling and support staff) words the invitation for patients to attend the DIGMA for their follow-up visits. For example, the provider and support staff can emphasize the many patient benefits that a well-run DIGMA offers, such as more time, support from others, greater patient education, answers to questions they might not have thought to ask, a warm and supportive atmosphere, snacks, etc.

Keeping DIGMA sessions full once same-day access has been achieved also depends upon naming the program in such a way that the patient can self-identify the DIGMA as being the appropriate venue of care for them to attend—so that they will likely go to the DIGMA instead of choosing to be seen individually. Therefore, calling the DIGMA something like "Dr. Smith's Refill Clinic," "Dr. Smith's Diabetes Program," or "Dr. Smith's Follow-Up Care DIGMA" will help the patient to recognize it as the appropriate venue of care for them.

DIGMAs Represent a Major Paradigm Shift and Pose Their Own Challenges

Third, it needs to be noted that, as previously discussed, DIGMAs (just like advanced access) represent a major paradigm shift that can create many of its own challenges—both operationally and otherwise. DIGMA and PSMA programs are not as easy to successfully implement as they at first appear to be. They require that all SMAs be carefully designed, appropriately supported, and properly run. The one disappointment that I have all too often experienced with my group visit models is how often healthcare organizations have failed to properly design, run, and support them. For example, healthcare systems all too often make one or more of the following mistakes in that they:

- Use the cheapest or most available SMA team rather than the best
- Launch prematurely without first carefully designing the DIGMA and securing the appropriate supports and facilities
- Fail to develop the quality marketing materials and to adequately promote the program to patients
- Do not ensure that all sessions are consistently filled, which is the greatest and most important failure of all with regard to the success of the program
- Lack understanding as to the many challenges needing to be addressed when making this important paradigm shift to group visits
- Fail to fully utilize and optimize the roles of behaviorists and nursing personnel
- Do not use Patient Packets, snacks, and other niceties that enhance the patients' perception of the SMA program
- Fail to provide the best possible champion and program coordinator (and give them the time necessary to conduct their vital functions)
- Do not provide all personnel associated with the DIGMA or PSMA with the appropriate training
- Fail to utilize dedicated schedulers to optimize attendance, etc.
- Fail to use an appropriately trained and skilled documenter
- Fail to utilize both a medical assistant and a nurse to increase efficiency and enjoyment
- Fail to understand the basics regarding the DIGMA model and how to implement it

Therefore, to be fully successful, you must recognize the extent of the challenges for this major paradigm shift—and then be seriously committed to addressing all such issues as they arise in order to make DIGMAs work for you and your organization. In addition, it is important to recognize that the increased productivity that DIGMAs engender can stress the system and exacerbate any pre-existing system problems—which can also introduce logistical and operational difficulties that will need to be addressed.

DIGMAs Enable Patients to Be Seen as Often as Needed—i.e., Without Follow-Ups Being *Stretched out*

On the positive side, this fourth point clarifies a philosophical difference that I have with some proponents of advanced access. These are the proponents who espouse the tenant that if there is not a strong best practices or evidence-based medicine rationale for continuing to see patients on the interval basis that you are using (e.g., such as seeing diabetic patients every 3 months), then why not *push out* their visits (say to every 4 months) and thereby experience a substantial reduction in demand by these patients?

As a former patient myself, one who was frustrated by traditional medical care and wanted both prompt access to care and more time with my doctors, I originally developed the DIGMA model in order to increase the amount of time that patients could have with their doctor and to provide them with prompt, barrier-free access to high-quality care. Because of this, I would prefer to see a different approach taken than to stretch out visits carte blanche. After all, DIGMAs are highly productive and efficient—so why not reinvest some of the benefit they provide into delivering the level of care to your patients that you would ideally like to offer?

Therefore my position would be the following: If you feel that you should ideally see that diabetic patient in 4 rather than 3 months, then fine—go ahead and *push out* their visit to 4 months. However, if you feel differently—such as that you ideally would like to see how that patient is doing in 2 weeks because you just recommended a dramatic change in their medication regimen during today's visit—then why not go ahead and schedule that patient into your DIGMA in 2 weeks (i.e., assuming the patient is willing to attend a group visit) rather than waiting 3 or 4 months? The same would be true for your noncompliant and/or *out of control* diabetic patients—i.e., why not see them more often rather than less and, at least in the case of noncompliance (where the group visit format can be superior), why not see them in your DIGMA rather than individually. After all, what difference will it make if you happen to see one extra patient in your DIGMA 2 weeks from now—say 16 patients instead of 15? Besides, doing so can help ensure that your future group sessions are filled.

However, let me be clear. I am not suggesting DIGMAs as a means of increasing inappropriate utilization of healthcare services. Rather, I am recommending that they be used for medically necessary visits and to appropriately enhance the care that we are able to deliver to our patients—so that we use some of the added capacity they provide to deliver the level of care that we would ideally like to offer (or, at least strive to be closer to this ideal than we were before as a result of our DIGMA group visit program).

Positive Patient Feedback About Better Access Persuades Even Reluctant Physicians

Physicians also appreciate the improved access that DIGMAs can provide, which can motivate some physicians to start one for their own practice, even physicians who are initially reluctant to do so. An illustrative example occurred not long ago when I received a telephone call from an internist who requested a meeting to discuss the possibility of starting a DIGMA for her practice. This physician had previously been adamant about not running a DIGMA because she felt that the individual office visits that she was already offering her patients provided the gold standard of care for her patients. When I asked this internist what the impetus was for her change of heart, she stated that she had been shopping that weekend in a local grocery store when she found herself waiting in the check-out line behind two women who were having an animated conversation that she could not help overhearing.

She overheard one woman say, "Can you believe it? We were able to get in right away, and then we had 90 minutes with our doctor—and we can come back into future sessions any week that we want to be seen! Wasn't that the most helpful and informative medical visit you've ever had? And we didn't even have to wait for months, like for a short appointment." The internist added, "It was like a running commercial for DIGMAs that did not stop until their groceries were bagged and these women finally left the store. As a result, I began to wonder if I might not be missing something by not running a DIGMA for my own practice. I couldn't believe how positive these two women were about their recent DIGMA experience, and how frustrated they had been by not previously being able to get in to see their doctor." As a result, this physician became motivated enough to try a DIGMA for her own practice—and to find out that she was actually quite good at running it.

Physicians See More Patients and Patients Experience a More Relaxed Pace

DIGMAs are counterintuitive in that physicians can see two to three (or more) times as many patients, yet patients feel that they have more time and a more relaxed, less pressured pace of care. This is especially true after the physician has been running the DIGMA for a couple of months and has gained some experience and comfort with group visits. Rheumatologist Thomas Abel, MD, comments on the efficiency benefits and more relaxed pace of care provided by his DIGMA as follows: "Because I am a rheumatologist, most of my patients have painful chronic ailments—conditions that require long-term follow-up care and, often, changes in medications. In my experience, a familiar and often repetitive pattern of educating patients and addressing their common concerns—for example, the role and potential toxicity of disease-modifying agents in rheumatoid arthritis and the impact of this chronic illness on home and work—can occupy a major portion of the medical appointment" (8).

He goes on to say, "After seven months of running my group, I have observed several positive results, not all of which I would have predicted. When one patient's medical treatment is discussed, other patients often bring up relevant concerns and helpful suggestions to share with the group. How often someone has said, 'You know, I had the same question, but forgot to ask!' Patients and family members who accompany them give emotional support and testimonials to others present. A trained psychologist present at the DIGMA can appropriately and expertly manage the emotional and psychosocial issues associated with chronic illness. All present at these sessions, including myself, found the DIGMA setting more open and relaxed than the traditional office setting, where limited time was available. The impact on my schedule and accessibility has been noteworthy" (8).

Some Efficiency Gains Come from the Group Milieu Itself

In part, these efficiency gains come from the group setting itself, because of the remarkable efficiency and time-saving benefits that all properly run group visits offer. Physicians do not have to repeat the same information over and over to patients individually, because the physician only needs to say things once to the entire group (often going into greater detail) while all present can listen and learn. Another efficiency benefit of the group experience itself is the help and support provided by other patients—as well as the multidisciplinary care delivery team—that is integrated into each patient's healthcare experience. Also, group visits can be overbooked according to the expected number of no-shows and late-cancels, thereby eliminating the waste of physician downtime due to this vexing problem for traditional individual office visits.

Other DIGMA Efficiency Gains Come from the Physician Delegating to the Team

Another, and even greater, source of efficiency gain in the DIGMA is that physicians can fully delegate to a specially skilled and trained multidisciplinary team, especially to the nurse/MA(s), behaviorist, and documenter. Also, physicians do not have to waste time looking for missing equipment, handouts, and forms because the group room and nearby examination rooms are to be properly equipped at all times, which is something that the SMA program coordinator looks after. In addition, physicians have 90 minutes of uninterrupted time with patients: they do not have to waste time going from examination room to office to examination room, or being distracted by various staff, telephone, and clinic demands.

Foster Some Group Interaction So Patients Feel They Are Spending 90 Minutes with You

Interestingly, based on extensive personal experience with over 20,000 patient visits in DIGMAs and PSMAs with more than 400 providers nationwide (and, more recently, internationally), it has been my observation that patients typically leave the session feeling that they have just been privileged to spend 90 minutes with their own doctor—and that they do not feel they only had 6 or 7 minutes with their provider. However, this perception requires fostering some patient interaction throughout the session so that patients are always attentive, engaged, and continuously learning from start to finish.

This was a surprising observation to me in 1996 and 1997 when, as champion and behaviorist, I first started running DIGMAs at the Kaiser Permanente Medical Center in San Jose, CA. I felt this to be an issue that was absolutely critical to the success of the DIGMA model. I would frequently ask patients, both during and after the session, how they felt about their DIGMA experience, including how much time they felt they had with their physician. In addition, I would debrief with patients individually afterward, have them complete detailed evaluations of the program, and telephone attendees at their homes afterward using structured interviews. No matter what method of inquiry I used, the result was almost always the same—patients most commonly reported feeling that they were spending 90 minutes with their doctor, including during the times that the physician was working with other patients, even if they had different medical issues—because they were able to listen, share personal experiences, and ask questions. It was not uncommon for patients to report that they even received answers to important medical questions that they did not know to ask because other patients did in fact ask these questions—questions that sometimes turned out to be of great interest and medical importance to the patient. Therefore, it is important to always foster enough group interaction in the DIGMA to keep patients actively involved, however not too much, as that would slow the group down and make it difficult to finish on time.

Physicians often have the exact opposite worry. They feel guilty about imposing on their patients by expecting them to stay for a full 90-minute DIGMA session, even though the cycle time for a brief 15- or 20-minute office visit (i.e., the overall amount of time it takes, from when the patient enters the clinic beforehand to when the patient eventually leaves after the visit) is often 90 minutes or longer. This is because it often takes more than 90 minutes to register for the individual visit; wait in the lobby until called; be roomed; have vitals taken; wait in the exam room until the physician enters; have the actual office visit; get dressed; schedule any necessary follow-ups; pick up prescriptions; and finally leave the clinic. On the contrary, what physicians often observe in the DIGMA is that many patients still want to stay longer even after the session is finished, which is why the physician needs to leave the group room promptly after the session is over. Similarly, the physician not infrequently observes that even patients who enter the group stating that they need to leave early often end up staying for the entire session because they are too interested and involved to leave.

DIGMAs Offer Drop-In Convenience

Patients really appreciate the fact that DIGMAs offer the convenience of simply dropping in for 90 minutes with their doctor and some other patients whenever they happen to have a medical need and want to be seen, without any barriers to care whatsoever. While not a necessary component of the DIGMA model (as some physicians prefer to have all patients preschedule their DIGMA appointments), it is recommended as it offers a convenience to patients and enables some patients experiencing last-minute medical needs to be accommodated in the highly efficient DIGMA setting. This drop-in convenience is available to the physician's patients on a weekly basis when DIGMAs are held weekly and on a daily basis when they are held daily. Patients are very appreciative of this barrier-free access to high-quality care, initially to the group visits themselves and ultimately (as evermore individual office visits are off-loaded onto highly efficient DIGMA visits, and individual visits are thereby freed up for patients truly needing them) to improved access to the physician's traditional individual office visits as well.

Despite the drop-in convenience that is offered, the vast majority of patients (perhaps 80–90% once the program is established, and virtually 100% initially when few patients know about the program and the fact that they can simply drop in) will preschedule DIGMA visits just as they do individual office visits. With DIGMAs, patients do not even have to schedule an appointment (but most do), although they are typically asked to telephone a business day or two in advance when they do drop in to let staff know that they are coming. In this manner, census can be monitored and charts can be ordered (i.e., for systems still using paper charts), and patients can confirm that the DIGMA will in fact be meeting that week, as the physician will occasionally be away at meetings, on vacation, out ill, or absent due to a variety of other reasons. It also permits them to be notified by staff in the unlikely event that the session needs to be canceled at the last minute for any reason, such as the physician being ill.

DIGMAs Address Mind and Body Needs

DIGMAs also offer the quality of care benefit of attending to patients' mind as well as body needs. This is because DIGMAs offer more time with the patient's own doctor, the professional skills of a trained behaviorist, the assistance of a multidisciplinary care delivery team, and the help and encouragement of other patients integrated into each patient's healthcare experience. Because of the additional time, plus the help provided by the behaviorist and other patients, DIGMAs excel in addressing the behavioral health, emotional, and psychosocial needs of patients—needs that often go under-diagnosed and under-treated in primary care settings, and which are known to drive a large percentage of all medical visits.

Properly addressing these *mind* needs of patients can substantially reduce demand for individual office visits, which improves access to the physician's practice. For example, appropriately diagnosing and treating patients' depression and anxiety symptoms would likely reduce their somatization, *doctor shopping*, and inappropriate utilization behaviors. Addressing the frequent psychosocial needs of patients (for which there is neither the time nor the behaviorist or other patients to help with during brief office visits) is the right thing to do for our patients and something that is often better handled in the DIGMA setting.

DIGMAs Treat Difficult and Demanding Patients

DIGMAs often work well with difficult, time-consuming, and demanding patients who are problematic to manage during brief individual office visits. Consider including the following types of patients in your DIGMA: inappropriate high utilizers of medical services; the worried well; patients who constantly telephone your office; patients who place unreasonable demands on you and your staff; information-seeking patients who bring numerous articles downloaded from the Internet (articles they expect the physician to read and comment on during their brief office visit); and patients who bring lengthy lists of questions to their visits that they want promptly answered. Also consider including patients who are non-compliant, anxious, depressed, angry, and distrustful of medical care or have extensive psychosocial needs that require much time, emotional support, and professional handholding (such as the lonely widow who views the high point of the week as being her doctor's visit). All of these patients have substantial mind needs that should be addressed, needs that will likely be better and more efficiently handled in the DIGMA (due to the added time and the help of the behaviorist and other patients) than in a brief office visit.

By way of contrast, traditional office visits offer barely enough time for addressing the body needs of patients, with little if any time left over for the time-consuming behavioral health, emotional, lifestyle, and psychosocial issues that patients so often bring to their office visits. Not only do you not have the time (and possibly the expertise) for dealing with such issues during traditional office visits, but you also do not have the benefits of a behaviorist and other patients to help with addressing them. This is but one of the many ways that well-run DIGMAs can both enhance quality and provide you with an effective practice management tool.

The behaviorist (often a psychologist or clinical social worker with group experience and interest in working closely with the physician and medical patients) can help in addressing patients' behavioral health and psychosocial needs, in triaging them into appropriate care, and in providing the physician with help in diagnosing depression, anxiety, and substance abuse, conditions that often go undiagnosed and can result in unnecessary suffering and high utilization of medical services. In addition, when time permits, the behaviorist can offer patients some brief training in stress management and relaxation techniques, especially during those brief intervals when the physician is drafting or modifying the chart note or has left the group room to provide a brief private discussion or examination.

On many occasions I have witnessed a skilled behaviorist detect a lifestyle, psychosocial, or mental health issue that the physician was hitherto unaware of and tactfully bring it to the physician's attention. When this happens, it is not uncommon for the physician to ask the behaviorist to discuss the resources that are available to the patient (e.g., smoking cessation program, diabetes education class, cognitive behavioral treatment program for depression, stress or anger management program, or community as well as internal resources) during the next break while the chart note is being completed, although the physician will sometimes instead choose to start the patient on an appropriate medication, such as an antidepressant.

Many Problematic Diagnoses Can Be More Easily Treated in DIGMAs

Many conditions that physicians often do not relish treating—such as fibromyalgia, headache, chronic pain, and irritable bowel—are frequently much more easily handled in the DIGMA setting, especially when there are related extensive psychosocial needs. Frankly, I have not found fibromyalgia, irritable bowel, etc., to be all that difficult to treat in the DIGMA setting (in fact, many behavioral medicine programs for headache, chronic pain, etc., are already group oriented), which is something that often surprises the physician. This difference can be so pronounced that I have begun to hypothesize that what we have here might not be groups of patients who are somehow inherently *difficult* to treat, but rather a mismatch between the needs of the patient and the type of service that we are offering (i.e., brief individual office visits alone), a situation that DIGMAs can help to rectify because of the unique combination of benefits they offer to such patient populations.

Patients Help Patients and Patient–Physician Relationships Can Be Enhanced

Other quality of care benefits offered by DIGMAs include the fact that patients help patients with suggestions and support, and the patient–physician relationship can be enhanced. Because of the enhanced accessibility and warm, relaxed atmosphere that properly run DIGMAs offer, plus the greater amount of time and patient education available, patients often report an improved relationship with their physicians. Patients sometimes comment that the DIGMA enhances the patient–physician relationship because it increases confidence in their doctor when they see how many different types of health problems and conditions they are able to successfully treat in the group setting. Not infrequently, patients will say something like, "I now know that no matter what happens to me, my doctor will be able to help me." The positive atmosphere of the DIGMA can be further enhanced by distributing Patient Packets filled with helpful information and by making healthy snacks available to patients.

As with all group visit models, DIGMAs provide the help and support of other patients. Patients share personal experiences, as well as hope and encouragement with one another. They share their knowledge of various internal and community resources that are available to them and also offer hard-earned pearls of wisdom and disease self-management skills that they have gradually gleaned over the years as a result of dealing with their own health problems. In addition, other patients are often most helpful in confronting noncompliant patients about the importance of following the doctor's medical advice and recommended treatment regimens. Feeling accountable to a peer group of fellow patients for improving one's lifestyle and adhering to recommended treatment regimens provides a very powerful incentive to other patients. In addition, patients gain perspective by recognizing that they are not alone, that there are others more severely afflicted, that things could be much worse, and that there is still much that they are able to do which others cannot.

DIGMAs Also Help Family Members and Caregivers

Patients often benefit from having a family member, caregiver, or support person accompany them to the DIGMA, and those support persons also benefit by coming because they can have their questions and concerns addressed by the patient's own doctor. In certain cases, such as the male diabetic with out-of-control blood glucose levels whose wife does the cooking, it is absolutely essential to reach the spouse. For this reason, DIGMAs are typically designed to include patients and their loved ones, caregivers, and family members, with patients generally invited to bring a support person to the session. However, be careful to make clear that while it is certainly permissible to bring a support person to the DIGMA, it is not acceptable to bring several (as they can be a group unto themselves).

Compliance Can Be Increased

In DIGMAs, the support and information provided by other patients, as well as the professional skills of the behaviorist, provide huge quality of care benefits to patients. In addition to their helpful tips, patients often provide an effective but gentle type of confrontation that is most helpful in getting a previously noncompliant patient to more fully comply with recommended treatment regimens. Others in attendance might have already experienced the same type of health problem for some time; taken the same type of medicine that is being recommended; undergone the recommended treatment or procedure; or made the lifestyle change that the physician is suggesting to the patient, but which the patient is not adhering to (quitting smoking, starting an exercise program, losing weight, starting on insulin or dialysis in a timely manner, etc.). Because of their own personal success stories, these patients—with whom the patient is able to identify—are often able to encourage and persuade the noncompliant patient to more fully accept the physician's treatment recommendations in a way that the physician simply cannot.

Patients also help other patients by making clear the potential risks that the patient faces through noncompliance and by pointing out that the recommendations which the physician is making are not as difficult or unachievable as the noncompliant patient might initially believe. It is amazing how influential another patient can be in relieving a noncompliant patient's anxiety and resistance when that patient has already successfully undergone the recommended treatment regimen or lifestyle change with benefit (e.g., insulin injections, chemotherapy, dialysis, thallium treadmill, diagnostic test or procedure, medication change, exercise, diet, smoking cessation).

Other patients can also be most helpful in persuading the resistant patient to comply with recommended treatment regimens by confronting them with the long-term consequences of noncompliance. This is especially true when these patients have themselves already suffered such deleterious consequences because they did not previously comply with the doctor's advice, such as the diabetic patient who has already suffered numerous laser surgeries and severe loss of vision as a result of not conscientiously adhering to the doctor's advice regarding diet, exercise, medications, and self-monitoring of blood sugars. When such a patient confronts a noncompliant juvenile diabetic (who is saying that he intends to live his life just like everyone else does, including eating, drinking, and smoking whatever and whenever he wants), the results can be remarkably effective. I have witnessed this type of interaction several times, for example, when another patient confronted a noncompliant juvenile male diabetic patient by lifting up an amputated foot and saying, "Boy oh boy, do you ever remind me of myself. Remember when I used to say exactly the same things to you, Doc? But don't be stupid like I was, or this could happen to you as well." This type of brief interaction, based on highly emotional shared personal experiences, can be more effective in persuading the noncompliant patient to comply with the physician's treatment recommendations than hours of theoretical reasoning and attempts at persuasion on the physician's part during traditional individual office visits.

Physicians Often Note Improved Compliance in Patients Who Attend Their DIGMAs

In discussing the impact of her DIGMAs on her practice, endocrinologist Lynn Dowdell, MD, addressed the benefits that the program offered to her noncompliant patients: "To optimize the utility of my DIGMA, I routinely invite every patient (for whom it is appropriate) whom I see during an individual appointment to have their follow-up visit with me be a group visit....I especially strive to refer my resistant and noncompliant patients (e.g., those who resist taking insulin or who have high HgA1C levels) to group because I have found it especially useful for helping these patients to make the lifestyle changes necessary to better control their diabetes. The health psychologist and the encouragement, support, and gentle confrontation of other patients in the group with similar conditions are invaluable for breaking through denial and persuading patients to comply with recommended medical advice. Overall, I have found my DIGMA group a valuable addition to my practice both by giving my patients more accessibility to me and by enabling me to deliver better service and follow-up care...Because more time is available and the setting is more relaxed, my DIGMA lets me answer questions more fully and for many of my patients at once...After individual consultations, I frequently use my DIGMA as a follow-up visit to discuss with patients the results of lab tests that I have ordered, to more closely monitor patients in a timely way, to order future tests, or to change medications as needed" (8).

Dr. Dowdell also adds, "In addition, patients in group frequently provide more helpful information to each other than I could. For example, one patient who had many questions about an upcoming adenosine thallium test was able to get a good idea about what it was like from others in group who had already undergone the same test. Similarly, many Type 2 diabetes patients who need insulin resist complying with medical advice out of fear. My DIGMA has proved especially helpful by providing these patients not only with the necessary information, encouragement, and support but also with reassurance from other patients already taking insulin that insulin injections are not as frightening as they might seem. Compliance with recommended medical regimens is thus improved….Similarly, an anxious male patient who was about to have pituitary surgery met another male patient in group who had the same procedure the previous month and gave a great deal of reassurance and firsthand information about the procedure and its aftermath. This help dramatically relieved the patient's worry and concern about the upcoming procedure" (8).

In another example, when one patient inquired in a DIGMA what needed to be done next regarding her angina, she strongly resisted the physician's suggestion that the next step should be a thallium treadmill. However, she was immediately persuaded to undergo this test when another patient explained exactly what it was like when she took it, pointed out that the doctor and nurse are there, and reassured her that it was not nearly as bad as she was imagining. This patient said, "The doctor's there. They'll talk you through it. You'll feel short of breath at first, but that only lasts around 30 seconds— and then it's OK. Everything will work out just fine, and it's not as nearly as bad as you might think." As a result, the patient promptly changed her mind and agreed to the recommended procedure in a timely manner. This is but one of countless examples that I have personally witnessed wherein the DIGMA group setting has helped to increase compliance with recommended treatment regimens.

The Group Can Provide Critically Important Reassurance

As an example of another type of benefit that the group setting has to offer, consider the inconsolable female patient who was tearful, despondent, and consumed by guilt over her belief that the medication she had taken for her rheumatologic pain caused her to miscarry a cherished and desperately wanted baby after years of trying unsuccessfully to become pregnant. Repeated efforts by the physician during previous individual office visits had failed to either assuage the patient's guilt or reassure her that miscarriage often occurs naturally for a variety of reasons. In addition, the physician had been unable to get the patient to understand that this was not an expected side effect of the medication she was taking. However, the needed reassurance was promptly forthcoming during the first DIGMA session that the patient attended when another patient told her that she had been on the same medication throughout adulthood, had borne three healthy children without a miscarriage, and did not believe that the medication caused the miscarriage. The patient's relief was dramatic, immediate, and almost palpable.

In discussing his rheumatology DIGMA, rheumatologist David Grannovetter, MD, said, "Simply put, its better care! The groups have a wonderful healing energy about them that is not only helpful to patients, but also gives me hope in general for our ailing healthcare system" (9).

In this same article, nephrologist William Peters, MD, states, "I believe that this model brings the human element back into healthcare. By providing a type of psychological management of medical illness that has not previously been available to physicians in traditional one-to-one office visits, the DIGMA more efficiently addresses psychological issues such as denial and noncompliance" (9). In a separate article, Dr. Peters adds that his nephrology DIGMA has "…benefited my patient population in substantial ways in terms of relieving their psychosocial stress related to their end-stage renal disease care, as well as providing them with the means to have closer contact with me in a therapeutically beneficial way…I would put this type of programs above the standard-of-care that the community offers" (10).

The Occasional Miracle Patient Provides Inspiration and Hope for All

Patients also appreciate another benefit of DIGMAs that is not easily provided by traditional office visits: the inspiration and realistic hope provided to the entire group by the occasional miracle patient. For example, the kidney patient attending the nephrology DIGMA who had been receiving dialysis treatment for more than 30 years and was still working and traveling, as well as the pancreatic cancer patient in an oncology DIGMA who was still living life fully and doing well a full 5 years after diagnosis and treatment, provided remarkable degrees of inspiration and hope to all fortunate enough to be in attendance. In fact, by the time this dialysis patient of 30 years finished talking about what dialysis was like in the early days (i.e., the long tubes filled with blood, the coldness of the returning blood and the hypothermia that one felt, and the lottery that one needed to first go through in order to have this cherished chance at survival), all present felt more accepting and less aggrieved by the inconveniences of the dialysis procedures that they were now undergoing.

Or consider the remarkably positive impact on the group that a patient can have who is: now living a relatively active life after receiving a recent liver transplant; able to discontinue dialysis after having received a kidney transplant; or doing well in her late 50s, despite dealing with type 1 diabetes throughout her life. All of these patients can provide a wonderful healing balm to all present at the DIGMA session.

DIGMAs Provide Greater Patient Education and Attention to Psychosocial Issues

One of the great patient benefits of a well-run DIGMA program is the remarkable amount of patient education that can be provided during this 90-minute shared medical visit. While the physician works with each patient individually in the DIGMA and PSMA group session, other attendees are able to listen, ask questions, and learn. Not infrequently, physicians will use educational props and materials, various anatomical models and charts, and an assortment of educational handouts to help get important points across to their patients in the DIGMA and PSMA settings (Fig. 3.1). Properly run DIGMAs provide effective medical treatment in a relaxed and informative setting—along with the information, encouragement, and support that patients and their families need for living their lives as fully as possible, despite their illnesses. As the physician goes around the group room sequentially addressing the unique medical needs of each patient individually, all present are able to listen, interact, ask questions, and learn.

Because others in attendance often have the same condition as the patient (often other patients who have already been dealing with the disease for a longer period of time), a unique opportunity is provided for the patient to meet, ask questions of, and discuss important issues with somebody else who is similarly afflicted—both within and outside of the DIGMA setting. DIGMAs also provide physicians with an opportunity to confront any misinformation that patients might have gleaned from the Internet or from friends and family. This is important because there sometimes are deeply rooted mistaken medical beliefs that are either cultural or familial in nature which need to be addressed, as they could otherwise deleteriously affect the patient's health.

The group setting releases patients from the isolation and power disparity of individual office visits. While incorporating most aspects of a traditional office visit, DIGMAs provide more integrated, holistic care by also dealing effectively with patients' psychological, emotional, and behavioral health needs—needs that are known to drive a large proportion of all medical visits and cannot usually be adequately addressed during the brief time span offered by an individual appointment (11–13). Everyone can benefit from the greater patient education and attention to psychosocial needs provided by the shared group experience, the additional time spent with the physician, the professional skills of the behaviorist, the advice provided by the nurse/MA, and the encouragement and helpful tips offered by other patients.

Physicians Can Glean a Different Type of Medically Important Information

It is not uncommon for physicians to leave the group commenting on how much they found out about their patients during the DIGMA session—information that they never knew, even for patients they had previously followed for many years. Because patients are often more open in the group setting than in traditional one-on-one office visits, which is quite surprising to many, it is not uncommon for patients to bring up and discuss certain types of issues in the DIGMA that they might not have previously disclosed to their doctor during prior individual office visits. This is especially true when other patients bring up subjects that the patient is denying or minimizing, or when they discuss their own highly personal issues (such as vaginal discharge, menstrual problems, erectile dysfunction, depressive symptoms) that the patient also happens to have, but has been reluctant or too embarrassed to bring to the doctor's attention.

Although physicians worry about missing something important in group, they often learn more. The question could be how much is already being missed during traditional office visits? Because a different type of information is often disclosed in the DIGMA setting than is revealed during individual office visits, physicians can sometimes receive different type of medically important information from the DIGMA than from traditional visits, the result being that physicians will likely learn the most about their patients when they offer both individual and group visits in their practice.

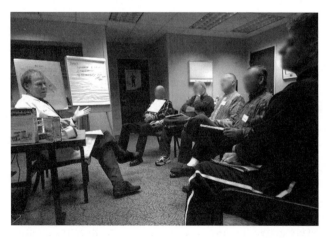

Fig. 3.1 In DIGMAs and PSMAs, the physician often enhances patient education by using a variety of educational materials, charts, anatomical models, and handouts while addressing each patient's health issues in turn so that all are able to listen, ask questions, and learn. (Courtesy of Dr. Thomas Morledge, Men's Primary Care Physicals SMA, Cleveland Clinic, Cleveland, OH)

DIGMAs Can Reveal Previously Undetected Symptoms That Are Denied or Minimized

Sometimes medically significant symptoms are minimized or denied by the patient (such as critically important cardiovascular symptoms), but are revealed to the physician for the first time after somebody else first brings them up in the group setting. Of course, not all patients will be as open in the group setting—and some will even opt to not attend. Furthermore, for patients to be so open during group sessions, it is imperative that the physician be comfortable with such personal discussions in the group. For example, if the physician is uncomfortable discussing erectile dysfunction or menstrual problems during the group, then this will certainly act as a damper to patient openness with regard to such discussions in the group setting.

It is not uncommon for a patient to say something in the group setting such as, "I didn't feel comfortable bringing this up in our last office visit, doc; however, I feel safe with these fine people here…" and then go on to discuss some of the most personal and intimate of topics. As a result, DIGMAs often provide physicians with a different type of information about their patients than is revealed during traditional office visits, additional information that can sometimes be medically important and most helpful to the medical decision-making process.

For example, when one patient recently discussed having chest pressure and shortness of breath on exertion during a PSMA for intake visits, another patient (who had already had his physical examination, and whose medical issues the physician had already addressed in the interactive group segment of the PSMA, which is basically a small DIGMA) chimed in by saying, "You know, now that you mention it, I've been having the same symptoms as you." Subsequent follow-up tests (which were ordered as a result of this belated disclosure during the group) revealed that one of this patient's major coronary arteries was 90% occluded. The physician later told me that, without the group, he would never have known this critically important medical information about this patient, and a heart attack in the not-too-distant future would have been the likely outcome.

Interestingly, during that same intake PSMA session, another patient whom the physician had already finished working with (a patient from out of the area who was new to the physician's practice) also disclosed for the first time that he had also previously experienced similar symptoms before he received his heart stents. Because this patient did not mention his heart stents to the physician (and had also failed to report them on the detailed health history form he had previously filled out), the patient was asked why he had cardiac stents. He replied that he had a serious heart attack 3 years ago—in fact, he had been unconscious for 3 days and was later told that he nearly died—but that he had *forgotten* to mention it to the physician.

In another example, one patient who had been quiet throughout most of a rheumatology DIGMA session casually mentioned (i.e., when others were complaining about the fatigue they were experiencing from their various rheumatologic conditions and from steroid withdrawal) that he would like the physician to prescribe a pep pill to give him energy. When asked about this request, the patient indicated almost indifferently that he had been fatigued a lot lately—especially with any minor exertion—and was having painful sensations in his chest and difficulty in breathing. As a result, this patient was given a stat cardiac work-up and not a pep pill. It turned out that he actually had advanced coronary artery disease; however, he had been in denial and was completely oblivious to the potential severity of the symptoms he was experiencing—symptoms that he had not brought up during his most recent individual office visits.

Similarly, another patient, who was noncompliant and in denial about her diabetes, nonchalantly entered an endocrinology DIGMA because of the excellent access it afforded. This patient sheepishly requested a prescription for glasses, stating that she hated to waste the doctor's time on such a trivial matter. She stated that she had come today only because it was so easy to just drop in, adding that she "…never would have bothered to schedule an appointment for something as minor as this." Because vital signs and finger stick blood glucose levels were routinely taken for all diabetic patients at the beginning of each endocrinology DIGMA session, this patient's blood glucose level was discovered to be over 900 mg/dL.

When confronted with this finding, she indicated that she had decided to live just like anybody else—to eat what she wanted, party when she felt like it, and drink when she was in the mood. While her out-of-control blood glucose levels were a complete surprise to the patient, detection of this condition allowed immediate emergency measures to be taken and for stern warnings to be given by the physician, the behaviorist, and the other patients. If it were not for the DIGMA, this patient would likely have gone for some time without realizing how out of control her diabetes was, possibly causing herself severe and irreversible damage.

Patients Sometimes Reveal Misuse of Medications

In a recent cardiology DIGMA, one patient was discussing how discouraged he felt because the angina he was experiencing was severely limiting his ability to function and enjoy his everyday life. He described how he used to relish jogging 4 miles or taking a 100-mile bike ride in the coastal mountains of northern California but lamented that he was now very frustrated because he wasn't even able to walk one city block without experiencing chest pains, shortness of breath, and fatigue. While he was speaking, another patient in attendance immediately broke into the discussion and asked, "If you want to take a walk, why don't you just go out and take one?" He said that he couldn't because of his severe chest pains.

The second patient went on to state that she also had angina, but loved to dance and therefore went dancing every weekend. In fact, she stated that she closed the bar down every Saturday night at 2 a.m. When asked by the behaviorist how she managed to go dancing each week despite being so physically limited by her angina, she responded that she simply took a nitroglycerine tablet on the drive over to the bar and that she then danced until her chest pains became too severe to continue dancing. When this happened, she would simply excuse herself and go to the ladies room, where she would take another nitroglycerine tablet and wait for the angina to subside, after which she would go back onto the dance floor and resume dancing until her chest pains re-emerged. She continued this process over and over throughout the evening but, as she noted with pride, she was able to continuing dancing until the bar closed at 2 a.m.

The cardiologist had no idea that the patient was using the nitroglycerine she had been prescribed in this manner and likely would have never known about it through individual office visits alone. Of course, on hearing this, the cardiologist was able to discuss how to take nitroglycerine more appropriately, plus was able to make other, less risky treatment recommendations to the patient regarding her lifestyle. This example illustrates the different types of information that physicians often obtain about their patients in the DIGMA setting. Because of the informal setting, the experiences being shared by other patients, and the greater amount of time available, some of the information gathered on patients during DIGMAs can be quite different from that which is disclosed during traditional office visits.

X-rays Can Be Ordered During Group on a Stat Basis

X-rays represent but another example of how DIGMA sessions can be max-packed for the patient's benefit and to reveal additional information promptly to the physician. Because of the extended length of the appointment, patients can sometimes be sent out of the DIGMA to have necessary X-rays taken during the session so that the physician can later read them before the session is over.

However, this approach will obviously only work in systems that can provide X-rays on a stat basis. A recent family practice DIGMA at which I was the behaviorist was quite unusual in that three different patients were referred out for X-rays during the early part of the session. All three of these patients returned less than 45 minutes later and had their X-rays read by the physician on a light box in the group setting (although some systems send X-rays electronically or just send the report), which was something that other patients also found very interesting, because patients seem to like seeing what their insides look like. In addition to X-Rays, other things (such as echocardiograms and removals of ear wax) can sometimes also be ordered during the DIGMA on a stat basis and reviewed before the session is over.

Patients Can Get Answers to Questions They Did Not Know to Ask

Another quality of care benefit that DIGMAs offer is that other patients in the session often ask questions that the patient never thought to ask, but the answers to which are medically important and helpful to the patient. Patients sometimes leave the DIGMA stating that the answers they heard to important medical questions they never knew to ask provided one of the most helpful benefits which they derived from the session. Patients often find this information to be both interesting and helpful and sometimes describe this aspect of their DIGMA experience as being similar to a mini-medical school class taught by their own doctor.

What types of issues are patients willing to discuss in a group? Patients often enter the group feeling alone and asking, "Why me?" However, they soon come to see that there are many others who share similar issues, some of whom are even much worse off than they are. While many physicians fear that patients will not be as open in the group setting as they are during traditional one-on-one office visits, actually the opposite is often true. A 2000 article in the Minneapolis Star Tribune quotes Dr. Mark Attermeier (a family physician at Luther Midelfort Mayo Clinic in Eau Claire, Wisconsin, who started a DIGMA in 1999) as follows: "Most doctors say the same thing: Nobody believes that it could possibly work…But it works very well… I'll talk about everything…People come in and talk about erectile dysfunction, sexual side effects…That's what groups do. They give permission for people to talk." The article goes on to say, "Colleen Skold, a psychologist who helps run group visits at Luther Midelfort, agrees. 'You'd just be surprised, I know I was, at how much patients are willing to talk in front of others,' she said." Pointing out that the DIGMA idea is catching on around the country, the article concludes by stating, "Attermeier says his patients do have something in common: humanity. They may have different problems, he said, but the issue of how to cope is the same. 'I want people to see that we're all in this mess together'" (14).

DIGMAs Can Help Underserved and Overlooked Patients

Physicians can use DIGMAs to reach out to underserved and overlooked patient populations, thus enabling them to provide important follow-up care to patients who have previously fallen through the cracks in the individual office visit paradigm. This is important because, due to backlogs, rushed visits, access problems, busy physicians, and overworked staffs, there is seldom the necessary time, inclination, energy, or capacity with traditional office visits to reach out and provide additional services to those high-risk patients whose needs are not being adequately met by the system.

For example, physicians can reach out to inappropriately low utilizers in their practices (one example might be those patients who have not been into the office for more than 2 years) by asking the dedicated scheduler attached to the DIGMA to telephone and invite enough such patients to fill a DIGMA session and have a "get to know each other and bring your injections and health maintenance current."

Along similar lines, the physician could ask the dedicated scheduler to telephone enough diabetic patients from his or her practice who have not been into the office for more than 6 months to fill a DIGMA session dedicated to "seeing how you are doing and checking your blood glucose levels." Likewise, patients that the physician has started on psychotropic medications—but who have not been back to the office for over a year—could be called by the physician's scheduling staff (or the dedicated scheduler) and asked to attend a DIGMA session to see how they are doing, so that they can be reevaluated and have their medications re-checked.

DIGMAs can also be designed to efficiently and cost-effectively reach out to other underserved or overlooked patient populations, such as the homeless, the uninsured, the urban poor, street or drug-involved patients, underserved minorities, inappropriate underutilizers, and possibly even some underserved geriatric patients on Medicare or Medicaid (because, as demand overwhelms supply, geriatric patients are likely to become increasingly underserved over time as baby boomers age and geriatricians continue to leave the field in droves). By enhancing capacity and reducing demand—and by promptly intervening

and better addressing the medical needs of these underserved patient populations—DIGMAs can increase quality to such patients by earlier detection, updated health maintenance, and readily accessible care (all of which can reduce the likelihood of adverse health risks in the future). By intervening in a timely manner and keeping a chronic health problem from escalating into a costly medical emergency, DIGMAs can help to reduce the future cost of care for these underserved, high-risk patient populations.

Some Things Can Be Done in DIGMAs That Cannot During Traditional Office Visits

There is no doubt that, for the most part, patients really like group visits, especially when they are properly run and supported. However, what is surprising to many is the fact that some things can be done in the group setting that cannot be done individually. Despite the fact that many physicians believe that the traditional individual office visit model of care in which they were trained and have been practicing is the best possible type of care, there are some things that can be done in a DIGMA that simply cannot be easily done during individual office visits.

Consider, for example, the busy, backlogged endocrinologist who has run DIGMAs almost daily in his practice, some of which are heterogeneous and open to most patients in his panel while others are quite homogeneous. Because he has such a large and busy practice, and one that covers a substantial geographic area, he is able to also run and fill some highly specialized homogeneous DIGMAs—such as a pediatric insulin pump group. These children often feel different. They might be ostracized or made fun of by other children because they cannot eat or exercise like other kids or because they are the only kids in school with an imbedded medical device. When he brings these children together from many schools covering three counties in his pediatric insulin pump DIGMA, there is instant bonding between them.

At the beginning of the DIGMA, he tells the parents to go to the lobby and have their own support group—and then tells the children to check their own blood glucose levels. Immediately afterward, he tells them, "I have a special surprise for all of you. Last night, I made homemade cinnamon rolls for each of you to enjoy. And, the one of you who is closest to 150 on your blood glucose level 1 ½ hours from now gets these two tickets to the theater this weekend." Well, that is an extraordinarily pleasant surprise for these young patients (for whom a doctor's visit has more often meant being stuck with a needle than a pleasant experience), who are suddenly and attentively calculating their carbohydrates and bolusing their insulin pumps. At the end of one session, a fifth-grade girl beat all the other patients, including some high school students.

The endocrinologist later commented that this was a quantum leap forward in the care that he was able to deliver because, in the rush of brief 15-minute office visits, he can barely say all that he needs to say. He does not know if the patients really understand what he is saying—and certainly cannot tell whether his patients are able to operationalize what he is telling them. However, in the pediatric insulin pump DIGMA he is able to see firsthand who understands (and is therefore able to keep their blood glucose level under tight control after a carbohydrate bolus) and who does not. He could even institute a buddy system wherein the young type 1 diabetic patient who gets it and is able to tightly manage his or her blood glucose level could be paired off with the child who does not. In fact, they could even contact each other outside of the group from time to time to help one another and see how the other is doing.

Furthermore, the patients in the group are all listening and learning throughout the entire session as the endocrinologist is sequentially working with one patient at a time in the DIGMA setting. How could you accomplish all of this during an individual office visit? Yet, all this can readily be accomplished in a well-run DIGMA with relative ease.

DIGMAs Offer More Timely Follow-Up Care

Patients can typically be seen in the DIGMA any week they have a medical need and want to be seen (or any day of the week, for physicians running daily DIGMAs), rather than being restricted to care by wait-lists, backlogs, and bottlenecks in the physician's regular office schedule. This improves access, at least for group visits, and translates into closer follow-up care being available to patients, as they can now schedule return appointments in a more timely manner. This improved access to group visits enables timely follow-up visits to be scheduled according to what the physician feels is best and most appropriate for the patient, without being limited by when the next individual follow-up appointment happens to be available on the physician's schedule, which might be weeks or months away. An additional benefit of this increased capacity on the physician's schedule is that continuity of care with one's own physician can often be increased because patients no longer need to be shunted off to mid-level providers in order to be seen.

In the extreme case of one heavily backlogged endocrinologist who began offering daily DIGMAs in his practice, he was able to offer his patients a 90-minute group visit any day they wanted to be seen as an alternative to initially waiting almost 6 months for the next available brief individual office visit. Soon, because so many follow-up visits were shifted to highly efficient group visits, individual office visits also became much more available to patients. Eventually, because access was improved and backlogs and wait-lists were eliminated, this physician was able to follow his patients as closely as he ideally wanted to. For example, he could even see them the following week if needed in order to see how they were doing after a major change had been made to their medication and/or treatment regimen.

DIGMAs Provide High Levels of Patient Satisfaction

Patient satisfaction has been repeatedly determined to be very high with the DIGMA model—often even higher than for individual office visits with the same physicians during the same time period. As a result of patient satisfaction being so high, physicians often witness a great deal of laughter among patients in their DIGMA (and PSMA) sessions (Fig. 3.2). The interested reader can find studies reflecting the high levels of patient satisfaction with DIGMAs in Chapter 9 on outcomes.

The following are but a few of the hundreds of examples of positive responses that I have received from patients over the years regarding their positive DIGMA experience:

- "I realize that I am not the only person with my type of problems. Dr.____ is very knowledgeable of each patient's problems and needs. Listening to other patients' questions helps me to remember questions that I forgot to ask."

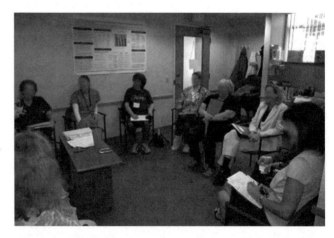

Fig. 3.2 Patient satisfaction with group visits is very high. Physicians often witness a great deal of laughter in their DIGMA and PSMA sessions. (Courtesy of Dr. Jan Millermaier, Women's Primary Care PSMA, ProMed Family Practice, Kalamazoo, MI)

- "It is very beneficial because questions you haven't thought of are addressed so that you'll know what to do if these things happen to you in the near future. It was very good and I was very satisfied."

- "Good to have both a doctor and a social worker present in order to better communicate in layman's terms. I like the 'teaching' of preventative medicine approach of these shared medical appointments. I give it a '10' overall."

- "You don't have to wait 3 months for an appointment with your own doctor. The doctor and staff were quick to resolve a problem with patient services that had been ongoing for a month. The visit overall was a comfortable experience with a more relaxed atmosphere than staring at four walls of a small room waiting for the doctor."

- "I was apprehensive about doing a two-part physical, but I enjoyed listening to others speak as well and thought of things that I wouldn't have thought of otherwise. I would definitely recommend this to other patients, friends, and family members. I got in right away and was pleasantly surprised considering I wasn't looking forward to it at all."

- "I recommend it for non-emergency, chronic health problems and plan to return. The presence of others with similar problems makes discussion with the doctor easier. I learned from listening to the others. An hour and a half seems just right. The atmosphere was relaxed and friendly."

- "We all had plenty of time to talk and share. There's a great benefit in sharing all the information. The appointment length was perfect. It is great sharing with others. One feels not alone with their issues."

- "My concerns were addressed very well. I went because of curiosity and with my several minor concerns. I was quite pleased that this type of service is available. I hope it continues."

- "I was so much better off than the rest of the patients that it improved my confidence...I learned a lot listening to the other patients. So I enjoyed the visit and learned a lot!"

- "If one is interested in overall health improvement for people, it is definitely educational. The fact that it is optional is good...It was helpful and something I would certainly try again. Great job of having information needed with no delay, using time well. Good preparation."

- "It was very nice to be with other people who have the same illness. I felt like the people there could understand my problems whereas other people have no idea what I'm going through. They are even on the same medicine. I also learned more than I would have in a short regular visit."

One example of how well the DIGMA model is able to meet patients' informational, behavioral health and psychosocial needs occurred when both rheumatologists at a large staff model HMO (one of whom specialized in fibromyalgia) simultaneously started rheumatology DIGMAs for their practices. Immediately after their inception, these two rheumatology DIGMAs drew virtually all of the patients from a previously successful fibromyalgia and chronic fatigue syndrome program—a behavioral medicine program that had been successfully running for over 2 years—which caused the program to fail immediately thereafter due to lack of census. In this program, which had previously been well attended by 10–15 patients each week, only 1 or 2 patients still attended once the rheumatologists started their DIGMAs.

These fibromyalgia patients simply preferred the venue of the DIGMA. When asked why, the answer they gave was a simple one: In the DIGMA they still received information about their condition, had the help of a psychologist, and obtained support from other patients—just as they had also received in the fibromyalgia and chronic fatigue syndrome program that they previously attended. However, they added, in the DIGMA they also had 90 minutes with their own doctor any week that they wanted to be seen and that, for them, this was the deciding factor.

Family practitioner Monica Donovan reports on her DIGMA as follows: "I believe that attending the group sessions can help people to build on their strengths, to pay closer attention to the positive aspects of their lives, and to make their medical care a more pleasant experience" (9). In another article, she states, "I actually enjoy the group more that I thought I would. Patients also enjoy the group. One patient who came to group was an obese lady with a traumatic hemipelvectomy and phantom limb pain. Because she was not highly educated, I was not sure how much of what transpired in group was directly relevant or understandable to her. To my surprise, she enjoyed the group very much. Perhaps the overall warm and accepting atmosphere was what she liked" (8).

DIGMAs Can Enhance Physician Professional Satisfaction

In an article in *The Permanente Journal,* Joseph Mason Jr., MD (who was then Subchief of Oncology in the Department of Medicine at the Kaiser Permanente Medical Center in San Jose, California, and Chair of the Northern California Kaiser Regional Chiefs of Oncology), reported on the enormous success of his DIGMA: "One of the biggest and most pleasant surprises of my medical career has been my experience with my Cancer DIGMA, which has provided a totally new type of service for my cancer patients. It is very popular among my patients, who receive a kind of support and education not easily possible within the confines of an examination room and brief individual visit. My patients routinely report to me their great satisfaction with the experience. As you can see, my DIGMA benefits my cancer patients in many ways. It improves their access to me by providing a weekly time when no barriers exist (not even a phone call) between them and me. It also gives my patients an opportunity to share their experiences and validate their predicament" (9).

In another article in which physicians actually running DIGMAs were asked to evaluate the overall impact that the program had on their medical practices (8), Dr. Mason stated still other unique benefits that his oncology DIGMA offered: "Emotional support is offered from the group's leaders and from other group members. Patients share much with each other—commiseration, helpful hints for coping with the burdens of treatment, recommended reading, and sources of supply for various items. Anger with, and distrust of, the health plan can be addressed and defused....At times, the group has made progress that probably would never have occurred in a private office session, no matter how much time was available. For example, one of my patients recently diagnosed with colon cancer was having a difficult time deciding about adjuvant chemotherapy. He had a clear understanding of the potential benefit of the treatment, but could not get a handle on the potential toxicity burden it might entail. Another patient was already receiving the same treatment and was able to provide a very helpful firsthand account. Their discussion allowed the new patient to make a better-informed decision than would have been possible otherwise."

Dr. Mason goes on to say, "Anger and frustration seem to be expressed more openly and naturally in my group because patients feel comfortable and safe there. This situation can often lead to accelerated resolution of related problems. For example, at one group session, two recently diagnosed cancer patients were both feeling considerable anger and were very vocal about expressing it from the very beginning of the session. By experiencing each other's anger and frustration—and by seeing the reaction of the group—they came to understand that their plight was common and that their anger about their misfortune was being displaced toward their physicians and healthcare system. What could have taken hours over multiple office visits was handled within about 20 minutes in the group" (8).

In an article in *The Permanente Journal*, neurologist Rajan Bhandari reported, "From a professional standpoint, I feel more satisfied in being able to meet both the medical and psychosocial needs of my patients in a very warm and relaxed environment. Having the drop-in format empowers patients by giving them freedom of choice" (9). In a different article, he reports on a professionally satisfying situation that actually occurred during one of his DIGMA sessions.

"One young woman had refractory complex partial and generalized major motor seizures since early adolescence. She had declined the epilepsy surgery offered to reduce the frequency and intensity of her major motor seizures. Her seizures had increased despite the patient's use of three antiepileptic drugs. Because she felt she could no longer work and feared that she would have a seizure in a public or social environment, she mainly stayed at home with her parents. When invited to attend my Neurology DIGMA, her initial reactions were panic and anxiety, but she and her very supportive mother eventually agreed to visit. About 20 minutes into the group visit, she had one of her fairly typical seizures, falling off her chair as several patients and I reached over to support and comfort her. After a few minutes, she became fully conscious albeit drowsy and confused. The silence in the room concerned me: What impact would this event have on her and the others? Did I do the right thing by inviting her? I could see the pained expression on her mother's face" (8).

Dr. Bhandari continued, "My fears were soon allayed as the patient rubbed her eyes, smiled quizzically, looked around the room, and said, 'I guess I won't have to tell you what I see Dr. B for!' The whole room burst into laughter. It was the best line she could have used to break the ice. The verbal and emotional support from other patients in the room, which she tells me has raised her self-esteem, clearly helped her overcome the fear and shame she felt about her illness. From my perspective as her neurologist, I can't imagine any other therapeutic endeavor—including prolonged psychotherapy—that could have achieved this outcome so quickly. From the perspective of the patient and her family, it would be hard to put a price on this group experience. She continued to visit the group about every four months and remained optimistic despite no clinically significant reduction in seizure frequency" (8).

With regard to the professional satisfaction that he derives from his DIGMA, C. Gregory Culberson, MD, states the following: "My neurology DIGMA has been the most satisfying new innovation brought to my practice during my 20 years with The Permanente Medical Group in San Jose....The results have easily surpassed my expectations. Patients' acceptance has been gratifying, both because of their expanded access to me as their neurologist and because of their positive experiences within the group…Patient satisfaction is high because patients and their caregivers leave with the knowledge that their medical issues have been addressed comprehensively, and without the time pressure that sometimes intrudes into the routine office visit…. Many patients have commented that the availability of my weekly group has given them the message that we are here for them and that they need not worry about receiving insufficient attention or about being a bother" (8).

Major Weaknesses of the DIGMA Model

In addition to its remarkable strengths, the DIGMA model also has its weaknesses. Most prominent among these are: (1) the model's reliance on the professional skills of the champion, program coordinator, and behaviorists; (2) the need to consistently meet pre-established census requirements; (3) the additional personnel requirements required (behaviorist, nursing personnel, documenter, and a dedicated scheduler); (4) facilities needs for a large group room capable of seating 20–25 and nearby examination room that is properly equipped; (5) the long list of additional support requirements (such as high-level administrative support, Patient Packets and snacks, quality promotional materials) that must be met for DIGMAs to yield full benefit; (6) DIGMAs represent a major paradigm shift that introduces much change and many operational challenges; (7) because of the dramatically increased productivity that they provide, DIGMAs can exacerbate any pre-existing system problems; and (8) physicians must adjust their care delivery style to best suit the group visit model (Table 3.4).

In addition, there are training requirements for a successful DIGMA. The DIGMA team as well as the physician and the physician's entire support staff must all be properly trained as to their roles and responsibilities. In addition, the physician must also be thoroughly trained in how to refer all appropriate patients into the DIGMA effectively, as well as how to overcome such program challenges as finishing sessions on time with all documentation completed (especially at first, during the initial sessions). Additional challenges include competing resource demands, the need for quality promotional materials, and the fact that DIGMAs are so counterintuitive that many beginner's mistakes (i.e., that can easily put the program at risk for failure) are commonly made. Failure to meet any of these needs could initially decrease census and ultimately undermine the success of the program.

Table 3.4 Greatest weaknesses of DIGMAs in practice

- Consistently maintaining targeted census levels is critical to success
- Selection of the best possible champion and program coordinator—and providing them with adequate time—are critically important (in larger systems)
- Successful DIGMAs require use of the most appropriate personnel, not the cheapest or most available
- Physicians must adjust their care delivery style to the group visit model
- DIGMAs can exacerbate any pre-existing system problems
- DIGMAs represent a major paradigm shift: they introduce change and many operational challenges
- The physician and entire DIGMA team must be skilled and trained
- The roles of nurse/MA(s) and behaviorist needs to be maximized
- A documenter should be utilized, especially when using EMR
- There are always competing resource demands
- The physician's entire support staff must be trained
- Effective promotion to patients is critical to success
- The physician must personally invite all appropriate patients during regular office visits
- DIGMAs are not appropriate for all patients and physicians
- Multiple operational challenges must be addressed
- It can be challenging to finish on time with documentation completed, especially during initial sessions
- DIGMAs are so counterintuitive that many beginners' mistakes are commonly made that can easily put the program at risk for failure
- Numerous support needs must be met
  - High-level administrative support
  - Personnel requirements—champion, program coordinator, behaviorists, nurse(s), documenters, and dedicated schedulers
  - An adequately sized group room is required
  - A nearby, properly equipped exam room is needed
  - Computers are needed for both the group room and exam room, and the IT infrastructure needs to be set up
  - Quality promotional materials are required
  - Patient Packets are highly recommended
  - Healthy snacks are recommended

Selection of Champion and Consistently Maintaining Census Are Critical to Success

Without question, the two greatest weaknesses of the DIGMA and PSMA models are (1) their critical reliance on a capable champion (and a rock-solid program coordinator to assist and support the champion) possessing a strong working knowledge of the DIGMA and PSMA models as well as exceptional professional and interpersonal skills (although a champion is only needed in larger integrated healthcare delivery systems) and (2) the importance of establishing, and then consistently achieving, targeted census levels in all sessions. Because the single most important key to a successful DIGMA is achieving consistently full sessions, *Physicians Practice* points out that "A DIGMA's success does not depend specifically on the size of a practice's patient panel, but on how the practice promotes group visits, so enthusiasm is important" (15).

Success of the DIGMA Rests on the Champion

The success of the entire SMA program rests on the highly skilled champion—plus the talented program coordinator, who works closely with the champion and attends to many administrative and operational details. The SMA champion typically needs to not only develop the initial pilot study but also move the DIGMA program forward from successful pilot project to organization-wide implementation. Because DIGMAs and PSMAs are census-driven programs, achieving full economic and psychodynamic benefit requires that *minimum*, *maximum*, and *targeted* census levels first be established for each and every DIGMA and PSMA that is launched (i.e., before each physician's first session is held) and that these census requirements be consistently met during all sessions thereafter. Staff at Harvard Vanguard Medical Associates/Atrius Health fondly puts it this way (and has even made T-shirts with this slogan on it): "Fill 'em or Kill 'em".

The responsibilities, prerequisite skills, and qualifications of the champion (and program coordinator) are discussed in considerable depth in Chapters 2 and 10, as is the importance of pre-establishing and then consistently maintaining minimum, target, and maximum census levels.

I have been to numerous medical groups who have failed to give sufficient attention to this issue of selecting the best possible DIGMA champion and program coordinator, and then to providing them with the necessary time to fully discharge their critically important responsibilities. As a result of not having a suitable champion (and the appropriate program coordinator to leverage the champion's time), and of not providing them with the required amount of available time each week, the group visit program fails to ever move forward from successful pilot to organization-wide implementation—in other words, the DIGMA and PSMA programs fail to thrive in such systems. The problem is that systems like these often have problems expanding their DIGMA program beyond a relatively small group of initial physicians. Instead of hundreds or even thousands of DIGMAs each week (which is where the organization could derive full benefit from their SMA program), the number of DIGMAs and PSMAs in such systems typically plateaus off at just a few (often less than 20 or 30). Furthermore, because the champion and program coordinator do not have the requisite time to carefully monitor the census of these SMAs, a secondary problem often also results in such organizations—i.e., inadequate group census.

Worse yet, many of these healthcare organizations have chosen to either have no champion at all or felt that the early adopters who initially started DIGMAs for their practices would somehow magically become champions later on. The problem with this is that these initial pilot physicians are often among the busiest and most backlogged providers in the organization and therefore the least likely to have the time and be able to take on this additional time- and skill-intensive responsibility. Furthermore, as discussed more fully elsewhere in this book, because physicians are often already fully committed to other duties within the clinic, they often do not make the best choice for DIGMA champion—except perhaps in the more limited role of overseeing the overall SMA program and reporting to the executive leadership team.

A Skilled Program Coordinator That Fully Assists the Champion Is Critical to Success

Another illustrative example clearly underscores the importance of also having a program coordinator to assist the champion and oversee group census in larger integrated healthcare delivery systems. I consulted with a large fee-for-service (FFS) healthcare organization with multiple medical centers for 18 months—flying out for 3 days once a month for an entire year and then for 3 days once a quarter for the next 6 months. I trained their physician champion and program coordinator, and helped to recruit various primary and specialty care providers at their various medical centers who were interested in running DIGMAs and/or PSMAs for their practices—and then helped these recruited providers in custom designing their programs. The DIGMA/PSMA program in this system initially took off well and continued to grow quite rapidly (and with relatively full group sessions) even after my services were no longer needed.

However, approximately 1 year later their program coordinator left the organization and was not replaced. Furthermore, they failed to secure the necessary dedicated schedulers. This resulted in two clear problems: (1) without a program coordinator to leverage his time, the physician champion now had to do everything, which bogged down his limited time dedicated to the program (limited because he also had a busy clinical practice to maintain within the organization) and ultimately resulted in a much slower rate of expansion of the program, if any, from that point onward; and (2) the group census began to drop off as a result of the program coordinator no longer being on top of group census on an ongoing basis to ensure that all sessions were consistently kept full (nor were there any dedicated schedulers to *top off* the census in these groups).

Meeting Predetermined Census Targets Is the Key to Success

Because different patients attend each DIGMA session, establishing and consistently maintaining three different census levels are absolutely critical to success. The *minimum census* level is simply the minimum number of patients in attendance that must always be achieved in order for the DIGMA to be successful, based on both medical economics and group dynamics. The *target census* (i.e., the number of patients that the physician would ideally like to have attend the DIGMA) is achieved through: personal invitations and referrals from the physician (which is most important); the physician's reception and scheduling staffs; and the dedicated scheduler attached to the program—as well as through use of high-quality, professional-appearing marketing materials. Thus, maintaining targeted census levels is critically dependent upon the DIGMA program being effectively promoted to patients. On the other hand, the *maximum census* is simply the maximum number of patients that the physician wants to have attend his or her DIGMA sessions, although the maximum number of patients may be somewhat larger due to the fact that sessions are typically overbooked according to the expected number of late-cancels and no-shows (less the anticipated number of drop-ins).

It is because of the critical importance of consistently maintaining pre-established census levels that so much effort in the DIGMA and PSMA models is expended upon ensuring that sessions are consistently filled. This includes all of the promotional materials used for the program (wall posters, program description fliers, announcement letters, invitations to attend, Patient Packets, and follow-up letters), the goal of which is to inform patients about the SMA and to persuade patients to attend at least one time—after which, experience has shown that the vast majority of patients (typically 85–95%) will be willing to return to the DIGMA setting, if they are only asked to return for their next follow-up visit. It is for this reason that so much effort goes into training the physician, the physician's reception staff, and the physician's scheduling staff (including on- and off-site scheduling staff, such as the call center) with regard to how to effectively and efficiently refer patients to the DIGMA or PSMA. It is also why the program coordinator generates weekly (or even twice-weekly) pre-booking census reports on all SMAs being held during the next 4–8 weeks, as well as an end of the week census report on the attendance that was actually achieved by each SMA held that week. This is also why a dedicated scheduler is attached to each DIGMA and PSMA in order to ensure that sessions are always kept full and *topped off* to desired capacity.

DIGMAs Require the Best Trained Personnel, Not the Cheapest or Most Available

Many initially believe that it is the behaviorist rather than the champion that is the critical factor in the success of the DIGMA model and consequently the weak link. As discussed previously, at least in the case of larger healthcare organizations, it is the champion—and the program coordinator that supports the champion—that are absolutely critical to the long-term success and growth of the shared medical appointment program. On the other hand, there are often several potential behaviorists that are available, at least in larger systems. However, in smaller group practices as well as solo practices, it is often the lack of an appropriate behaviorist and the required group room space that create the greatest problems for the DIGMA and PSMA programs. However, the lack of a group room can sometimes be overcome in such situations by using any other space that might be available, such as using a staff break room or the lobby during off-hours.

With appropriate training from the champion, there are many psychologists, social workers, diabetes nurse educators, nurse practitioners, Pharm.Ds, nurses, health educators, etc., who can occupy the important behaviorist position—although they will often require additional training with regard to fostering group interaction, managing group dynamic issues, addressing psychosocial issues, pacing the group, etc. Although experienced mental health professionals with a history of running large groups and working with chronically ill medical patients are often the preferred choice for behaviorists in DIGMAs, it is important to note that many mental health professionals (perhaps as many as two out of three, or so) will not have the motivation or skill set to successfully make this transition from mental health to the front line of delivery of medical care.

The role of the behaviorist in a DIGMA or PSMA is dramatically different from the behaviorist's role in traditional mental health groups because it is a more active, directive, structured, fast-paced, and self-disclosing role than is the case for most psychiatry and behavioral medicine groups. In addition, the behaviorist's role is focused upon helping and supporting the physician in every possible way, rather than on the behaviorist being the leader or doctor in the group.

It is equally true that many healthcare organizations around the country undermine and sabotage their DIGMA and PSMA programs by making poor choices for behaviorists—often by using the cheapest or most available personnel, rather than the most appropriate persons for the job. For example, I have personally observed healthcare systems choose a social worker instead of a psychologist, a counselor instead of a social worker, a nurse instead of a counselor, a medical assistant or health educator instead of a nurse, or even an unlicensed administrative assistant or clerical person on the physician's staff rather than the most appropriate person as behaviorist—all in the interest of trying to save money or using the most readily available personnel. I strongly urge you to avoid this beginner's mistake, one that can frustrate the physician (because the needed behaviorist support is not being provided), greatly reduce the productivity gain of your DIGMA or PSMA program, jeopardize the success of your entire program, and actually end up costing you more in the long run.

Because of their intense personnel and resource demands, SMAs are an expensive and complex form of care to deliver, although, when they are properly run and after experience is gained, one quickly finds out that they are perfectly doable and that they are not rocket science. As discussed in the financial analysis section at the end of Chapter 2, they should end up costing less per patient visit because of their dramatically increased productivity—as well as the long-term financial benefits that can accrue from improved accessibility, quality, service, education, continuity, satisfaction, and max-packing of visits. I say continuity because DIGMAs have been demonstrated to improve access, yet some systems are using other means that involve follow-up care being with other providers than the patient's own (such as mid-level providers) to improve access to care.

Physicians Must Adjust Their Care Delivery Style to the Group Visit Model

DIGMAs are quite different from the individual office visit model in that physicians must: (1) make optimal use of the behaviorist, nurse/MA(s), and documenter through delegating fully to them; (2) coordinate seamlessly with all members of the entire DIGMA team; (3) run the DIGMA or PSMA throughout as a series of individual office visits with observers; (4) keep the group focused upon the care that is being delivered to each patient in turn; (5) shift to delivering medical care properly for the group visit format without inappropriately bringing vestiges of the old individual office visit model into this new setting; (6) foster a certain amount of group interaction, but not too much; (7) remain cognizant at all times of the fact that there is now an entire group of patients and support persons (rather than just a single patient) to treat, educate, and always keep involved; (8) maintain ideal group census throughout all sessions, which involves personally inviting all appropriate patients seen during regular office visits; and (9) pace themselves to finish sessions on time, despite the fact that care must be delivered to multiple patients and that all documentation needs to be completed during group time.

These are issues that physicians do not need to worry about with traditional individual office visits. Physicians are often tempted to carry over various elements of the individual office visit into the DIGMA group setting; however, when they do, they often do so at their own peril. To be fully effective in the DIGMA and PSMA settings, physicians must adjust their care delivery style to optimally fit these group visit models (Fig. 3.3).

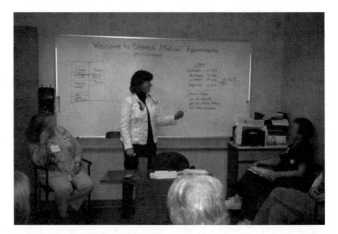

Fig. 3.3 Providers must adjust their care delivery style to optimally fit these group visit models, such as by addressing the unique medical needs of each patient individually in the group setting during DIGMA and PSMA sessions. (Courtesy of Dr. Jan Millermaier, Women's Primary Care PSMA, ProMed Family Practice, Kalamazoo, MI)

It is often best to start DIGMAs with physicians having busy practices and heavily backlogged schedules. This is because those physicians who feel hopelessly backlogged, and whose patients must wait weeks or even months to be seen, will typically have an easier time filling their groups and meeting census targets. This, of course, is provided that these busy, backlogged physicians remember to invite all appropriate patients seen during regular office visits to have their next visit be in a future DIGMA session. Such physicians can easily forget to invite patients because, prior to starting their DIGMA program, all that they needed to know about filling their schedule was to simply go to work—and their schedule for the day would automatically be full. In addition, physicians who are constantly repeating the same types of information and advice to different patients individually throughout the workweek are certainly able to benefit from a SMA, as that same advice can be given to numerous patients simultaneously in the group setting, and often in greater detail because of the greater time available. On the other hand, physicians with unfilled schedules and numerous unfilled appointments will have a hard time filling a DIGMA, and physicians unwilling to either invite their patients or put the necessary effort into designing and running their group will likely fail.

Two Contrasting Examples of Diabetic DIGMAs

I recently had the opportunity to sit in on back-to-back Diabetes DIGMAs (which also included a couple of pre-diabetic and cardiac patients) for two physicians whom I had previously trained and helped custom design their DIGMAs. These two highly talented and concerned physicians are among the most capable and kindest providers that I have ever been privileged to work with. I can safely say that their patients were very fortunate to have them as their physicians.

The first DIGMA, which had 11 patients in attendance, was a fast-paced, information-packed, cohesive, lively, interactive, and fun group experience that was enjoyed by patients, physician, and DIGMA team alike. Interestingly, a wealth of information regarding recent laboratory findings was well covered, but in a manner that was focused, succinct, highly informative, and interesting and never seemed to drag on or become boring. Having heretofore had a couple of months experience in running her DIGMA, this physician had already developed a talent for delivering care in the group setting, pacing her DIGMA, and fostering just the right amount of group interaction. She also coordinated with her behaviorist and documenter and succinctly presented

education points to group (i.e., in the context of working with each patient individually) in such a manner that all patients were kept interested and involved throughout.

Despite the fact that this physician was initially somewhat skeptical and resistant to the DIGMA concept (and had initially given herself only a "C" grade for her earlier DIGMA session efforts just a couple of months before), she now found herself enjoying the group immensely and giving her DIGMA a "B+" to "A" grade. Clearly, this physician had successfully made the transition from the traditional individual office visit model to the DIGMA group visit setting.

On the other hand, despite the fact that the second group had certain advantages over the DIGMA session discussed previously (such as the behaviorist starting the group 25 minutes prior to the physician's arrival, warming up the group, and writing down what each patient wanted to get out of today's session), the second physician's DIGMA, which used the same behaviorist and documenter, suffered from four major deficiencies which deleteriously impacted the session. First, this very conscientious physician (who was always willing to give her patients all of the time they wanted or needed and who was still very new at running her DIGMA) sequentially delivered the lengthy list of lab results from A to Z to each person in turn, without extracting commonalities and presenting them to the group as a whole and stimulating some group discussion. Second, she delivered these results and talked to each person in the group much as she did when she saw them individually, without fostering much group interaction, looking at the other patients, or asking such questions as "Who else has had this problem?" or "Have any of the rest of you found a solution that might prove helpful to others when they face this same type of problem?"

Third, she only had six patients in her group, which was significantly lower than the suggested DIGMA group size of 10–16 patients, which made for a group that was not only economically unsustainable but also boring (especially because the few patients in attendance had little in common and were not talkers). Interestingly, DIGMAs with far fewer patients do not seem to finish any sooner than larger groups of the recommended size, i.e., the work appears to expand to fill the time available. Fourth, because patients were bored, frequent distracting side conversations occurred between patients that the behaviorist failed to promptly address, with the result being that these side conversations persisted and made the session noisy and chaotic.

Because the same type of information was being repeated over and over to each patient individually (and without any group interaction being fostered), this latter approach, which was appropriate for individual office visits but not for the DIGMA group setting, came across as highly repetitive, somewhat disjointed, and unable to hold the attention of other group members. In short, the entire process soon became boring, tedious, and monotonous. It was made even worse by the small group size and the fact that over 40 minutes' time was spent with the first patient, who always seemed to have one more question and to whom this physician kept returning over and over (a group dynamic flaw that the behaviorist should have promptly addressed, but failed to do so). In other words, this physician failed to adapt her style to the DIGMA setting and instead carried too much over from individual office visits—and, in combination, this deleteriously impacted her DIGMA and threatened its success.

This was unfortunate because, if there was ever a physician who tried hard to give her DIGMA everything that she had to ensure its success, this physician was it. However, despite being extremely sensitive to her patients' needs and very giving of herself, her DIGMA was far from optimal. Even though much of the work that it would take to make for a highly successful DIGMA had already been done, this DIGMA session could hardly be described as successful, so more work was needed to resurrect and save this DIGMA program.

Fortunately, these problems were able to be resolved with relative ease. First of all, in order to be economically viable and have a workable group dynamic, the group size needed to be increased to at least 10 patients. Second, the physician and DIGMA team needed some additional training with regard to fostering the proper degree of individual focus vs. group interaction, which was easy to provide. Third, the behaviorist was given some additional training regarding techniques for promptly (yet tactfully) addressing distracting side conversations that might occur in the group setting. And fourth, it was recommended that whenever such Diabetes DIGMA sessions were held in the future (i.e., which involved discussing the results of numerous different lab tests), the information would be organized by having the nursing staff prepare a wall chart beforehand listing all of the patients' names and their lab values—and by having all abnormal findings circled in red. In this manner, the presentation of such tedious data can be briefer, better organized, more interesting, and in a format that identifies patients having similar issues and thereby encourages group discussion.

Each of the patient's names could be shown as a separate row on this chart, which would also include all of that patient's test results depicted in the various columns—total cholesterol, HDL, LDL, triglycerides, creatnine, fasting glucose, hs-CRP, ALT, TSH, homocysteine, insulin, C-peptide, HbA1C, etc. (Fig. 3.4 depicts an example of such a chart). Furthermore, all of the abnormal findings shown on the chart were to be circled in red. In this way, the test results could be efficiently covered for each patient in turn during the DIGMA session, but in a manner that would foster

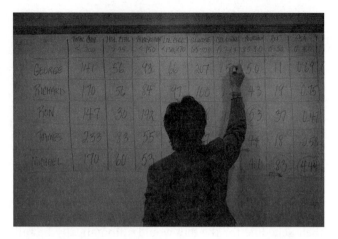

Fig. 3.4 To better organize data, and to involve all patients in the DIGMA, each patient's name and test results can be depicted in the various rows and columns of a wall chart mounted in the group room, with abnormal findings circled (typically in a contrasting color, such as red, so as to stand out). (Courtesy of Dr. Thomas Morledge, Men's Primary Care PSMA, Cleveland Clinic, Cleveland, OH)

some group interaction yet be much more focused, succinct, and informative—and with abnormal findings clearly standing out and catching the eye of affected patients.

Foster the Right Amount of Group Interaction

Furthermore, all of this could be accomplished while fostering some group interaction and making the entire presentation more stimulating and interesting to all in attendance—and without the need of repeating the same information to different patients individually. For example, let's assume that the first patient that the physician addresses in the group setting (whom we will call John) has a low HDL but high LDL, total cholesterol, and triglyceride levels. Then the physician could start off with that patient by saying something like, "As you can see, John, your good cholesterol (HDL, with the 'H' standing for healthy) is low, your bad cholesterol (LDL, with 'L' standing for lousy) is high—and your total cholesterol and triglycerides are also high. OK, listen up Steve, Mary, Linda, Paul, and Bill because you have the same problems. Notice that you have these same columns of numbers circled in red as well, which indicates that your findings are abnormal. Most of the rest of you have at least some of these problems, or else you soon might because these are common accompaniments of diabetes. Therefore, what I am about to say applies to all of you—so, listen up."

Then, while all of the patients are paying close attention, the physician goes on to explain the relevant medical issues to all of the patients at once—only one time, but often in greater detail. As the physician continues going around the group addressing each person's medical needs in turn, there might be some different nuances or distinctions from this more general discussion that happens to apply to particular patients in the room, and these issues can be discussed when the physician later deals with these patients in turn. However, the entire cholesterol spiel would only need to be made one time, but with greater detail than in an individual office visit.

In other words, while the physician addresses the unique medical needs of each patient individually in the group setting and others listen, it is important that some group interaction be fostered so that all attendees stay attentive and actively involved. However, too much interaction would slow down the SMA to the point where it does not finish on time, which would be counter to one of the important goals of all DIGMA and PSMA sessions, i.e., to finish on time with all documentation completed.

DIGMAs Can Exacerbate Pre-existing System Problems

Another weakness of DIGMAs and PSMAs is that they introduce considerable change, which can stress the system and exacerbate any pre-existing problems that might exist, especially given the dramatically increased volume of patient visits they introduce. These changes require proper facilities, personnel, training, promotional materials, and attention to a myriad of operational and administrative details in order for the SMA program to be fully successful, as well as an adequate budget and high-level administrative support. Also, these changes often prove to be more difficult to achieve in actual practice than they might at first appear to be.

For example, a slow receptionist might be marginally acceptable when one patient is registering at a time for a traditional office visit. However, when 10–15 patients arrive close together to register for a DIGMA at the front desk, such a receptionist can quickly become overwhelmed, the solution to which will likely require additional training, extra help during the registration process, preplanning, or a shift in personnel.

Similarly, if paper charts are only sometimes arriving on time for individual appointments (i.e., in systems still using paper charts), they will most likely also not be on time when 15 are ordered at once for a DIGMA. And when there are operational problems in the office, disgruntled staff who feel overworked, or communication problems between the physician and staff during individual office visits, these problems can deteriorate even further as a result of the added workload that accompanies seeing three times as many patients in a shared medical appointment.

Because of the added patient volume and the fact that SMAs do tend to exacerbate any pre-existing system problems, there is a need to both (1) make the necessary adjustments that would be required with any new program and (2) make the additional efforts required to address and rectify these pre-existing system difficulties that are already present (but to a lesser degree with traditional office visits) in the physician's practice. The good news here is that by solving such pre-existing systems problems, the entire remainder of the workweek (i.e., for group and individual visits alike) can often flow better for the physician's office, because these problems most likely had already been surfacing to some degree during normal clinic hours. However, the bad news is that if you fail to take the necessary corrective action, these pre-existing system problems could frustrate patients and staff alike, undercut the efficiency and effectiveness of your group visit program, and possibly even cause your DIGMA or PSMA to fail.

DIGMAs Are Not Appropriate for All Patients and Physicians

While appropriate for most patients, as discussed earlier, DIGMAs are not appropriate for all patients. For example, DIGMAs are generally unsuited for patients not speaking the language in which the DIGMA is being conducted, patients too demented or hearing impaired to benefit, patients who refuse to maintain confidentiality, patients experiencing medical emergencies, patients with serious contagious illnesses, those who refuse to attend a group session, and patients too shy, anxious, or inhibited in a group setting to benefit. Similarly, DIGMAs are not for all physicians, such as those who: are not willing to invest the necessary time; are unwilling to personally invite all appropriate patients seen during regular office visits; have unfilled practices and many open appointment slots; or are so resistant to the group visit concept that they are not willing to voluntarily run one. However, what is surprising is just how many physicians can successfully run a DIGMA program and how large the percentage of patients who can benefit is.

SMAs Introduce Change and Many Operational Challenges

DIGMAs, CHCCs, and PSMAs represent a major paradigm shift, introduce much change, and can present substantial operational challenges. They introduce change not only because they involve a shift from individual to group visits, but also because they represent a transition to a team-based approach to care. Physicians worry, "What if I say something stupid in front of 20 of my patients at once?" "What if I am asked a question that I can't answer?" "What if I lose control of the group and it spirals negatively out of control?" and "What if this whole thing is a mistake and I end up with egg all over my face?"

Billing Issues

In addition, billing issues for group visits are by no means completely resolved and CPT codes for group visits do not yet exist. However, with certain restrictions, many systems are billing—at least for DIGMAs and PSMAs—according to the level of care delivered and documented (as discussed in Chapter 10). Such systems are taking the view that DIGMAs and PSMAs (but not necessarily other types of group visit models) are being run throughout as a series of one patient–one physician encounters, with observers attending to each patient's unique medical needs individually. Billing for these two group visit models is thus being done according to the level of care delivered and documented using existing CPT codes—but not billing for either counseling time or the behaviorist's time (for reasons already discussed).

Physician Recruitment, the Multidisciplinary Team, and Running the Group

The entire DIGMA team must not only be well trained in their individual responsibilities but also coalesce into an efficiently functioning team. In addition, as has just been discussed above, DIGMAs must be run quite differently from the traditional individual office visit model in order to be fully successful. There are numerous operational steps involved in physician recruitment and in the design, planning, implementation, and evaluation phases of each and every DIGMA that is launched (See Chapters 10 and 11). Each step takes planning and time, and each step poses its own operational challenges and training requirements. However, all of these steps must be appropriately taken before the final product can be expected to fully achieve the multiple benefits that the DIGMA model was originally designed to achieve. It is for these reasons I say that, while achievable and by no means rocket science, DIGMAs and PSMAs have numerous operational, planning, personnel, facilities, physician recruitment, and support requirements that must be met in order for success to be fully achieved—therefore, implementing a DIGMA or PSMA program is not as easy as it might at first appear.

Change in the Culture of the Organization

The healthcare organization's culture can also be an issue when implementing a DIGMA program. For systems that are already using a multidisciplinary team-based approach to care, the operational challenges posed by DIGMAs and PSMAs will be less dramatic. However, in systems for which the culture is one of physician autonomy and not of a team-based approach to care, and where the individual office visit is the only modality used, the operational issues introduced by SMAs can be more challenging. Other such issues include the level of productivity already being achieved by providers throughout the organization (where providers in organizations with lower levels of productivity often find themselves having a more difficult time adjusting to the patient volume demands of the DIGMA model) and the organization's propensity toward innovation and change, such as whether it has already made the transition to advanced access, electronic medical records, patient-centered medical home, etc.

By instituting a SMA program, the organization is choosing to make an important long-term commitment to change in how care is to be delivered to its patients and how their business is going to be run. However, at the same time, it is important to note that SMAs are meant to always be voluntary to patients and physicians alike, so that patients preferring individual appointments should always be able to have them—in fact, because so many individual visits are off-loaded onto highly productive DIGMA visits, traditional office visits should also become more available to patients as a result of the DIGMA program (i.e., so that they end up benefitting from the program anyway). Similarly, physicians preferring to not run SMAs should not be compelled to do so, otherwise an angry physician and a lousy group visit will be the likely result.

Administrative, Personnel, Training, and Facilities Support

A weakness of the DIGMA model is the additional administrative, personnel, training, and facilities support requirements they entail; however, this is the case for virtually all innovations. Introducing any new healthcare delivery innovation that differs as much as DIGMAs do from traditional office visits will require high-level administrative support, without which the program will almost certainly fail. In addition, there are facilities requirements for a successful DIGMA program, which includes a comfortable, fully equipped group room of sufficient size to hold 20–25 people (with adequate ventilation, comfortable furnishings, and enough chairs) and a properly equipped exam room located nearby. Finally, there are significant personnel and training requirements as well as computer, electronic medical record, and IT requirements.

However, it is important to recognize that enough patients can be seen in DIGMAs and PSMAs to dramatically increase productivity and more than cover these additional costs (see the financial analysis in Chapter 2). It is important not to skimp on the required extra personnel (behaviorist, nurses, documenters, dedicated schedulers, champion, and program coordinator) as they enable the program to move forward throughout the organization and allow for sufficient patients to be seen to leverage existing resources and dramatically increase physician productivity. Because many sites and smaller practices lack the necessary group room space, they will need to either look off-site for appropriate space or make use of whatever space happens to exist within their facilities. No group room space translates into no DIGMA; however, a Physicals SMA might still be possible (due to their substantially lower census requirements and consequently to the fact that they can often use a correspondingly smaller group room). However, do not despair if at first you do not believe that the appropriate group room space is available to you, because one can often locate such space if one only searches available resources closely enough—which can include the possibility of using the staff lounge, cafeteria, storage space, or even the lobby during off-hours.

Every DIGMA Must Be Promoted Effectively

Because consistently maintaining full group sessions is the key to a successful DIGMA or PSMA program, to fully achieve the benefits for which the DIGMA model was originally designed, the program must be effectively promoted to patients—which, in turn, requires that high-quality marketing materials be employed. It is important that all promotional materials be appealing to the eye, have a professional appearance, and be of high quality, i.e., in order to accurately reflect the high-quality care that patients can expect to receive when they attend this innovative new type of care delivery modality called a DIGMA. An example of a particularly well-done wall poster is depicted in Fig. 3.5, and a good example of a program description flier is shown in Fig. 3.6. It is certainly not enough to simply photocopy a hastily drafted poster or flyer for the DIGMA program, scotch tape it onto the physician's lobby and exam room walls, and then expect this to draw sufficient patients into the program to meet predetermined census requirements. (Please note that examples of all the important forms and promotional materials required for a successful DIGMA and PSMA program are included in the DVD attached to this book.)

Because DIGMAs represent a team-based paradigm for delivering medical care in a supportive group setting, they differ dramatically from the traditional individual office visits that patients have come to expect. Consequently, an effective promotional effort is required to persuade patients to attend for the first time—for which the physician, staff, DIGMA team members, and all promotional materials must be properly aligned if success is to be achieved. Although it is an ongoing challenge to get patients to attend a properly run DIGMA the first time, once patients do in fact attend they almost invariably like it—and there is a high probability that they will be willing to attend a future DIGMA session the next time they have a medical need (16).

Failing to develop quality promotional materials for the DIGMA program in order to keep costs down is the wrong way to save money, because it will dramatically reduce the likelihood of full groups and success. Instead, initially invest in the development of high-quality marketing materials from the very start—but save money from that point onward by developing all such promotional materials in template form, so that these materials can be used over and over at minimal cost with all new DIGMAs that are subsequently implemented. See Chapter 10 for more details on the promotional materials.

If the Group Size Is Large, Focus Must Remain Upon Highest Priority Concerns

Although there is considerable time available during the session and much help is provided by other patients as well as the entire SMA team, it is nevertheless important for the physician and behaviorist to remain focused and succinct throughout the DIGMA as the time—while substantial—is nonetheless limited. Another weakness of the DIGMA model can be that, when the group size is large, the physician may not be able to address all of the multiple medical problems on the *laundry lists* that the various patients bring into the DIGMA session; therefore, the focus will need to remain on the highest priority items. However, as the physician then goes around the group and continues to sequentially address each of the remaining patient's high priority health concerns in turn, there is a good chance that at least some of these lower priority concerns will be addressed anyway. Also, if there is some time remaining toward the end of the DIGMA session, the physician can come back to the patient's unresolved concerns.

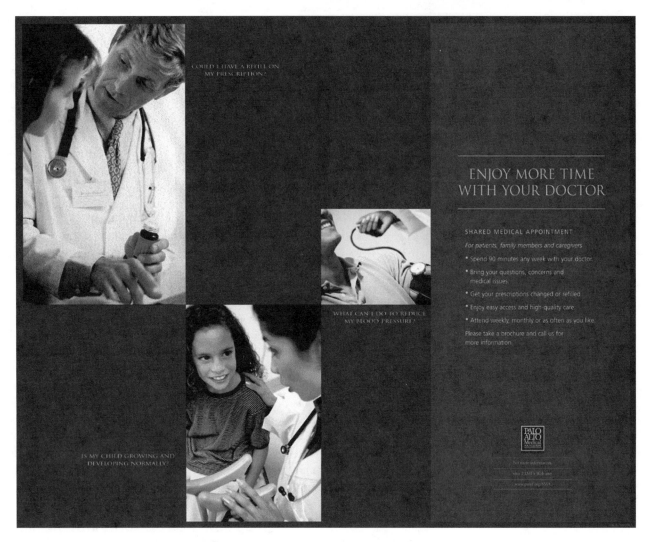

Fig. 3.5 All promotional materials for DIGMA and PSMA programs should be of high quality, such as this professional appearing wall poster. (Courtesy of Palo Alto Medical Foundation, Palo Alto, CA)

However, should some patient health concerns remain unaddressed at session's end, an advantage of the DIGMA is that any patients who might still have unaddressed medical issues after the session is over can always be invited to return to the next session to deal with these remaining issues. In reality, I have found that this situation seldom happens in actual practice (in fact, the far greater concern in general is that not enough patients will attend all sessions, not that patients' medical issues will end up going unaddressed). Nonetheless, it is heartening to realize that, in the event that the physician is not able to address all of these lower priority medical concerns during the DIGMA session, patients can always be encouraged to return to a subsequent session so that these remaining issues can also be promptly attended to.

Another heartening feature of DIGMAs is that, as the program continues to run over time and evermore of the physician's patients attend the group to have their *laundry list* of medical issues *whittled down*, patients eventually tend to come in more often for single-issue, focused visits. This is because such *laundry lists* are often symptomatic of poor access—i.e., since patients end up storing up many medical issues for their visits by the time they are able to get in and be seen—with the natural result being that, over time, these extensive lists are worked through in DIGMAs because of the improved accessibility that they provide.

Outcomes Studies Are Difficult to Obtain

Another weakness of the DIGMA model comes from the fact that, because patients only attend when they have an actual medical need, different patients typically attend each DIGMA session. Also, the DIGMA is open to most or all patients in the physician's practice or chronic illness program and could therefore include thousands of

Fig. 3.6 An example of a nicely done program description flier (one that is both informative and eye appealing) is depicted. (Courtesy of Harvard Vanguard Medical Associates, Boston, MA)

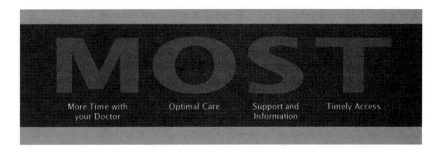

A SPECIAL INVITATION

**Patients can now attend a
MOST Shared Medical Appointment for their next medical visit.**

In a well-organized session with other patients, a MOST Shared Medical Appointment allows you to:

- Experience a complete medical visit...and more
- Spend 90 minutes with your own doctor
- Be seen promptly
- Receive personal attention from your medical team and others
- Feel listened to in a relaxed setting with other patients

Bring your questions, concerns, and medical issues to be addressed. Brief private examinations and private discussions are provided as needed. Participants are asked to maintain confidentiality for any information discussed in the group. The cost of a MOST visit is the same as a regular office visit. Your family member or caregiver is welcome to join you at no additional charge.

MOST visits are held weekly on Monday from 3:30 to 5:00 p.m. in Conference Room B.

To schedule a MOST shared medical appointment with Dr. XXX call Internal Medicine at XXX-XXX-XXXX.

When you arrive at the practice, please check in as usual, and you will be directed to your appointment.

Personalized care from your doctor in a supportive group setting

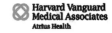

**Harvard Vanguard
Medical Associates**
Atrius Health

patients. Therefore, outcomes studies for the DIGMA model typically take longer and need to be larger than is required for CHCCs, where the same 15–20 patients attend each monthly session, and outcomes studies relative to a matched control group are relatively simple and straightforward. This is especially true of the heterogeneous DIGMA model in primary care, where the relatively healthy patient who comes in for a sprained ankle today might not return to the DIGMA for a year or more, and could then be coming in for an unrelated medical issue (such as sinusitis, tennis elbow, or an earache)—which could make outcomes studies considerably more time consuming and challenging than for CHCCs.

Outcomes studies are less of an issue with the homogeneous DIGMA subtype that is frequently used in chronic illness population management programs. This is because, even though different patients typically attend sessions, they all still have the same chronic disease or condition, which can make outcomes studies much easier

to successfully conduct. For example, because all patients attending DIGMAs in a diabetes population management program would have diabetes, measuring such outcomes over time as improvements in blood pressure, lipids, or blood glucose control—and then comparing these results to a control group receiving traditional care only—would be a comparatively simple matter (albeit not as easy as for the CHCC, where outcomes for only the same 15–20 patients who consistently attend need to be measured and compared to a matched control group). Outcomes studies regarding the mixed DIGMA subtype will likely prove to be of intermediate difficulty, falling somewhere in between the heterogeneous and homogeneous subtypes; however, such studies will likely be hampered by the fact that mixed DIGMAs often evolve into heterogeneous DIGMAs over time. Despite these challenges, outcomes studies are just now beginning to appear in the literature—many of which are included in the outcomes chapter (Chapter 9) of this book.

A Concluding Comment Regarding the Strengths and Weaknesses of DIGMAs

As can be seen from the foregoing discussion, DIGMAs have many strengths—but they also have their share of weaknesses. In this chapter we have discussed many of the strengths and weaknesses of the DIGMA model, often using real-life examples drawn from the author's professional experiences with DIGMAs and PSMAs in a variety of healthcare settings during the past decade and a half. Although they offer a remarkably potent additional tool in the doctor's *black bag* for better managing both chronic illnesses and large, busy, and backlogged practices, they must be carefully designed, appropriately supported, well promoted, and properly run to be fully successful. All of the DIGMA's strengths and weaknesses pose issues that must first be addressed in order to run a successful SMA program. Only then will DIGMAs completely succeed in achieving the multiple productivity, access, quality, economic, outcomes, service, and patient as well as physician professional satisfaction benefits that they were originally designed to achieve.

References

1. Murray M, Berwick DM. Advanced access: reducing waiting and delays in primary care. *Journal of the American Medical Association* 2003;289(8):1035–1040.
2. Armstrong B, Levesque O, et al. Reinventing veterans health administration: focus on primary care. *Healthcare Quarterly* 2006;9(2):80–85.
3. Green LV, Savin S, Murray M. Providing timely access to care: what is the right patient panel size? *Joint Commission Journal on Quality and Patient Safety* 2007;33(4):211–218.
4. Murray M, Bodenheimer T, et al. Improving timely access to primary care: case studies of the advanced access model. *Journal of the American Medical Association* 2003;289(8):1042–1046.
5. Murray MM, Tantau C. Same-day appointments: exploding the access paradigm. *Family Practice Management* 2000;7(8):45–53.
6. Noffsinger EB. Enhance satisfaction with drop-in group visits. *Hippocrates* 2001;15(2):30–36.
7. Noffsinger EB. Solving departmental access problems with DIGMAs. *Group Practice Journal* 2001;50(10):26–36.
8. Noffsinger EB, Mason JE Jr., Culberson CG, et al. Physicians evaluate the impact of Drop-In Group Medical Appointments (DIGMAs) on their practices. *Group Practice Journal* 1999;48(6):22–33.
9. Noffsinger E. Will Drop-In Group Medical Appointments (DIGMAs) work in practice? *Permanente Journal Fall* 1999; 3(3):58–67, with permission from The Permanente Press.
10. Noffsinger EB. Increasing quality of care and access while reducing costs through Drop-In Group Medical Appointments (DIGMAs). *Group Practice Journal* 1999;48(1): 12–18.
11. Cummings NA. Behavioral health in primary care: dollars and sense. In: Cummings NA, Cummings JL, Johnson JN, editors. Behavioral health in primary care: a guide for clinical integration. Madison, WI: Psychosocial Press, 1997. pp. 3–21.
12. Mechanic D. Response factors in illness: the study of illness behavior. *Social Psychiatry* 1966;1:11–20.
13. Mechanic D. Strategies for integrating public mental health services. *Hospital Community Psychiatry* 1991;42:797–801.
14. Lerner M. You, your doctor and a room full of strangers. Minneapolis Star Tribune. Sunday, November 26, 2000. pp. A1 & A18.
15. Donato S. Docs dig the DIGMA (Drop-In Group Medical Appointment). *Physicians Practice* 2001;11(3):A1–A8.
16. Bronson DL, Maxwell RA. Shared medical appointments: increasing patient access without increasing physician hours. *Cleveland Clinic Journal of Medicine* 2004; 71(5):33–37.

Chapter 4
The Cooperative Healthcare Clinic Model: Following the Same Group of Multi-Morbid Geriatric Patients over Time

CHCCs were associated with increased self-efficacy; better communication between participants and physicians; better quality of life; fewer health plan terminations and switching to non-study physicians; and lower emergency, hospital, and professional services utilization. There were no significant changes in function or health status. Although the only statistically significant difference in cost was for fewer ED visits by CHCC patients, the overall cost savings for CHCC patients over the 24-month study was $41.80 per member per month. CHCC participants also expressed significantly greater patient satisfaction in a number of areas than did controls.

From Scott JC, Conner DA, Venohr I, et al. Effectiveness of a group outpatient visit model for chronically ill older health maintenance organization members: a 2-year randomized trial of the cooperative health care clinic. *Journal of the American Geriatrics Society* 2004;52(9):1463–1470.

The CHCC Model

The Cooperative Health Care Clinic (CHCC) model was originated by Dr. John C. Scott at Kaiser Permanente in Colorado in 1991 and was the first of today's three major group visit models to be developed. I say "today's three major group visit models" because, whereas there are other SMA models out there (and undoubtedly will be many more in the future), these three appear to me to be the most widely recognized, essential, and basic ones—with such other less well known models seemingly being largely combinations, specialized applications, or offshoots of these three basic models. The DIGMA, CHCC, and PSMA models are the original and basic models upon which many others can be, have been, and will be built. The CHCC model instills deep social bonds as it offers exceptional continuity of care for the 15–20 patients fortunate enough to receive it, (although the actual CHCC group census achieved is often considerably less), because, in the CHCC, the same group of patients (typically high-utilizing patients as that is where maximum cost offset occurs) sees the same doctor and nurse at regular intervals. The CHCC was developed with the desire to improve the quality of care provided to high-utilizing, non-frail older patients. Although establishing homogeneous patient groupings by disease was considered initially, this plan was quickly abandoned as impractical due to the multiple chronic conditions that older patients so often experience. As with the DIGMA, it is built on the premise that care should be delivered by the most appropriate member of the care team, which allows much costly physician time to be off-loaded onto less costly members of the multidisciplinary team. Like other group visit models, patient satisfaction with CHCCs is very high. Patients enjoy socializing with others dealing with similar issues; like the amount of education and helpful information they gain; appreciate having more time to get their questions fully answered; enjoy getting to know their doctor better; and feel that their psychological and emotional issues are better attended to. Some patients even say that the friendships they form are closer than family, and that their CHCC visit is one of the things they most look forward to each month.

Both the CHCC and DIGMA models focus on return or follow-up appointments for established patients and provide a new model for the physician's office visit, although DIGMAs are occasionally used for initial intakes as well (especially when the intake examination does not involve disrobing and can be conducted in the

E.B. Noffsinger, *Running Group Visits in Your Practice*, DOI 10.1007/b106441_4,
© Springer Science+Business Media, LLC 2009

group setting, such as is the case for podiatry). Both of these group visit models are extremely effective at what they are designed to accomplish i.e., to improve quality, outcomes, education, support, cost-effectiveness, and patient and provider satisfaction. While the DIGMA and CHCC are both major contemporary group visit models, they could hardly be more different (both theoretically and operationally) in terms of their structure, staffing, flow, focus, strengths, weaknesses, and outcomes. It is interesting to note from the outset that these three independently conceived group visit models (DIGMAs, CHCCs, and PSMAs) are mutually supportive and enhancing rather than mutually exclusive.

Origins of the CHCC

In developing the CHCC model, Dr. John C. Scott (and internist and geriatrician), a pioneer in group visits and a personal friend for whom I have the greatest respect, used a group visit format to provide efficient, high-quality healthcare to high- utilizing, multi-morbid geriatric patients. This chapter, which has been read and approved by Dr. Scott to ensure that it reflects his views throughout, draws not only from his publications with colleagues (1–6) but also articles we have published together (7–10). It also draws from numerous personal conversations that we have had over the years, including during many presentations that we have made together to, international, national and regional healthcare audiences.

The CHCC Was Born Out of Professional Frustration

Born out of professional frustration, the CHCC model was developed by Dr. Scott in order to find a better way of cost-effectively meeting the complex and time-consuming mind/body medical needs of multi-morbid geriatric patients—needs he found himself unable to meet during the time constraints of the traditional office visit. He found that the group format not only provided an ideal venue for increased efficiency and patient education (since many patients could be learning from the educational presentation and group components of the visit at once, thus avoiding repetition) but that the group also made it much easier to gain a patient's trust and compliance, i.e., when treatment recommendations are reinforced by others in the group who have already successfully undergone the recommended treatment or lifestyle changes. He also found that a successful CHCC program requires real

and meaningful administrative support; however, in return for this support, the program provides a host of benefits. Like myself, Dr. Scott views group visits as being extended office visits that better address patients' educational, social, and psychological needs as well as their immediate physical needs—and notes that that group support enhances patients' well-being. Dr. Scott has also pointed out that group visits are designed to emphasize self-care and patient empowerment, and that in the process of interactively sharing information with patients, doctors often end up learning as much as patients.

What the CHCC Was Designed to Accomplish

The CHCC model was originally designed to provide better and more ongoing care for the same group of 15–20 high-utilizing, multi-morbid geriatric patients being followed over time, with the overall objective of reducing resource utilization and the associated costs of delivering care. As discussed in this chapter, enhancing patient education and preventative medicine, increasing self-efficacy, improving patient and physician satisfaction, decreasing referrals to subspecialists, and reducing costs (particularly major costs involving hospitalizations, emergency department visits, urgent care utilization, and skilled nursing care) are all goals of the CHCC model that have been achieved.

These older patients experiencing multiple chronic health problems are complex patients, and they often bring to their medical visits an extensive laundry list of mind–body needs that cannot be fully met during the brief amount of time allocated to a relatively short individual office visit. These wide-ranging patient needs can often be better met during the CHCC because of the greater amount of time available, the extensive patient education provided, and the help and support provided by both the care team and other patients. As with patients in DIGMAs and PSMAs, seniors in CHCCs have proven to be quite open to sharing experiences and to discussing highly personal issues in the group setting (including disability, loss of independence, feeling a burden to friends and family, death and dying, and end-of-life decisions), which has actually enhanced the patient–physician relationship.

In His Own Words: A Personal Communication from Dr. John C. Scott

Dr. Scott wanted to make a contribution to this book, which he has done very nicely in the following statement:

For the last 30 years the American College of Physicians has said that 90% of all diagnoses are made on the basis of history alone. During that time we have witnessed an amazing explosion of diagnostic and therapeutic technology. Ultrasound, CAT scans, MRIs, PET scans, gamma knifes, lasers, and a myriad of new drugs have resulted in the ACP now saying that 87% of all diagnoses are made on history alone. In other words, accurate diagnosis requires a good history of the illness, and that, in turn, requires good communication.

Unfortunately, the current model of medical care delivery is not structured to facilitate good communication. Everyone involved in medical care today is in a rush. If you are a physician who feels rushed in your day-to-day practice (or a patient who has been rushed), you need to read this book and put what it says into practice.

We now have the most expensive medical system in the world, tens of millions of uninsured, and outcomes for many disease states that rank far below countries that spend half of what we do in terms of gross national product on medical care. The Institute of Medicine has identified what they refer to as a "quality chasm" between the state of our knowledge and the day-to-day application of that knowledge. Patients are unhappy and, according to the Institute for Health Care Improvement, many patients are frankly unsafe—even in our hospitals. Physicians are unhappy in what should be a noble and rewarding profession. Burnout is rampant, beginning as early as the second year of residency, as reported in an article in the *Annals of Internal Medicine* (11).

What is the core of the problem? *Time*. There simply is inadequate time to communicate with patients. There are multiple factors at play: an aging population, the increasing burden of chronic disease, and a reimbursement system that seems to value procedures far more than history, education, counseling, and medical decision-making. As a result, the average primary care office visit in this country is now between 14 and 18 minutes, and often less than half of that time is spent face to face with the physician.

Research shows that four out of five people over 65 have at least one chronic condition and that the risk of disability increases with age. Furthermore, chronic disease accounts for 90% of all morbidity, 80% of all mortality, and 80% of all healthcare dollars. Yet we continue to try to meet the healthcare needs of our resource-intensive geriatric patients through the same old, rushed and inefficient, one-on-one doctor–patient dyad—a model that was designed for acute rather than chronic care, and for younger rather than older patients. Consider instead the many quality, cost, and preventive medicine benefits that group visits can offer to this challenging multi-morbid geriatric patient population: more time; better teaching; ongoing access and care; improved efficiencies; lower costs; improved outcomes; and a multi-disciplinary team of professionals.

In 1991, a group of six internists working in a small Kaiser Permanente clinic in Denver, Colorado, experimented with a concept, new to internal medicine but practiced for decades in psychiatry—the group doctor office visit (CHCC). Two randomized controlled trials found better outcomes, lower costs, and most importantly, improved satisfaction for both patients and physicians, and this concept began to take root in disease management programs around the nation. As a result, the disease-specific Specialty CHCC was eventually born, which expanded to various medical subspecialties what had been learned with CHCCs for geriatric patients in primary care.

The author of this book, Dr. Ed Noffsinger, developed another completely different model of group care in 1996 while working independently at the Kaiser Permanente Medical Center in San Jose, California—i.e., the Drop-In Group Medical Appointment (or DIGMA) model. He subsequently developed the Physicals SMA (or PSMA) model for efficiently delivering private physical examinations in 2001 at the Palo Alto Medical Foundation. All of these group visit models result in increased time for communication with patients and, more importantly, provide a forum for patients to communicate with each other on the subject of living with chronic medical problems.

The models have now expanded, encompassing medical issues from pediatrics to geriatrics. A quick check of the Internet regarding the CHCC, DIGMA, and PSMA models will give the reader an idea of the range of possible applications of group visits. Data regarding these group visit models exist (much of which is discussed in this book), and more is being generated every day—on enhanced quality, improved efficiencies, increased patient education, greater patient satisfaction, better clinical outcomes, and lower costs. These visits should continue to expand and play an ever-increasing and important role in the future of medicine.

Over the last decade, Dr. Noffsinger and I have both worked in multiple venues (American College of Physicians, American Academy of Family Physicians, Institute for Healthcare Improvement, American Medical Group Association, etc.), in multiple systems (HMOs, Veterans Administrations, military, academic, public, and fee-for-service systems) and in several countries (the United Kingdom, Canada, Belgium, Sweden, Holland, etc.) We have been delighted to watch the reception of the group visit concept evolve from hostility to healthy skepticism—and then to curiosity, and ultimately to enthusiasm. Research projects are planned or under way in areas as diverse as diabetes, Parkinson's disease, and hypertension. We anticipate more data will continue to be generated in the near future, and that this data will underscore the quality, efficiency, and economic benefits of group visits—and the role they can play in the future of healthcare delivery.

Ed and I both feel that group visits can play a major role in correcting many of the current deficiencies of our healthcare system. However, neither of us is so presumptuous as to believe that group visits are the only answer to our current dilemmas. E-mail, phone visits, interactive electronic medical records, advanced access, and other healthcare innovations still to come will all play a part in the coming changes to our delivery system. However, it is important to note that all of these other processes are still based on one-to-one communication. None of them takes advantage of the multiple efficiencies offered by the group; nor do they allow for the mutual support, education, patient empowerment, and adjustment of expectations that regularly occur in the group setting. It is group visits that accomplish that.

Group visits are truly redesigning the doctor office visit in a way that is exciting to patients, physicians, and healthcare administrators alike. Those of you who are reading this book—and are about to put group visits into practice—will probably agree that the rewards of our profession are more closely linked to our humanity than to our technology. As you are seeing in the pages of this book, there is a fairly large subset of patients who—once they have experienced the group visit process—actually prefer it to the traditional one-on-one office visit model. Physicians who have done group visits almost uniformly feel that it is the highlight of their practices. Medical and nursing schools need to modify their curricula to include the appropriate training and knowledge base needed for the emerging roles of these health professionals to facilitate and manage group visits. The physician–patient relationship is enhanced and, once mastered, the group visit process is far less strenuous than racing from exam room to exam room—i.e., to encounters that are all-too-often truncated and repetitious.

Is there a downside? Yes. First of all, group visits can be abused, and this potential abuse must be strenuously guarded against at all times—a topic covered fully in Chapter 8 of this book. Second, there are challenges in the area of reimbursement, especially with regard to CMS (Center for Medicare and Medicaid Services). Despite the accumulating evidence regarding the quality, effectiveness, and efficiency of group visits, Medicare will currently pay only for care delivered "one on one." They fear "fraud and abuse" (which some would say is the hallmark of the current system).

Both Dr. Noffsinger and I fervently believe that, because it is always looking for better ways of delivering quality medical care more efficiently (and with less cost) in order to leverage its own resources, no one has more to gain from group visits than Medicare. No organization, including organized medicine, will change from within. External pressure is the only force that produces change. Be that force. Read this book carefully. Implement its recommendations. And help to change our healthcare delivery system for the better (John C. Scott, MD, personal communication 3/2/2002).

Strengths

CHCCs are ongoing groups for older patients that are not time-limited. The CHCC model is the most intuitively appealing of all three of today's major group visit models because the same group of 15–20 high-utilizing medical patients is followed over time on a monthly basis, so that outcome measures can be made with comparative ease (i.e., by simply using a matched control group receiving traditional care for these 15–20 patients). Because the same patients attend regularly (some CHCC groups have already been meeting for more than 10 years), patient bonding can be very intense—bonds that are sometimes described as being stronger than family. Another strength of the CHCC model lies in bringing routine health maintenance current for these patients, and in the high levels of both patient and physician satisfaction. The many strengths of the CHCC model are depicted in Table 4.1.

Patients

In the CHCC model, the same group of 15–20 high-utilizing, multi-morbid geriatric patients is followed periodically over time in order to better and more efficiently meet the complex mind-body needs of this challenging, resource-intensive, high-risk, and time-consuming patient population. Because many elderly patients have difficulty driving at night, daylight hours are much preferred, if not essential. The CHCC format permits patients to share personal experiences, support one another, learn from each other (as well as from the multidisciplinary team), and to receive medical care that addresses existing medical needs while bringing routine health maintenance current. As with DIGMAs and PSMAs, one of the goals of a CHCC is to inform and empower patients, and to teach them to be partners in their own disease self-management—such as in taking their own blood pressures and blood glucose levels. Unlike DIGMAs, patients are generally not invited to bring a spouse or support person with them to the CHCC; however, because many elderly couples often see the same doctor, there are often many

Table 4.1 Strengths of the CHCC model

- *Continuity of care* since the same group of 15–20 patients is followed periodically over time by the same physician and nurse
- *Greater patient education and attention to psychosocial issues* in this multidisciplinary team-based approach to care
- *Therapeutic benefit of the group dynamic* as the help and support of other patients is integrated into each patient's healthcare experience
- *Increased patient empowerment and disease self-management skills* as patients learn how to take better care of themselves and to better utilize the resources available to them within the healthcare system and community
- *Decreased rate of decline* of independent functioning has been reported
- *Strong patient bonding* as the same patients meet monthly and the group can meet for many years
- *More time for the physician's other patients* because, by effectively dealing with some of your highest maintenance and utilizing patients in the CHCC, these patients do not need to occupy many 15–20 individual appointments—which frees up some individual appointments for your other patients
- *Improved doctor–patient relationships* due to the relaxed atmosphere, amount of social support, and greater amount of time available
- *Improved independence* and functional ability, together with improved perception of quality of life, have been reported
- *Increased patient and physician professional satisfaction*, with the anticipated consequences of better patient retention and decreased physician burnout
- *Reduced costs* (especially the big ticket costs) due to the reduced number of referrals to medical specialists and to reduced emergency department, hospitalization, and skilled nursing costs for these 15–20 high-utilizing, multi-morbid geriatric patients that are participating and being followed
- *Patient retention* because CHCCs have been shown to result in not only a high level of patient satisfaction but also a higher likelihood of patients staying with the healthcare system (thus making group visits not only good medicine but also good business)
- *Outcome studies are relatively easy to conduct* as one only needs to study the same group of 15–20 patients over time and then compare their results to a matched control group receiving usual care (which is a much easier study than for DIGMAs, where most of the physician's practice often qualifies to participate and different patients typically attend every session)
- *The CHCC model is evidence-based*, which is one of its greatest strengths, making the demonstrated outcome benefits of the CHCC not only important but also reproducible

spouses in attendance at a CHCC (as they are the doctor's patients as well).

Because it is specifically designed for serving high-utilizing, non-frail seniors with multiple medical conditions, the CHCC model seeks to achieve better clinical outcomes by enlisting patients as primary caregivers in their own care as well as for other group members. An essential ingredient to the CHCC's success is the tight bonding and close ongoing relationships that develop between patients. This is a natural result of having the same small group of 15–20 multi-morbid geriatric patients, who have much in common, meeting together on a monthly basis—sometimes for many years. It is these supportive relationships that contribute toward patients sharing information and coping skills, encouraging and helping one another, communicating more effectively with their physician and nurse, and developing very close interpersonal bonds.

Group Size

Much experience with the CHCC model has demonstrated that the ideal group size is 15–20 patients for three reasons: (1) groups having more than 20 participants tend to lose their group dynamic and the personal interactions that are so critical to success; (2) groups with fewer than 15 patients require too much energy from the

physician and nurse to keep the group dynamic lively and interactive; and (3) fewer than 15 patients translates into groups that are not economically viable due to the fact that there are overhead costs to the CHCC program (including 2 ½ hours of physician and nursing time as well as some preparation and post-session work). Since attendance has been found to be often between 70 and 80%, group membership must be a few patients larger—perhaps 20–25—in order to ensure that the ideal number of 15–20 patients in fact attends each session. This is because there is some attrition over time due to drop-outs, frailty, moving, and death—all of which requires a plan for occasionally recruiting and integrating additional patients into the group. Therefore, when you set up your CHCC, always strive to meet this ideal census target of 15–20 patients as it is critically important to the overall success of the program. The physician and nurse are encouraged to monitor census on an ongoing basis and to add additional patients as necessary to maintain both desired census levels and the economic viability of the program.

Confidentiality

The format of a typical CHCC session consists of an initial structured 90-minute group segment (with warm-up, educational presentation, working break/care delivery, Q&A, and planning for the next session components), which is followed by an individual care segment of approximately 1 hour's duration—i.e., for the approximately one-third of patients in attendance who actually need to be seen individually. While confidentiality is available to patients seen during the hour of individual care open to patients at the end of the group time, the same is not true for the 90-minute group segment of the CHCC—where patients medical concerns and issues are discussed both in front of other patients (especially during the educational and Q&A segments) and within earshot of other patients in the group room (as in the working break). Dr. Scott has found confidentiality to be less of an issue with CHCCs than for DIGMAs because: (1) the same small group of 15–20 patients attends all sessions; (2) patients make their own rules for the CHCC; and (3) because of the close social bonds that form between patients over time. While confidentiality is admittedly probably more of an issue for DIGMAs and PSMAs than for CHCCs, being conservative by nature, I would still personally recommend having all attendees sign a formal confidentiality release drafted by your medical risk department or corporate attorney—and then follow their guidance as to how often it should be re-signed (at the beginning of every monthly session, every 6 months, annually, etc.).

Staffing

The CHCC is usually staffed by a physician, a nurse, and outside speakers as needed, plus, in larger systems, a program coordinator to oversee the program and handle both operational and administrative details. Because physicians and nurses have typically not received specialized training in the skills reqired to facilitate and manage groups, they need to receive specific training in conducting CHCC sessions, especially in fostering patient participation and group interaction—and in not turning sessions into a class. In order to minimize costs, tasks are delegated to the most appropriate member of the CHCC care team.

Outside speakers (such as pharmacists, nutritionists, physical therapists, and health educators) are also brought in as part of the multidisciplinary team on an as-needed basis. For example, many CHCCs have added a pharmacy intervention component in which the pharmacist can talk about medications and their interactions, review the medications that patients are taking (which patients are invited to bring to the session), ensure that patients understand how to take their drugs properly, identify and resolve potential drug-related problems, and discuss how to appropriately store their medicines.

In addition, the nurse works collaboratively with the physician to monitor the care provided to CHCC patients outside of the monthly sessions. There can also be a physician champion in larger systems charged with the responsibility of moving the program forward throughout the organization.

When first starting out with CHCCs, the *see one, do one, teach one* minimal preparation method will likely work reasonably well. However, when more than five or six CHCCs are up and running (especially when they are in various facilities throughout the system), another approach is required. In this case, formal orientation and training of the providers and patients becomes more important—as does ongoing monitoring in terms of both quality and effectiveness. Experience has shown that a nurse administrator is often the best person to perform these training and monitoring functions, and that one such appropriate person can manage numerous CHCCs, especially with the help of a monitoring checklist.

It is also important to include administrative support staff and clinic managers in the CHCC, so that they become champions and ensure that the necessary nursing and physician resources are available to the program. If CHCCs are not fully integrated into clinic operations, and if key administrative leadership is not included in the CHCC decision-making process, then the necessary resources (personnel, supplies, and facilities) might be directed toward other clinic programs and needs.

Structure

The CHCC addresses routine healthcare needs through an interactive process of education, social relationships, and shared experiences, as well as care from the physician and multidisciplinary care team. Whereas routine care needs (such as injections and vital signs) are provided during CHCC sessions, urgent and emergent medical needs are still obtained as before between CHCC sessions. This expectation needs to be occasionally reinforced by the physician and nurse, who must monitor the group's utilization between sessions to ensure that patients are behaving accordingly and to offer appropriate coaching as needed.

First Select and Recruit the Appropriate Patients

Before the first CHCC session is held, the physician's practice needs to be searched for high-utilizing, multi-morbid geriatric patients. From these, patients will need to be recruited for the CHCC, either by personal invitation from the physician and staff during regular office visits or by sending them an advanced written invitation to attend. Dr. Scott recommends that you be certain to speak frankly to patients regarding your reasons for running the CHCC as they are bright, intelligent people who are now more informed than ever. They are fully aware of our healthcare system's shortcomings and that many of these are the result of financial concerns. Because many patients are seeking more satisfying alternatives to our current medical system, physicians may find it surprisingly easy and refreshing to openly acknowledge such issues as rushed visits, poor access, inadequate staffing, poor communication, less than ideal follow-up, etc.

Dr. Scott has found that physicians need not be afraid to state either their own goals for the group visit program or the organization's insistence that the CHCC be economically viable—which requires their full participation for the program to continue—as this motivates patients accepting the invitation to join to become allies by attending regularly and demonstrating the program's effectiveness. However, when inviting patients to attend, the physician must be certain to also explain the many patient benefits that the program is expected to provide (extra time, greater patient education, closer follow-up care, answers to questions you might not have thought to ask, the help and support of others dealing with similar issues, etc.), i.e., in addition to the cost savings that will enable the program to continue. It should also be explained that, whereas patients are encouraged to seek routine care within the CHCC, participation in the program is completely voluntary and traditional follow-up visits are always allowed—plus, emergency and urgent care should be sought between sessions as needed through normal channels.

Choose Only Those Patients Who Commit to Attend

Past experience demonstrates that approximately 40% of high-utilizing, multi-morbid geriatric patients from a physician's practice accept the invitation to attend, 20% are indecisive, and 40% decline to participate. Because these patients must make the commitment to attend sessions regularly on a monthly basis, the focus turns to the 40% who accept the invitation. Clearly, the greatest economic benefit will be realized by selecting patients with an unqualified willingness to participate in group sessions; therefore, it is best to

focus upon this group of patients. Regular attendance needs to be encouraged because of both its economic impact upon the program and the effective group dynamic and emotional support it creates. It needs to be explained that those who fail to attend regularly will be replaced by other patients from the physician's practice who are more committed to the program. This is because, unlike DIGMAs (where patients only need to be sufficiently motivated to attend a single session), patients attending a CHCC must commit to attend sessions on a periodic, ongoing basis—i.e., potentially, for many years.

Hold an Initial Session to Explain the CHCC and Have Patients Develop Their Own Rules

An initial session is then held to explain the program and to have patients develop the norms and rules they want for their group—as an important tenant in the CHCC is that the patients participate not only in their own healthcare decision-making but also in the development of the program. It is here that regular attendance should be encouraged and the rules regarding attendance fully explained. In addition, while not mandatory, the patients' active participation in group discussions should be openly sought. Patients need to know that their experiences, questions, and knowledge are not only helpful to other group members but also a key to the CHCC's success.

Structure of Subsequent Ongoing Sessions

Subsequent to this initial session, ongoing CHCC sessions typically have an initial 90-minute interactive group segment that is followed by an additional 60-minute segment of individual care in which patients needing to be seen are provided with an individual appointment (typically four to seven patients are seen individually each month). This structure therefore involves 2½h of the physician's time per monthly CHCC session. During the group, the physician can educate, foster interaction, increase patients' awareness of important symptoms (shortness of breath, chest pressure or pain, etc.), and teach patients how to more appropriately utilize the system, such as same-day appointments, urgent care, and the emergency department. The group component of these sessions is structured into several distinct segments; however, there is much flexibility as to how these segments are run and how much time is spent on each.

- **The initial 90-minute group segment**

  - *Warm-up* and socialization (approximately 10–15 minutes)
  - *Educational presentation* on a topic preselected by patients during the last session (approximately 30 minutes)
  - *Working break* (this is an approximately 20- to 30-minute-long working break during which snacks are served while vitals signs are taken, prescriptions are refilled, medical charts are updated (patients are given their own medical chart summary to take with them), medical care is delivered to patients individually by the physician and nurse, and the four to seven patients needing to be seen individually during the hour of one-on-one care that follows the group are identified
  - *Question and answer* time (approximately 10–15 minutes)
  - *Planning for the next session* (approximately 5–10 minutes).

- **The subsequent 60-minute individual care segment**

  - Once the 1½-hour group is finished, all patients are invited to leave except those that need to be seen individually during the approximately hour-long individual care segment that follows—typically, it is only approximately one-third of the patients (i.e., four to seven patients) that need to be seen individually.

Flow of a CHCC

In the CHCC, it is imperative that the physician, nurse, and multidisciplinary team foster group interaction and participate in group discussion in order to keep it from turning into a class. Patients typically sit in a U-shaped seating arrangement (i.e., a horseshoe seating arrangement that fosters group interaction) so that the educational presentation can conveniently be delivered by the speaker, and so that the physician and nurse have easy access to patients—as this arrangement allows the physician and nurse to go around the group from opposite sides during the working break to deliver medical care. During all monthly CHCC sessions, the same 15–20 patients attend the initial 90-minute interactive group segment—and, of these, approximately four to seven patients stay on an *as-needed* basis to be seen individually during the subsequent 60-minute individual visit segment.

Unlike DIGMAs (i.e., in which all care that can possibly and appropriately be delivered in the group setting is provided there, so that all in attendance can listen and benefit), in the CHCC, the actual medical care is still presented to patients individually—i.e., outside of the group setting, for both the *working break* and *individual care* segments. It is important to keep in mind that the CHCC was independently developed some 5 years earlier than the DIGMA model, so that the fact that it retains some vestiges of the traditional office visit model (which the DIGMA does not)—such as delivering medical care to patients one-on-one and in private, rather than delivering as much care as possible and appropriate in the group setting—is not surprising. The typical format and flow of a CHCC session is discussed below; however, it is important to keep in mind that there is ample flexibility as to how to structure the CHCC session.

Warm-Up

At the start of each CHCC session, there is an introduction and welcome where participants can meet each other, socialize, and attend to any group business and announcements. During the warm-up, patients are often paired off and given an exercise to stimulate discussion, a process that tends to become less formal over time—as groups become more cohesive and patients become more comfortable in conversing with each other. At early meetings, planned icebreakers appropriate to the group can even be used. Patients can be asked to discuss any of the following questions. "Where were you when Pearl Harbor was attacked?" "Describe the first Christmas or birthday that you can remember." "What was your most memorable trip?" This warm-up serves as glue that helps to keep the group bonded. It has been observed that as patients bond through the sharing of life experiences, they become more open to sharing their medical issues and personal concerns. Over time, the socialization time gradually becomes less formal and more informal, so that vacation stories or even favorite jokes can be told. During these 10–15 minutes that are spent developing a tightly knit group and a sense of community, you can hear the intensity of the discussion escalate as patients get to know each other better.

I have personally witnessed this phenomenon several times during joint presentations that John and I have given together in which we had the healthcare audience participate in mock CHCC, DIGMA, and PSMA sessions. When Dr. Scott started his CHCC demonstration, he would often ask the audience to pair off and discuss what college was like for them—or what they remember about what Christmas was like when they were a child. While the room would often be relatively quiet at first, the noise of people talking would slowly but steadily rise until it hit a crescendo within approximately 10 minutes, after which we would actually have a difficult time getting these healthcare professionals to stop talking, because they were enjoying themselves so much.

Educational Presentation

The warm-up is followed by an educational presentation that is approximately 30 minutes long—and on a topic that has been selected by the patients during the previous session (although there are several core topics that are covered during the first year and repeated as needed thereafter). It is here that possible solutions and coping strategies for the patients' medical issues and concerns are discussed. The educational presentation (which often includes topics not always discussed during traditional office visits) can be given by the physician, nurse, or a guest speaker—such as a pharmacist, nutritionist, physical therapist, audiologist, occupational therapist, or individuals representing community resources. For every CHCC, there is a formal core set of topics that is covered at various times during the first year: patient care notebooks; routine health maintenance; pharmacy brown bags; living wills and advanced directives; use of emergency services; long-term care; etc. During the pharmacy brown bag presentation, patients are asked to bring all of their medications (including any over-the-counter drugs) in a brown bag so that the pharmacologist who comes in as the guest speaker for the session can individually go over the contents of each patient's brown bag.

Later on, patients begin to select their own topics, such as: how to avoid falls; proper medication use and storage; how to eat properly during holidays; cardiovascular signs and symptoms among the elderly; nutrition and exercise; Medicare policies and coverage; control of chronic pain; stress, depression, and relaxation techniques; grief and loss; sleep disorders; and end-of-life issues. Patients are encouraged to share personal experiences and coping strategies during this time, and to bring their own unique thoughts and solutions to the group. The group leader (physician, physician assistant, nurse practitioner, pharmacist, health educator, social worker, nutritionist, etc.) fosters interaction, draws together and organizes what is being said, emphasizes important points, tactfully corrects any misinformation that is being shared, and adds additional information as appropriate. Patients can also work on commitments to their own disease self-management and specific lifestyle goals (such as regular exercise, smoking cessation, or dietary changes). They can also write down their goals and keep a log or journal to bring into subsequent sessions—i.e., containing specific behavioral changes that they are committed to making, and how well they are doing at keeping their commitments.

Working Break (and Delivery of Medical Care)

Next comes the most active and essential part of the group segment of the CHCC, which is inappropriately referred to either as the *break* or the *working break*. During this coffee break and socialization period, snacks are served for all to enjoy—often snacks brought in by the patients themselves (by designated members of the group). During this approximately 20- to 30-minute working break and care delivery segment, the nurse or medical assistant goes down one side of the U-shaped gathering, while the physician goes down the other, delivering care to patients individually. Any of the following can be done with regard to all patients at this time (i.e., while other patients are eating snacks and talking with one another): vital signs can be taken; injections given; prescriptions refilled; body mass index measurements taken; urine samples collected; routine tests ordered; any lab and X-ray results discussed, certain referral forms signed; medical records updated; forms filled out for everything from durable medical equipment to parking stickers; and certain medical issues addressed individually by the physician and nurse (such as those all-too-common "Oh, by the way, doc" issues).

Thus, a good half hour of the CHCC session is dedicated to one-on-one care within the group (during the working break and care delivery segment), with care thus being given and documented during the group session; however, this medical care is delivered to patients individually, while others are socializing—i.e., not in front of each other in the group setting (like DIGMAs and PSMAs), where efficiency can be gained, repetition avoided, and all present can simultaneously listen and learn. Individual medical records are available and updated, along with everyone's personal care notebooks (as every patient is given a personal care notebook which is updated during each session). The personal care notebook is a mini-chart that should be part of any CHCC model. It contains the problem list, medication list, last EKG, disease management guidelines when appropriate, health maintenance chart, and advance directives. Patients are asked to keep this record themselves and to update it as appropriate. It is really a part of the "Cooperative" in "Cooperative Health Care Clinic" as it involves patients in the monitoring of their care.

The physician and nurse also make note of any patient questions and address them during the 10- to 15-minute question and answer period that follows—so that all present can benefit from the answers and discussion that ensues. It is at this time (i.e., during the working break segment of the visit) that the determination is made as to which patients will need to be seen individually during the hour of individualized care that will follow the group session. Although patients might occasionally be asked to schedule a traditional individual office visit with the physician, most of the time patients' medical issues can be appropriately addressed during the hour of individual care that follows the 90-minute group session.

Question and Answer Period

The working break is followed by a highly interactive question and answer period that addresses such topics as issues presented during the educational presentation, the latest pharmaceutical ads, medical stories in the mass media, and any personal questions that patients might have. This is an informal 10- to 15-minute question and answer period led by the physician during which patients' questions are answered in the group setting—where all can listen and learn—while group interaction between patients is fostered. Typically, there are many questions that focus upon the educational topic presented earlier in the CHCC session.

Planning for the Next Session

Immediately after the question and answer portion, the patients spend approximately 5–10 minutes setting up the next meeting. They discuss who will be responsible for bringing snacks as well as what topic they would like to have addressed during the educational presentation of the next session. The subject to be covered can include any of a number of core topics that each CHCC strives to cover during the first year, or it can focus upon any subject of mutual interest to the various group members.

The Individual Visit Segment (Which Follows the Group)

The 90-minute group segment of the CHCC session is then followed by up to 60 minutes of individual care for the four to seven patients in attendance needing it, while other patients, who only need to attend the group segment, leave once the group is over. It is here, during the final hour of the typically 2½-hour CHCC session that the physician provides individual medical visits—i.e., for those patients the physician deems appropriate to be seen, patients expressing the need to be seen, and patients due for their routine health maintenance visit. During this individual care segment, the exact same care is typically provided (i.e., but only to approximately one-third of the patients attending the group while the others go home) to one patient at a time in the CHCC setting as is delivered during a traditional office visit. The intent is for each patient to be seen individually in the CHCC approximately four times a year. Roughly half of these patients are seen for intervening illnesses or flares in chronic conditions, with the other half being seen for routine health maintenance (e.g., routine checks for diabetes, heart disease, or for physical examinations). As with traditional office visits, care is delivered to patients individually during the individual visit segment—i.e., apart from the other group members.

In a 2004 article in *Private Practice Success*, Dr. Scott discusses the individual visit segment of the CHCC in the following manner. "'At that point, it's back to just the plain old doctor visit except you don't have to redo the social piece and you've got all the questions answered already,' Scott says. 'And since patients know that they're coming back, they don't bother you with a laundry list of worries and concerns.'.... 'CHCC takes you off the treadmill and gets you thinking about your patients,' Scott says. 'This is one way to enrich and enliven your practice and bring back some of the joy of practicing medicine'" (12).

The Specialty CHCC Subtype

Just as the DIGMA and PSMA models have their heterogeneous, mixed, and homogeneous subtypes, the CHCC model (which was designed for high utilizing, multimorbid geriatric patients) has its own unique subtype as well—i.e., the Specialty CHCC, which shares many of the characteristics of the original CHCC model, but is used in the various medical specialties. In addition to multi-morbid geriatric patients in primary care, the CHCC model has proven to be versatile and adaptable to many disease states and conditions, and has also been used in the management of various chronic illnesses. The CHCC model has thus evolved to include the Specialty CHCC subtype, which is generally applied to the medical subspecialties. There is considerable flexibility in how one designs their CHCC or Specialty CHCC, for example, by having some individual care prior to the group as well as after. Nothing is *set in concrete*, so you have a great deal of freedom to design your CHCC or Specialty CHCC in such a way that it best meets your—and your patients'—needs. In the Specialty CHCC subtype of the CHCC model (which is sometimes referred to as the disease-specific CHCC, and is used in various medical subspecialties) the patients in attendance are usually experiencing the same diagnosis or health condition (e.g., diabetes, asthma, hypertension, hyperlipidemia, congestive heart failure, COPC, fibromyalgia, well baby checks, depression, orthopedic pre- and post-op visits, and irritable bowel syndrome).

Specialty CHCCs and CHCCs Share Many Similarities

Like the original CHCC model, Specialty CHCC sessions follow the same group of patients over time and have a similarly structured format: (1) a 90-minute group segment (with warm-up, educational presentation, care delivery, question and answer, and planning for the next session segments); followed by (2) approximately 60 minutes of individual care for those needing it. Like CHCCs, Specialty CHCCs often focus upon high-utilizing patients because that is where the maximum economic cost offset occurs—and thus where optimal financial benefit can be realized. Like other group visit models, CHCCs and Specialty CHCCs also offer a multidisciplinary team-based approach to care as well as the help and support of other patients integrated into each patient's healthcare experience. Furthermore, they provide a venue that can be most helpful in eliciting critical missing pieces of medical history, in addressing key lifestyle and disease self-management issues, in prioritizing medical interventions, and in tracking health maintenance and disease management protocols.

Specialty CHCCs and CHCCs Also Have Important Differences

However, Specialty CHCCs differ as to the types of patients in attendance (patients in the various medical subspecialties vs. multi-morbid geriatric patients in primary care), the duration of the program (which might be time-limited with the Specialty CHCC as opposed to ongoing monthly sessions with the CHCC), the frequency with which sessions are held, and possibly even as to content. In the Specialty CHCC, the sessions might be held irregularly according to best practices guidelines (i.e., rather than monthly, like CHCCs), and a provider other

than the patient's own physician might be used. Despite these differences, the disease-specific CHCC still resembles the geriatric CHCC group in many ways. However, there is considerable flexibility as to how the Specialty CHCC is structured (such as the individual care being delivered at the beginning, rather than at the end, of the session).

For example, a Specialty CHCC for hypertension might be designed to meet monthly for the first 3 months, then to meet again in 6 months, and finally to have follow-up meetings after 1 and 2 years. While older patients with multiple medical problems might enjoy ongoing monthly meetings and benefit from interacting frequently with other patients and the CHCC healthcare team, younger and healthier working patients will likely not need this intense level of contact and support. Unlike traditional CHCCs for high-utilizing seniors, Specialty CHCCs are generally designed for patients of any age having a specific medical condition.

Another difference is that, with the Specialty CHCC, continuity of practitioners or patients within the group is not essential to improved outcomes like it is for the traditional CHCC model. In addition, the emotional support provided is often less important than the educational component. Instead, the primary purpose of the Specialty CHCC is to deliver disease- or condition-specific care and information to patients as efficiently as possible. Specialty CHCCs can be used to address the quality assurance mandates of health plan administrators, which Dr. Scott points out is important because disease management guidelines sometimes seem to be proliferating faster than physicians' can read—let alone implement—them, and reporting requirements (such as Healthcare Effectiveness Data and Information Set) are proliferating rapidly as well.

Because they are run by medical subspecialists (or else including specialists as guest speakers), the Specialty CHCC can be an excellent venue for implementing these guidelines—as well as for involving patients in their own disease self-management and monitoring their own compliance. While the Specialty CHCC format might vary according to the needs of various diagnostic groups (so that frequency, content, staffing, and duration may differ accordingly), the key components of the CHCC program still apply and can result in improved quality of care, increased patient and physician satisfaction, and contained costs.

Charting

A goal of all group visits, including the CHCC and the Specialty CHCC subtype, is to start and finish on time—and, whenever possible, to have all charting completed by the end of the session. Therefore, when starting any new group visit program, it is important to consider how an individual progress note will be completed for each patient during group time. For CHCCs and Specialty CHCCs, charting is often a relatively straightforward matter because the personal charts provided for each patient are individually updated during the working break of the session—i.e., while the nurse circulates among the patients checking vital signs and providing injections, and the physician goes around the group determining who needs to be seen individually during the hour that follows the group. Individual care delivered to patients during the hour-long individual visit segment (i.e., which follows CHCC and Specialty CHCC group sessions) is typically documented for patients just as it is for traditional office visits.

Outcome Data for CHCCs

CHCCs can improve quality, patient education, patient satisfaction, and the bottom line. They can also reduce redundancy and utilization, and accomplish all this while simultaneously enhancing outcomes. One of the advantages of the CHCC model is that it is evidence based, with two independent clinical trials having been published that confirm better outcomes, lower costs, increased patient and physician satisfaction, and higher retention (1,4). I have had the pleasure of personally co-presenting to various medical audiences with Dr. Scott many times, during which he discussed the major positive advantages of the CHCC as well as the impressive results of these two research studies. As previously mentioned, the fact that the same 15-20 patients are followed over time makes it a comparatively easy matter to compare utilization and clinical outcome data on these CHCC/Specialty CHCC patients with a matched control group receiving ordinary care.

The First CHCC Randomized Control Study

This initial CHCC study was a 1-year randomized controlled research study that was funded by a Kaiser Permanente Garfield research grant (4). The objective of this study was to compare the impact of CHCC group outpatient care to traditional office visit care for non-frail, chronically ill, older adults who were high utilizers of healthcare services—i.e., by looking at health services utilization, cost, self-reported health status, and physician as well a patient satisfaction. For the CHCC experimental group, the pilot randomly selected 160 non-frail geriatric

patients with chronic conditions who were over 65 years of age and high utilizers of both inpatient and outpatient services during the past 12 months—e.g., one or more outpatient visits per month and one or more calls to the nurse or physician every 2 months. The control group consisted of another 161 patients over age 65 who received traditional care.

Important Statistically Significant Results Were Obtained

Statistically significant outcome measures obtained after 1 year of follow-up showed fewer emergency room visits (0.41 for the CHCC group vs. 0.67 for the control group), specialist MD visits (3.22 vs. 3.95), and repeat hospital admissions (1.43 vs. 1.89). They also showed more phone calls to the nurse (8.7 vs. 7.89) and fewer physician calls (1.4 vs. 2.53), a larger percentage of CHCC patients receiving influenza (81 vs. 64%) and pneumonia (20 vs. 4%) vaccinations, as well as greater patient and physician satisfaction with CHCC vs. traditional care—all of which were statistically significant at the $P = 0.05$ level. There were no differences between groups on self-reported health and functional status; however, the overall cost of care was reduced by \$14.79 per member per month for the CHCC group—a reduction in cost largely attributable to the high cost items of ER visits as well as repeat hospitalizations and SNF utilization (3 vs. 7%, although this SNF utilization result was not statistically at the 0.05 level) (4).

These Results Have Important Public Policy Ramifications

With baby boomers rapidly emerging as geriatric patients, there is a great need to develop innovative new methods of care delivery that are effective, highly efficient, and cost-effective for this rapidly growing elderly patient population. What is needed is a realistic alternative to the traditional individual office visit, as these office visits lack the benefits of a multidisciplinary team, the help and support of other patients, and the ability to efficiently deliver health information to chronically ill geriatric patients—all of which are clear benefits of the CHCC. Furthermore, the rushed individual office visit is viewed by many as not being that well suited to addressing the multiple, time-consuming medical needs of an aging patient population during the allotted time. Pointing out that the rapidly growing population of multi-morbid geriatric patients already consumes a disproportionate share of outpatient and inpatient healthcare dollars, the authors make clear the importance of this study. As a result of this study, the authors conclude that CHCC care for high-utilizing, chronically ill, non-frail geriatric patients can simultaneously reduce ED visits, visits to subspecialists, repeat hospitalizations, and the cost of care as compared to traditional office visit care—while also delivering some preventive services more effectively, and increasing both patient (with 49% of the CHCC group vs. 27% of controls rating their visit as *excellent*) and physicians satisfaction (4).

There Are Two Concerns with This Study

There were two items of concern to me with regard to this study, both of which undoubtedly reduced the overall economic benefit of the CHCC program in this study. First of all, the average attendance in CHCC groups was only eight patients, which is a far cry from the targeted ideal group size of 15–20 patients. Second, the no-show rate was very high, with patients only attending approximately 55% of the scheduled CHCC sessions—which is a problem for CHCCs, as they are designed for consistent attendance and ongoing continuity of care (4–6). In fact, 13% of patients randomly assigned to the CHCC group never attended a single session, and another 12% dropped out before the 1-year study ended. Clearly, since the success of group visit programs ultimately rests in large part on consistently meeting predetermined census targets, every necessary effort must be expended to ensure that you have full group sessions at all times.

The Second CHCC Randomized Control Study

Dr. Scott and his team next conducted a larger study using a sample of just under 300 patients that were studied over a longer period of time (2 years) in order to validate the results of the earlier 1-year pilot study discussed above (1). The goals of this study were to compare the effectiveness of the CHCC with usual care for pre-frail, older patients with chronic conditions. This replication study was larger in scale, involving 19 (vs. 6) physician-led CHCC groups and a 2 (vs. 1)-year time period. The results reported were for that subset of 294 patients (i.e., 37.1% of the 793 patients who agreed to participate in the study, of whom 145 were in the CHCC experimental group whereas 149 were in the usual care group) who, before enrollment and randomization, expressed "strong interest" in participating in a CHCC. A computer-generated random number sequence was used to randomize the study patients between CHCC and usual care, with randomization being done within each of the 19 participating physicians' group of patients in order to control for differences in practice styles. CHCCs were employed in which study patients met with their own primary care provider and nurse on a monthly basis. No significant differences existed on any of the demographic and baseline measures for the experimental and control groups.

The Results of This Second Study Also Demonstrated Important Findings

This study demonstrated that—whereas the CHCC did not impact outpatient utilization, health, or functional status—it did reduce hospitalizations and emergency department visits, and did so while increasing several patient satisfaction, quality of life, and self-efficacy measures.

Group Size and Attendance Were Concerns in this Study as Well

A concern to me (in that it undoubtedly reduced the potential overall favorable economic impact of the CHCC in this study) is that the average attendance during the 459 group sessions held during the study period resulted in a mean of only 7.7 patients attended CHCC sessions (again, far short of the recommended CHCC group size of 15–20 patients). Another concern is that the mean number of group meetings attended per patient was just 10.6, or 40.8% of the total number held during this 2-year study. There was a wide variability in rates of attendance, with 25.5% attending two or less meetings during the 24-month study. Table 4.2 depicts the utilization of CHCC experimental vs. control patients during this 24-month study, with probability values being based upon chi-square adjusted for physician.

Several Important Conclusions Were Made by the Researchers

The authors concluded, "CHCCs were associated with increased self-efficacy; better communication between participants and physicians; better quality of life; fewer health plan terminations and switching to non-study physicians; and lower emergency, hospital, and professional services utilization. There were no significant changes in function or health status. Although the only statistically

Table 4.2 Utilization at 24 months for CHCC and control patients

Type/unit of service	Mean ± standard deviation		
	CHCC ($N = 145$)	Control ($N = 149$)	P-value
Clinic visits/patient	33.0 ± 21.4	34.0 ±/ 22.6	0.48
Pharmacy fills/patient	45.0 ± 40.4	48.0 ±/ 49.1	0.53
Hospital admissions/patient	0.44 ± 0.89	0.82 ± 1.7	0.013
Hospital observation admissions/patient	0.16 ± 0.45	0.38 ± 2.2	0.26
Hospital outpatient visits/patient	0.92 ± 3.7	0.72 ± 2.2	0.81
Professional services/patient	5.9 ± 10.1	10.3 ± 17.9	0.005
Emergency visits/patient	0.66 ± 1.3	1.1 ± 1.5	0.008
Skilled nursing facility admissions/patient	0.15 ± 0.68	0.28 ± 1.20	0.28
Home health visits/patient	0.8 ± 2.5	1.3 ± 3.1	0.06

Probability values being based upon chi-square adjusted for physician, From Scott JC, Conner DA, Venohr I, et al. (1), with permission of J Am Geriatr Soc.

significant difference in cost was for fewer ED visits by CHCC patients, the overall cost savings for CHCC patients over the 24-month study was $41.80 per member per month. CHCC participants also expressed significantly greater patient satisfaction in a number of areas than did controls.... Although there were likely to be additional factors at work, fewer terminations from the health plan and switching to non-study physicians by CHCC members may also reflect higher satisfaction with their healthcare. These outcomes may be the result of benefits inherent in the CHCC group model: a multidisciplinary team approach to medical care, regularly scheduled monthly meetings, enhancement of the provider–patient relationship, increased health education, and the therapeutic benefit of group interactions between patients and between patients and their providers.... The CHCC model provides regularly scheduled opportunities for patients to see their primary care providers. Regularly scheduled visits allow providers to monitor patients more closely and recognize geriatric syndromes that evolve slowly over time." However, the authors do caution: "CHCC may not be a substitute for the regular office visit in pre-fail seniors because clinic use did not change. Service utilization savings came from the prevention of more costly ED visits, hospital admissions, and professional services" (1). However, the savings from hospital admissions and professional services (as well as cost of termination from health plan) were not significant at the $P = 0.05$ level—although they were significant at the $P = 0.10$ level.

Limitations of the Second Study

In discussing the limitations of this study, the authors point out that the CHCC requires periodic monitoring to keep it from turning into a class, that any financial benefit requires a sufficiently large group size, that group care is not appropriate for patients who are uncomfortable with the group setting, that CHCCs are not suitable for physicians not comfortable with leading group discussions, and that CHCCs may not be as effective in dealing with other patient populations than pre-fail geriatric patients. Another limitation they point out is that the savings tend to be downstream (e.g., for reduced hospital admissions, professional services, and ED usage), which makes the CHCC model most suitable for integrated healthcare delivery systems. Finally, the authors comment that it is often difficult to get clinic support because many benefits of the CHCC are invisible to clinic staff.

A Related Article also Demonstrated Important Findings

In a related article using the same patients but coming at the data in a different way, Coleman et al. also demonstrated that monthly CHCC group visits reduced emergency department utilization for CHCC participants who participated in the 2-year randomized control study. The patients for this study were 295 older adults (60 years of age or older) who were high utilizers of outpatient services and had one or more chronic illnesses. They found that the CHCC patients in the intervention group had fewer emergency department visits than the control group (0.65 vs. 1.08 ED visits) and were less likely to have any ED visits at all during the 2-year study (34.9% vs. 52.4%), results that were statistically significant at the $P = 0.05$ level (even after controlling for co-morbid conditions, functional status, demographic factors, and prior utilization). These authors explained the context for their study as follows: "Emergency department utilization by chronically ill older adults may be an important sentinel event signifying a breakdown in care coordination. A primary care group visit (i.e., several patients meeting together with the provider at the same time) may reduce fragmentation of care and subsequent emergency department utilization." They attribute this reduced ED utilization among elderly patients attending CHCCs to coordination of care, improved continuity of care, and earlier identification of health problems—but add that this hypothesis requires further study (13).

A Brief Sampling of Other CHCC Studies

There are numerous other published studies involving the CHCC model, and such studies are continuing to appear; however, due to limited space, the results from a sampling of just two of these studies (which address less-studied types of patient populations) will be briefly discussed here. In a study conducted at the Adult Primary Care Center at the Medical University of South Carolina at Charleston that was meant to evaluate use of group visits in delivering care to uninsured or inadequately insured patients with type 2 diabetes, the authors randomly assigned 120 patients whose diabetes was uncontrolled into CHCC (59 patients) and usual care (61 patients). Ages ranged between 22 and 83 (with the average age being 54.0), and 78.3% of these patients were female. The authors evaluated the suitability of the CHCC (involving a primary care internist and a diabetes nurse educator) for this patient sample using attendance records, the Trust in Physician Scale, and the Primary Care Assessment Tool—with measurements being made at baseline, 3 months, and 6 months. They reported that: (1) the level of patient attendance at CHCC sessions indicated acceptance of the CHCC care delivery modality; (2) CHCC patients showed improved trust in their physician compared to those receiving traditional care; and (3) the CHCC group tended to report better coordination in their care, better community orientation, and care that was more culturally competent. They concluded that group visits were appropriate for these uninsured and under-insured patients, and that the group fostered an improved sense of trust in their physician (14).

Another study, published in 2006, describes a pilot program at the University of Washington that extends the CHCC model to patients with dementia, and reports on the results of three Cooperative Dementia Care Clinics (CDCCs) that met monthly for as long as 1 year. It involved patients and caregivers drawn from a dementia clinic roster who had required specialty care for at least 3 months. Although this work is still in its early stages, the authors concluded that the CHCC could work for high-risk dementia patients and their caregivers (15).

"In CDCCs, responsive sharing of ideas, especially about difficult or painful subjects, was often quite lively, and the process helped alleviate families' reluctance to adopt new ways of managing care at home. Some of the most difficult subjects, including fear of the future; disappointment with thwarted life plans; and feelings of grief, anger, and frustration, fostered group cohesion and support for meeting the challenges of the present and those yet to come. This open exchange of ideas contrasted with expectations at the outset of the program....For the providers, the opportunity to witness dementia patients offering understanding, caring, and sound advice to one another and to caregivers was one of the most surprising and meaningful parts of the experience. The CDCC format revealed cognitive and empathic capacities in dementia patients that are generally invisible in traditional medical visits and gave patients a chance to experience their contributions as valuable....The therapeutic elements of group experience in general include recognition of the universality of experience, instillation of hope, imparting of information, direct advice from other members, and the opportunity for members to give to one another. All of these aspects of the group experience contributed significantly to the care of CDCC participants and were recognized by them over time" (15).

With CHCCs, the Frequency of Sessions Is Critically Important

CHCCs, which are designed to accommodate follow-up visits for high-utilizing, multi-morbid geriatric patients, can be held as frequently as every 2 weeks or as infrequently as every 6 months; however, they are typically held on a monthly basis. On the other hand, Specialty CHCCs are generally held at more variable time intervals, depending upon best practices and the specific needs of each patient population by diagnosis. It is important to note that, with CHCCs, the frequency with which sessions are held appears to be critically important to success. Appropriate frequency of contact with patients is not only clinically important, but also permits timely identification of health problems before they become medical crises. A 2-year study of a quarterly group intervention that was only held every 3 months in a frail elderly population failed to show any beneficial effect on utilization, incontinence, falls, etc. (16).

On the other hand, experience at the Cooperative Health Care Clinic in Colorado has demonstrated that when monthly CHCC sessions are canceled for any reason, many of the patients will make appointments for traditional office visits during the weeks following the canceled session. However, it has not yet been determined whether these added individual appointments are medically necessary or if they are just motivated by a psychological need to *touch base* with the physician. Although other interpretations of the data could be made, it is possible that the explanation lies in monthly CHCC sessions being sufficient to meet the needs of these high-utilizing geriatric, multi-morbid patients whereas quarterly sessions are not (9).

Do I Have The Skills Needed to Run a Group Visit?

For the most part, providers need to essentially have the exact same professional skills to successfully conduct a CHCC that are required to conduct a traditional office visit, e.g., empathy, the desire to deliver high-quality care, a broad knowledge base, necessary training and experience, and the continuing education required to address patients' multiple and varied medical needs. With traditional office visits, the topics of conversation often change several times, which is something that physicians are comfortable with but rarely have adequate time to fully discuss or analyze. Basically the same thing happens in a group visit, although the topics may change a little more frequently. However, there are a couple of major differences in that the group setting provides: (1) enhanced efficiencies in which physicians are better able to effectively communicate a great deal of important information to their patients; (2) plenty of time to enter into these discussions in sufficient depth and detail for physicians and patients alike to be satisfied; (3) the opportunity to deliver information to many patients at once (so that the repetition that is so common with traditional office visits is thereby obviated); and (4) a venue in which sessions can be overbooked according to the expected number of no-shows and late-cancels (thus avoiding expensive physician downtime and making group visits immune to this problem that is so vexing and costly for traditional individual office visits).

Active listening skills, multitasking abilities, critical diagnostic skills, medical decision-making skills, and the ability to prioritize issues are all skills that physicians exercise daily in the individual office visit setting, and which are readily transferable to the group visit setting. However, because they offer more time and a more relaxed pace of care, group visits have the potential to provide greater patient education, closer attention to patients' psychosocial needs, and a more satisfying overall healthcare experience for patients and physicians alike. Like other group visit models, CHCCs and Specialty CHCCs also offer a multidisciplinary team-based approach to care as well as the help and support of other patients integrated into each patient's healthcare experience. Furthermore, they provide a venue that can be most helpful in eliciting critical missing pieces of medical history, in addressing key lifestyle and disease self-management issues, in prioritizing medical interventions, and in tracking health maintenance and disease management protocols.

It is important that physicians feel free to be themselves—i.e., rather than feeling that they somehow need to be artificially professorial or entertaining. Because patients generally select their doctor based upon the physician's personality, skill set, practice style, ability to communicate, and how she/he normally interacts with patients, patients just want their physician to be themselves in the CHCC—or in any other type of group visit model, for that matter. Patients in the CHCC have already selected and bonded with their physician, and therefore do not expect (nor do they want) their physician to be different in the group than they are in traditional office visits. Patients just want quality medical care, good service, and more time with you as their physician.

Keep in mind that patients will leave the group visit setting with their medical needs met and with a great deal of helpful information. They will receive much of this information from the physician and nurse; however, a great deal of it will also come from interacting with the other patients. All patients want in a group visit is for the same doctor that they have grown to like and trust during traditional office visits to show up in the group room. In other words, you only need to be yourself in the group—the same person you normally are during regular one-on-one office visits. Nothing more is required (other than some training in group dynamics and fostering group interaction), so do not fret needlessly that you somehow might not be the right person—nor have the right personality—for a group visit as, simply put, this has never proven to be an issue. Now that you know that you can do it, why not try a group visit for your practice?

Notice the Differences Between CHCCs and DIGMAs—Including Billing Differences

As can be seen, CHCCs differ from DIGMAs in many ways. One important difference is that medical care is delivered to patients individually during CHCCs while other patients are not listening—both during the initial *working break* of the group segment and during the individual visit segment. In other words, in CHCCs, the medical care is not delivered to patients in front of one another in the group setting (where efficiency can be gained, repetition can be avoided, and all present can listen and learn from what the doctor is saying)—which, from start to finish, is a defining characteristic of DIGMAs. Also, the actual delivery of medical care is the focus during only certain portions of the CHCC visit (i.e., the *working break* and individual visit segments), whereas it remains the central focus throughout the entire DIGMA session—which, as a result, is best conceptualized, from start to finish, as a series of individual office visits with observers. In addition, whereas DIGMAs cover most or all patients in a physician's practice (or in a chronic illness treatment program), CHCCs represent a continuity model in which the same group of 15–20 patients is followed over time—typically high utilizers only, as that is where the major economic advantage lies (but only 40% or so of these high-utilizing patients will likely make the necessary commitment to attend the CHCC regularly).

Another major difference is that the patient education occurs in the form of a formal educational presentation in the CHCC, whereas it comes in the context of the physician sequentially working individually with one patient after another in the group setting in a DIGMA—i.e., while others listen, interact, ask questions, and learn. In addition, the CHCC is typically a 2½-hour session that is broken down into a 1½-hour group segment followed by approximately 1 hour of one-on-one care for approximately one-third of the patients in attendance. In a typical CHCC, approximately two-thirds of the patients attend the group portion of the session only. By way of contrast, DIGMAs are typically 90 minutes long, have only a group segment (although any patients needing a brief private discussion or exam are provided one in the nearby exam room, typically toward the end of the session), and consists from beginning to end of the physician delivering one-on-one medical care to each patient individually in the group setting—i.e., while others listen, interact, and benefit.

DIGMAs are best viewed from start to finish as being a series of individual office visits with observers that provides the same medical services as traditional office visits—in other words, they are run throughout as a series of one doctor–one patient encounters addressing the unique medical needs of each patient individually. However, this is not the case for CHCCs and Specialty CHCCs because of the substantial amount of group time spent on the warm–up, educational presentation, question and answer, and planning for the next visit segments. Therefore, it is anticipated that these differences are likely to be reflected in the form of important billing differences between these models in the fee-for-service world, especially for those CHCC/Specialty CHCC patients that only attend the group segment.

What Outcome Measures Should I Use?

In evaluating any group visit model, it is important to keep the distinctions between these SMA models clearly in mind when developing the outcome measures that you will use.

This enables you not only to select appropriate measures for the DIGMA, CHCC, or PSMA that you intend to use, but also to avoid developing unrealistic expectations as to what each model can achieve. For example, one would expect CHCCs to reduce utilization of ER, hospital, and nursing home services among the same group of high-utilizing, multi-morbid geriatric patient being followed over time; however, productivity and access (which are fortes of the DIGMA and PSMA models) would likely not be improved—and those CHCC benefits that do occur will likely be greatest for high-utilizing patient, but much less for lower utilizing patients. Disease-specific Specialty CHCCs would be expected to improve care delivery and satisfaction among patients in the medical subspecialties; however, they would not be expected to increase physician productivity or to improve access (which are specific strengths of the DIGMA and PSMA models). Therefore, the selection of proper evaluative measures is critical to monitoring the success of any SMA program.

Weaknesses

As is the case with all group visit models, CHCCs and Specialty CHCCs also have their own particular weaknesses, which are depicted in Table 4.3.

Foster Group Interaction and Keep CHCCs from Becoming a Class

CHCC and Specialty CHCC sessions should be interactive, not lectures. As Dr. Scott points out, there is a world of difference between delivering a lecture on angina and heart disease vs. asking the group: "Has anyone present ever had a heart attack?" and "What was it like for you, and what did you do about it?" Interactive group process involves several patients responding to these questions with their own special stories—and with the physician not only delivering medical care and counsel but also acting as a facilitator (i.e., while adding information and elaborating as appropriate). In a *Modern Healthcare* article, Dr. Scott underscored the need to keep groups from turning into lectures (17).

Physicians need to view patients as *primary caregivers* who are learning to help themselves and each other better manage their own health problems. Furthermore, physicians also need to recognize that much of the benefit of a group visit comes from patients interacting with and helping each other. Therefore, it is extremely important to foster some group interaction from time to time

Table 4.3 Weaknesses of the CHCC model

- Unless group interaction is constantly fostered, the CHCC can easily turn into a class
- Therefore, CHCCs will not be appropriate for approximately 60 percent of invited patients
- Because the economic cost-offset is greatest, CHCCs are typically designed for high utilizing patients
- Therefore, low- to mid-utilizing patients might not result in the same economic gain
- Patients must commit to attend regularly (but only approximately 40% do commit)
- For the most part, other patients do not benefit when medical care is delivered privately in a CHCC
- Only a small (albeit costly) part of the physician's practice is covered
  - CHCCs and Specialty CHCCs are primarily for 15–20 high-utilizing patients
  - All other patients in the physician's practice are largely unaffected
- 2.5 hours of the physician's time is required
- Patients attend prescheduled sessions whether they have a medical need or not
- Unlike DIGMAs and PSMAs, CHCCs do not leverage physician time, increase productivity, or improve access
- Because benefits of the CHCC are largely *downstream*, they are greatest in managed care organization but less for individual physicians
- Real and meaningful administrative support is required
- The CHCC's benefits are largely invisible to staff in the clinic
- They require up-front skill building in group process
- Initial physician and patient resistance needs to be overcome
- Because only 15–20 patients in the physician's practice are affected, CHCCs are of limited value in managing a busy, backlogged practice
- Documentation can be problematic, especially when electronic medical records are used
- There are billing concerns, especially for the approximately two-thirds of patients who attend the largely educational group only (i.e., who are not seen individually afterward)

throughout the session. As can be seen, doing a CHCC group well requires up-front skill building around group process along with appropriate coaching and monitoring—especially in the areas of fostering both group interaction and the perception that this is a medical visit and not a class.

Even well-intentioned physicians, when left to their own devices, will often slip into the professor or authority figure role. This is because these roles are typically more familiar and comfortable for physicians than that of being the facilitator of an interactive process. This interactive facilitator role contrasts sharply with a lecture-type format in which there is a one-way delivery of information from the physician to the group, yet the latter is exactly what can happen if care is not taken to avoid this problem in the CHCC (or Specialty CHCC subtype of this model). It is important to always keep in mind that this interaction validates participants as legitimate sources of information for one another in coping with their health problems. Patients are thereby reinforced by each other as well as by the physician and nurse, and everyone benefits from this interactive and therapeutic process of the group. We must realize that patients often have more direct, *hands on* experience in coping with their illnesses and the aging process than their medical caregivers do. Therefore, we must appreciate that the patients themselves are often their own primary caregivers and that they need to be validated for the important role that they play as caregivers in their own lifestyle management and personal well-being. But to draw patients out so that they share

this valuable, hard-earned information with one another—i.e., which they have gained from firsthand experience by adjusting to, and coping with, their own health problems—it is important for the provider to run the CHCC in a manner that fosters group interaction, and not as a formal lecture or class.

Because they most likely have not been trained in conducting group visits during medical school (and have probably had little or no experience in leading groups), SMAs can be intimidating and anxiety provoking to physicians—especially when first starting their group visit program. This can in turn be self-defeating because when experiencing the discomfort of anxiety, physicians can easily turn to the lecture-type format with which they are more comfortable—which can undermine the interactive process that is required for a successful CHCC. By interaction, we are referring to all of the important sharing of information, mutual support, and dynamic social interaction which all group visit models are designed to achieve. Physicians must therefore guard against this tendency to lecture rather than to foster interaction during the CHCC or Specialty CHCC session—i.e., so that the group maintains a lively, healthy, and interactive nature wherein much information and emotional support is exchanged. Trust me, this type of group will prove to not only be maximally beneficial to patients but also be much more professionally satisfying to the physician as well.

While CHCCs and Specialty CHCCs are intuitively appealing because the same group of 15–20 high-utilizing patients is followed over time, constant vigilance must nonetheless be paid to fostering group interaction and—because of their substantial educational format—to keeping patients from viewing the CHCC as a class rather than a medical appointment. This is because, although medical care is delivered, the group segment of the CHCC is structured in such a way that it has a considerable amount of socialization and education time built in (i.e., through its warm-up, educational presentation, question and answer, and planning for the next session segments). Therefore, without being careful in this regard, it is possible for CHCCs and Specialty CHCCs to be viewed as classes rather than group medical visits. This is especially true for those patients who happen to attend the group segment of the visit only (i.e., for approximately two-thirds of the patients attending any given session), and who do not need to be seen for individual care afterward during the subsequent individual treatment segment of the session.

Patients Must Commit to Attend Regularly

One of the challenges for the CHCC model and its Specialty CHCC subtype is that patients must make the commitment to attend ongoing, periodically scheduled sessions on a regular basis, regardless of whether or not they happen to have a medical need at the time. Having to make this extended commitment to attend can be a turn-off to many. Because patients need to make an ongoing commitment to the program (which stands in stark contrast to DIGMAs and Physicals SMAs, where patients only need to commit to a single session in order to attend), CHCCs are particularly inappropriate for patients who are new to the system and do not yet have an established relationship with their doctor—or for patients who are uncomfortable in a group setting and unwilling to commit to attending on a regular basis. For high-utilizing patients having a lower level of commitment (as well as for the vast majority of patients who less frequently utilize healthcare services), DIGMAs therefore often make a better choice—as maximum economic benefit and cost offset for CHCCs typically occurs with high-utilizing patients who strongly commit to attending regularly.

Other Patients in the Group Do Not Benefit when Care Is Delivered Individually in a CHCC

With the CHCC, only a portion of the medical care is delivered in the group setting; the rest is presented to patients one-on-one during the individual care segment

that follows. Because the individualized medical care is actually delivered during the *working break* of the group segment of the CHCC (i.e., while patients are enjoying snacks and socializing with one another), only the handful of patients within earshot get to listen, learn, and benefit from this one-on-one care that is being delivered by the physician to patients individually. Worse yet, others are not able to listen and benefit during the hour of individual care that follows, which is delivered to approximately one-third of the patients after the group is over—as it is delivered one-on-one to patients in private, after most of the patients have already left. Thus, unlike DIGMAs, any efficiency benefit that the group setting could have offered at the time that this medical care is being delivered is thereby lost (i.e., during both the group and individual visit segments of the CHCC), so that we are largely left with the same inefficiencies here as with traditional individual office visits.

This is dramatically different from the DIGMA model, which (except for truly private discussions and exams) is run like a series of individual office visits from start to finish, but almost always in the group setting and in front of all the other patients. In this way, all of the patients attending the DIGMA can listen, learn, ask questions, interact, and benefit while the physician is sequentially addressing the unique medical needs of each patient individually. In this sense, the CHCC does not fully benefit from all of the potential efficiencies that the group visit format can offer; however, it does instead offer the benefit of a formal, interactive educational presentation during each session. While beneficial to patients, this has the potential of creating billing problems for CHCCs and Specialty CHCCs, and of fostering the impression that this is a class rather than a medical visit.

Most of the Physician's Practice Is Not Covered and 2.5 Hours of Time Is Required

Because basically the same 15–20 high-utilizing patients are followed over time on a monthly basis (i.e., regardless of whether or not they happen to have a medical need to be seen at the time), excellent medical care and close monitoring can be provided to this small but costly cohort of patients—and strong patient bonding can occur. However, it must be kept in mind that: (1) the CHCC model is primarily for high-utilizing patients (i.e., not for the far more frequent low- or moderate-utilizing patients) as this is where maximum economic gain is achieved; (2) only 40% of high-utilizing patients will make the required degree of commitment to attend the CHCC regularly on a monthly basis (thus making

CHCCs largely inappropriate for low and medium utilizing patients, as well as for approximately 60% of high utilizers); (3) unlike DIGMAs, the CHCC does not impact the vast majority of the physician's practice (nor does it improve access in any substantial way for the physician's other 1200–2500 patients); and (4) it is for established patients only and not for new patients.

In addition, because CHCCs involve 2½ hours of physician time (1½ hours for the group, followed by 1 hour of individual care) rather than the 1½ hours required for most DIGMAs or Physicals SMAs, a correspondingly larger number of patients must be seen consistently during every session in order to cover the cost of the program. Additionally, because only a small but costly subset of the physician's practice is covered (rather than most or all of the practice) and because CHCCs have not been shown either to increase the physician's productivity or to improve access to the physician's practice (all of which are great strengths of the DIGMA model), CHCCs do not provide the effective practice management tool that DIGMAs do for better managing busy, backlogged practices. The CHCC does, however, provide exceptional care for this small but costly group of 15–20 high utilizing, multi-morbid geriatric patients fortunate enough to participate.

Benefits Are Greatest in Managed Care Organizations, Less for Individual Physicians

Dr. John Scott recently pointed out to me that one of the limitations of the CHCC is that all of the demonstrated savings are *downstream*, so that unless you have a closed system like the VA, Kaiser Permanente, or the military, the savings are difficult to measure. Because the major financial benefits of the CHCC model lie in the *big ticket* items (such as in reduced emergency department, hospitalization, and nursing care costs), its dramatic economic success will be most enjoyed by integrated healthcare delivery systems rather than by the physicians running them. In other words, the individual physician in a solo practice will likely not enjoy this financial benefit in his/her own practice—although running a CHCC could certainly be a professionally rewarding endeavor for the physician. Furthermore, unlike DIGMAs, the CHCC does not improve either the individual physician's overall productivity or access to the physician's practice. Because it is not meant to be a practice management tool that covers the physician's entire practice, the CHCC's major physician benefits will be more along the line of the improved quality, education, physician–patient relationships, and ships satisfaction benefits that the model

provides for established patients. It is these benefits that will likely be of greatest interest to the solo practitioner—i.e., as opposed to any immediate financial, practice management, or access benefits (for which the DIGMA model would be the SMA model of choice).

Real Administrative Support Is Required

It is critically important that administrators and clinic managers understand the multiple benefits that CHCCs can offer, and that they support and become champions of the program. Unless there is real and meaningful administrative support, the physician and nursing resources required for a successful CHCC program may not be available—and the goals of the program will thereby not be achievable. As clinic administrators are challenged to stretch existing resources ever further in the face of proliferating and competing resource demands, the necessary ingredients for a successful CHCC may not always be available—especially with the necessary degree of priority assigned to the program, so that the physician and nurse will consistently and reliably be available. Therefore, CHCC groups need to be integrated into normal clinic operations, with CHCC sessions being viewed by all as an important part of the entire clinic's overall approach to care delivery.

The CHCC's Benefits Are Invisible to Staff in the Clinic

Unfortunately, the benefits of the CHCC model are often invisible to the staff, which can result in necessary resources being diverted to more visible demands—and can undercut nursing and administrative support for the program, despite the long-term favorable results that a properly run CHCC program can provide. As Dr. Scott has pointed out during many of the presentations that we have given together over the years, the fact that its benefits are largely invisible to staff in the clinic providing care can create a major roadblock for CHCCs. Frontline nursing supervisors can be overwhelmed meeting the here and now imperatives of emergency care, prompt access, and unscheduled walk-ins. In striving to meet the quality and service mandates of managed care, nursing staffs are often stretched to the breaking point providing accessible care for a host of minor complaints that need to be addressed. As a result, it all-too-often happens that critical staff is frequently diverted to more visible demands within the clinic, despite their awareness of the long-term favorable benefits of CHCCs. Therefore, it is important to note that, with CHCCs and Specialty CHCCs, dedicated nursing support is essential and that, in and of themselves, upper-level administrative support and the blessing of organizational leadership are not sufficient. Therefore, when you consider establishing CHCCs (or any other group visit program for that matter) at your organization, be sure to first consider the support requirements necessary for success—and then be certain to consistently meet them so that full benefit can be attained (18).

CHCCs Require Up-Front Skill Building in Group Process

Using the CHCC model to best effect requires more up-front skill building in group process (fostering group interaction, managing group dynamics, handling various problems that can occur in the group, etc.) than can often be provided. As Dr. Scott has pointed out to me, even though it is sometimes the case that no special skill building is provided, it would nonetheless be valuable to have the appropriate training, even though it might not be essential. Nonetheless, the CHCC is a model that requires adequate coaching and monitoring in order to be maximally effective, and this might not be readily available. However, Dr. Scott has reported that when an appropriate program coordinator is available who is properly trained as a trainer (and when provided with the necessary time and training protocols), this person might be able to oversee as many as 40 CHCC and Specialty CHCC groups (10).

Practice Management Limitations

CHCCs and Specialty CHCCs provide great care and a pioneering tool for more effectively managing the same group of 15–20 high-utilizing patients over time—a small but costly portion of the physician's total practice. However, because they do not affect the other 1200 to 2500 patients on the physician's panel, neither CHCCs nor Specialty CHCCs improve access for the other patients in the provider's practice—nor do they provide an effective practice management tool for better managing busy, backlogged practices (i.e., since they do not typically increase either the physician's productivity or access to care). Similarly, they do not provide an effective tool for more efficiently reducing overall patient phone call

volume, for reducing patient complaints about poor access, or for optimizing the physician's schedule—all of which are strengths of the DIGMA model. Nonetheless, what the CHCCs and Specialty CHCCs do accomplish, they do exceedingly well.

Physician and Patient Resistance

As is the case for all shared medical appointments, CHCCs provide a venue for care that is dramatically different from the traditional office visit—one that is largely unknown to physicians and patients alike. Therefore, it introduces a great deal of change and can engender both physician and patient resistance, especially initially—i.e., at the beginning of the CHCC program. This can make it difficult to get the program *off the ground* and *up and running*. The good news here is that—because patient and physician professional satisfaction with the program are very high—once some CHCCs have been successfully launched (and patients as well as physician colleagues begin to hear positive reports about them and their many benefits), these resistances can slowly but steadily be overcome.

Documentation (when Electronic Medical Records Are Used)

The issue of documenting all patients' individual chart notes in the CHCC group setting can prove challenging for systems using electronic medical records (EMR). The issue of data entry and retrieval can prove challenging for CHCCs now that we are in the computer age. As originally employed, the CHCC featured patients sitting with their personal paper medical chart in front of them, which made it easy for chart notes to be updated during the *working break* (i.e., as the nurse and physician moved from patient to patient around the group room, entering pertinent data). Here, notations were made in the medical chart both during and after the group session. However, transitioning to a fully computerized medical record will require new formats for transferring information in the CHCC—as well as use of functional laptop or desktop computers in the group room. However, as Dr. John Scott recently noted in a personal conversation, Kaiser Permanente transitioned to EMR 10 years ago with no apparent impact on their CHCC group visit program.

Billing Concerns with the CHCC and Specialty CHCC Models

Finally, for those patients who attend the group but are not seen afterward during the individual care segment, there could be billing issues in a fee-for-service environment due to the highly educational structure of the CHCC group segment. CHCCs certainly differ dramatically from DIGMAs, which are run like a series of individual office visits from start to finish (but almost entirely in the group room rather than an exam room), i.e., delivering the exact same types of care, and often more, as traditional office visits. The question of billing in the fee-for-service world is particularly acute for those CHCC patients not taken out of the group room and seen individually once the group segment is over.

It seems to me that taking each patient out of the room during the group presentation just to be able to bill for the visit presents a case of *the tail wagging the dog*. I say this for two reasons: (1) because the idea of seeing each patient individually represents a holdover from the same old individual office visit model of care (a system that we know has serious efficiency, access, cost, and quality problems); and (2) because it undermines the very essence and value of a well-run group visit program in that patients are thereby deprived of much education from (and much time spent with), their own doctor. In addition, patients are missing part of the group/educational presentation by being taken out of the group room.

Whereas a physician might think that, by taking patients out of the group room and delivering care to them one at a time they are somehow providing each patient with highly personalized care—after all, that is what they are used to doing in the exam room during routine office visits—what they are really doing from the standpoint of the group visit is depriving the other 15 patients in the group room from listening to, and learning from, what they are saying. As a result, repetition is not avoided, efficiency is not gained, and the multiple benefits that group visits are known to offer are undermined.

Some might counter with the argument that a health educator or some other speaker (nutritionist, physical therapist, psychologist, smoking cessation program representative, etc.) could be presenting to the group while the doctor is taking patients out of the group room one at a time. However, this misses the point that patients have come to the group visit for a medical visit with their own doctor, not for a class. Remember that a SMA is first and foremost a group medical appointment that is meant to efficiently and effectively deliver medical care—and to provide patients with more time to learn from their own doctor. Therefore, it is not a class, support group, psychiatry group, health education program, or behavioral medicine program.

Concerns regarding billing in the CHCC might depend to some degree—during both the working break and the individual care delivery segments of the session—on specifically what care is delivered, how it is provided, and what is documented. Another complicating factor is that, unlike the DIGMA model, the group segment of the CHCC model does not closely resemble the traditional individual office visit model of care—at least for those patients who attend only the group segment of the CHCC visit (i.e., for all the 15–20 patients attending the group, except for the four to seven patients typically seen one-on-one during the individual care segment that follows the group).

Another billing concern for the CHCC model and its Specialty CHCC subtype is that the group sessions are held according to some type of prearranged scheduling sequence (e.g., such as monthly visits for the multi-morbid geriatric patients being seen in a typical CHCC)—i.e., rather than being based upon true medical need. Whereas those patients having a real medical need to be seen during any given monthly session would likely pose no billing problem, those without a legitimate medical need (i.e., who are only coming in because they had committed to do so) might very well pose a billing issue.

A final point that needs to be emphasized, even though it has been discussed elsewhere, is that there are no existing CPT codes for group visits at the present time. For a variety of reasons such as those discussed previously, it appears that the issue of securing an appropriate CPT code is an especially important one for CHCCs and Specialty CHCCs (although less so for DIGMAs and PSMAs). However, obtaining such group visit billing codes can be a long and arduous process, and one which must include safeguards against abuse. Because DIGMAs and PSMAs are run from start to finish like a series of individual office visits with observers, they are often billed using existing billing codes according to the level of care delivered and documented—except for the billing of counseling time (as many patients might simultaneously be benefiting from this counseling and it would be egregious, if not outright fraudulent, to bill several times over for the same counseling) or for the behaviorist's time, which is treated as an overhead expense to the program. Because of this, it is not only patients, physicians, and healthcare organizations that can benefit from a well-run DIGMA or PSMA program, but also third-party insurers. The latter can benefit both by getting accessible, efficient, and high-quality care for those they do insure, and by not being billed either for counseling time or for the behaviorist's time.

The Center for Medicare Management has stated that, generally, a physician may only bill for a face-to-face encounter with one patient during any one visit. There are exceptions for group psychotherapy sessions and medical nutrition therapy. Also, under Medicare Part B, outpatient diabetes self-management training sessions are allowed. In group medical appointments, a physician can provide care to one patient, while others observe, with the physician only billing for the care directly given to each patient individually, and not to any benefit derived by the other group members who happen to be observing and learning from this encounter (John Scott, personal communication, Center for Medicare Management, March 2007).

Because DIGMAs and PSMAs are run from start to finish like a series of one doctor–one patient encounters with observers (i.e., like a series of individual office visits with observers), this would seem to imply that these visits are billable according to the level of care delivered and documented to each person individually; however, counseling time could only be charged to the individual patient being addressed at any given time, and not to other patients who happen to serendipitously benefit by observing, listening, and learning.

Chronic Disease Management Applications

Group visits have a very important and positive role to play in managing chronic illnesses, both for the chronically ill patients that happen to be in the physician's own practice and for the many patients being treated in chronic illness population management programs (see my chronic illness paradigm that makes full use of group visits that is discussed in Chapter 7). Unfortunately, at the very time that our glut of baby boomers is reaching Medicare age and incurring an accelerating host of chronic illnesses, we are losing our geriatricians, increasing our patient panel sizes, facing ever-shorter office visits, and discovering the multiple inadequacies of the individual office visit in effectively meeting this rapidly increasing demand. We are now witnessing a growing mismatch between supply of medical services and the multiple demands being placed upon them. More than ever, we currently need the multiple benefits that properly run group visits can offer. When it comes to chronic illness treatment programs, like other group visit models, CHCCs need to be evaluated for such applications based upon their relative strengths and weaknesses—which must therefore be understood prior to embarking on such applications.

Strengths and Limitations of CHCCs in Chronic Illness Treatment Programs

Certainly, a couple of great strengths of the CHCC in chronic disease management applications are the frequency with which patients can be seen and the remarkable patient bonding that can occur over time. The amount of patient education that can be provided in the educational segment of the CHCC is also a plus, as is the fact that CHCCs are ideally suited for some of the highest utilizing patients within the population management program.

Although they can provide great care for the 15–20 patients being followed, having all patients start at one time—and then following the same group of high-utilizing patients periodically over time at preset intervals—can limit the value of the CHCC model and its Specialty CHCC subtype when it comes to applications in chronic illness population management programs. This is especially true:

1. for larger population management programs in which a great number of different chronically ill patients (perhaps thousands or even tens of thousands) need to be followed over time, whenever they need care—and the 15–20 patients being followed monthly in the CHCC will likely prove to be *a drop in the bucket*.
2. where all levels of disease severity and utilization of healthcare services are being included (such as many low- and mid-utilizers, along with some high utilizers)
3. where patients have highly variable healthcare needs, so that periodically scheduled CHCC sessions (or even irregularly scheduled Specialty CHCC sessions) may not be ideally helpful

Strengths of DIGMAs in Chronic Illness Management

All three of the above are strengths of the DIGMA model, where almost all patients in the chronic illness program would be included (i.e., regardless of disease severity or utilization behavior)—and where patients would only need to come in when they have an actual medical need rather than according to some preset schedule (in fact, they could just drop-in). As it turns out, DIGMAs are particularly well suited to chronic illness treatment programs because of the many specific advantages that they offer—including the facts that productivity and access are improved, that almost all patients in the chronic illness program can attend any time that they have a medical need, and that DIGMAs are widely used in fee-for-service systems (although the entire issue of billing for group visits is still evolving and not yet completely resolved).

CHCCs, DIGMAs, and PSMAs Not Only Work Well Together But Also with Other Group Programs

As can be seen, DIGMAs, CHCCs, and PSMAs (which are discussed in Chapter 5) are all important and solid group visit models; however, they are very different—and each model (as well as its subtypes) has its own particular advantages and disadvantages. These models differ in design, accomplish different ends, and have different strengths and weaknesses. They are open to dissimilar groups of patients, are run quite differently, require different staffing, achieve different purposes, and appear to have different billing issues. These models have many theoretical and operational differences, yet they complement each other very nicely and can work well together in actual practice—I am fond of saying: "It's a case of one plus one equals three."

As but one example of how these models can work together, take high-utilizing patients—which normally are a forte of the CHCC model. However, even among these high utilizers of healthcare services, only approximately 40% will make the necessary commitment to attend a CHCC on a regular basis—the rest will either equivocate, demure, or refuse the invitation. This focus is complemented nicely by DIGMAs, where almost all patients are free to attend (regardless of whether or not they are high utilizers) and where patients only need sufficient motivation to attend a single session—i.e., rather than needing to make an ongoing commitment to attend periodically. Because of this, many of the 60% of high utilizers unwilling to commit to a CHCC might be willing to attend a DIGMA for a single session—or even occasionally, on an *as-needed* basis. However, the level of patient bonding will likely be less for the DIGMA than for a CHCC, and greater attention will likely need to be paid to consistently filling all sessions.

These differences which DIGMAs, CHCCs, and PSMAs possess are such that they provide complementary (not competing) SMA models—models that work well together in actual practice. Equally important, these group visit models also work well together with the judicious use of individual office visits, which they were designed to complement and were never meant to totally replace. Furthermore, the DIGMA, PSMA, and CHCC models do not just work together with both each other and individual office visits, they also complement (i.e., rather than compete with) virtually every other type of successful group program that the healthcare organization might already have put into place—e.g., health education programs, nutrition groups, smoking cessation programs, support groups, psychiatry groups, substance abuse programs, and behavioral medicine groups. In other words, if you already have other types of group programs in place at your system, then do not view CHCCs, DIGMAs, and PSMAs as competitors. Instead, view these SMA models as something that will complement, enhance, and work well with any such programs that you might already have worked hard to put into place.

The Future of the CHCC Model

In an article that I co-authored with Dr. Scott (18), we said the following regarding what we felt the future held for the CHCC model. Our thoughts then hold equally true today—not only for CHCCs and Specialty CHCCs but also for DIGMAs and Physicals SMAs as well. "The future for the CHCC model looks bright. Reflect at first only on the geriatric population. This population, currently about 12% of the whole, will double in the next two or three decades. It does and will control the majority of wealth in the country and thus, for better or worse, will influence federal healthcare policy. Medicare will not be allowed to languish, and 7 ½ minute doctor office visits (long predicted, currently not uncommon, and surely the scourge of the future) will not be tolerated, even under the rubric of 'computer-assisted quality time' or 'institutional memory.' People want to talk to doctors about aging, death, and dying. WWW.DEATH.com will not suffice—not for today's elderly population, and not for their children and grandchildren. The same is true for virtually every chronic disease in every age group. People's thoughts, beliefs, fears, and expectations about their medical issues cannot be bundled into simple guidelines and checklists. Human reactions to illness are often the major determinants of outcomes, regardless of prescribed interventions. It takes time to address these issues, and the CHCC model provides both the time and the environment to do this. The current one-to-one doctor–patient paradigm is not only economically unsustainable as a sole delivery system, but lacks the power and the therapeutic benefit of the group dynamic" (18).

References

1. Scott JC, Conner DA, Venohr I, et al. Effectiveness of a group outpatient visit model for chronically ill older health maintenance organization members: a 2-year randomized trial of the cooperative health care clinic. *Journal of the American Geriatrics Society* 2004;52(9):1463–1470.

2. Houck S, Kilo C, Scott J. Improving patient care. Group visits 101. *Family Practice Management* 2003;10(5):66–68.

3. Scott JC, Robertson BJ. Kaiser Colorado's Cooperative Health Care Clinic: a group approach to patient care. In: Fox PD, Fama T, editors. Managed care and chronic illnesses: challenges and opportunities. Gaithersburg, MD: Aspen; 1996.

4. Beck A, Scott J, William P, et al. A randomized trial of group outpatient visits for chronically ill older HMO members: the cooperative health care clinic. *Journal of the American Geriatrics Society* 1997;45(5):543–549.

5. Scott J, Gade G, McKenzie M, Venohr I. Cooperative health care clinics: a group approach to individual care. *Geriatrics* 1998;53(5):68–70, 76–78, 81; quiz 82.

6. Scott JC, Robertson BJ. Kaiser Colorado's Cooperative Health Care Clinic: a group approach to patient care. *Managed Care Quarterly* 1996;4(3):41–45.

7. Noffsinger EB, Scott JC. Practical tips for establishing successful group visit programs. Part 1: leadership skills and guidelines. *Group Practice Journal* 2000;49(6):31–37.

8. Noffsinger EB, Scott JC. Practical tips for establishing successful group visit programs. Part 2: maintaining desired group census. *Group Practice Journal* 2000;49(7):24–27.

9. Noffsinger EB, Scott JC. Preventing potential abuses of group visits. *Group Practice Journal* 2000;49(5):37–38, 40–42, 44–46.

10. Noffsinger EB, Scott JC. Understanding today's group visit models. *The Permanente Journal* 2000;4(2):99–112.

11. Shanafelt TD, Bradley KA, Wipf JE, et al. Burnout and self-reported patient care in an internal medicine residency program. *Annals of Internal Medicine* 2002;136(5):358–367.

12. McLeod L (ed.). Multitask in the exam room: three shared-appointment models help physicians see more patients. *Private Practice Success*, July 2004;6–8.

13. Coleman EA, Eilertsen TB, et al. Reducing emergency visits in older adults with chronic illness: a randomized control trial of group visits. *Effective Clinical Practice* 2001;4(2)::49–57.

14. Clancy DE, Cope DW, Magruder KM, et al. Evaluating group visits in an uninsured or inadequately insured patient population with uncontrolled Type 2 diabetes. *The Diabetes Educator* 2003;29(2):292–302.

15. Lessig M, Farrell J, Madhavan E, et al. Cooperative dementia care clinics: a new model for managing cognitively impaired patients. *Journal of the American Geriatric Society* 2006;54(12):1937–1942.

16. Coleman EA, Grothau LC, Sandhu N, et al. Chronic care clinics: a randomized controlled trial of a new model of primary care for frail older adults. *Journal of the American Geriatric Society* 1999;47:775–783.

17. Thompson E. The power of group visits: Improved quality of care, increased productivity entice physicians to see up to 15 patients at a time. *Modern Healthcare* 2000;30(23):54, 56, 62.

18. Noffsinger EB, Scott JC. Understanding today's group visit models. *Group Practice Journal* 2000;49(2):46–58.

Chapter 5
The Physicals Shared Medical Appointment Model: A Revolutionary Access Solution for Private Physical Examinations

Group medical appointments provide patients with prompt access to care, greater attention to their psychosocial needs, and increased time with their medical team.... A group medical visit model, called a Physical Shared Medical Appointment (PSMA), was employed because this uses individual patient examinations followed by a group meeting. On the day of the visit, brief physical examinations were performed on each patient...At completion of the 2-hour visit, patient surveys indicated an extremely high level of satisfaction and the preference to attend a future PSMA. Issues discussed during the group meeting were pertinent to all transplant recipients, regardless of diagnosis. The PSMA model allows the patient to spend extended time with their care providers while providing the care providers an opportunity to discuss health issues with numerous patients during 1 appointment. The Dartmouth Transplant PSMA model is expanding to pretransplantation and postallogeneic transplant recipients.

Kenneth R. Meehan, et al. Group medical appointments: organization and implementation in the bone marrow transplantation clinic. *Supportive Cancer Therapy* 2006;3(2):84–90.

Introduction to Physicals Shared Medical Appointments

After 2 years of conceptualization and trial and error, I completed development on the physicals shared medical appointment model (PSMA) in 2001. I originally developed this model of care delivery in recognition of an existing healthcare need: timely access to high quality, private physical examinations in primary and specialty care was becoming increasingly challenging for patients in many healthcare systems nationwide. Long waits for physical examinations and new patient intakes were commonplace, but unacceptable from the standpoint of providing good service to our customers—i.e., our patients. The PSMA model represents an important healthcare innovation because it provides quality care, solves access problems to physicals, enhances patient satisfaction, and leverages existing resources to dramatically increase physician productivity in the delivery of physical examinations in primary and specialty care.

Meant to enhance patient satisfaction and maintain appropriate privacy at all times, I developed PSMAs to offer patients the benefits of: (1) prompt access to private physical exams; (2) more time with their doctor; (3) max-packed visits; (4) greater patient education and attention to psychosocial needs; (5) the professional skills of a behaviorist; and (6) the help and support of a care delivery team as well as other patients integrated into each patient's healthcare experience. Although I originally started the PSMA model in primary care as a means of improving access to care, enhancing quality, improving patient and physician professional satisfaction, and increasing the efficiency of delivering complete physical examinations in internal medicine and family practice, the model has since been expanded into numerous applications in many medical subspecialties. I first published upon the PSMA model in a series of four articles in the American Medical Group Association's *Group Practice Journal*, and have drawn from that material from time to time throughout this chapter of the book (1–4).

Where the PSMA Model Began

The first clinical applications of the PSMA model in actual practice occurred in 2000–2001 at the Palo Alto Medical Clinic (PAMC), which is a part of the larger Palo Alto Medical Foundation, and a Sutter Health affiliate. PAMC is a large multispecialty medical group of approximately 225 primary and specialty care physicians in Northern California conducting approximately 700,000 outpatient visits per year with $200 million annual revenues with a payer mix at that time that was approximately 60% fee-for-service and 40% capitated (and overall, about 10% of patients were Medicare). I was then their Director of Clinical Access Improvement as well as the originator and head of their Shared Medical Appointment Department, which was responsible for launching 18 DIGMAs and PSMAs per year throughout the organization in primary and specialty care.

The PSMA model was originally implemented in primary care at PAMC to address significant access problems for physical examinations, as some family practice and internal medicine physicians had backlogs in those days as large as 200+ physicals. David Drucker, M.D., who was then the president and CEO of the Palo Alto Medical Foundation, put the case for PSMAs this way: "Patient access is far and away our biggest concern—particularly in the area of primary care. Our access problems are based on a number of different factors, including difficulty recruiting physicians and staff, the demise of other medical groups in the area, tremendous patient demand, etc. In many ways this is a happy situation—to have this level of patient demand. On the other hand, it does produce these access problems and service issues. So, we are looking at ways to improve our access while maintaining our quality and we think that SMAs—particularly in the area of physical examiniations—are a way to address this. Access is a problem, and the Physicals Shared Medical Appointment is a way to address this problem—both solving the access issue and achieving the highest level of quality and patient satisfaction" (1).

The Medical Necessity of Physical Examinations Is Variable

Some might question the medical necessity of providing physical examinations at all, an issue that is complicated by the fact that patients request physicals for a large number of different reasons. While some requests for physicals are demands of questionable medical necessity, others entail necessary prevention, vague or specific symptoms, or chronic illnesses that can involve multiple organ systems and need to be closely monitored. The appropriateness of, the medical need for, and the ultimate benefit of physical examinations will undoubtedly differ considerably for differing types of patient demands. Nonetheless, one thing is clear: When a physical examination is medically necessary and appropriate, it is a benefit to all if such appointments are accessible and readily available to our patients—which is what the PSMA model has been designed to help achieve. Look at it this

way: As long as primary and specialty care physicians are going to provide some types of physical examinations, why not utilize the PSMA model to have them provide these exams more efficiently and with higher levels of patient satisfaction?

Distinguishing Characteristics of PSMAs and Why They Are Used

PSMAs are used for efficiently delivering physical examinations, especially when the physicals need to be conducted individually and in private, such as when disrobing is involved. Otherwise, if privacy is not required and disrobing is not involved so that the exams could be provided in the group setting (such as in podiatry), then the DIGMA model could instead be employed. In addition, because new patient intakes often involve a private physical exam, the PSMA model is often used in both primary care and numerous medical subspecialties for bringing new patients in—i.e., either into the system or into the individual provider's practice. It can similarly be used in any chronic illness population management program where timely access to private physical examinations is an important consideration.

In other words, the PSMA model can provide: (1) better physician management of busy, backlogged practices (by dramatically increasing the efficiency of, and access to, private physical examinations); (2) better management of chronic illnesses through effective treatment programs for the chronically ill (especially when a private physical examination is needed either to intake patients into the program or as part of the ongoing recommended treatment regimen); and (3) for new patient intakes as well as for private physical examinations for established patients in both primary and specialty care. Productivity is gained in PSMAs in several ways (for example, by the physician avoiding unnecessary repetition and delegating to members of the treatment team), and inefficiency is avoided by overbooking sessions (just like the airlines do) according to the expected number of no-shows and late-cancels—thereby avoiding expensive physician *downtime* due to unfilled physical examination slots, which are often the greatest time sinks in the physician's practice. However, one of the PSMA's greatest productivity gains lies in deferring almost all discussions, except truly private matters and what needs to be discussed in order to conduct the exam, from the inefficient one-on-one exam room setting to the highly efficient group setting—where all present can listen and learn, and repetition can be avoided. The distinguishing characteristics of the PSMA model are detailed in Table 5.1.

Table 5.1 Distinguishing characteristics of the PSMA model

- The only group visit model to specifically focus upon private physical examinations, not follow-up visits
- Improved access to physical examinations
- Dramatically increased physician productivity (typically 200–300% or more) in delivering physical examinations
- Equally applicable to physicals in primary care and the various medical and surgical subspecialties
- Provides the same types of medical care as traditional individual physical examinations
- Run as a series of one doctor–one patient encounters throughout, focusing upon the unique medical needs of each patient individually
- Can be used by all types of primary and specialty care providers delivering physical exams (physicians, nurse practitioners, osteopaths, podiatrists, etc.)
- Sessions are overbooked according to the expected number of no-shows and late-cancels
- The PSMA is used for physical examinations deemed to be medically necessary
- A "Patient Packet" is sent to patients 2–3 weeks in advance so that patients can complete a detailed health history form as well as all appropriate lab tests prior to the visit
- Someone on the physician's staff usually enters data from the completed health history forms returned to the office into each patient's PSMA chart note prior to the session
- The provider's nurse typically writes down all patients' lab results on a group room wall chart prior to the session
- Actual visit consists of two components—the physical examination segment (typically done first) and the interactive group segment (which is basically a small DIGMA)
- Minimal talk occurs in the inefficient exam room setting (only that which is necessary to actually conduct the physical and truly private matters)
- Almost all discussion is deferred to the interactive group segment that follows—where repetition can be avoided, efficiency can be gained, and all present can interact and learn
- Typical group size in primary care is seven to nine male or six to eight female patients, but is somewhat larger (often 10–13 patients) in the medical and surgical subspecialties, where exams are typically of a more limited nature and can be done faster
- A multidisciplinary, team-based approach to care that typically involves two nurses/MAs, a behaviorist, and a documenter—plus a dedicated scheduler to ensure sessions are full
- Integrates the help and support of other patients into each patient's healthcare experience
- Greater patient education and attention to psychosocial issues are usually provided
- A relatively small group room plus four fully equipped exam rooms are usually employed
- Two nurses/MAs are typically employed during the first half of the PSMA session, with each responsible for two of the four exam rooms (i.e., rooming patients and completing vitals and all nursing duties) – or else, one can room patients and take vitals while the other cleans up the exam room immediately after each patient's physical is completed (i.e., as the patient is being escorted back to the group room)
- In order to have the typical four exam rooms available for the PSMA, it is often the physician's own two exam rooms that are used–along with another two exam rooms of a colleague who is consistently not in the clinic at the time that the PSMA is held
- The exam rooms can be in the physician's own office area, rather than nearby the group room)
- There are heterogeneous, homogeneous, and mixed subtypes of the PSMA model
- The mixed .PSMA subtype is most commonly used in primary care–i.e., in which patients are divided up according to sex and age group
- Used extensively in many areas of primary and specialty care—i.e., whenever a private physical exam is needed (for intakes as well as physicals for established patients)
- Appropriate privacy is always maintained
- Patients are not nude together, or herded en masse from station to station to gain efficiency
- Visits are max-packed by fully expanding the nursing personnel and behaviorist's duties
- While the physician is conducting the private physicals during the first half of the session, the behaviorist is in the group room with the rotating group of unroomed patients—writing down the medical issues that each patient wants addressed during today's visit, educating, and fostering group interaction
- Documentation support is almost always provided throughout
- There are high levels of patient satisfaction and physician professional satisfaction

Many Consider PSMAs to Be "No Brainers"

Some healthcare administrators have referred to the PSMA model as a *no brainer* because, as they put it: "Any time you can triple the productivity of the physician in delivering complete physical examinations while also having happier patients and physicians—and can accomplish this while simultaneously eliminating the waste and physician downtime of no-shows and late-cancels—then that is a no-brainer." When properly designed, supported, and implemented, PSMAs can also be of greatest economic benefit to physicians and healthcare organizations (i.e.,

among all group visit models) because they are tripling the efficiency of delivering physical examinations rather than follow-up visits (like DIGMAs and CHCCs)—and physical examinations represent one of the greatest time sinks in the physician's practice.

Up to nine primary care physicals can be provided in the same amount of time that it would normally take to deliver just two or three, or up to 13 physicals in specialty care in the amount of time that it would usually take to deliver just two to six physicals (Table 5.2). In the case of one plastic surgeon that I consulted with having 1 hour intake appointments for breast reduction surgeries, we

Table 5.2 Why the PSMA model is so efficient

1. It provides a multidisciplinary team-based approach to care that off-loads as much as possible and appropriate from the physician, and instead delegates these responsibilities to the various, less costly SMA team members
2. It enables providers to conduct the actual physical exam in a streamlined fashion by using a documenter, along with two nurses/MAs and several properly equipped exam rooms, during the first half of the session—without the delays, interruptions, and inefficiencies that so often accompany traditional physical examinations
3. It defers almost all discussions from the inefficient individual exam room setting (except for what needs to be discussed in order to conduct the exams and truly private matters) to the more productive group room setting that follows—where repetition can be avoided and all present can simultaneously listen, interact, and benefit
4. As the physician goes around the group room focusing upon each patient individually in the interactive group setting, efficiency is gained because patients begin to say: "I had five things I wanted to discuss with you today, but you already covered three of them"
5. Detailed health history forms as well as all lab tests are completed by patients prior to the visits, and entered beforehand into patients' PSMA chart notes (plus, test results are written on a wall chart by a nurse or MA prior to the session, with abnormal results circled in red)
6. During the first half of the session, the behaviorist ferrets out each patient's medical issues that they want to have discussed today and writes them down on a flip chart or erasable whiteboard (often with grid lines on it), thus saving the time that it would otherwise take the physician to do so
7. A documenter is typically provided throughout the entire session (i.e., in both the private exam and interactive group segments), which greatly enhances the physician's productivity—and can result in a superior chart note that is both comprehensive and contemporaneous
8. Sessions can be overbooked according to the expected number of late-cancels and no-shows, thus making PSMAs immune to these costly problems—i.e., by eliminating expensive physician downtime experienced with individual physical exams when patients do fail to attend)

were actually able to increase her productivity by approximately 800% during her first PSMA session (and to accomplish this with increased levels of patient satisfaction)—which was the highest increase that, at least to my knowledge, has ever been achieved by either the DIGMA or PSMA models.

Of All SMA Models, the PSMA Is the Most Counterintuitive and Misunderstood

Yet there is probably no other group visit model that is so counterintuitive, so misunderstood, and so frequently poorly designed in actual practice as the PSMA model. When done properly, PSMAs can be a huge success; however, when incorrectly designed and improperly run, they can be extremely frustrating and quick to fail. Therefore, this chapter is specifically dedicated to enabling you to understand the *nuts and bolts* of designing and conducting PSMAs correctly in your practice so that you too can enjoy the multiple benefits that this remarkable and innovative group visit model can offer when successfully applied.

The concept of delivering private physical examinations in a group visit setting is completely counterintuitive and conjures up images of old World War II physicals in which patients were nude together and ushered en masse from station to station in order to gain efficiency. Yet the PSMA model is nothing like that, as it gains its efficiency through a simple observation—i.e., what takes almost all of the time in a physical examination is not the exam itself, but rather all the talk that accompanies it. So why not gain efficiency by conducting rapid but thorough physical examinations individually in the privacy of the exam room, and defer all of the talk (except for what needs to be discussed in

order to conduct the exam and truly private matters) to an interactive group segment that follows immediately afterward (basically a small DIGMA)—where all present can listen and learn, and repetition can be avoided?

Full Sessions Are the Key to Success

The most important key to a successful, lively, and highly interactive PSMA is to maintain desired census levels during all sessions—i.e., to consistently achieve the target census of six to eight female or seven to nine male patients in primary care (or of 10–13 patients in most of the medical and surgical subspecialties, where the exam itself is often of a more focused and limited nature). This is important both for effective group dynamics and the economic viability of the program. Because of the relatively small number of patients in attendance (i.e., when compared to DIGMAs and CHCCs), I would recommend that you design your PSMA to be toward the high side of the recommended census range rather than toward the low side in order to achieve effective group dynamics. Maintaining census targets is best accomplished by effectively promoting the program, by personally inviting all appropriate patients seen during regular office visits to have their next physical in a PSMA, and by overbooking sessions according to the expected number of no-shows and late-cancels. Of course, it is equally important that the physician and treatment team be properly trained, clearly understand their respective roles and responsibilities, and gain sufficient experience in actual practice to efficiently see this number of patients during a 90-minute PSMA session—i.e., while delivering quality care and still finishing on time with all documentation completed.

PSMAs Are Already Gaining Widespread Attention in Primary and Specialty Care

Originally designed for primary care, PSMAs are now being expanded widely into many of the medical and surgical subspecialties in such applications as digital rectal exams in urology; prenatal exams in obstetrics; pelvic exams in gynecology; foot exams in podiatry; well-baby exams and school, camp, and sports physicals in pediatrics (Fig. 5.1); intakes for breast reduction and for carpal tunnel surgeries in plastic surgery; intakes and follow-ups for knee and hip replacement surgeries in orthopedic surgery; intakes and follow-ups for bariatric surgery and benign fibrocystic breast disease in general surgery; follow-ups for bone marrow transplants in hematology; vaccinations for long- and short-term travelers in travel medicine; pacemaker interrogations in cardiology; cosmetic issues, acne, and skin cancers in dermatology (i.e., when full-body skin exams are needed); pre-surgery cataract physicals in ophthalmology; and intaking combat vets from Iraq and Afghanistan into the VA. For example, Kaider-Person et al. recently found that they were able to use the PSMA model at Cleveland Clinic's Bariatric Institute to provide high-volume follow-up and offer bariatric patients prompt access to care, and to accomplish this with high levels of patient satisfaction (5).

More and more, the PSMA model continues to be refined, adapted, and expanded into new areas of application in both primary care and the various medical subspecialties. Many medical specialists doing procedures and surgeries appreciate the fact that the PSMA model enables them to off-load many time-consuming individual intake and/or follow-up appointments onto highly efficient PSMA visits—which allows them to open up more procedure and surgery time on their master schedules, and to therefore to do more of what they often love to do most while simultaneously enhancing their bottom lines.

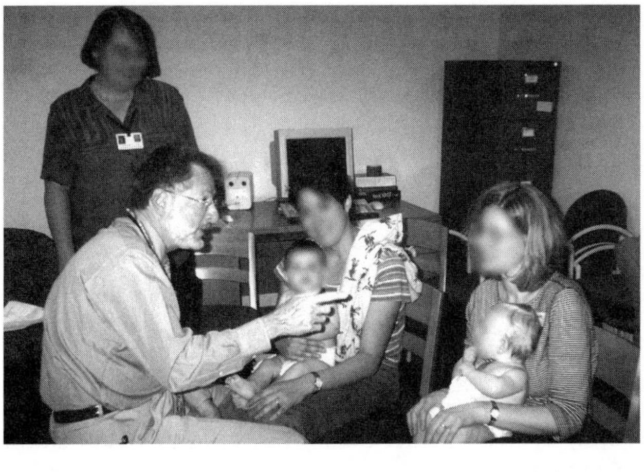

The Role of PSMAs in Chronic Illness and Geriatric Programs

Like DIGMAs, PSMAs can play an important role not only in better managing busy and backlogged practices (by solving access problems to physical examinations, and by enabling many individual physical exam appointment slots to be converted into follow-up or other visit types), because so many physical exams can be off-loaded onto highly efficient PSMAs each week), but also in the care of geriatric and chronically ill patients due to the crucial role they can play in both geriatric programs and chronic illness care pathways. For example, PSMAs can be used both in intaking patients into a chronic illness population management program (i.e., whenever a private physical exam is required as part of the intake process), and for providing private physicals for routine follow-ups on patients already enrolled in the disease management program. Although still quite new and unfamiliar to many, the PSMA model has already been successfully employed with several chronic illnesses and health conditions in a wide variety of primary and specialty care applications. Like DIGMAs, PSMAs have been successfully used by many types of providers (physicians, nurse practitioners, physician assistants, etc.) having a wide variety of personalities and practice styles—and in a wide variety of settings (e.g., in fee-for-service, capitated, PPO, HMO, IPA, military, and public hospital settings).

Fig. 5.1 This Well Baby Checks Pediatrics PSMA for infants was enjoyed by all (courtesy of Dr. Richard Green, Well Baby Checks PSMA, Palo Alto Medical Foundation, Palo Alto, CA)

PSMA Patient Sources

Although patients for the PSMA are typically drawn from the physician's own practice, this is not necessarily the case. Whenever possible, it is wise to draw patients from your own practice as that enhances continuity of care; however, there are also many situations in which this is not possible or appropriate. For example, in chronic illness treatment programs, patients are often referred according to diagnosis by many providers. Therefore, physicians attached to the chronic illness population management program will often see patients having a particular chronic illness for that component of their care—even though these patients are typically being followed by different physicians throughout the system for other aspects of their care. In addition, sometimes providers on a particular team, module, pod, etc., will share patients between themselves, so that when such providers run a PSMA they might very well include the patients from the other providers in their group.

Another example of physicians seeing patients outside of their own practice was provided by a primary care provider who was struggling to keep his PSMA sessions full once he had caught up with his own backlog of patients waiting for physicals—i.e., as a direct result of the productivity gains that he achieved through his PSMA. This challenge of filling subsequent PSMA sessions persisted even after he cut back substantially on the number of individual physical examinations that he offered each week on his master schedule. He therefore asked his busy physician colleagues who also had access problems for physical examinations whether he could also include their wait-listed patients in his PSMA. Although a couple of colleagues refused this generous offer, others were all too happy to accept it—and ultimately found that doing so helped them to solve the access problems they had to physical exams in their practices as well.

An Access Solution for Physical Examinations

The contemporary healthcare challenge of providing prompt access to physical examinations represents a significant and pressing healthcare delivery problem for numerous medical groups around the country. For example, Al Fisk, M.D., Medical Director of The Everett Clinic stated: "One of our biggest problems is access. We have a huge demand for primary care appointments—for physical exams, new appointments, same-day visits, and re-checks. We also have a huge demand for specialty appointments. We are unable to grow fast enough to meet these needs" (1).

Simultaneously maintaining desired levels of access to both physical examinations and follow-up appointments through use of existing resources presents a significant and ongoing challenge to many integrated delivery systems in today's rapidly changing and highly competitive healthcare environment. Many group practices and managed care organizations simply lack the necessary resources to hire enough physicians and associated support staff to achieve and maintain good access to both physical exams and return appointments in primary and specialty care through sole use of the traditional individual office visit model. Furthermore, when emphasis is placed upon improving access for return appointments, it sometimes results in deteriorating access for physical examinations and vice versa.

As reported in the January 2002 issue of *Group Practice Journal*, David Hooper, M.D., senior administrator of clinical services at the Palo Alto Medical Foundation, states: "The PSMA and DIGMA programs are the only methods I have ever seen that simultaneously improve M.D. morale, improve patient satisfaction, improve access, improve the healing experience for patients with chronic symptoms, and make money. The Physicals Exam SMA is even more important to this organization than DIGMAs are for return visits. This is because the single most expensive service we provide in the outpatient setting is the annual exam. We don't have enough M.D. capacity to do the preventive services that our patient population needs from us. We have to get creative about how to provide these services more efficiently. We will not be able to hire enough doctors to keep up with the growth of our practice" (1).

Benefits of a Well-Run PSMA Program

In this section, we address some of the multifarious benefits that properly run PSMAs can offer. Despite the additional personnel and facilities requirements that they entail, PSMAs can so greatly increase a physician's productivity in delivering private physical examinations that they are nonetheless able to offer a substantial net economic benefit to those providers who choose to use them.

Increased Time with One's Physician, Greater Patient Education, and the Help and Support of Other Patients

As with all SMA models, properly run PSMAs can increase both the amount of patient education and the amount of time that patients have with their physician—plus they integrate the help and support of other patients into each patient's healthcare experience.

Quality Care and a Multidisciplinary, Team-Based Approach to Care

Like other SMA models (although they are directed at follow-up visits rather than physical examinations), the PSMA model provides quality medical care and a multidisciplinary, team-based approach to care. In the case of PSMAs, the multidisciplinary team typically includes two nursing personnel; a behaviorist who—unlike DIGMAs, where the preferred behaviorist is often a psychologist or social worker due to the large group size—is often a nurse; a documenter; and a dedicated scheduler to ensure that all sessions are consistently kept filled to the desired capacity. In addition, larger healthcare systems typically also have a SMA champion and program coordinator in order to move the group visit program forward throughout the entire system as rapidly as possible. In addition, everything possible is done to enhance the quality of care within the PSMA—i.e., Patient Packets that include relevant educational materials, max-packed visits, prompt access, more time, greater patient education, etc.

Greater Efficiency, Improved Access to Physicals, and High Levels of Patient and Physician Satisfaction

Key features of the PSMA model include dramatically increased physician productivity in delivering physical examinations; improved patient access to physical exams; high levels of patient and physician satisfaction; greater attention to psychosocial issues; and a series of one physician–one patient encounters throughout focusing upon delivery of individualized medical care from start to finish.

New Physicians Can Grow Their Practices—Plus Help Solve the Organization's Access Problems

In addition to the multiple benefits for which PSMAs were originally designed, there are many additional potential benefits that are less obvious. For example, consider the new physician whose schedule is not yet full who happens to work at a facility with access problems—i.e., a facility having some very busy physicians with established practices and long wait-lists for physical exams. By starting a PSMA for his/her practice and including new patient intakes, this physician can both grow a practice plus immediately benefit from the increased productivity and efficiency of the PSMA model—and do so while simultaneously helping the facility to enable new patients to get into the system without waiting.

This physician can also help to improve access to physical examinations at the facility by asking backlogged colleagues for permission to have their patients who are wait-listed for physical exams given the opportunity to attend the physician's PSMA within a couple of weeks. Although this decreases continuity of care, it does enable wait-listed patients to be seen promptly for a physical examination—and many patients will prefer this option to waiting, especially once the patient benefits of the program are explained. Although some colleagues might not agree to this arrangement, others very likely will—plus appreciate both the improved access to physicals that this approach will ultimately provide to their own practice and the increased service that will be offered to their patients.

Patients Sometimes Bring Up Medically Significant Symptoms for the First Time

There are many other potential benefits to a carefully designed and properly run PSMA program. For example, take the patient who denies, minimizes, or fails to report medically important information to the physician—such as cardiovascular symptoms, which are known to often go under-reported in the primary care setting. Whether this occurs out of ignorance or psychological defenses, the results of keeping the physician uninformed can ultimately be catastrophic to the patient. However, this under-reporting of important medical symptoms can be less likely to happen in the PSMA setting. When another patient brings up symptoms, risk factors, or health problems during the interactive group setting that also apply to the patient, experience demonstrates that the patient will often let the doctor know that this discussion also applies to him/her—which permits this medical issue to then be properly addressed, even though it might not have been previously disclosed to the physician.

In one recent Primary Care PSMA, a patient only brought to the doctor's attention that he had been having shortness of breath and chest pain upon even the slightest exertion because another patient brought these issues up in his own case. As a result, the physician was able to arrange for prompt follow-up cardiac testing, which subsequently revealed a severe blockage in one of the patient's major coronary arteries. This is not an uncommon event in a PSMA, and should help to allay the fears of physicians who are concerned that they might miss something important in the PSMA group setting. The truth is that, despite their own best efforts, they will likely occasionally miss things in the group setting; however, what surprises many is how often they are already missing important things during traditional office visits. Because patients often reveal a different type of information in group visits than they do during traditional office visits, my belief has always been that the physicians who will end up knowing the most about their patients are those who offer both individual and group visits in their practices.

Improved Compliance with Recommended Treatment Regimens

Another hidden benefit of the PSMA program is improved compliance with recommended treatment regimens. Other patients in the group will often support the physician in getting noncompliant patients to rethink their position and follow the doctor's treatment recommendations—often doing so in a kind and gentle (albeit firm) manner. Patients refusing to make the treatment or lifestyle change that is being recommended by the physician can often be persuaded to comply by other group members who have already made such changes—such as those who have already quit smoking, begun exercising, lost weight, started insulin, began to watch their diet, or started dialysis. Patients who were once similarly noncompliant with the physician's treatment recommendations—patients with whom the noncompliant patient can readily identify—can be particularly effective in this regard. Similarly, patients who are reluctant to take a medication or to undergo a recommended diagnostic procedure (such as a colonoscopy or thallium treadmill) can often be persuaded to do so by other patients who have already taken the medication or undergone the procedure. These patients frequently encourage the reluctant patient to do likewise, often by indicating that it is not as difficult as it sounds—or else by pointing out what the consequences of not following through on the doctor's treatment recommendations could be.

All Types of Providers of Physical Examinations Can Benefit—Not Just Physicians

Analogous to our discussion of the DIGMA and CHCC group visit models, although the term *physician* will usually be used in this chapter on PSMAs, all types of providers of physical examinations (such as nurse practitioners, physician assistants, osteopaths, surgeons, and podiatrists) can also run PSMAs for their practices with the similar benefits—i.e., by using the same types of program design, staffing, facilities, and promotional materials. I only use *physician* here because that is the term that I am most used to employing in the numerous presentations to medical groups that I have made over the years—i.e., because most of the audience is typically physicians and because many of them object to the term *provider*.

PSMAs Can Benefit the Entire Department

Another medical group had five obstetricians at one of their facilities, all of whom had access problems for prenatal exams in their practices. Therefore, I encouraged each of these five obstetricians to start a weekly 90-minute PSMA for prenatal exams in their practice—with each obstetrician's SMA being held at the same time in the morning, but on five different days of the week. The first obstetrician's Prenatal PSMA would be on Mondays at 8–9:30 AM, the second on Tuesdays from 8 to 9:30, etc. In addition to including their own patients, all five obstetricians agreed to also open their Prenatal PSMAs to patients from their colleagues' practices as well—i.e., patients needing or wanting an immediate appointment, but unable to get in to see their own obstetrician in a timely manner. Figure 5.2 shows a Prenatal PSMA.

This approach provided three clear and important benefits to the entire Obstetrics Department at that facility. *First* of all, this Prenatal PSMA design offered the added benefit of providing a useful tool for handling the *bumps* that so often occurred in each obstetrician's practice—i.e., when they had to cancel a couple hours of office visits in order to go and deliver a baby. This was important as these bumps had become the *bane* of their existence—especially when the patient being bumped had already been bumped before (or had waited weeks for the appointment that was being bumped) and there was nowhere else on the obstetrician's schedule in which to put the bumped patient during the next couple of weeks.

Because each of these five obstetricians designed their PSMAs as they did, all prenatal patients who were bumped from any obstetrician's regular office visit schedule could thereafter be given the following choice when

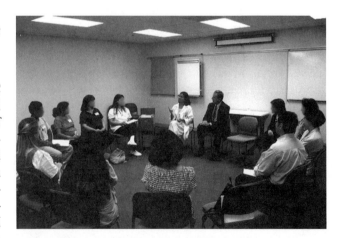

Fig. 5.2 As the behaviorist, I found this Obstetrics Prenatal Exam PSMA to be a delight to participate in (courtesy of Dr. Mary Ann Sarda-Maduro, Obstetrics Prenatal Exam PSMA, Palo Alto Medical Foundation, Palo Alto, CA)

being rescheduled: (1) they could be scheduled either into their own obstetrician's next available brief individual appointment, which might be weeks away; or (2) they could instead be scheduled into the 90-minute Prenatal PSMA the very next morning (or else into the first such PSMA that the patient was able to attend). The patient would then be promptly scheduled into whichever choice they made. Even if they chose the individual appointment weeks away, having this choice tended to diffuse their anger over the fact that they had been bumped and now needed to wait for weeks in order to get back in to see their own obstetrician—i.e., because they could have instead made the choice to be seen in the 90-minute PSMA the very next morning. Furthermore, the patient—instead of opting to attend another obstetrician's PSMA the next day or to wait for an individual appointment that might be weeks away—could choose instead to attend the next session of their own obstetrician's PSMA, which would be held within a week.

Second, in four out of five such cases, attending the Prenatal PSMA the following morning would also provide the secondary benefit of providing a "*get to know you*" visit with one of the other obstetricians in the department, who might in fact be the obstetrician who ultimately delivers the patient's baby if it occurs after hours, depending upon who happens to be on call at the time. This saved many individual office visits within the department as, prior to instituting this Prenatal PSMA program, each patient had to be scheduled for an individual visit with each of the other four obstetricians—some of which no longer needed to be made due to the patient having already met that provider through their Prenatal PSMA.

Third, it solved the department's access problems regarding prenatal exams. Initially, the Obstetrics Department's access problems were solved for group visits, because a prenatal exam PSMA visit could immediately be offered to all of their patients any day that they wanted to be seen. Soon, the department's access problems were solved by the PSMA program for individual prenatal exam visits as well—i.e., because so many individual prenatal exams were being off-loaded onto highly efficient PSMA visits, so that they too eventually became more available (i.e., as a result of the increased capacity that the PSMA afforded). In other words, many individual office visits were also saved in the Obstetrics Department because patients liked the PSMA program due to the many benefits that it offered to them. Therefore, each of the obstetricians was able to invite many of their own patients back to their Prenatal PSMA for many of their regularly scheduled prenatal follow-up visits—an offer that numerous patients accepted in lieu of traditional follow-up office visits, which opened up even more individual prenatal exam visits.

Additional individual office visits were saved because patients were invited to attend a Prenatal PSMA in a timely manner whenever they wanted to be seen—i.e., rather than scheduling and waiting for a brief individual office visit that might be days or weeks away when they had a question or medical need in between their normally scheduled visits. In this case, they could simply pre-schedule or drop-in to the next available Prenatal PSMA that best fit their own schedule. However, when patients did drop in, they were asked to telephone the office at least a day in advance for two reasons: (1) to confirm that the group would in fact be meeting that day (and that the obstetrician was not out ill, on vacation, or attending a meeting); and (2) to let the office staff know that they were coming so that census could be monitored and paperwork organized.

Overview of the PSMA Model

PSMAs are generally held weekly for 90 minutes, although they could be of either shorter or longer duration and could be held either less or more frequently. Patients only come when they need a physical examination—i.e., these are medically necessary visits. Frequently divided by sex and age group using the mixed subtype, Primary Care PSMAs most frequently contain between 7–9 male patients (or 6–8 female patients); however, the census in the various medical subspecialties is often somewhat larger (typically between 10–13 patients) because the exams are of a more limited nature and can be completed faster. In general, these patients are due or past due for a physical examination, and typically meet certain selection criteria—such as position on the wait-list, age range, sex, and diagnosis. Because these physical exams would normally require 20–45 minutes each when provided individually—plus would include some no-shows and late-cancels—the PSMA result is typically a 200–300% or more increase over the physician's productivity for traditional individual physicals in the primary care (with 300% being the most common goal), and sometimes 300–400% (or even more) in the various medical and surgical subspecialties. Exceptions to this are pediatrics, obstetrics, and dermatology, where productivity can often only be doubled through the PSMA due to the fast pace that these providers so frequently have in delivering individual physical examinations. The major component parts of the PSMA are discussed in more detail later in the chapter.

The PSMA Team

Because PSMAs represent a multidisciplinary team-based approach to care in which the various nonphysician team members contribute to all aspects of the visit (including identifying and rectifying any relevant personnel, facilities, promotional, IT, operational, administrative, and organizational problems that could impact the program), the key to success lies in assembling a skilled and compatible team that enables the physician to delegate as many responsibilities as possible and appropriate onto other, less costly members of the team. As depicted in Table 5.3 (on the behaviorist's responsibilities), Table 5.4 (on the champion and program coordinator's

Table 5.3 Various duties of the behaviorist during the initial physical examination segment of the PSMA (while alone with the rotating group of unroomed patients)

- Arrive a few minutes early to welcome patients, introduce staff, and warm the group up
- *Write important patient health concerns down* on a flip chart or whiteboard. First and foremost, tactfully ask each patient: "What are the one or two (or else, two or three) most important health concerns that you would like to discuss with the physician today"—i.e., during the interactive group segment. The behaviorist then writes all of these issues down next to each patient's name on a flip chart or whiteboard, along with any other significant issues that the patient may have reported on the health history form that they previously completed and sent to the physician's office. Then, upon later entering the group room after completing all of the private physical examinations, the physician can see in a glance what all of the health concerns are of the various patients. This saves the physician time. These issues, along with important findings from the physical exam and any pertinent lab test results depicted on the wall chart in the group room, are discussed as the physician sequentially addresses each patient during the interactive group setting that follows.
- Give the *introduction* to all patients in attendance (see Chapters 2 and 10, as well as the behaviorist training video on the DVD attached to this book to see how I recommend giving the introduction to a DIGMA or PSMA). In this introduction, the behaviorist: (1) welcomes patients and explains the benefits that the PSMA is intended to offer to patients (prompt access, more time, greater patient education, answers to questions they may not have thought to ask, etc.); (2) discusses what to expect during today's session and how to make the best possible use of the interactive group segment and the time being spent with the physician (for example, by focusing immediately upon those issues of greatest importance to them, and by sharing helpful personal experiences with other patients); (3) addresses all relevant aspects of confidentiality and the need for patients to sign the confidentiality release form; (4) encourages patient participation; (5) points out that individual physical exams are still available to patients in the future, just like before (although patients are also welcome to return to the PSMA setting for future physical exams if they prefer); and (6) covers housekeeping and personal comfort issues (such as where the bathrooms are, the need to turn cell phones off, and the fact that coffee, healthy snacks, and water are available on the table for patients to enjoy whenever they would like during the session). This usually means giving the introduction twice during the first part of the PSMA session (i.e., while the behaviorist is alone with patients) so that all patients are able to hear it, including those who were initially roomed in exam rooms when the introduction was given the first time. It is true that the behaviorist could avoid this duplicity by waiting until all patients have had their private physical examinations completed, and then giving a 3- to 5-minute introduction once all patients are present in the group room at the start of the interactive group segment. However, the interactive group segment is always packed with patient–physician interactions and is just 45 minutes or so in duration. Therefore, giving the introduction twice to patients before the physician enters the group room for the interactive group segment gives the physician additional time and increases the physician's productivity during the session.
- Ensure that all present have *signed the confidentiality agreement/release* form for the session and then collect signed forms from any attendees who might not yet have signed and turned it in when previously asked to do so by the receptionist and/or nurse.
- *Distribute and discuss informational handouts* preselected by the physician to patients with various health conditions such as: educational handouts on community and internal resources; healthy lifestyles (exercise, nutrition, weight loss, smoking cessation, etc.); screening tests (such as those for colon cancer screening); and medical topics of common interest (such as on cholesterol, hypertension, diabetes, breast self-exam, osteoporosis, PSA and prostate health, heart disease, etc.). This only occurs after the various patient concerns discussed above have first been written down on the flip chart or whiteboard, and when the behaviorist still has additional time remaining (while the physician is outside of the group room providing the private physical examinations with a minimum of discussion). The behaviorist is alone with the rotating group of unroomed patients for approximately the first 45 minutes of the session, so it is wise to have a backup plan to avoid awkward silences should the behaviorist run out of things to say. However, in these discussions, the behaviorist does need to stay within his/her skill set and scope of practice under licensure
- *Discuss behavioral health and psychosocial issues of common interest* to the patients who are present, assuming that the behaviorist is a mental health professional, although the issues discussed will likely be quite different if the behaviorist is a nurse. The behaviorist could possibly even provide handouts as appropriate (on such issues as brief stress reduction and relaxation exercises, sleep problems, depression, anxiety, substance abuse, stress etc.) that are of relevance to the group–or on various medical and nursing issues, if the behaviorist is a nurse. It is important that the behaviorist be tactful when bringing up and discussing psychosocial issues, keeping in mind that the patients are here for a physical examination from their physician
- *Warm the group up by fostering some group interaction* during this time when patients are in the group room with just the behaviorist—as, they can often interact with each other in a helpful, supportive, and encouraging manner. Also, other patients may add health-related issues to their own list on the whiteboard or flip chart, i.e., because other patients bring them up first as issues that they would like to discuss with the physician. This can be especially important with cardiovascular symptoms, which are known to frequently be minimized or denied by patients and often go under-reported to physicians. Patients might also share personal experiences (or coping and disease self-management strategies) that have worked for them during this segment of the PSMA visit
- *Perform all of the normal behaviorist responsibilities for a DIGMA* during the subsequent interactive group segment—i.e., just as soon as all private physical examinations are completed and the physician enters the group room for the interactive group segment of the PSMA session (which is essentially a small DIGMA). When the physician first comes into the group room, the behaviorist can take a minute to briefly bring the physician up to date on any important issues that might have been brought up during the time that the behaviorist has just spent alone with the patients—especially those issues that need to get into patients' chart notes

Table 5.4 What the champion and program coordinator can do to help you

- Custom design the PSMA to the physician's specific needs, goals, and patient panel
- Arrange to have all forms, promotional materials, and enclosures for the Patient Packet (as well as a chart note template) customized and developed from existing templates and materials in the SMA program—i.e., for the physician's review, modification, and ultimate approval
- Help to secure the team members that will be attached to the physician's PSMA—nurse/MA/nursing tech(s), behaviorist, documenter, and dedicated scheduler
- Develop a computer code for the physician's PSMA program, and change the master schedules of the physician and the entire team to include the PSMA on an ongoing basis
- Mail announcement letters to all appropriate patients in the physician's practice prior to launching the PSMA program
- Train the physician's reception, nursing, and scheduling staffs as to their respective roles and responsibilities in supporting the program—and in effectively referring all appropriate patients into the PSMA
- Train the behaviorist, documenter, and nursing personnel attached to the PSMA, although it is advisable for the physician to also play some role in this training to ensure that their respective duties are conducted in the PSMA as the physician wishes
- Set up the necessary procedures and pre-booking census reports to ensure that the appropriate number of patients are consistently scheduled into each session
- Secure and schedule the group room and exam rooms for the PSMA on a regular basis, except, of course, for the physician's own exam rooms
- Ensure that all the necessary equipment (including working computers, printers, and telephones as needed) is properly installed in the group and exam rooms—and that these rooms are properly set up for the PSMA sessions (forms, medical equipment, furnishings, proper IT infrastructure, etc.)
- Order wall posters, and have them framed and prominently mounted on the physician's lobby and exam room walls—along with a dispenser (to be mounted next to the framed wall poster) capable of holding 100 or more program description fliers
- Make sufficient copies on an ongoing basis of all promotional materials (fliers, invitations, handouts, Patient Packets, etc.) to be used by the physician (or else delegate this to SMA site champion)
- Address all of the logistics surrounding the Patient Packet (and assign appropriate personnel to them) so that these materials are sent to—and received back from—scheduled patients in a timely manner
- Prior to the session, arrange to have a motivated person from the physician's support staff enter data from completed health history questionnaires returned by patients into their respective PSMA chart notes
- Arrange to have physician's MA or nurse enter the lab test results for each patient entered on the lined whiteboard in the group room prior to the start of the PSMA session
- Handle any operational, system, or administrative issues that might need to be addressed in order to launch and run a successful PSMA program
- The champion and/or program coordinator can also sit in on two or three of the physician's initial PSMA sessions, observing and measuring the amount of time consumed by each physical (and in working with each patient in the interactive group segment)—plus join the physician and PSMA team (behaviorist, nursing personnel, and documenter) as they debrief after sessions for 15–20 minutes during the first 2 months of implementation—focusing upon fine-tuning and improving the program to make it even better and more efficient in future weeks
- They can help keep all sessions filled to capacity by issuing a weekly pre-booking census report on how full all sessions are for the next 4 sessions, and then by alerting the physician and staff regarding any insufficiently filled sessions—as well as by having the dedicated scheduler *top off* any unfilled sessions by calling lists of appropriate patients selected by the physician and inviting them to attend
- Once launched, they can evaluate the PSMA program on an ongoing basis and issue periodic reports to keep both the physician and management updated on the program, how it is progressing, and whether or not it is meeting its goals

responsibilities), and Table 5.5 (on the nursing personnel's responsibilities), all members of the PSMA team provide vital support functions and play critically important roles in the overall success of the program.

A characteristic feature of the PSMA (and DIGMA) is the *behaviorist* (often a nurse in PSMAs, but sometimes a specially trained mental health professional such as a psychologist or social worker with group experience and interest in working with medical patients) who, like the physician, is present throughout the entire session. The behaviorist discharges a myriad of responsibilities during both the initial physical examination (as depicted in Table 5.3) and interactive group segments (as discussed in Chapters 2 and 3, on DIGMAs, as this is essentially a small DIGMA) of each and every PSMA session. The

behaviorist assists the physician in a multitude of ways: (1) by running the small, revolving group of unroomed patients during the initial physical examination segment while the physician is providing the private exams (warming up the group, giving the introduction, identifying patients' health concerns and writing them down, distributing handouts, collecting any signed confidentiality waivers that have not yet been turned in, addressing psychosocial and behavioral health issues, etc.); and (2) by keeping the interactive group segment of the session running smoothly and on time (facilitating the group, handling group dynamic issues, addressing psychosocial issues, temporarily taking over the group while the physician is reviewing and modifying the chart note immediately after working with each patient, etc.).

Table 5.5 Fully expand the nursing role (RN, LVN, MA) to be all that it can be

- Usually two MAs (or nurses) and four exam rooms are used in the PSMA to ensure that enough patients are always roomed to make certain that the physician never catches up with the nurses—and, therefore, is never left waiting in the hallway for a patient to be roomed and for vitals to be completed
- They will usually divide up their duties in either of two ways: (1) so that each one is responsible for two of the four exam rooms; or (2) so that one rooms patients and completes vitals while the other cleans up the exam room after each physical examination is completed.
- Room all patients in turn into the exam rooms being used in the PSMA
- Take all standard vital signs, plus any extra vitals as requested by the physician
- Update and bring all injections current (flu shots, tetanus, pneumovax, etc.)—again, if it is within the nursing personnel's skill set and scope of practice under licensure
- Perform any other *special duties* requested by the physician—such as checking the peak flow and pulse oximetry (pO_2) levels of any patients with asthma
- Ensure that all patients have signed the confidentiality release form for the session, and have any patients who have not yet done so sign it at this time
- Give patients any appropriate handouts that the physician might want the nurses to distribute
- Search the patient's medical chart for routine health maintenance that is due and update it—pulling and partially completing any appropriate referral forms (i.e., the patient information parts of these forms)
- According to the physician's wishes, the nursing personnel can review and update each patient's personal and family medical history (drug allergies, health habits, high-risk behaviors, current medications, changes in health status, any health concerns they might be having, etc.), and then document these items into the patient's chart note for the PSMA session
- Assist in the documentation support for the PSMA session by entering into the patient's chart note any germane information related to the functions that the nursing personnel have just performed—usually in a separate section of the chart note template that has been set aside for entering all nursing functions performed (which can later be reviewed by the physician either in the exam room or when completing the chart note after working with each patient in the interactive group setting)

The *champion* (used in larger systems only) is the critically important, pivotal person who is charged with overall responsibility for the entire PSMA program (see Table 5.4)—from developing the PSMA program and helping newly recruited physicians to design and implement their PSMAs, to moving the program forward throughout the system as rapidly as possible from pilot study to facility- and organization-wide implementation.

The *program coordinator* (also used primarily in larger systems only) is responsible for: assisting the champion in every possible way; supporting all physicians running PSMAs in their practices on an ongoing basis; monitoring census regularly; managing the dedicated schedulers and behaviorists; producing periodic evaluations and reports for the program; and handling most of the PSMA program's operational and administrative details (see Table 5.4).

The *nursing personnel* (usually two nurses/MAs/nursing techs—and typically including the physician's own nurse or MA—with each responsible for two exam rooms) play a much expanded role in the PSMA—much as they do in a DIGMA (see Table 5.5). They not only room patients and take vital signs but also update injections, help keep routine health maintenance current, update performance measures, document the nursing duties that have been performed on each patient, and perform additional *special duties* as requested by the physician. In addition, one of the nurses/MAs typically prepares the large wall chart depicting all of the patients' previsit lab test results prior to the visit—typically with findings that the physician considers to be abnormal circled in red and borderline findings circumscribed by a dotted red line. Sometimes, rather

than each MA being responsible for two exam rooms, one MA will room patients and take vital signs while the other cleans up the exam rooms after each exam is completed. A nurse or MA can also make confirmation phone calls a couple of days prior to the PSMA to confirm the appointment, ensure that pre-visit labs have been completed, check that the detailed health history form has been completed and returned to the office, and conduct a medication reconciliation.

The *dedicated scheduler* is charged with the responsibility of *topping-off* sessions and ensuring that every session is completely full. The dedicated scheduler is typically a clerical person with scheduling and telemarketing skills who has been specially trained to telephone and invite patients that the physician wants invited (from the waitlist for physicals, from other lists selected by the physician, or from those already scheduled for individual physicals weeks or months into the future), and then sends the Patient Packet to patients who agree to attend the PSMA.

Administration and *the physician's entire support staff* also play crucial roles in supporting the program, inviting and scheduling patients, and in making the PSMA program a success. For example, a motivated volunteer from the physician's support staff is typically recruited to enter into patients upcoming PSMA chart notes the information that was completed by the patient and returned to the office—i.e., information written onto the detailed health questionnaire form that was included in the Patient Packet originally sent to the patient. It is worth noting that some systems are trying to address firewall problems so that this information could be entered directly by patients into their own upcoming PSMA chart note. The

MA or nurse frequently enters each patient's previsit lab results on the lined whiteboard in the group room prior to the session. It is worth noting that it is often quite helpful, when enlisting the support of the physician's support staff, to have them actually sit in on a PSMA session as soon as possible—perhaps one or two at a time, starting with key members of the scheduling staff, then the reception staff, and finally any other members of the nursing, administrative, and clerical staffs.

The *documenter* plays a critically important role in PSMAs, a function that is especially important for systems using EMR—as it generally takes considerable time to document an appropriate EMR chart note on physical exams, although systems still using paper charts can sometimes develop a PSMA chart note template that is sufficiently efficient for physicians to complete on their own (i.e., because it is largely preprinted and in check-off form). The documenter increases the physician's efficiency by minimizing the outlay of physician time in the extensive charting responsibilities that physical examinations entail. The documenter is usually a specially trained medical transcriptionist, nurse/MA, nurse practitioner, Pharm.D., medical resident or fellow, clerical staff member, etc.

The documenter, who is also present throughout the entire session, uses the physician's own chart note template to create a real-time, comprehensive, and contemporaneous chart note on each patient—i.e., for the physician to then review, modify, and sign immediately after working with each patient in turn during the interactive group segment of the PSMA. Always present in the group room during the interactive group segment, the documenter can either shadow the physician (in which case, the documenter must be qualified to be in the room with disrobed patients) or remain in the group room documenting what the behaviorist is doing during the preceding physical examination segment—depending upon what the physician wants. In some cases, the provider prefers to briefly jot down physical findings on a crib sheet while conducting physical examinations in the privacy of the exam rooms, and then gives these notes to the documenter upon exiting the exam room (as, in this case, the documenter remains outside of the private exam room setting, but has access to a computer in the area) to complete the physical findings portion of each patient's PSMA chart note.

Being Contemporaneous And Comprehensive, PSMA Chart Note is Often Superior

Also, because a specifically trained documenter using the physician's own chart note template can draft a comprehensive and contemporaneous chart note in vivo and in real time during the PSMA session, superior chart notes for medical services delivered can thereby be generated—which can optimize billing for all medical services rendered. During traditional individual physical examinations in the clinic, the physician would normally forget some of what transpired during the session by the time the chart note was drafted—simply because the chart note would be generated some time later (i.e., immediately after the appointment, during lunch, at the end of the day, by coming in on Saturday morning to wrap up loose ends, etc.). In general, the more delayed the writing of the chart note, the more that will likely be forgotten—and the more likely that the medical services actually provided will be under-billed.

The Documenter Must Learn How to Draft a Good Chart Note Beforehand

Prior to the start of the PSMA, the documenter will need to familiarize himself/herself with the physician's own unique style of writing chart notes. This is accomplished by: (1) reviewing many chart notes previously drafted by the physician beforehand, in order to get a feel for the template that the physician is using; (2) getting the necessary training from the IT department as to charting templates that are already available on the EMR system employed by the organization, and in selecting the one that most closely matches the physician's own charting template; (3) obtaining any needed training from the organization's billing and compliance officer to ensure that all elements important to billing are always entered into chart notes; and (4) shadowing the physician for a couple of days, if necessary, drafting the chart notes for these individual office visits until both the documenter and physician are comfortable with the chart note being generated. The important point here is that the documenter needs to have a good working knowledge in drafting the type of chart note that the physician wants prior to the start of the PSMA—even though this learning process will be ongoing in the PSMA as the physician reviews and modifies each patient's chart note in turn.

The Documenter's Responsibilities During a PSMA

The physician needs to decide what to have the documenter do during the first half of the session—i.e., when the physical examinations are being conducted. In particular, whether to have the documenter: (1) accompany the physician from one exam room to another and enter physical findings into the record while the physical exams are being performed (in which case, the documenter must be a nurse or somebody licensed to be in the exam room with disrobed patients); or (2) whether to have the documenter stay in the group room during the initial physical examination segment to document what is occurring there between the behaviorist and the small rotating group of unroomed patients (an approach which will slow physicians down because they will then need to enter the physical findings into the chart notes themselves). Sometimes, physicians will write the physical findings down on a crib sheet—and then give it to the documenter to enter into the chart note when the physician emerges from the exam room after each physical exam is completed. Although this is less efficient than having the documenter present in the exam room and documenting the physical findings, it can be used whenever it is best (for whatever reason) for the documenter not to be in the exam room.

However, in return for having a documenter, the provider should be willing to (1) consistently achieve targeted census levels for the PSMA and (2) see an additional patient in the PSMA setting (i.e., beyond the pre-established PSMA census level) in order to cover the added overhead cost. Having a documenter to handle 70–90% of the documentation responsibilities for the session is a strong motivator for physicians to run a PSMA in their practice, and therefore to maintain the targeted census level. Many physicians look at chart notes as a necessity, but as drudgery as well. I have yet to meet the physician who states: "You know, the main reason that I went into medicine was to draft chart notes, because that's what I most enjoy doing." Certainly, being able to offer a documenter to the physician who is considering a PSMA for his/her practice will make the champion's job of moving the DIGMA and PSMA program forward throughout the system (and to maintaining desired census levels) a much easier one—because many physicians will otherwise choose to not run a SMA due to concerns regarding the drafting of so many individual chart notes.

Consider Having a Documenter Contingent upon the Physician Maintaining Census

Providing a documenter can also align the interests of the physician with those of administration. Consider, for example, the physician who concludes that even though they can see the pre-established targeted number of patients in their PSMA, they would prefer to see several fewer patients—because it is easier and more relaxing to do it that way. This could undermine the economic, productivity, and access benefits of the entire SMA program, but administration might feel helpless to *hold the line* on census in such a case—especially in systems that are physician run.

However, by offering a documenter—but making the documenter contingent upon achieving targeted census levels on average—administration is offering the physician a strong incentive for consistently maintaining pre-established census levels out of self-interest. Personally, I would gladly see several more patients in my DIGMA or PSMA if it meant that most of my charting responsibilities would be handled for me—especially when I understood that a superior, comprehensive, and contemporaneous chart note that employed my own chart note template would be drafted.

What Skill Set Is Required of a Documenter?

Who can serve as documenter in a PSMA? Clearly, the documenter must have computer skills, be a fast typist, have good grammar and spelling skills, and understand medical terminology. Furthermore, the documenter should be able to work closely with the physician, be a good learner who is able to multitask, and be willing and able to generate the precise type of individualized chart note that the physician wants documented on each patient in the PSMA—i.e., from the chart note template that has been developed for the program. Documenters must also have enough self-confidence to feel comfortable about interrupting the physician in the group setting whenever they have a question that needs to be answered about the chart note—such as how to spell the term that the physician just used (or the medication that was just prescribed). It is also helpful for the documenter to calm and unflappable at all rimes.

Depending upon available resources, the documenter can come from any number of possible disciplines. For example, the documenter could be a nurse, medical assistant, or medical transcriptionist specifically trained for this duty. The documenter could also be a medical resident (who would simultaneously be learning not only how to draft a good chart note but also how to run a group visit), a Pharm.D., or a nurse practitioner. It is important to note that using another provider (such as a nurse practitioner or PA) is seldom recommended—as they could instead be seeing their own patients and generating their own RVUs in the clinic. However, it is one way that such providers can become more comfortable with the PSMA concept by gradually introducing themselves to the PSMA by temporarily being a documenter—i.e., if their intent is to start their own DIGMA or PSMA shortly thereafter. Or else, the documenter could be a highly motivated clerical person drawn from the physician's front- or back-office staff. However, the ultimate choice of documenter will probably depend more upon who happens to be available—and upon the skill set and personality of that individual—than it will upon their particular professional discipline.

Do keep in mind that, in the event the physician wants to have the documenter follow him/her from exam room to exam room during the physical examination segment of the PSMA to document the physical findings that the physician is saying out loud (i.e., rather than staying in the group room and documenting what is occurring between the behaviorist and small rotating group of unroomed patients), then being in the exam room with disrobed patients will need to be a part of the documenter's scope of practice under licensure. Also keep in mind that having another provider (nurse practitioner, PA, Pharm.D, physician, etc.) as a documenter during the PSMA is usually a bad idea as—unless their overhead is costed out according to their hourly wage—this will reduce the productivity gain of the PSMA by half because that provider could also have been seeing patients individually during the 90 minutes of group time.

Subtypes of the PSMA Model

The PSMA model has the same three subtypes as the DIGMA model: homogeneous, heterogeneous, and mixed—of which the mixed subtype tends to be most frequently used in primary care while the homogeneous subtype is most commonly used in the medical and surgical subspecialties. Each subtype has its own strengths and weaknesses; however, together they provide one of the many available options that enable PSMAs to be customized to the specific needs, goals, practice styles, and patient panel constituencies of individual physicians.

The Homogeneous Subtype

In the intuitively appealing homogeneous subtype of the PSMA model, only patients meeting specific diagnostic, condition, age, sex, utilization, risk, etc., criteria qualify to be seen in any given session—so that some commonality exists among the patients, which encourages patient bonding and enables the physician to reach many patients at once while avoiding repetition.

In the Homogeneous Subtype, Patients Can Be Grouped for PSMAs by Diagnosis

The homogeneous subtype is often used for particular diagnoses and conditions in the medical and surgical subspecialties, as well as in chronic illness population management paradigms, such as for diabetes, COPD, CHF, or asthma. It can also be used to better manage large, busy practices—typically by either focusing upon one type of grouping of patients or by seeing different homogeneous groupings of patients in a sequence during successive weekly sessions. In other words, this can be either for just a single condition, diagnosis (or cluster of diagnoses, such as *hyperlipodiabesity*), etc., that happens to be predominant in the physician's practice—or it can occur for one homogeneous grouping after another, until the entire sequence of groupings is completed (after which the entire sequence can be repeated over and over). In the latter case, the criteria used for homogeneous PSMA sessions could be based upon a sequence of diagnoses—for example, diabetes, kidney stones, COPD, and hyperlipidemia. Thus, an internist could provide physical examinations in a weekly homogeneous PSMA in the following sequence of sessions: diabetic and pre-diabetic (i.e., endocrine syndrome) patients during the first weekly session; asthmatics the next week; followed by headache patients, irritable bowel, obesity, women's health issues, etc.—until the entire sequence is completed. After completing the entire sequence of homogeneous weekly groupings, the sequence would then be repeated over and over.

Although intuitively appealing, this approach has considerable operational difficulties as staff and patients lose track of the sequence, especially when the physician is absent for a session, and may therefore resist scheduling patients into homogeneous PSMA sessions for that reason—i.e., for fear of being reprimanded for putting the wrong type of patient into any given session. Similarly, having a single diagnosis as a focus for all homogeneous PSMAs may prove problematic in terms of keeping all group sessions full—i.e., unless the physician's practice consists almost entirely of that diagnosis or if the homogeneous PSMA is being conducted within a chronic disease management program (in which case there would likely be a sufficiently large pool of patients with that particular diagnosis to ensure that all PSMA sessions can be kept full).

Patients Can Be Grouped by Age and Sex

For example, a busy family practitioner providing physicals for large numbers of both female and male patients might conduct a homogeneous PSMA for his/her practice according to sex and age criteria—e.g., by providing physicals in a weekly sequence of sessions first for women and then for men of specific age ranges. Thus, session 1 could be for women 21–40; session 2 for women 40–60; and session 3 for women over 60; which could then be followed by a similar sequence of sessions for men on the fourth, fifth, and sixth sessions in the sequence. Once completed, the entire sequence of weekly sessions would then be repeated over and over during subsequent months. While intuitively appealing, in using this model, one would need to make certain that staff and patients clearly understand what will happen in the event that the physician misses a session due to illness, vacation, meetings, etc.—so that there is no confusion or misunderstanding as to the subsequent sequence of sessions. For example, in the event that the physician misses a session due to a last minute illness, would the patients that are scheduled for that session be rescheduled into the next appropriate PSMA session in the sequence? Or else, would all subsequent sessions be postponed by a week so that the patients from the canceled session could be scheduled into the next week's session, which would require calling and rescheduling all patients who have prescheduled into future sessions in order to postpone them by a week—which certainly does not seem like a viable option.

Patients Can Be Grouped by the Type of Surgery or Procedure Being Faced, as well as by Condition or Situation

Similarly, the homogeneous PSMA sessions could be grouped in specialty care according to the type of surgery or procedure that patients are currently facing or have already undergone. This could include breast reduction and carpal tunnel intakes in plastic surgery; benign fibrocystic breast disease follow-ups in general surgery; hip and knee replacement surgery intakes and follow-ups in orthopedic surgery; pre- or post-bone marrow transplant patients in hematology; pre-surgical physical exams for cataract surgeries in ophthalmology; whole body skin exams for melanomas in dermatology; prostate cancer or incontinence intakes and follow-ups in urology; etc. Homogeneous PSMA sessions could also be condition or situation specific—such as for prenatal exams in obstetrics or for well-baby checks as well as school, camp, and sports physicals in pediatrics.

While Intuitively Appealing, Homogeneous PSMAs Are Seldom Used in Primary Care

Although intuitively appealing, the homogeneous PSMA subtype is most commonly used in the medical subspecialties and in chronic disease management programs. It is much less frequently used as a practice management tool

in primary care due to the diversity of their practices: (1) sessions can be harder to keep full—especially as the criteria for each homogeneous session becomes more selective and restrictive—so that fewer patients within the primary care physician's practice qualify to attend each of the narrowly defined sessions; (2) if different homogeneous groupings are seen in a sequence, then the sequence of sessions can be difficult for both patients and staff to keep track of, especially after the physician misses a session due to illness, meetings, or vacation; (3) scheduling staff might not schedule patients appropriately into sessions for fear of being reprimanded for placing patients into the wrong session; (4) there could be so many different groupings in the sequence that it could be too long of a wait before the patient having a particular diagnosis could attend the next appropriate session; and (5) patients might appropriately schedule the correct homogeneous PSMA session based upon their primary diagnosis, but then bring up a laundry list of diverse, unrelated medical needs into the session that are individualistic and not relevant to the focus of that session.

There Are Many Difficulties with the Intuitively Appealing Homogeneous Subtype

As regards this final point of patients frequently bringing a lengthy list of medical concerns to the visit, this certainly happens quite often during traditional physical examinations. As this continues to occur in a homogeneous PSMA (especially once the physician sees that such diverse issues can be successfully addressed during the session), there tends to be a natural evolution for the homogeneous primary care subtype of the PSMA model to become more heterogeneous over time.

There are other difficulties as well with the homogeneous model. For example, patients could be mistakenly scheduled into the wrong session. Along similar lines, the scheduling staff might be hesitant to schedule patients into homogeneous PSMAs for fear of mistakenly scheduling the wrong type of patient into any particular session— and then being punished as a result. Therefore, they might (indeed, they often do) instead choose to simply not schedule any patients at all into the homogeneous PSMA. As is the case with DIGMAs, the support of the scheduling staff is critical to the success of the PSMA program due to the key role they can play in keeping all sessions filled. Also, in the case of a sequence of sessions, patients who have to wait too long for the next appropriate session might instead schedule an individual physical examination appointment—a situation that runs counter to the intent of the PSMA program (which is to off-load individual physical exams onto more productive, accessible, and cost-effective PSMAs whenever possible and appropriate, and to thereby improve accessibility to physicals).

The Heterogeneous Subtype

In the heterogeneous subtype of the PSMA model (which is at the opposite end of the homogeneous–heterogeneous spectrum), sessions are designed in such a way that most or all types of patients (typically of a given sex in primary care) can attend each and every session—regardless of age, diagnosis, condition, etc.

Although not intuitively obvious, this model minimizes operational problems, is relatively easy to administer, often works well in actual practice, and is therefore sometimes used (although not nearly as often in primary care as the mixed PSMA subtype). The heterogeneous PSMA design offers the advantages of: (1) being easy for patients and staff to keep track of, and to schedule into (as all sessions are open to the same large group of patients); (2) being relatively easy to keep sessions full, as most patients qualify to attend each session; (3) patients having little wait time until the next appropriate session; (4) scheduling staff not having to worry about scheduling the wrong patient into any given session; and (5) being able to address the *laundry list* of diverse mind–body issues that different patients bring into the heterogeneous PSMA setting.

As an example of a heterogeneous PSMA design in primary care, consider an internist who performs mostly male physicals. In this case the internist might choose a 90-minute weekly heterogeneous PSMA design in which every session is open to physical examinations for all male patients from the internist's practice—regardless of age, health status, diagnosis, or utilization behavior. Of course, the issues brought up in such heterogeneous groupings could be quite diverse. Because they are diverse does not mean that the issues being discussed are not of interest to other patients, especially when some group interaction is fostered.

Similar to the case for heterogeneous DIGMAs, patients report that they find it interesting when the physician is addressing diverse medical issues brought up by other patients (i.e., even when these issues do not directly apply to them) for several reasons: (1) while these issues might not apply to them now, they could end up facing these very same issues in the future should they ever develop similar health problems; (2) these issues might apply to other people they know (parents, relatives, neighbors, friends, etc.); (3) they find having the physician discuss so many diverse medical issues "like being in a mini-medical school class taught by my own doctor"; or (4) "it's better than watching ER!". Also, because of the amount of press regarding prostate problems and breast cancer, younger men in a heterogeneous PSMA for men might find it interesting when the physician is addressing older patients with BPH or prostate cancer—and younger women in a female heterogeneous PSMA could similarly find it interesting when the physician was addressing breast disease and breast cancer with some of the older women in attendance.

In This Subtype Patient Groupings Can Be Too Diverse

Although the heterogeneous model has been successfully employed in some primary and specialty care applications, it must be used with caution due to the small group sizes of PSMAs—and because the heterogeneous PSMA model can result in patient groupings that are too diverse to achieve maximum benefit and efficiency. Here, patient groupings could be too diverse to be able to avoid repetition and redundancy in discussing issues, and to achieve high levels of patient bonding and sharing. In other words, the heterogeneous model can sometimes result in patient groupings that are too diverse to optimize patient bonding and commonality of issues—which, due to their relatively small group sizes, is much more of a problem for heterogeneous PSMAs than for heterogeneous DIGMAs.

As a result, the heterogeneous PSMA subtype tends to be less frequently utilized than either the mixed subtype or the homogeneous subtype (which can be widely used in the medical subspecialties and chronic disease management programs). On the other hand, some heterogeneous PSMAs (especially in the medical subspecialties) are sufficiently homogeneous by their very nature to work well in practice—such as heterogeneous Obstetrics PSMAs for prenatal exams, which are open to all of the obstetrician's pregnant patients (i.e., regardless of age, trimester, health status, marital status, utilization behavior, or number of previous pregnancies) or heterogeneous Endocrinology PSMAs—because most of the patients in them will likely have diabetes (and most commonly, type 2 diabetes). Actually, this terminology can be a little confusing as one might argue that the aforementioned "heterogeneous obstetrics PSMA for prenatal exams" is in fact a homogeneous PSMA for prenatal patients.

The Mixed Subtype

Although the homogeneous model (with its disease and condition specific focus) is frequently employed in medical specialties and population management programs for chronic illnesses, the mixed subtype of the PSMA model is also very popular—and is probably the most frequently used PSMA subtype in actual practice in primary care.

In the mixed subtype of the PSMA, the physician's practice is typically divided into four large groupings of patients—with one being the focus of the PSMA during each of the 4 weeks of the month, and with the same sequence of sessions being repeated over and over during future months. In the mixed subtype, patients are usually separated into large, relatively homogeneous groupings containing similar ages, sexes, diagnoses, medical conditions, or healthcare issues. In this subtype, patients and staff can easily remember which week of the month contains the PSMA session that has the focus which is most relevant to each patient. It is important that the patient groupings for each of the four weekly sessions that are held each month be designed to be sufficiently broad so that all sessions can consistently be kept full. In addition, the four categories of patients must also be sufficiently inclusive to ensure that all patients that the physician wants the PSMA to cover do indeed qualify for at least one of the four weekly sessions held each month.

As is the case for DIGMAs, for the couple of months each year containing five weekly mixed PSMA sessions, the fifth session of the month could either be closed or be designed to include whatever group of patients the physician wants covered—for example, backlogged patients of a certain type on the wait-list or those types of patients having the greatest access problems to physicals in the physician's practice. Similar to the case for the mixed subtype of the DIGMA model, mixed PSMAs also often have the proviso that—in the event that a patient's schedule makes it difficult or impossible to attend the most appropriate session for them that month—the patient would then be invited to attend another appropriate session which better meets the patient's scheduling needs (i.e., even if the focus of that session was not the best fit for that particular patient). This proviso is made because, whenever possible and appropriate, the goal is for patients to choose a highly efficient and productive PSMA for their physical examination rather than a more costly individual physical examination (with the restriction that the patient must be appropriate for the alternative session being attended, which would not be the case for a male patient who finds it more convenient from a scheduling point of view to attend the PSMA session focusing upon some grouping of female patients).

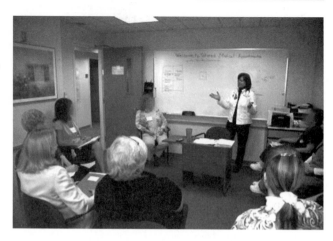

Fig. 5.3 The mixed subtype of the PSMA model is most frequently used in primary care, because it allows patients to be divided according to large sex and age groupings—thus ensuring some commonality of issues, so that appropriate patient education can be efficiently provided (courtesy of Dr. Jan Millermaier, Women's Primary Care PSMA, ProMed Family Practice, Kalamazoo, MI)

divided according to large sex and age groupings—so that patients attending any given session will share some common medical issues and concerns (Fig. 5.3). The same is true for the various medical and surgical subspecialties, although the homogeneous subtype is also frequently used here (e.g., for diabetes, arthritis, cardiovascular problems, and breast reduction intakes). This commonality fosters a certain degree of patient bonding while enabling the provider to gain efficiency by discussing some issues of common interest to many patients at once, thereby avoiding the need for time-consuming and costly repetition. The following are examples of the mixed PSMA subtype, i.e., in which each of the four weekly sessions is divided into patient groupings that are sufficiently broad (while still being somewhat homogeneous) to, in combination, cover all the types of patients that the physician wants included in the PSMA.

Some Primary Care Examples of the Mixed PSMA Subtype

For example, a female internist doing mostly same-sex physicals on female patients might employ a mixed PSMA to deliver physicals to women 40 (or 45) and over on the odd weeks of the month (addressing peri-menopausal and age-related health concerns such as HRT, osteoporosis, and cancer) and women under 40 or 45, respectively, on the even weeks—focusing upon birth control, infertility, PMS, STDs, child-rearing issues, etc. Or, if this internist had approximately equal numbers of physicals for females of all ages, she might design her mixed Primary

In Primary Care, the Most Frequently Used PSMA Is the Mixed Subtype

In primary care, the mixed subtype of the PSMA model is most frequently used because it allows patients to be

Care PSMA to provide physicals to females 18–29 on the first week of the month; women 30–44 on the second week; women from 45 to 59 on the third week; and women 60 and over on the fourth week of the month.

Similarly, a male family practitioner who predominantly provides physicals to male patients of all ages might select a mixed PSMA design that delivers physicals to men 50 and over on the even weeks of the month—and to men under 50 on the odd weeks. However, the four male groupings of the month could also be for males 21–34 on the first week; 35–49 the second; 50–64 the third; and 65 and over on the fourth week of the month. The exact ages used for these dividing points should take into account not only the different medical issues that various groupings of patients face but also what ages should be used in order to have enough patients of each category in order to keep all sessions consistently full. In other words, the exact breaking points of these age groupings (and consequently the patient mix) would be determined by the physician—but would depend upon patient demand (i.e., the volume of patients needing physical examinations by sex and age groupings) and upon the needs of the patients, the physician, and the physician's practice. Ideally, these dividing points would be selected so that there was some commonality of issues between patients in any particular grouping in order to foster some patient bonding and to avoid needless repetition—and so that the various patient groupings were themselves large enough to ensure that all sessions could be consistently kept filled to desired capacity.

As an additional example of the mixed PSMA in primary care, consider internists, family practitioners, and nurse practitioners with busy practices who provide numerous physicals each week to male and female patients of all ages. These providers could utilize the following type of mixed Primary Care PSMA design: physical examinations for adult females under 40 on the first week of the month; women 40 and over on the second week; adult males under 50 on the third week; and men 50 and over on the fourth week of the month. For those months having five sessions, the mixed PSMA could either be closed on the fifth session or be open to whatever group of patients the physician wants included—which would typically be that group of patients most severely backlogged for physical examinations (i.e., for whom the patient demand for physical exams is greatest). The proviso here would be that a male under 50 could also attend the session for men 50 and over if it better fits his schedule, just as the female patient 40 or over could attend the session for women under 40 should that better fit her schedule. However, neither sex would be invited, in this mixed PSMA example, to attend a session for the opposite sex—as this could be inappropriate and interfere with open discussions on the patients' part.

In Primary Care PSMAs, the Sexes Are Usually Kept Separate

This latter decision was reached during the very first mixed Primary Care PSMA session ever held—which was designed for men 50 and over. One of the male patients in attendance pointed out that his wife, who was also one of the doctor's patients, had asked him if she could also attend the session with him because she needed a physical examination as well. When I asked the other men in the group how they would have felt about it if she had attended, they all initially agreed that it would have been all right; however, one of the quieter men in the group then added that—although it would have been fine by him—he "probably wouldn't have talked." Others in the group then admitted that they felt the same. For this reason and others (for example, some issues might be awkward to discuss in front of the opposite sex, whereas other issues might not be relevant to the opposite sex), all agreed that keeping PSMA sessions uniform as to sex was a wise policy for primary care physical examinations. However, this issue of keeping the sexes separate is often less of an issue in the medical subspecialties, such as for diabetic or cardiac patients. Figure 5.4 shows an over-50 men's primary care PMSA.

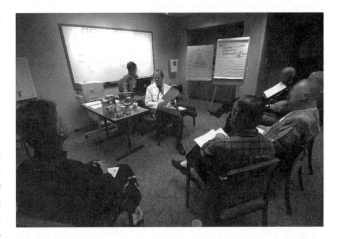

Fig. 5.4 Primary Care PSMAs are usually segregated according to sex and age, as in this PMSA for men over 50. Notice documenter on computer behind physician and lab test results on wall chart (courtesy of Dr. Thomas Morledge, Men's Primary Care PSMA, Cleveland Clinic, Cleveland, OH)

Patient Privacy in PSMAs

The PSMA model is the least intuitively obvious of the three major group visit models, as it is difficult to imagine how physical examinations can be efficiently conducted in a shared medical appointment format. Just like the case for DIGMAs, the issue of confidentiality is treated very seriously in all PSMAs. All attendees are asked to sign a confidentiality waiver at the start of each session. In addition, confidentiality is also thoroughly covered in the behaviorist's introduction to each session. Recall that the behaviorist's introduction is often given twice in the group room during the initial physical examination segment of the PSMA, so that all patients get to hear the introduction—including the four patients that might have been roomed in exam rooms when it was first given. Also, it is very important that the fact that part of the PSMA occurs in a group setting be made clear to patients in all promotional materials as well as by the physician's scheduling staff, so that there are no surprises—and no patient feels that a *bait and switch* tactic had been used upon them.

Billing for PSMAs and DIGMAs

Throughout the entire session (i.e., throughout both the physical examination and interactive group segments), PSMAs are run as a series of one doctor–one patient encounters that address each patients unique medical needs individually. Like DIGMAs, PSMAs focus upon the delivery of quality medical care to one patient at a time from start to finish, i.e., there is no educational class-like presentation, no formal question and answer period, no planning for the next session, and no separate behavioral health or support group component. As with DIGMAs, all patient education occurs during the interactive segment of the PSMA in the context of the physician working with one patient at a time while others in the group are privileged to listen, learn, interact, and benefit. Also like the case for DIGMAs (but not for other group visit models that are more class-like or psychosocial in nature), many fee-for-service (FFS) systems bill for PSMAs just like individual office visits—i.e., according to the level of care delivered and documented, using existing E&M codes (except that they do not bill either for counseling time or for the behaviorist's time, which is treated as an overhead expense to the program).

In a 2001 article in Modern Physician, Sutter Medical Group discussed their approach to billing, since group visits are not specifically addressed in the current CPT manual. As in individual office visits, physicians provide all the care they normally would, but in the group setting, and then bill by standard procedures (6).

Although I am an expert in group visits and not in billing and compliance, there is one integrated healthcare delivery system—one that billed based upon the level of

care delivered and documented—that took an approach to billing that I found particularly appealing (7). Their approach was to first notify all insurers about what they were doing and why. They notified all of their insurers, including Medicare, that they were starting a DIGMA and PSMA program in order to improve access, offer patients more time with their physicians, provide greater patient education, enhance patients' care experiences, integrate the help and support of other patients into each patient's healthcare experience, etc.

They also told them exactly what they would be doing in terms of billing: that they would be billing for DIGMAs and PSMAs exactly like individual office visits, according to the level of care delivered and documented using existing E&M codes. However, they would not be billing either for counseling time (as many patients could be benefiting at once and it would be egregious, and most likely outright fraudulent, to bill several times over for the same block of counseling) or for the behaviorist's time—which was instead treated as an overhead expense to the program because, to do otherwise, would result in patients getting two bills (and consequently two co-payments) for a single visit, which would anger patients and obviously be problematic.

Clearly, not billing for counseling time or the behaviorist's time provides a benefit to insurers, which is in line with the previously mentioned goal of patients, physicians, healthcare organizations, insurers, and corporate purchasers all simultaneously benefiting to some degree from the group visit program. In addition, this organization reviewed all billings for the first 2 months after each new DIGMA or PSMA was started—and spot-checked them for compliance thereafter in order to ensure that all outgoing SMA bills were supported both by the level of care delivered and by appropriate documentation.

Although billing issues for group visits are still evolving and are not yet completely resolved (and because no E&M codes currently exist that are specific either to group visits in general or the various types of group visit models), many healthcare organizations in the fee-for-service world are therefore currently offering DIGMAs and PSMAs—and billing according to the level of care delivered and documented using existing E&M codes (but not billing for counseling time or the behaviorist's time). Many question whether separate group visit billing codes are even necessary for the DIGMA and PSMA models, as they are run from start to finish as a series of one doctor–one patient encounters with observers—i.e., attending in turn to each patient's unique medical needs (which is not the case, however, for other types of group visit models).

They treat DIGMAs and PSMAs in this manner because they feel that this is the best that they can do within the existing rules and current billing and compliance guidelines. At least this appears to be the case for

DIGMAs and PSMAs in particular, as these are the two group visit models that are run from start to finish just like a series of individual office visits with observers—and with the same medical care (and often more) being delivered. However, these organizations stand ready to adapt to any future changes in regulations and billing requirements that may occur for the various group visit models, which they can only hope will be carefully thought out and reasonable so as to not undermine the multitude of patient, physician, and organizational benefits that well-run SMA programs can offer.

Census Targets for PSMAs

As with DIGMAs, there are three types of census levels that need to be predetermined for each PSMA program before it is actually implemented. The *target census* (or ideal census) for a PSMA is typically seven to nine male patients or six to eight female patients for most 90-minute sessions in primary care. An additional patient (or occasionally even two) would typically be added to this number to compensate for the expected number of no-shows and late-cancels—i.e., by doing like the airlines and overbooking sessions accordingly. In the case of the medical subspecialties, where the physical exam is often more limited in scope and therefore quicker to perform, the target census is often higher than for comprehensive physical examinations in Primary Care PSMAs—with 10–13 patients being a relatively common target census in the various medical subspecialties. On the other hand, the *maximum census* is set to be the most patients that the physician is willing to see in a fully attended PSMA; however, it is actually set to be slightly higher than this as it must take into account the likely number of no-shows and late-cancels per session.

While the target census for a PSMA is typically set to at least triple the physician's productivity in delivering physical exams (although there are a couple of exceptions for physicians who are already extremely productive in delivering physical examinations, and for whom the PSMA model may only be able to double their productivity), the *minimum census* is often set somewhat lower than the target census—such as to at least double the physician's productivity (or perhaps more). However, for reasons of effective group dynamics as well as the economic viability of the program, I personally prefer to set the minimum census at a considerably higher level than this. In actuality, I almost always prefer to set the minimum census for almost all PSMAs in primary and specialty care to at least triple the provider's actual productivity (as opposed to potential scheduled productivity) in delivering physical examinations through individual office visits alone.

There are three exceptions that I have found in practice wherein the PSMA model can only double the physician's productivity—all of which are the result of extremely high initial levels of physician productivity in providing individual physical examinations. These exceptions are prenatal exams in obstetrics, full baby skin exams in dermatology internists and family practitioners offering only 15 or 20 minute physical examinations, and well-baby checks as well as school, camp, and sports physicals in pediatrics.

The Chart Note Template

In addition, when custom designing the PSMA program, the physician needs to develop the chart note template that will be used for the program—i.e., that the documenter will use for drafting the real-time individualized chart note on each patient. For systems still using paper, the chart note template to be used in the DIGMA or PSMA should be largely preprinted and in check-off form whenever possible in order to increase efficiency. For systems using electronic medical records (EMR), physicians can either choose to use a chart note template that has already been developed for the SMA program (i.e., selecting the existing SMA program template closest to their own needs, and then customizing it to their own specific requirements) or continue with a chart note template similar to that which they are already using during individual physical examinations. In any case, the documenter needs to be specifically trained (e.g., by reviewing 20–40 of the physician's normal individual office visit chart notes to get a sense of the format being used, and by shadowing the physician for a couple of days thereafter and documenting individual physical exams) in efficiently documenting the chart note through the use of the selected template according to the specific desires and requirements of the individual physician – i.e., prior to the actual launch of the PSMA. This training will continue on an ongoing basis after the PSMA is implemented because the physician will review and modify the chart note generated by the documenter on each patient immediately after working with that patient during all future PSMA sessions. This provides the documenter with immediate and ongoing feedback from the physician, which makes for a quick learning curve.

PSMAs Have Three Basic Components

The PSMA model can best be conceptualized as consisting of three basic components—two of which constitute the PSMA session itself, whereas the "Patient Packet

Segment" precedes the actual session. The actual session is divided into two parts: (1) the *physical examination segment* during which the physical exams are provided by the physician to all patients individually in the privacy of an exam room (but with a minimum of talk), while the behaviorist meets with the small and rotating group of unroomed patients in the group room; and (2) the *interactive group segment* which typically occurs immediately afterward in the supportive group setting (with the physician, behaviorist, documenter, and patients present throughout), where all present can listen, learn, and encourage one another as the physician sequentially addresses the unique medical issues of each patient individually. The physical examination segment of the PSMA can likewise be divided into two parts: (1) the *private part* of the physical examination consisting of those components of the physical which involve disrobing and require privacy (e.g., prostate, rectal, and testicle exams for men; pelvic and breast exams for women) as well as any other components of the exam that either the physician or patient prefers to have conducted in private and; (2) the *non-private part* of the physical (i.e., the remaining components of the physical examination, which do not need to be conducted in private) which could in theory be provided during the interactive group setting if so desired. The flow of a typical PSMA session is presented in Table 5.6.

The Initial "Patient Packet" Segment

When patients are scheduled into the PSMA appointment (unlike DIGMAs, patients are typically prescheduled and do not generally drop-in), the person from the physician's support staff who has been assigned this responsibility sends a *Patient Packet* to each patient that has been scheduled into the PSMA—typically 2–3 weeks in advance of the session. The Patient Packet can include any number of items, and is customized to the particular needs and requirements of the individual physician. However, it typically contains the following items: (1) a personalized one-page cover letter, signed by the provider, that welcomes patients, thanks them for signing up, and describes all important details about the program (including its patient benefits and what to expect); (2) a program description flier that is specifically designed to describe and promote the program; (3) any important informational handouts and educational materials that the physician might want to select for inclusion (e.g., a recommended health maintenance screening schedule by sex and age group; diagnosis or condition-specific educational handouts); (4) a detailed health history

questionnaire (usually similar to the form already being used by the physician for individual physical examinations, but often more detailed and including sections on personal and family health histories, recent health changes, current medications, allergies, any special medical concerns, etc.) which the patient needs to complete and return to the office (by mail, e-mail, web site, or personally delivering it) at least a couple of business days prior to the session; and (5) forms for any needed routine and special lab tests (especially blood screening tests) that need to be completed prior to the appointment.

The goal is to schedule patients into the PSMA 2–4 weeks in advance of the session, and then to promptly send the Patient Packet to patients by mail, fax, or electronically (e-mail; web site; etc.). The patient is instructed (when scheduling the appointment as well as in the cover letter) to complete the enclosed forms as soon as possible and to promptly return them to the office once completed—either personally or by mail, fax, or electronically (i.e., assuming that firewall problems can be overcome). The goal is to schedule patients far enough in advance to allow sufficient time for patients to complete the routine health maintenance and screening tests in advance of the visit—and to complete and return the detailed health history form contained in the Patient Packet to the office at least a few days prior to the PSMA session that they are to attend. If the lab tests are not done prior to the session, or the detailed health history questionnaire is not completed and returned to the office 3–5 days prior to the visit, then someone from the physician's office needs to promptly follow-up with any such patients and strongly encourage them to do so immediately. Some physicians even make it a policy to postpone seeing any such patients in the PSMA until they have completed the health form and lab tests.

Some physicians also have their nurses complete a large wall chart before the PSMA session—one that contains all of the patients' names in the rows and all of their lab test results in the columns, and with any results that the physician considers abnormal circled in red. In addition, physicians often have someone from their staff abstract and enter the information contained in the completed health history questionnaire (that has been returned to the office) into patients' medical charts prior to the scheduled session. This will help to organize the physician's discussions with patients during the interactive segment of the PSMA session—plus add considerably to the physician's efficiency in conducting the group, as the physician will be able to see the lab test results on all patients in a glance (with abnormal findings highlighted in red) upon entering the group room for the interactive group segment.

In addition, physicians will have the relevant information from the completed health history forms already entered into patients' chart notes by a member of their

Table 5.6 Flow of a typical Primary Care PSMA

2–3 Weeks prior to the session: the Patient Packet segment
- Patient Packet is assembled and mailed to all pre-registered patients

2 Weeks to 3 days prior to session
- Patients complete detailed health history form and return it to the physician's office
- Patients complete all blood screening tests (and anything else the physician has ordered)
- Avoid emergency interruptions during PSMA by arranging clinic coverage in advance

2–4 Days prior to the session
- Staff member follows up with any patients who have not yet completed form or tests
  - Patients are told to get these done ASAP
  - If not done prior to session, patients will be postponed until they are completed
- Staff member enters data from completed forms and tests into PSMA chart note
- Nurse/MA makes confirmation phone calls to all scheduled patients—doing a medication reconciliation, confirming that detailed health questionnaire, and pre-visit labs have been completed, reviewing HEDIS measures, and checking for any injections or routine health maintenance that is due
- Beforehand, nurse/MA prepares a large wall chart (typically an erasable whiteboard with grid lines on it) containing each patient's test results
  - Display all screening test results as columns (and all patients' names in rows)
  - Circle in red any findings that the physician considers abnormal
- Once completed, chart is displayed in group room (temporarily covered for privacy)

15–45 Minutes before PSMA session
- Seven to nine male (or six to eight female) patients start arriving and registering for PSMA session
  - Each receives a name tag (first name) and is asked to sign confidentiality release
  - Any support person accompanying patient also signs release, which is collected
- Patients are either asked to sit in lobby or are directed to the group or exam rooms
  - Two nurses/MAs and four exam rooms are usually used (each nurse/MA handles two exam rooms)
  - First four patients to register are typically individually roomed in the exam rooms
    - Nurses/MAs take vital signs, give injections, update health maintenance, and provide special duties on each patient as they are roomed
    - Nurses/MAs prepare patients for physical exam (gown, etc.)
    - Nurses/MAs enter what they have done on the patients' chart notes
    - Nurses/MAs pull out and complete patient identifying information on any referral forms for physician's signature
- The remaining patients (other than those in exam rooms) are directed to the group room after they register
- If physician arrives early, exams can be started on roomed patients with vitals completed

From 10–15 minutes beforehand until the start of the session
- Behaviorist arrives into group room (can escort unroomed patients from the lobby)
- Behaviorist welcomes patients, gets patients talking, and asks each patient what they want to discuss with the physician today
- Each patient's first name and medical concerns are written on flip chart or whiteboard,
- Behaviorist usually gives same introduction as for DIGMA (but twice so all can hear it)
- Behaviorist explains benefits, confidentiality, and encourages patients to participate

First half (∼45 minutes) of the PSMA: The private physical examination segment
- The physician provides physical examinations to one patient at a time in the exam rooms
  - These are complete exams, but are performed rapidly with a minimum of talk
  - Most male physicals take 3–6 minutes, and female physicals a minute or so more
  - Only private matters and that which needs to be said for the exam are discussed
  - All other talk is tactfully deferred to the interactive group segment that follows
  - The documenter can follow provider from one exam room to another
    - The documenter would document physical findings spoken by provider
    - Preferred by most physicians, but documenter must be a nurse, MA, or somebody licensed to be with disrobed patients
    - Or else, documenter can stay at a computer outside of exam rooms (but nearby) to enter physician's *crib sheet* notes into each patient's PSMA chart note just as soon as physician finishes exam on that patient
    - Or else, documenter can stay in group room charting what occurs there
    - In latter case (which is generally not as desirable), physician documents own physical findings in chart note
  - When physician finishes an exam, the patient dresses and is taken back to group
  - MA/nurse cleans exam room
  - The nurse/MA immediately calls out and rooms another patient from the group
  - Enough nurses/MAs and exam rooms are used to ensure the provider is never held up
  - This process continues until all physical examinations are completed
  - This process usually takes the first half of the session (i.e., around 45 minutes)
  - Upon rooming and completing expanded PSMA nursing duties on all patients, nurses/MAs return to normal clinic responsibilities
  - Once all physicals are done, one MA can stay to recheck elevated blood pressures and then become care coordinator

Table 5.6 (continued)

- Meanwhile, the behaviorist runs the small rotating group of unroomed patients
  - As each patient returns from the exam room, their health concerns are noted
  - Behaviorist continues writing down medical concerns (while fostering some group interaction) until all patients are done
  - Behaviorist can discuss handouts and psychosocial issues during any extra time
  - Discussions continue as patients return from exam room while others are roomed
  - Provider is briefed upon any such discussions upon later entering the group room
  - Behaviorist gives introduction a second time (including confidentiality briefing)
    - When patients who did not hear first introduction return to group room

Second half of PSMA session (i.e., last ~45 minutes): The interactive group segment
- Last half of the PSMA session (interactive group segment) is basically a small DIGMA
  - Physician enters group room just as soon as all physical examinations are done
  - PSMAs are run like a series of individual office visits from start to finish
  - Throughout, medical care is provided in a series of one doctor–one patient encounters
  - Provider runs this segment like DIGMA, starting with any needing to leave early
  - The provider sequentially addresses each patient's unique medical needs
  - Physician discusses results of physicals, labs, and completed health history forms
  - Physician addresses each patient's medical concerns on flip chart or whiteboard
  - For each patient, physician also refers to lab test results depicted on wall chart
  - History, risk assessment, medical decision-making, counseling, etc., are provided for each patient in turn
  - While each patient is treated individually, some group interaction is fostered
  - When finished with a patient, the provider reviews chart note with documenter
- The behaviorist handles group dynamic and psychosocial issues, keeps group running smoothly and on time, and temporarily runs group while provider steps out of group room (for brief private discussions or exams) of finishes each chart note
- The documenter generates individualized, contemporaneous, and complete chart notes
- The two segments combined make PSMAs complete individual physical examinations
- The PSMA goal is to always to start and finish on time—and end with chart notes done
- One MA or nurse, rather than returning to regular clinic duties, can become the care coordinator—calling patients out of group room to schedule any follow-up appointments or referrals, and to give them their PSMA chart note after visit summary (AVS)—which includes treatment plan, medications, etc.)
- Provider steps out to discuss any private issues arising in group interactive segment—typically toward end of interactive group segment so as to not interrupt flow of group

At the end of session
- Physician formally ends session (hopefully on time) by thanking patients for attending
- Physician needs to leave as soon as session is over, or else patients will also stay
- Documenter also leaves as soon as session is over
- Patients (plus any support persons) anonymously complete patient satisfaction form
  - Some systems ask all attendees to complete patient satisfaction form after group
  - Do this anonymously—have patients put completed form in a box without any patient identifying information
  - Other systems prefer to later send patient satisfaction form by mail

Behaviorist stays 10–15 minutes late to clear and straighten up group room
- Behaviorist stays a few minutes late to answer logistical questions, clear the room, and straighten up group room

SMA Team debriefs after sessions for first 2 months
- For first 2 months, provider and SMA team (behaviorist, documenter, and MA/nurse(s)—sometimes with the champion and program coordinator) can debrief after sessions to improve the PSMA program and make future sessions better and more efficient
- After first couple of months, debriefings will only need to occur on an as-needed basis

staff—i.e., rather than having to do it themselves. By so doing, the physician will be in possession of both results from the lab tests that were ordered and the latest health history form information that has been abstracted into the patients' medical records prior to the PSMA session. Having this latest updated information at their fingertips at the time of the visit enables physicians to treat patients based upon the most recent information and test results available—which can enhance the quality of care delivered in PSMAs. This is particularly true for healthcare systems where such information and screening test results are typically not available for traditional individual physical exams. Having the list of each patient's medical concerns (i.e., that were written down on a flip chart or whiteboard

in the group room by the behaviorist earlier during the initial physical examination segment of the PSMA) further adds to the physician's efficiency in the PSMA setting.

The PSMA Visit Typically Begins with the Physical Examination Segment, Which Is Conducted Thoroughly but Rapidly with a Minimum of Talk

On the actual day of the PSMA visit, the patients are registered, sign confidentiality releases, and are taken to a group room as for a DIGMA (so that information will not be repeated here), except that nursing personnel enter early enough to (1) room approximately four early arriving patients into exam rooms for physical examinations and (2) complete all nursing duties on these patients prior to the arrival of the physician. Immediately upon entering the PSMA session, the physician typically begins providing physical examinations on those patients who have been roomed into the exam rooms first—and upon whom all nursing duties have been completed. As with DIGMAs, the behaviorist similarly enters the group room a few minutes early to warm up the small, rotating group of patients—and begins conducting the previously described behaviorist's duties, such as welcoming patients, giving the introduction, and writing down the issues that patients want to discuss during today's visit.

It is during the physical examination segment of the PSMA that patients are roomed (typically two to four at a time in separate exam rooms), that vital signs are taken, that injections and routine health maintenance are updated, and that expanded nursing duties are performed. It is also when the physician sequentially delivers physical exams to all patients individually in the privacy of the exam room—much as they would for traditional individual physicals, except for minimizing the amount of talk in the exam rooms (and tactfully deferring it to the interactive group segment that follows). The physical examination segment typically takes approximately half of the time that is allocated to the entire session (e.g., approximately 45 minutes in the case of a 90-minute PSMA). It typically consists of the physician sequentially conducting individual private physical examinations in rotation on all patients in attendance, usually with four patients being roomed at a time in four different exam rooms (although two to six exam rooms have been variously employed at one time or another).

Depending on the physician's preference, vital signs could also be taken at other times during the session by the nurse/MA. However, taking vitals in the privacy of the exam room when rooming patients does offer certain advantages, such as (1) patients can talk to the nurse without disturbing the group, which could be a problem if vitals were taken in the group room and (2) patients' weights can be taken in private, as patients are sometimes reticent to share their weight and age with others. Depending upon the physician's preference, the documenter can either shadow the physician as physical examinations are being given (assuming that the documenter's scope of practice includes being able to be with disrobed patients) or stay in the group room documenting what the behaviorist is doing.

One important difference between the PSMA and traditional physical examinations is that exams in PSMAs are conducted thoroughly but rapidly, with an absolute minimum amount of talking between the doctor and patient—which definitely involves a learning curve for participating physicians. It might take a couple of months of actual experience (and of debriefing after sessions with the PSMA team) for providers to become comfortable and efficient with this new approach.

As a SMA champion, I often stand outside of the exam rooms during a physician's initial PSMA session with a stop watch, timing how long each physical exam takes and listening for any unnecessary talk and laughter inside the exam room—which will certainly slow the PSMA down and make it difficult to finish on time. To the maximum extent possible and appropriate, all discussions (except those which are truly private or needed to conduct the exam)—as well as answers to questions posed by patients—are tactfully deferred from the inefficient one-on-one exam room setting to the subsequent interactive group component of the PSMA session—where all present can benefit, repetition can be avoided, and efficiency can be increased. This is accomplished tactfully and without the physician appearing to be rude or disinterested in the patient's issues, for example, by the physician saying something like: "Oh, that's a great point! Why not write that question down for now and bring it up in the group that follows where everyone can benefit from the answer?" The patient is simply told that, rather than having such significant questions and health concerns addressed individually in the exam room, such discussions are so important that they should be deferred to the group that follows—where all present can listen, interact, and learn.

The main point here is that, by removing almost all the time-consuming talk and discussion from the inefficient exam room setting, the physical examination segment is conducted with great efficiency—typically only taking $3\frac{1}{2}$–6 minutes for a complete primary care physical on men, and a minute or two longer for women. Actually, only the private part of the physical examination needs to be performed in the physical examination segment, whereas the non-private part can be completed in either the physical examination segment or in the interactive group segment—although most physicians prefer the former, as they find it to be more convenient and efficient to provide the non-private parts of the physical in the exam room rather than the group room in the PSMA model.

The Interactive Group Segment

The third component of the actual PSMA session is the interactive group segment, which is basically a small DIGMA. Together with the physician and behaviorist (and frequently a documenter), all of the patients are simultaneously present in the group room for the interactive group segment. Occasionally, the physician's own nurse will also attend—sometimes acting as documenter—although the nurse/MA(s) more commonly return to normal clinic duties as soon as their nursing duties on all patients have been completed in the physical examination segment. Quite often, either a MA or nurse stays to then become the care coordinator—i.e., to retake elevated blood pressures, schedule all recommended referrals and follow-up appointments, and to individually give patients their after visit summary (AVS). Typically lasting between 45 and 60 minutes in a 90-minute PSMA, it is during this interactive group segment that almost all of the discussion between the physician, patients, and behaviorist occurs as the physician sequentially works with each patient individually—and, in that context, discusses such topics as diabetes, treatment options, medication side effects, exercise, nutrition, and community and organizational resources.

The physician does not give a *class-type* presentation during the interactive group segment of the PSMA. Instead, as is the case for DIGMAs, all of the patient education occurs in the context of the physician working with each patient individually while others listen, interact, ask questions, and learn. During the interactive group segment, the physician can often go into more detail because efficiency can be increased and repetition avoided—and because of the extra time that is available. By deferring topics of common interest to the group room (which are made clear in the group room from the flip chart listing all of the patients' concerns and from the wall chart depicting all of the patients' lab test results), where everyone can simultaneously listen and benefit, internists and family practitioners can discuss issues only once but often more comprehensively. This is especially important for those issues that they normally would find themselves repeating over and over to different patients individually throughout the workweek.

For example, the physician can discuss such issues of common interest as cholesterol, hypertension, breast self-exams, prostate problems, diabetes, osteoporosis, GERD, HRT, asthma, sun protection, irritable bowel, incontinence, fungus toenails, stress management, sleep problems, depression, alternative medicines, information patients glean from the Internet or direct pharmaceutical ads, and internal and community resources. It is during the interactive group segment that almost all of the talking, social interaction, history taking, risk assessment, patient education, and attention to psychosocial aspects of the physical examination visit occur. Questions are answered, health concerns are addressed, important healthcare information is provided, healthy lifestyles are encouraged, diseased self-management strategies are explained, noncompliance is addressed, prescriptions are changed or

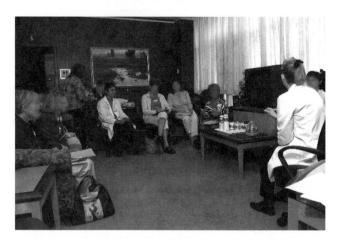

Fig. 5.5 In the interactive group segment of this Women's Health PSMA, healthcare information is provided, questions are answered, healthy lifestyles are encouraged, disease self-management strategies are discussed, noncompliance is addressed, prescriptions are changed or refilled, referrals are made, and many tests and procedures are ordered (courtesy of Dr. Holly Thacker, Women's Health PSMA, Cleveland Clinic, Cleveland, OH)

refilled, many tests and procedures are ordered, and internal as well as outside referrals are made (Fig. 5.5).

As in a DIGMA, the physician works individually with one patient after another in the interactive group segment but also fosters some group interaction (but not too much so as to finish on time). Group discussions are frequently stimulated by various patients' questions and health concerns—and helpful suggestions are often made by other patients. As with DIGMAs, the goal of every PSMA is to address the unique medical needs of all patients individually; to provide quality care with high levels of patient and physician professional satisfaction; to start and end on time; and to have all documentation completed during the session. Also like DIGMAs, the physician will need to leave the session as soon as it is over, or the patients will continue to stay as long as the physician does. On the other hand, the behaviorist should stay 10–15 minutes afterward to answer any last minute questions that patients may have (such as where to go for their colonoscopy or diabetes program), to clear the room, and to quickly straighten the group room up for the next group that will use it.

Three Ways as to When to Conduct the Physical Examination Segment

There are three possibilities as to when to conduct the physical examination segment during the PSMA session—i.e., during the first part of the session; ongoing throughout the session; and during the last part of the session. Together, these three approaches represent but one of the many options that the robust PSMA model makes available to individual physicians for customizing the program to their exact needs, goals, preferences, practice styles, and patient panel constituencies.

Option 1: Conduct Physicals During First Part of the Session (Most Common Choice)

In this option, the physician conducts the physical examinations individually in the privacy of the exam rooms (which always includes the *private part* of the physical exam, plus often much or all of the *non-private part* as well) during approximately the first half of the PSMA session—i.e., while the behaviorist temporarily leads the small, revolving group of unroomed patients.

Here, the physician first completes the private physical examinations individually on all patients with a minimum of discussion, and then immediately goes to the group room afterward to conduct the subsequent interactive group segment of the PSMA session. Experience with numerous primary care physicians as well as medical and surgical subspecialists in healthcare systems nationwide has demonstrated that this option of completing the private exams first tends to be the most productive and efficient—as well as the least disruptive of the group process. It is therefore the approach that typically works best in actual practice. In this option, as well as the other two options that will be discussed shortly, because the charting requirements for physical examinations tend to be quite extensive, it is strongly recommended that a documenter be used throughout the PSMA session—in order to not only optimize the physician's efficiency, but also to generate a superior real-time chart note that is both comprehensive and contemporaneous.

Option 2: Provide Physical Examinations Throughout the Interactive Group Segment

Here, physical examinations are delivered throughout the interactive group segment, which constitutes the entire PSMA session. In this option, the physician steps out of the group room with each patient in turn during the interactive group session to conduct a brief private exam in a nearby exam room (i.e., if there is a private component to the physical examination), or else the exam can be conducted in the group setting if there is no private component—in which case you basically have a DIGMA rather than a PSMA. Stepping out of the group room to conduct a physical examination typically happens after the physician has finished working with each patient in turn in the interactive group setting, and involves going to the exam room to complete any components of the physical examination that the physician might prefer to provide in private. Unfortunately, doing this can not only be inefficient (as patients need to disrobe, etc., prior to the actual exam) but also disruptive of the group process. Of the three options being discussed here (i.e., for providing the physical examinations segment before, during, or after the interactive group segment of the PSMA session), this approach of providing the physical examinations during the interactive group segment of the PSMA is the least used—and the most difficult to perform successfully in actual practice.

This option actually represents a common beginner's mistake as physicians often initially prefer to start their PSMA sessions with a brief introduction by the behaviorist that is promptly followed by the interactive group discussions—i.e., during which the physician would individually take each patient out to a nearby exam room for the physical exam immediately after working with that patient in the group setting. However, providers will quickly find that, although intuitively appealing (because it so closely resembles what they normally do with individual physical exams), this approach is replete with difficulties. Actually, this approach represents a common beginner's mistake often made by physicians who are new to group visits—physicians who are clinging to elements of the individual office visit model of care to their own peril when they shift to group visits. In this case, they are sequentially leaving the group room with each patient individually to conduct the private exam—i.e., with the mistaken belief that this is somehow better for billing purposes or for providing a more personalized, better form of care for their patients.

I Do Not Recommend This Option For Several Reasons

If patients are indeed being shuffled back and forth between the group and exam rooms by sequentially being taken out of the group room for a private physical examination (i.e., after the physician has finished talking to them in the group room), then this approach is too wasteful of time and full of patient flow difficulties to be efficient. This is because the nursing personnel must somehow first room and complete all nursing functions on each patient in turn—and get each patient gowned and prepared—by the time the physician leaves the group room and enters the exam room for the patient that has just been worked with in the group setting. The same types of inefficiencies and group disruption also occur after the exam because the physician immediately returns to the group room, whereas the patient is somewhat delayed in doing so because they must first get dressed—

at which time they then enter and disrupt the group. As can be seen, completing the physical examination segment first (and keeping it separate from the interactive group segment) is usually a far better and more efficient option.

Because stepping out of the group room with one patient at a time to do the private physical examination can be so inefficient and disruptive of the group dynamic (plus, can so drastically undercut the amount of time patients spend with the physician, and consequently the amount of patient education that they can derive from the session), this approach tends not to be used very often. Simply put, I seldom recommend this approach. Nonetheless, some systems are making this mistake—for example, by having a diabetes educator as the behaviorist running the group as a diabetes education class while the physician steps out with one patient after another to perform the physical examination. However, this mistaken approach greatly reduces the amount of direct contact time that each patient is able to spend learning from their own physician in the group setting—which therefore dilutes the entire PSMA program down to being less medical and more educational in nature, which can have negative billing implications as well.

Such an Approach Can Often Result in a DIGMA Rather than a PSMA

On the other hand, if one tries not to step out of the group room to conduct private exams, what one has is a DIGMA. This approach of just having an interactive group setting during which the physical examinations are delivered—i.e., without any separate physical examination segment—tends to only be used in circumstances where there is no private component to the exam (i.e., when patients do not need to disrobe, so that the exams can be efficiently conducted in the group room). For example, such an approach can be used in the case of pacemaker interrogations in cardiology, foot exams in podiatry, and diabetic foot exams in endocrinology. However, when this happens, you basically have a DIGMA rather than a PSMA—i.e., other than the fact that the focus of the SMA session might happen to be upon a physical examination rather than a follow-up visit.

Option 3: Perform the Physical Examination Segment During the Last Part of the Session

Although providing the private physical examinations during the last part of the PSMA session (i.e., after the interactive group segment) is intuitively appealing—and was in fact the first approach that I used in actual practice—experience has repeatedly shown that it is not nearly as efficient as Option 1 (i.e., as performing the private examinations during the first part of the PSMA session, before the interactive group segment).

In Option 3, the session typically begins on time with the behaviorist's introduction, which emphasizes the fact that all Q&A and group discussions are to occur during the interactive group segment that immediately follows—and not later on during the time that the physician is providing private physical examinations to patients individually in the exam rooms. As soon as the behaviorist's introduction is finished, the physician immediately begins to lead the interactive group segment of the PSMA visit like a DIGMA—i.e., by sequentially focusing upon the unique medical needs of each patient. This often involves using the wall chart with lab test results written on it (as well as the flip chart upon which the behaviorist has already written down each patient's health concerns) as a guide.

Only afterward, during the last 30–45 minutes of the Option 3 PSMA session, does the physician leave the group room to provide the exams individually in the privacy of the exam rooms for all of the patients attending the session. While the physician is working with the last one or two patients in the interactive group segment, the nurse/MA(s) call out two to five patients (depending upon the number of exam rooms available) from the group room and escort them into the exam rooms to begin vitals, etc. That way, by the time the physician has finished working with the last patient in the group room, the first cohort of patients will have been roomed and prepared with all of their nursing duties completed. While the physician is providing private physical examinations to the patients in the exam rooms, the behaviorist takes over leading the remainder of the group. The behaviorist typically discusses any handouts preselected by the physician as well as any behavioral health and psychosocial issues of interest to those patients who happen to still be present in the group room—unless the behaviorist happens to be a nurse (which is often the case in a PSMA), in which case issues more appropriate to the skill set of the nurse might instead be discussed at this time. Once their private physical exam is complete, each patient can then choose to either go home or return to the small group being led by the behaviorist. As always, the goal is to finish on time with all chart notes completed.

In Option 3, Keep the Number of Patients Roomed for Physicals to a Minimum

Because PSMAs are relatively small (with the census typically being 6–9 patients in primary care and 10–13 patients in the medical subspecialties), it is recommended that when Option 3 is used, the nursing personnel only room two patients at a time toward the end of the session.

Otherwise, if three or more patients are roomed at a time in different exam rooms, the number of patients that are left remaining in the group (i.e., which is being led by the behaviorist) rapidly becomes quite small—so that the group dynamic can be quickly lost. For the same reason, once their private exams have been completed, patients should be encouraged to return to the group room to gain additional benefit—i.e., rather than just going home (as this keeps the group size larger and the psychodynamic more productive).

Option 3 Is Seldom Recommended Because It Is Difficult to Finish on Time

Unfortunately, despite being intuitively appealing, Option 3 suffers from one major drawback—but it is a critically important one (i.e., physicians often finish late and sometimes quite late). This happens because—no matter how much the physician and behaviorist emphasize that all discussion is to occur in the initial interactive group segment, and not later in the exam room—patients almost always still want to ask the physician a few additional questions during their private physical examinations toward the end of the session. Sometimes, they even *store up* their questions to ask the physician later during their private physical exam.

As a result, the patients end up engaging the physician in further discussions while they have the physician alone to themselves in the privacy of the exam room. In part, this is habit and is based upon what patients have grown to expect as the result of a long history with traditional individual physical exams. However, regardless of the reason, the net result is that the physician is now stuck with answering all of these questions in the inefficient one-on-one exam room setting, which ultimately undercuts the productivity gains of the PSMA and results in the physician not finishing sessions on time.

Because this approach was so intuitively appealing to me, the first PSMAs that I ever ran were of this type; however, I quickly found it to be a beginner's mistake because the physicians using it were so frequently finishing late—and often very late. In fact, starting with Option #3 almost cost me the PSMA model as the first three physicians to try it were so frustrated about finishing late that they wanted to quit—and two did.

Weaknesses of the PSMA Model

Although the PSMA model is unique among today's major group visit models because it alone focuses upon the efficient delivery of private physical examinations rather than follow-up appointments, it is nonetheless closely related to the DIGMA model—i.e., with approximately half the session, the group interactive segment, essentially being a small DIGMA. Therefore, PSMAs suffer from most of the same disadvantages as the DIGMA model. Like DIGMAs, PSMAs must be carefully designed, adequately supported, well promoted, and properly run—plus consistently have all sessions filled to pre-established target census levels. Both models suffer from the weaknesses of having substantial personnel and facilities requirements (which are similar, but somewhat different)—as well as the need for high-quality, professional appearing promotional materials. In larger systems, like DIGMAs, PSMAs also require a champion, a program coordinator, and dedicated schedulers to ensure that the PSMA program is rapidly moved forward throughout the system and that all sessions are consistently filled. These are personnel resources that might not be readily available within the system, and for whom there will likely be competing demands.

Personnel Requirements

Although both group visit models require a behaviorist, the preferred behaviorist in a DIGMA is typically an experienced psychologist or social worker with group skills who enjoys working with physicians and medical patients, whereas the preferred behaviorist in a PSMA is often a nurse. Although having two nursing personnel (rather than one) and a documenter are helpful in a DIGMA, they are almost a necessity in a PSMA. Two nurses/MAs are also needed, typically with each being responsible for managing two of the four exam rooms, in order to expeditiously dispatch all of the expanded nursing duties that PSMAs entail. In addition, having two nurses allows them to always stay ahead of the physician in their rooming of patients and performance of expanded nursing duties—which is critical as efficiency dictates that the physician must never be left waiting in the hallway for a patient to be roomed and to have all nursing functions completed.

Because of the extensive documentation requirements that physical examinations entail, having a documenter is even more important for PSMAs than for DIGMAs—yet, it is sometimes challenging to find an appropriate person available within the system to act as documenter. Like DIGMAs, PSMAs also require a champion, program coordinator, and dedicated schedulers in larger organizations to expeditiously move the SMA program forward throughout the system and to consistently meet predetermined census targets.

Facility Requirements

Just like DIGMAs and CHCCs, PSMAs have their own facilities requirements—which can also be a weakness for PSMAs because the appropriate group and exam room space might not be readily available to the provider. Because physical examinations and new patient intake appointments are usually of longer duration than return or follow-up appointments for established patients, it generally takes fewer patients in attendance for PSMAs to triple a physician's productivity than is the case for DIGMAs. Therefore, PSMAs generally have the advantage of needing a smaller group room than do DIGMAs and CHCCs (especially if support persons are not included). A group room only half a large as that required for a DIGMA can often be used because only six to nine patients typically attend a Primary Care PSMA—i.e., rather than the 10–16 patients that is common for a DIGMA or the 15–20 patients (plus additional support persons) recommended for a CHCC. Another reason that a smaller group room is needed for PSMAs is that, unlike DIGMAs and CHCCs, spouses and support persons are often not invited to attend. When equipping a group room, in addition to making it a warm and comfortable environment with enough chairs, consider having a large wall clock on at least two (if not all four) of the walls so everyone remains cognizant of the time at all times—which helps to keep the group moving along so that it finishes on time.

DIGMAs typically require only one exam room—i.e., one that is located nearby the group room. However, PSMAs do have the disadvantage of requiring two to five exam rooms (with four exam rooms typically being ideal)—although these multiple exam rooms can often be in the provider's own office area rather than adjacent to the group room (as is preferred for the DIGMA exam room). Although only two to four exam rooms might be required in a Primary Care PSMAs dedicated to male patients, as many as four or even five exam rooms might be needed for efficiently dispatching female physicals in primary care.

Many Physicians Do Not Find PSMAs to Be Intuitive

Although PSMAs work well in both primary and specialty care, many providers do not find this model to be at all intuitively obvious—and therefore fail to consider implementing PSMAs in their practices. This is especially unfortunate because a large number of physicians actually running them for their practices find their PSMAs to

be professionally satisfying and a *no brainer*. They say this because of: (1) the dramatic increases in relative value units (i.e., RVUs) and productivity that this model can provide in the delivery of physical exams; (2) the improved access to physical exams that they so often experience in their practice once a PSMA has been started; (3) the fact that costly physician downtime as a result of patient no-shows and late-cancels can virtually be eliminated for physical exams by correspondingly overbooking PSMA sessions; and (4) the high levels of patient and physician professional satisfaction engendered by the PSMA model.

Filling All Sessions to Targeted Census Levels Can Prove Challenging

Another weakness is that the great efficiency and productivity gains provided by PSMAs can create a different type of challenge—i.e., where to draw the patients from in order to keep sessions filled once the physician's own backlog of patients that are wait-listed for physical examinations has been brought current and eliminated. It is surprising how efficient this model is at providing physical examinations, and at how quickly it can work down backlogs and wait-lists for physicals. Like DIGMAs, the key to a successful PSMA session is to consistently keep all sessions filled to the desired capacity. Once the physician's own wait-list for physical examinations has been brought current and eliminated, the physician will somehow need to create additional demand for PSMA physicals in order to keep all future PSMA sessions filled to targeted census levels.

When this does happen (i.e., once wait-lists and backlogs for physicals are brought current), here are five steps that providers can take to put pressure on—and increase demand for—PSMA appointments. *First*, they can reduce the number of individual physical examinations that they offer each week, perhaps by restructuring the provider's master schedule to shift many individual physical examination time slots to other appointment types (such as by creating additional return appointments or extra time in the schedule for procedure and/or surgeries). *Second*, providers can increase their panel sizes so that more patients need physical examination appointments each week. *Third*, providers can accept new patient intakes for their practice (i.e., for new patients who need a private physical examination as part of their intake) directly into the PSMA, so that both established and new patients needing a physical exam are included in the PSMA. *Fourth*, the provider can try to recruit patients from elsewhere in the clinic—such as by including wait-listed patients from other providers' practices who are unable to schedule timely physical exams (but only for providers who agree to this arrangement). Or else, such providers might be able to draw some patients into their PSMA from chronic illness population management programs—i.e., for patients willing to attend who need a timely physical exam. The problem with this fourth approach is that, while it can improve access to physical examinations, it reduces continuity of care with patients' own providers. *Fifth*, the provider can also increase demand for PSMA sessions by reducing the number of hours spent in the clinic each week, especially by reducing the number of individual physical examination appointments offered each week.

The Behaviorist's Job Is More Difficult in PSMAs

In Option 1 (which is the most common type of PSMA), the provider is typically absent from the group room for approximately the first half of the session—i.e., while delivering individual, private physical exams on all patients in the various exam rooms (one patient at a time but with minimal discussion). As a result, another weakness of the PSMA model is that it typically places greater pressure upon the behaviorist than does the DIGMA model because, throughout almost all of the DIGMA session, the physician is present in the group room delivering medical care. However, in the Option 1 PSMA, the physician is absent from the group room for the entire first half of the session while the behaviorist is left alone in the group room with a small, revolving group of unroomed patients—which puts considerable pressure on the behaviorist. It can be challenging for the behaviorist to keep this small, revolving group of patients moving along, and to make the best use of this time spent alone with patients. The challenge for the behaviorist is to keep the group productive, interactive, and interesting to all patients present in the group room at any given time— and, at the same time, to try at all times to not run out of things to talk about and be doing things that will ultimately prove helpful to patients and the physician.

During this time, the behaviorist has several jobs to do: (1) welcoming patients and warming up the group to get patients interacting with one another; (2) distributing nametags and collecting signed confidentiality release forms from any patients for whom this has not already been done; (3) giving the introduction to the PSMA session, usually twice so that all can hear it, including any late arrivers and the four or so patients who happened to be roomed in the exam rooms when it was initially delivered (thereby later saving precious interactive group

segment time, because patients are able to hear the introduction prior to when the physician joins the group after completing all of the physical exams); (4) asking patients what medical concerns they would like to discuss with the provider today; (5) writing these issues down on a flip chart or erasable whiteboard next to each patient's name, along with any other medically important issues that the patients might have reported on the health history form that they previously completed and returned to the office (i.e., for the physician to promptly see, upon later entering the group room for the interactive group segment); (6) distributing and reviewing handouts preselected by the provider (which can be discussed along with any other contents in the Patient Packet that was sent to patients when they scheduled today's PSMA visit); and (7) performing any other duties the provider and behaviorist might want to have provided during this time.

At the same time, the behaviorist must avoid any possible perception of appearing self-serving—for example, by promoting the behaviorist's own private practice, a book they might have written, or a program they might be involved with. The behaviorist must at all times maintain a focus upon optimal patient benefit, and avoid any possible patient perception regarding potential conflict of interest or personal gain.

Behaviorists Must Have Specific Qualifications and Stay Within Their Scope of Practice

In addition to being professionally competent, experienced in running groups, possessing a strong working knowledge regarding the PSMA model, and understanding the medical and psychosocial needs of medical patients and their families, it is also helpful if the behaviorist is friendly, warm, compassionate, and congenial in their style of relating to patients. Unlike the DIGMA model (where the preferred behaviorist is often a mental health professional, such as a psychologist or social worker with group experience and expertise), in the case of the PSMA model, a gregarious nurse who knows the patients is often a preferred choice for the behaviorist role. This is because the group size is typically much smaller in the PSMA than in the DIGMA—especially during the initial physical examination segment, and because this small group of patients often pumps the behaviorist for medical information—often of a type that the nurse can readily give but the mental health professional cannot do to not being either within their skill set or scope of practice under licensure.

A nurse practitioner would certainly also provide an excellent choice for behaviorist in the PSMA—in which case the census must be correspondingly larger to compensate for the increased overhead cost of using two providers (unless, of course, the nurse practitioner or PA chooses to work a couple of extra hours in the clinic so that his or her overhead cost to the PSMA is clearly the hourly wage, and not the revenues that the nurse practitioner or PA would have produced to the system by seeing patients themselves during 2 hours of clinic time). Therefore, when a nurse practitioner is used, it is very important that the time spent as behaviorist in the PSMA be viewed as extra hours in the clinic. In this case, the financial model used to assess the overhead cost of the behaviorist to the PSMA program would then only charge for the nurse practitioner's time according to the nurse practitioner's hourly wage. This would result in a much smaller overhead cost to the PSMA program than if the nurse practitioner's time were to be billed out according to the revenues that could have been generated for the system had the nurse practitioner instead been acting as a provider seeing patients individually during this amount of clinic time. If the latter were to be the case, the high overhead expense charged to the SMA program would unfortunately make the nurse practitioner too costly to be a realistic choice for behaviorist in a PSMA. (For a detailed financial analysis of the PSMA and DIGMA models, see the last part of Chapter 2.)

It is imperative that, just as is the case for DIGMAs, the behaviorist used in PSMAs stay at all times within their scope of practice under licensure—as well as within their skill set and level of professional competence. This can sometimes prove to be challenging to the behaviorist, especially when alone with the rotating small group of patients during the first half of the session—particularly when being pressed for medical information outside of their scope of practice. At such moments, the behaviorist can always tell patients that they will need to discuss that matter with the physician during the interactive group segment that will be following. However, if the physician has preselected any handouts on the topic being asked about, then the behaviorist can certainly distribute such handouts to interested patients in the group and go over some of the information contained therein—i.e., while pointing out that these handouts were preselected by the physician and limiting their comments to such information as is contained in these handouts.

Logistical Challenges in the PSMA's "Patient Packet"

One additional weakness of the PSMA model is that there are logistical and operational issues posed by the Patient Packet that is initially sent to patients when they schedule a PSMA appointment. First of all, the physician for whom the PSMA is being custom designed must decide precisely what items will be included in the Patient Packet—although the contents usually include such items as a cover letter (signed by the physician) welcoming patients and describing the program; a health maintenance schedule by age and sex; a detailed health history form to be completed by the patient and returned to the physician's office prior to the visit (typically similar to the health history questionnaire already being used by the physician for physical examinations, but more detailed); a form for lab tests (typically blood and urine tests) to be completed prior to the visit; and any handouts selected for inclusion by the physician.

Once the contents of the Patient Packet are determined, it must then be decided how far in advance of the appointment that it is to be sent to patients (e.g., 2 or 3 weeks ahead), and in what manner will it be sent (mail, e-mail, web site, etc.). It must also be determined how the completed health history form will be returned to the office by patients, and whether a self-addressed, stamped envelope should be included in the Patient Packet for this purpose. It will also need to be decided how far in advance of the session the completed health history form will need to be received by the physician's office.

Although it will typically be a receptionist, scheduler, MA, volunteer, or motivated clerical person on the physician's staff, it also needs to be planned who will: (1) assemble and mail the Patient Packet to all patients when they initially schedule the PSMA appointment; (2) take primary responsibility for receiving the completed health history forms from all patients registered to attend each week (and ensure that all such completed forms are returned to the office in a timely manner); and (3) follow-up with patients who have not returned their completed health history form or had their routine blood screening lab tests done a couple of days prior to the session—explaining that patients must return their completed health history form and get their lab tests done prior to attending the PSMA session. If the physician feels strongly about this matter, then it could also be added that otherwise the patient will be postponed until the next appropriate session after these two items have been completed (but only if another patient can be located at the last minute to replace such a patient who is late in getting their labs or form completed so that PSMA sessions are kept full).

In addition, someone on the physician's support staff needs to abstract and enter the relevant information from the completed health history forms (i.e., that have been returned to the office) into patients' chart notes for the upcoming PSMA session. And finally, someone (typically a nurse) also needs to transfer patients' lab test results onto a wall chart in the group room prior to the PSMA session—i.e., depicting each patient as a separate row and circling findings that the physician considers abnormal in red.

How to Maximize Productivity and Efficiency in a PSMA

Let us next examine the various techniques and resources that physicians can use effectively to maximize their productivity and efficiency in running a PSMA for their practice.

Stay Succinct and Focused

The single greatest challenge that physicians face in running a PSMA for their practice lies in staying focused and efficient throughout the entire session, in delivering the level of quality care that they hope to provide their patients with, and in finishing on time with all documentation completed. It is very important to start and end on time, and to make every reasonable effort to consistently do so. Keep in mind that there are temptations to linger at every turn—temptations that you must resist if you are to be efficient and stay on time throughout the session. It is tempting to enter into social chitchat and inefficient individual discussions when alone with patients in the exam rooms. There is certainly a learning curve associated with becoming comfortable with tactfully deferring all possible conversation (except that which is truly private or necessary in order to complete the exam) to the more efficient interactive group segment that follows. There is also a tendency for physicians to take too long with the first couple of patients addressed during the interactive group segment of the PSMA session (as well as with the first couple of physical examinations provided). In addition, there can also be a natural tendency to take too long in the interactive group segment when discussing treatment recommendations, medications, recommended lifestyle changes, diabetes, heart disease, hypertension, cholesterol, HRT, osteoporosis, etc., especially when those topics are of particular interest to the physician.

The behaviorist can contain the talkative or dominating patient, help to draw out the quiet patient, and facilitate getting group discussions back on track when distracting side conversations occur in the group—or when tangential comments derail the focus of the group. Most physicians grow to appreciate having their behaviorist tactfully intervene when discussions are overly lengthy and no longer productive for patients, or when they are starting to become tangential or purely academic—especially because of the help it provides in getting finished on time. Virtually all physicians find this to be preferable to not having the behaviorist intervene at all, with the result being that discussions can become lengthy and continue past the point of being of practical value to the patients—and, as a result, of finishing late. However, it does take some time and experience in actually running the PSMA for the physician, behaviorist, nursing personnel, and documenter to learn to seamlessly coordinate their efforts throughout the session so as to be optimally efficient in finishing on time with all work completed.

Physicians Must Fully Delegate to the PSMA Team

In order to double or triple their productivity in delivering physical examinations, physicians must learn to effectively delegate as much as possible to other members of the PSMA team. Simply put, the census of the PSMA (and therefore the ultimate productivity and efficiency benefits of the program) can be maximized only by having the physician delegate as many time-consuming responsibilities as appropriate and possible to other, less costly members of the PSMA team. This allows the physician to do much less, but that *much less* is what the physician alone can do—i.e., that for which the physician has gone through extensive medical school and residency training in order to provide, and the type of care that physicians generally most enjoy delivering.

In Larger Systems, Delegate Fully to the Champion and Program Coordinator

In larger systems, the champion for the DIGMA and PSMA program (who is given overall responsibility for the entire SMA program) plays a critical role in designing and implementing first the pilot study, and then—assuming that the pilot is successful—in moving the SMA program forward throughout the system to full-scale, organization-wide implementation. The program coordinator, who works closely with and assists the champion, handles most of the operational and administrative details associated with starting, running, expanding, and evaluating the SMA program.

During the planning and start-up phases of every new PSMA, the physician can delegate most of the associated time-consuming tasks to the champion—who, in larger systems, might in turn delegate many of these duties to the program coordinator. Although the physician will undoubtedly need to invest some time and energy into designing and setting up their PSMA program, the champion and program coordinator can minimize the extent of the physician's time commitment. The physician's participation in the PSMA launching process can typically be limited to: (1) four to five planning and training sessions, some of which will be between the physician and champion whereas others will include the physician's support staff and the various team members (behaviorist, nursing personnel, documenter, and dedicated scheduler) selected for the physician's PSMA, sessions which should be held outside of normal clinic hours whenever possible to avoid costly clinic downtime; and (2) customizing forms, handouts, promotional materials, the chart note template, and the Patient Packet for the program according to the physician's particular needs and practice (typically from templates and materials already developed for the SMA program by the champion, program coordinator, and other physicians).

Although most of the initial planning meetings will usually include only the physician and the champion, subsequent meetings will likely be larger and include, at various times, the entire PSMA team and occasionally all of the physician's support personnel (scheduling staff, receptionists, office manager, etc.) necessary to make the PSMA successful. In order to save the physician time, some of these larger information and training meetings may be conducted by the champion and program coordinator without the physician needing to be present. Therefore, these meetings can variously include the physician, nurse/MA(s), behaviorist, documenter, dedicated scheduler, champion, program coordinator, office manager, the physician's receptionists and schedulers, and the supervisors for the physician's nurses, receptionists, and schedulers. There are three goals for these meetings: (1) to custom design each PSMA so that it best meets the needs of the physician and the physician's practice; (2) to minimize the physician's time commitment to getting the PSMA designed and implemented; and (3) to do everything possible to ensure that the PSMA program is successfully launched and properly run.

The champion and program coordinator, not the physician, should oversee most of the time-consuming tasks associated with the planning and start-up phases of each new PSMA that is launched. Since many of these tasks are repetitive with the launch of every new PSMA, the champion and program coordinator can usually dispatch them more efficiently and at lower cost than would be the case if the physician were to do them—e.g., using the *pipeline* (see Part 2, Chapter 11) established by the champion and program coordinator for systematically launching all new

DIGMAs and PSMAs. Also, delegating these tasks to the champion and program coordinator whenever possible will minimize any physician time away from normal clinic duties during the planning, designing, training, launching, and evaluating stages of every new PSMA that is implemented. With the assistance of the physician, the champion and program coordinator will ensure that all operational details for the PSMA program are attended to in a timely manner. The many ways that the champion and program coordinator can help the physician are presented in Table 5.4.

Maximize the Behaviorist's Role

It is surprising how much of the physician's valuable time can be spent on psychosocial and behavioral health issues during the interactive group segment of the PSMA session. Experience has shown that it is often just as effective (and sometimes more so), and definitely far more expedient, for such issues to be handled whenever possible by the behaviorist when alone with the group during the initial physical exam segment of the visit—and during the brief amount of time that the behaviorist has when temporarily leading the interactive group segment while the physician is completing the chart note on each patient. However, for this approach to work, it is required that the behaviorist: (1) understands what the behavioral health and psychosocial issues of these medical patients are likely to be; (2) has the skill, training, and experience to successfully address these issues within the limits and confines of the PSMA setting; (3) has a relationship of trust developed with the physician so that this teamwork can be effectively coordinated; and (4) is fully utilized by the physician— who must be willing to delegate such duties to the behaviorist, and to correspondingly relinquish a certain degree of control in the PSMA setting.

Making full use of the behaviorist throughout each PSMA session certainly means delegating fully to the behaviorist during both the physical examination and interactive group segments of the PSMA session. This includes having the behaviorist pace the interactive group segment so that it runs smoothly and finishes on time, even if this means having the behaviorist occasionally intervene with tact to truncate any lengthy discussions that the physician might be entering into (i.e., before they become lofty, completely academic, and of minimal practical value to the patients).

Just as with DIGMAs, full use also means accepting the help of the behaviorist in numerous ways throughout the interactive group segment of the PSMA session: (1) in managing group dynamic issues (such as drawing out the quiet patient, containing the controlling or dominating patient, tactfully dealing promptly with two patients who might start up distracting side conversations in the group room as such side talk can quickly become an annoyance to patients and slow the group process down, etc.); (2) in briefly addressing patient's behavioral health and psychosocial issues as they arise, typically more to bring these issues to the attention of the physician for treatment (e.g., who might opt to start such patients on a psychotropic medication) or to triage patients into the appropriate internal and external programs of the physician's choosing (e.g., cognitive behavioral treatment programs for depression or anxiety, smoking cessation classes, stress management programs, community support groups, etc.) rather than having the behaviorist actually treat these issues in the PSMA setting (for which there is not sufficient time); (3) in temporarily running the group alone for a couple of minutes while the physician is completing the chart note immediately after working with each patient (or should the physician have to step out of the group room briefly in order to have a brief private discussion with a patient or to attend to a clinic emergency); etc.

As can be seen, in order to effectively dispatch these duties, the behaviorist will need to play a relatively structured and active role in the PSMA, be knowledgeable of internal and external resources available to the patients, and remain focused and succinct throughout. The behaviorist will often need to focus more on stimulating group interaction and discussion than on being the educator himself/herself, and on speaking to the group in a warm and succinct manner—i.e., in sound bites rather than extended explanations.

Maximize the Role of Nursing Personnel

Optimizing physician efficiency in the PSMA setting also requires making the best possible use of the nursing personnel (typically two nurses, medical assistants, nursing techs, etc.) assigned to the PSMA—plus expanding their role to max-pack visits by completely utilizing their skills, capabilities, and scope of practice under licensure. Because nursing personnel are so often under-utilized in ambulatory outpatient settings in healthcare systems around the country (often repetitively performing such mundane functions as rooming patients and taking a small set of vital signs), they typically very much enjoy working in DIGMAs and PSMAs. In these SMA settings, nurses can: (1) develop professionally; (2) showcase their skill set; and (3) have the professional satisfaction of maximizing their contribution to this multidisciplinary team-based approach to care. In addition, consider having them enter into each patient's chart note the nursing services that they have rendered in the PSMA setting (as well as their findings). One of the

nurses utilized in the PSMA could also be assigned the responsibility of entering the lab results just obtained on all patients onto a wall chart in the group room prior to the session.

Sit down with your nurse/MA(s) beforehand and ask them what all they can do in the PSMA setting to fully contribute to making the program all that it can be—based not on what they are currently doing in the clinic, but upon what they ideally could do in the PSMA. For example, consider having the nursing personnel attached to the PSMA perform such duties as are depicted in Table 5.5 (plus have them volunteer what else they could do to make the PSMA even better). With DIGMAs and PSMAs alike, there is often a sense of excitement and positive team building that occurs because all members of the SMA—team including the MAs and nurses—recognize that they have contributed in a meaningful way to the overall success of the program.

Delegate to the Documenter

Although the physician will ultimately be held responsible for the content and quality of the chart note, it is important that the physician also gain efficiency in the PSMA setting by delegating a great deal of the responsibility for drafting a comprehensive chart note onto the documenter. The need for documentation support is particularly critical in the PSMA model because physical examinations generally impose far greater documentation demands upon the physician than do return visits—which are the focus of DIGMAs and CHCCs. Despite ultimately being the physician's responsibility, the amount of time and energy required to complete chart notes on all patients attending the PSMA session can be reduced considerably through use of a documenter. In return, it is recommended that the physician agree to consistently meet targeted census levels—plus one additional patient in order to cover the added cost of having a documenter.

In addition, because the chart note drafted by the documenter is both contemporaneous and comprehensive (and uses the physician's own documentation template), it can provide a superior chart note as compared to that which the physician might generate on their own after working with each patient individually in the PSMA setting. This is because some of what has been done with that patient would likely already have been forgotten by the time that note was written, even though it would be drafted by the physician immediately after working with each patient in turn in the group setting—a situation that would be much worse for those physicians choosing to complete chart notes on all patients in attendance after the session is over (which is something that I never recommend doing).

An additional benefit of having a documenter is that, unlike physicians (who seldom enjoy drafting chart notes), the documenter volunteers for the job because they believe that they will enjoy doing the documentation on all patients—which can add to the quality of the chart note. In addition, as the documenter continuously gains experience over time, their chart note will likely only get better. I recently heard independently from two different physicians at different sites in a larger healthcare system—physicians who share a couple of patients with a specialist that runs a DIGMA—to the effect that they were just reviewing the most recent chart note on their shared patient (which happened to be a DIGMA chart note) and found it to be the best that they had ever seen from this specialist. Needless to say, upon later hearing about this positive feedback regarding the quality of the DIGMA chart note, the documenter was exceedingly proud.

Only through such documentation support will the physician be able to efficiently complete the lengthy documentation requirements that physical examinations entail within the time constraints of the PSMA. This is especially true for systems using electronic medical records (EMR), and goes a long way toward ensuring that the physician does not get the common complaint that: "My doctor never looked at me. He/she just looked at the computer the whole time." Although having a documenter remains helpful for optimizing physician efficiency in healthcare systems still using paper charts, physicians are sometimes able to get by without one—either through use of a chart note template that is largely preprinted and in check-off form, or by dictating chart notes into a microcassette. If the physician does dictate the chart note into a recorder, then it is recommended that the physician use this as a teaching point during the session by dictating loudly into the recorder immediately after working with each patient individually during the interactive group segment—so that the entire group can listen and learn. The physician can even say something like the following to the group: "OK, listen up everybody. I am going to dictate the chart note on Tom, so listen carefully and let me know if I leave anything out". Patients often learn a lot by listening intently to both how the physician summarizes their case and to the physician's treatment recommendations. Nonetheless, even in the case of systems still using paper charts and physicians who dictate into a microcassette, having a documenter can still increase physician efficiency as there would then no longer be any transcribed chart notes coming back later from the system's medical transcription that the physician would be required to go through and correct long after the PSMA is over.

Depending upon what the physician wants the documenter to do during the initial physical examination segment of the PSMA session, the documenter will either (1) shadow the physician by going from exam room to exam room and entering the data into each patient's chart note as the physician is stating all physical findings out loud while conducting the physical examinations (in which case the documenter will need to be a nurse or someone qualified to be in the room with disrobed patients) or else (2) stay in the group room with the behaviorist and small group of unroomed patients entering the reasons for today's visit into each patient's chart note (as well as anything else that the behaviorist might be covering). In a variant of the first approach (i.e., when the physician prefers to not have the documenter in the exam room), the physician could also quickly write the physical findings down briefly on a *crib sheet*—and then give it, as soon as the exam is over, to the documenter (who is using a nearby computer outside of the exam room) to enter into the patient's PSMA chart note. I generally recommend the former as it adds to the physician's efficiency during the PSMA; however, some physicians are so used to entering their own physical findings into the chart note when conducting physical exams that they prefer the latter. Then, during the interactive group segment, the documenter will obviously be in the group room scribing into each patient's chart note what is transpiring there in real time—i.e., as the physician is delivering care to that patient in the PSMA session, exactly as is done in DIGMAs.

Involve the IT Department to Simplify the EMR Documentation Process

For healthcare organizations that are already using EMR, another key area of documentation support is to have the IT Department work on making the EMR documentation process for PSMAs as *user friendly* as possible. Among other things, such help from the IT Department can include all of the following points:

- Help in developing the basic PSMA documentation template developed for each medical subspecialty
- Have the ability to preprint (to the maximum degree possible, through simple keystroke shortcuts) a complete *normal* physical examination chart note template for each patient in attendance, so that only changes, updated information, and abnormal findings regarding the patient need to be entered into the PSMA chart note
- Have the ability to drop large preprinted sections into the chart note through simple keystroke shortcuts (such as paragraphs on hypertension, diabetes, cholesterol,

and PSA) for various diagnoses and conditions—i.e., along with any pertinent abnormal findings

- Adapt the EMR in every possible way to maximally accommodate it to the specific documentation requirements of the PSMA physician, and to make it as *user friendly* as possible

Involve the Organization's Documentation and Billing and Compliance Experts

Similar to involving IT in the planning and implementation phases of the PSMA program, I likewise recommend including the documentation as well as billing and compliance officers in the organization—as their contributions can often be invaluable in optimizing both chart notes and billing. The billing and compliance officer can also be involved in training the documenter for the PSMA, with an emphasis upon making certain that all of the key elements for billing purposes are indeed included in the chart note. I remember one time in particular when, as the billing and compliance officer pointed out, by including two rather simple additional components in the PSMA, we could bill at a considerably higher level—which gave us an opportunity to explore including those two components, as they were beneficial to the patients anyway. In effect, we would essentially have been delivering a much higher level of care than we would have been able to bill for if we had not involved billing and compliance in the planning process for this PSMA. Similarly, on several occasions, I have found it to be invaluable to involve the organization's documentation officer in the PSMA planning process because the end result was often a superior chart note.

Despite Delegating As Much As Possible to Others, the Physician Must Still Personally Invite All Appropriate Patients

Despite all of the champion and program coordinator's efforts during the planning and start-up phases, as with DIGMAs, there is one important responsibility that every physician running a PSMA must commit to undertaking on an ongoing basis. Physicians must take approximately 30 seconds during every office visit with all patients needing a physical examination (who meet the criteria for their PSMA) in order to: (1) briefly explain the program to all appropriate patients in positive terms; (2) personally invite them to attend the PSMA the next time they need a private physical examination; and (3) promptly book all patients accepting this invitation into the appropriate upcoming PSMA session.

There is nothing more important in persuading them to attend a PSMA the next time they need a physical examination than a positively worded, personal invitation from their physician, who must, by the way, personally believe in their PSMA program in a heartfelt manner if they are to expect patients to accept this invitation and actually attend.

How the Physician Words the Invitation Is Important to Its Success

When inviting patients, the physician should first briefly describe a couple of the program's key selling points for the patient—prompt access, more time together, greater patient education, the help and support of other patients, etc. Then, the physician can add something like: "It's also fun, plus you'll get answers to questions that you might not have thought to ask because others will ask them. And you will have the opportunity to meet some other patients of mine dealing with similar issues, who will likely share some helpful hints. We even serve some snacks. Would you like to give it a try and come to my PSMA for your upcoming physical exam?" Such a positively worded statement is often helpful in persuading an ambivalent patient to attend a PSMA for the first time. On the other hand, success is hardly to be expected with a bland invite like: "You are due for a physical examination. You can have either an individual physical or you can come to my group. Just schedule whichever you like when you leave." In this case, the patient will almost certainly go out and schedule what they are familiar with—i.e., a traditional individual physical examination—thus putting the PSMA program at high risk for failure.

While patient satisfaction with properly run PSMAs is very high for those patients who do attend, the challenge lies in getting patients to attend for the first time—as patients are used to the old way of receiving traditional individual physical examinations. However, once there, patients almost always like this new venue of care and are willing to return to it the next time they need a physical examination—or to a DIGMA for their next return appointment, in the event that the physician also happens to run a DIGMA for their practice.

Thirty Practical Tips for Making Your PSMA Program a Success (Table 5.7)

Table 5.7 depicts 30 practical tips that will help you to make your PSMA program a success, some of which are discussed here while others are discussed elsewhere in this book. These are but a few hard-earned pearls that have

Table 5.7 Thirty helpful tips for making your PMA program a success

1. First secure administrative support, as group visits represent a major paradigm shift from traditional individual office visits and require real and meaningful support from administration in order to succeed.

2. Secure the budgetary, personnel, promotional, and facilities resources required for success.

3. In larger systems, secure the best possible champion to oversee the entire program and rapidly move it forward throughout the organization—plus secure the best available program coordinator to assist the champion in handling many of the program's operational and administrative details.

4. Start by adhering closely to the PSMA model as it is presented here in order to avoid making many beginners' mistakes.

5. Promote the program effectively to all appropriate patients by utilizing high quality, professional appearing promotional materials; however, try to develop all such materials for the PSMA program in template form in order to minimize costs.

6. Have all attendees sign a confidentiality release during each session—patients as well as any support persons accompanying them.

7. In both primary and specialty care, always try to increase physician productivity for physical examinations by 200–300% or more—preferably 300% in most cases.

8. Establish and consistently meet targeted census levels (typically between 7 and 9 male patients or 6–8 female patients per 90 min PSMA in primary care, and 10–13 patients in most medical subspecialties) during all sessions to optimally leverage the physician's time and simultaneously have the best possible group interaction. Generating weekly pre-booking census reports on all sessions for the next 2 months (plus using a dedicated scheduler) can be most helpful in achieving census targets.

9. Do like the airlines do and overbook sessions according to the expected number of late cancels and no-shows—i.e., to make yourself immune from this otherwise vexing and costly problem of physician downtime.

10. Be certain that the PSMA program is completely voluntary—both to the patients who attend and the physicians who choose to run them in their practices.

11. Carefully select all handouts to be used in the program, as well as all of the enclosures for the Patient Packet.

12. Carefully design and work out the logistical details around the Patient Packet: what will be included in the contents; who will assemble them; how far in advance will they be mailed; who will receive the completed health history questionnaires returned by patients; how will they be returned to the physician's office; who will abstract this information beforehand into the chart notes for the session; who will follow-up with patients who fail to return their completed health history forms or to complete their lab tests in a timely manner; will patients who fail to do so be postponed until a later session; etc.

13. Use skilled, trained, motivated, and compatible PSMA team members—the best available rather than the cheapest.

14. Try to secure 2 nursing personnel (nurses, MAs, nursing techs, etc.) who are enthusiastic supporters of the program and able to perform the expanded nursing duties of the PSMA.

15. Prior to the session, have one of the nurses gather all of the new lab test data from all of the patients and enter it onto a wall chart that will then be posted in the group room and used in the PSMA—circling abnormal findings in red.

16. Carefully select an appropriate, well-trained behaviorist (often a nurse, but sometimes a psychologist or social worker) with the necessary skills for the program—one who is compatible and able to work closely with the physician—and then make full use of the behaviorist throughout the entire PSMA session.

17. To optimize physician's productivity, secure the necessary documentation support via a specifically trained documenter who is a good typist, facile on the computer, knowledgeable about medical jargon, unflappable, able to multitask, compatible with the physician, and capable of generating an excellent chart note—one that is both in line with the physician's wishes and uses the physician's own chart note template.

18. Assign a dedicated scheduler to the PSMA and allow adequate time each week (usually up to 2–4 hours, or as needed) to call lists of patients selected by the physician for the PSMA so as to ensure that all sessions are consistently filled to capacity.

19. Delegate fully, maximally utilize the skills of the entire PSMA team, and fully expand the roles of the behaviorist and nursing personnel.

20. Adequately train the entire PSMA team, as well as the physician's reception and scheduling staffs, so that all can fulfill their roles in making the program a success. Here is point 21 to 30 of Table 5.7, which would not fit on the previous yellow "Sticky Note":

21. Secure the necessary facilities, which typically include a small group room capable of seating 10–16 persons and 2–5 exam rooms (with 4 often being optimal).

22. Solve any operational or system problems as they arise.

23. Whenever possible, try to provide the private physical exams first and the interactive group segment afterwards—which is usually the best and most efficient design for the PSMA model.

24. Conduct the private physical examinations thoroughly but rapidly by minimizing all unnecessary talk in the inefficient exam room setting—and by limiting any such talk to truly private matters and those which need to be discussed in order to conduct the exam. Tactfully defer all other discussions and Q&A to the interactive group segment that follows.

25. Stay focused and succinct throughout the PSMA session, but be certain to foster some group interaction during the interactive group segment.

26. Provide any simple procedures that might be needed either during the private physical examination or towards the end of the session—unless the physician chooses to do them during the group, such as dermatologists sometimes do when freezing skin tags.

27. Always strive to start and finish on time—and to complete all documentation during the session—so that when the PSMA session is over, all of the work is done.

Table 5.7 (continued)

28. Expect that you will likely finish late and not have all charting completed during your first few sessions, and that you will be tempted to make your group smaller for the next session. However, do not yield to this temptation because the reason you are finishing late is that you and your team are still learning and not yet fully coordinated. Instead, maintain your census and debrief with your team for 15–20 min after sessions for the first 2 months (and from time to time thereafter), focusing upon how to make subsequent sessions even better and more efficient.
29. In larger and mid-sized systems, strive to launch the targeted number of Physicals SMAs per year—perhaps as many as 12–18 programs annually.

been gained through the trials and tribulations of my personal experience in working with over 400 physicians (and over 20,000 patient visits) in DIGMAs and PSMAs that I have helped to launch nationwide. Hopefully, these pearls regarding keys to success and pitfalls to avoid will prove helpful to others who are considering a PSMA program for their practices—so that they can learn from, and not have to repeat, my previous mistakes (upon which these pearls are quite often based).

Whenever Appropriate, Defer Discussions from the Exam Room to the Group Room

A common beginners' mistake is unnecessarily entering into social chitchat or inefficient individual discussions with patients in the exam room. Although this is something that physicians are accustomed to doing during traditional individual physical examinations, it is very wasteful of time. This is a mistake because doing so ends up reducing the amount of time that the physician can spend in the highly efficient interactive group setting—as the entire PSMA visit, including both the physical examination and interactive group segments, has only a fixed amount of time allocated to it (typically 90 minutes). All of the promotional materials for the PSMA program, as well as the behaviorist (during the introduction) and physician, need to make it very clear to patients that the private physical examination segment of the session is only for the physical exam—and for occasional brief private discussions, as necessary—and that almost all discussion will occur in the group segment that follows.

Remain Concise and Focused Throughout

Failure to stay succinct and focused throughout the session (i.e., during both the physical examination and interactive group segments) is one of the most common mistakes made in practice by physicians running PSMAs for their practices. Avoid social chitchat and as much talk

as possible while alone with patients in the exam room—while at the same time, being certain not to come across as disinterested or rude. Whenever possible, tactfully defer as much discussion as possible from the inefficient exam room setting to the highly efficient interactive group segment that follows. However, even during the interactive group setting, limit yourself to succinct and focused discussions that will be helpful to the patients in attendance—avoiding any theoretical or tangential discussions that are not directly pertinent to the medical needs of the patients who are present, no matter how interesting they might be.

Whenever Possible, Limit the Amount of Time Spent on the First Couple of Patients

Spending too much time on the first couple of patients—in either the exam room or the group room setting—is a common error frequently made by many physicians when they first start a PSMA in their practices. Be careful to not take too much time with the first couple of patients that you work with in both the physical examination and interactive group segments. Instead set a pace with the first patient or two that you can sustain throughout the remainder of these segments and still finish the PSMA session on time. Keep in mind that if you should happen to fall into this common trap, you will likely end up finishing late—and possibly even quite late.

Be Sure to Foster Some Group Interaction, but Not Too Much

It is important to foster some group interaction during the interactive group segment in order to keep discussions in the group lively, engaging, and interesting to all, but too much interaction can be problematic. View group interaction as like using spices in cooking—a little bit can go a long way toward making a superior dish, but too much can ruin it (in the case of PSMAs, by taking up so much time that the physician cannot finish on schedule).

As with DIGMAs, during the interactive group segment, physicians sometimes make the common mistake of falling into the individual exam room model of just talking to the patient that they are focusing upon—and forgetting to involve the rest of the group in the discussion. When this happens, other patients will then quickly become disinterested—and might even start distracting side conversations among themselves or, worse yet, leave the group altogether. A sure sign that this is happening would be if patients were to get up, one by one, and leave the session immediately after their medical needs have been addressed by the physician in the interactive group setting. It is imperative that the physician always keeps in mind that a group visit is an entirely different venue of care delivery—i.e., one in which considerable attention must be paid to the group itself as well as to the individual patients within it. For this reason, foster some group interaction from time to time throughout the interactive group segment—and be certain to not go over and quietly speak privately to one patient while turning your back to the rest of the group. Also, be sure to speak loud enough at all times so that all present can hear you and learn from what you are saying.

While Appropriate for Most, PSMAs Are Not Meant for All Patients

Although PSMAs are appropriate for most types of patients needing a physical examination, they are not meant for all patients—nor are they intended to completely eliminate the need for individual physical examinations. For example, it is usually best to try to exclude the following types of patients from your PSMA program.

- Those who do not speak the language that the PSMA is being conducted in; however, if enough monolingual patients speaking that language exist to ensure full sessions, then certain sessions each month could actually be conducted in that language—providing that the physician speaks that language or an appropriate translator is available
- Those who are too hearing impaired or demented to benefit
- Patients with serious contagious illnesses (such as SARS, bird flu, or TB)
- Patients who refuse to maintain confidentiality
- Patients experiencing a medical emergency (such as severe, acute chest pains)
- Patients who refuse to attend because they prefer a traditional individual physical examination

As regards patients who do not speak the language and those who are too hearing impaired or too limited in their comprehension to benefit, these patients can often be seen either individually or in a PSMA that has been specifically designed for such patient populations. For example, one could hold Spanish-speaking PSMAs for monolingual Spanish-speaking patients; utilize microphones and loudspeakers for the hearing impaired (while the physician, behaviorist, and documenter wear earplugs); or encourage appropriate caregivers to accompany patients having significant cognitive impairments. However, before starting highly specialized homogeneous PSMAs like these, first make certain that you are seeing enough patients of that particular type to keep such sessions consistently full. Certainly, PSMAs are not for patients who will not maintain confidentiality, nor are they for patients who refuse to attend because they strongly prefer traditional individual physical examinations.

Strive to Increase Productivity by 300%

The goal is always to have the PSMA session end on time with all documentation completed, and to accomplish this while seeing enough patients during each session to leverage the physician's time by 200–300% or more—with 300% being the most common goal. Furthermore, the goal is always to accomplish this while delivering quality care, improving performance measures and outcomes, maintaining appropriate privacy, keeping the program voluntary to patients and physicians alike, and achieving high levels of both patient and physician professional satisfaction.

A 200–300% Increase in Productivity Can Only Be Achieved by Delegating Fully to the Entire PSMA Team

As previously discussed, the physician needs to effectively delegate as many responsibilities as possible and appropriate to other, less costly members of the PSMA team—initially to the champion and program coordinator during the planning and start-up phases of the program, and later to the behaviorist, nursing personnel, documenter, and dedicated scheduler attached to the PSMA on an ongoing basis. Delegating so much to others leaves the physician with much less to do (i.e., that which the physician alone can do), and this in turn enables the census and productivity in PSMA sessions to be optimized. While the group itself adds somewhat to the efficiency of the PSMA session (because things only need to be said once for the benefit of all so that repetition can be avoided, and because sessions can be overbooked according to the expected number of late-cancels and no-shows), this is not the main reason that PSMAs are so efficient.

As with DIGMAs, the major reason that PSMAs are so productive is because they have the opposite effect of almost every other change that has occurred in medicine during the past decade or two—which seem to always be putting evermore responsibilities and work onto the shoulders of the physician. The secret to the PSMA's success (as well as to the success of the DIGMA model before it) is that it does just the opposite—i.e., by taking as many duties and responsibilities as possible off the physician and placing them instead onto the shoulders of a less expensive and specifically trained multidisciplinary care delivery team.

If Predetermined Census Levels Are Not Consistently Met, Track Down the Problem and Solve it Promptly

Carefully work out the details of promoting the program and scheduling enough appropriate patients into every PSMA session so as to ensure that predetermined target census levels are consistently met. Everybody involved in inviting, referring, and scheduling of patients into the PSMA must understand their roles and responsibilities—and be held accountable for fulfilling these functions (or be given additional training should they fail to perform). Are there framed wall posters prominently displayed on the physician's lobby and exam room walls, and is a dispenser capable of holding at least 100 program description fliers attached next to it? Are these dispensers being kept full, and who is responsible for doing so (as well as for ordering new fliers before they run out)?

Is the physician's reception staff giving out invitation letters and saying a few kind words about the PSMA program to all appropriate patients as they register for their regular office visit appointments (so that the patients can read the flier while waiting in the lobby)? Is someone responsible for replenishing these invitations before they run out at the reception desk? Are the physician's nurses promoting the program to all appropriate patients seen during normal office visits, and making certain that each patient gets a program description flier to read while waiting for the physician to arrive in the exam room? Is the physician's normal scheduling staff appropriately trained to refer patients into the PSMA when they need a physical examination, and have the guidelines and sample scheduling scripts necessary for doing so been put into place?

Try to have a dedicated scheduler attached to the PSMA program to ensure that all sessions are consistently filled to capacity. Will the dedicated scheduler be inviting patients by phone, or doing so by mail and e-mail as well? Will the dedicated scheduler be allocated adequate time each week to fulfill this vital function—typically 2–4 hours on weeks where their assistance is needed, although no time is needed when the physician and staff are able to keep upcoming PSMA sessions filled? If a call center (either on- or off-site) is to be involved with scheduling patients into the PSMA, how will accountability for scheduling patients into the PSMA be introduced and maintained within the call center? For example, will there be a couple of specially trained *scheduling angels* within the Call Center to whom all incoming calls from patients wanting to schedule an appointment with the PSMA physician will be referred, so as to increase the likelihood of successfully referring and scheduling patients into the PSMA?

What patients are to be invited and, if patients' names are coming from lists (such as lists of the physician's patients by age, sex, or diagnoses; lists of patients already scheduled for individual physicals beyond a certain point in the future; lists of patients provided by the physician; and existing wait-lists), who will be responsible for generating and updating these lists of patient's names? Who will be responsible for securing the physician's approval as to which patients on the list are to be called and not called? Also, if patients are to come from other physicians' wait-lists as well, which physicians have and have not agreed to this arrangement—and for what types of patients?

Secure the Necessary Documentation Support

If physicians are to increase their productivity by 200–300% or more, then they will need to secure the necessary documentation support for their PSMA program to efficiently complete the PSMA chart notes on so many patients during the allotted time. Having documentation support translates directly into increased physician productivity during the session. This documentation support includes: (1) somebody to abstract the information from the completed health history forms (i.e., the form contained in the Patient Packet originally sent to the patient upon scheduling the PSMA, and that was subsequently completed by the patient and returned to the office prior to the session) into patients' PSMA chart notes prior to the session; (2) the help of the nursing personnel in documenting all of the information and data they collect (as well as the expanded services they are performing) into the nursing section of the chart note; and (3) actually having a documenter present throughout the PSMA session (i.e., in both the physical examination and interactive group segments), which is especially important for systems already using EMR.

Schedule Patients into PSMAs 2–3 Weeks in Advance

Scheduling patients into PSMA sessions at least 2–3 weeks in advance appears to be ideal. The Patient Packet could either be sent to patients as soon as they schedule their PSMA appointment or approximately 2–3 weeks before the session. The Patient Packet needs to be sent to patients far enough in advance of the visit for the patient to complete the required blood and urine screening tests and to also complete and return the enclosed health history form. Keep in mind that the health history questionnaire is quite detailed and can be time-consuming for the patient to fill out—and that it will take some time for a staff member to abstract this information from the completed forms that have been returned to the office (as well as the new lab test results that have been gathered) into each patient's chart note prior to the session.

Prescreen New Patients

Be cautious about including patients in your PSMA with whom you are completely unfamiliar—i.e., without first at least doing a little basic prescreening. If, as some physicians do, you accept either new patients or patients from other physicians' practices into your PSMA, then try to first find out a certain minimum amount of basic screening information about such patients. When physicians accept other physician's patients—or patients new to their own practice—into their PSMA without any prescreening whatsoever, they run the risk of having unexpected situations occur that could slow their PSMA down and make it impossible to finish on time.

This situation occurred in a Family Practice PSMA designed for adult women when a new patient the physician had never seen before attended the session. She was in her mid-30s and a recent immigrant. She had never been sexually active, and had considerable difficulty speaking and understanding English. She had come from a country where healthcare services were far below Western standards, and had never previously had either a pap smear or a pelvic exam. Therefore, these procedures needed to be explained to the patient in considerable detail in the exam room—which proved to be especially time-consuming because of the language barrier. The end result was that the private physical exam for this patient took much longer than the few minutes normally allotted for an adult woman in a PSMA.

To make matters even worse, this patient's friend also attended the same session as a new patient. As it turned out, her circumstances were similar—but even more challenging to the physician because, although she previously had one pelvic exam in her nation of origin, she described it in broken English as the worst experience she ever had in her entire life. It therefore took the physician even more time in the exam room to comfort and reassure this patient—and to complete the physical examination—than it did for her friend.

Needless to say, this physician ended up finishing the PSMA session quite late—and also felt pressured and frustrated by the experience. It is important to note that this problem could have been completely avoided by simply instituting a very basic prescreening procedure for patients new to the physician wanting to attend the PSMA. For example, by only accepting patients who speak fluent English and have previously had a pelvic exam that went relatively well (two basic prescreening questions that could be quickly asked by either the physician's scheduling staff or by the specifically trained dedicated scheduler), this problem could have been avoided. Patients who fail to pass such a basic prescreening test (and therefore do not qualify for the physician's PSMA) could instead be scheduled into a traditional individual physical examination.

If You Finish Late At First, Do Not Immediately Cut Back on Your Targeted Census Level

Expect that you will likely finish late and not have all of your charting completed during your first few sessions. When this happens, one of the first thoughts that you and your behaviorist will likely have is the temptation to make your group smaller for the next session by immediately reducing your targeted census level. However, it is very important that you do not yield to this temptation, because the reason you are finishing late is likely due to the fact that you and your team are not yet well coordinated and are still learning. Instead, maintain your census and debrief with your team for 10-15 minutes after sessions for the first 2 months (and, as needed, from time to time thereafter), focusing upon just 2 things: (1) how to make future sessions more time efficient; and (2) how to make subsequent sessions even better.

If, after a couple of months, you find that you are still finishing quite late (yet that you have tried everything possible to get done on time), then go ahead and reduce your target census level—but only by one patient, and then try again to finish on time during the next 2 months. If you give into the temptation of reducing group size prematurely, you will never grow to truly appreciate how much better a full group can be not only economically, but psychodynamically as well—as you will likely find that a full group is also a more lively, fast-paced, interactive, and interesting group.

Have Patients Stay for the Entire Session

Because important medical care, information, and support are provided during all parts of the PSMA session, patients should be encouraged to stay for the entire visit whenever possible. This is especially true when the private exams are provided during the first part of (or even during) the session—because there is so much to learn throughout the interactive group segment, even after the physician has addressed the patient's particular individual medical needs in this setting. Undoubtedly, there will be occasional patients who will need to return to work as soon as possible (or return home to care for children). Nonetheless, whenever it is possible, patients should be encouraged to stay for the entire session so as to gain full benefit from the PSMA experience.

Ten Common Beginner's Mistakes When Starting a DIGMA or PSMA Program

Physicians and healthcare organizations often make many beginners' mistakes when starting a DIGMA and/or PSMA program of which, ten of the most common are discussed here. Remember that group medical appointments are often counter-intuitive, involve much change, stress the system, and are a major paradigm shift–all of which can lead to many beginner's mistakes.

First Prove That It Works, and Then Administration Will Support It

The first common mistake is when the organization tells the physician who has an interest in starting a DIGMA or PSMA program to first do one and demonstrate that it works—and then administration might support it. The problem here is that DIGMAs and PSMAs represent a major paradigm shift and require administrative support as well as significant personnel, facilities, and promotional resources in order to succeed. It is foolhardy to expect motivated physicians to somehow go out and develop a successful group visit program on their own, without any meaningful administrative support. Such an approach will almost certainly result in unnecessary frustration, numerous design and operational errors, inadequate census, and a program that has a high likelihood of failure—even in systems where group visit programs could otherwise be very successful.

Launching the SMA Program Prematurely

Another common error is for physicians, upon hearing about DIGMAs, CHCCs, or PSMAs, to become so excited about starting one that they launch their group visit without first securing the necessary supports for a successful program. First of all, the physician must read up on these different group visit models and thoroughly understand them in order to select the best one for meeting his or her own particular needs—and then, the physician must design and run it properly. This book is an ideal resource for accomplishing these ends. In addition, the physician will need to first secure administrative support, and then obtain the necessary promotional materials (notice that examples of all necessary promotional materials and forms for DIGMAs and PSMAs are included in the DVD attached to this book). The physician must then carefully select all the patient education materials and informational handouts for the program, obtain and schedule the required facilities, and then secure and train the necessary personnel for the SMA team. The physician will also need to develop the chart note template, have the medical risk department or corporate attorney develop an appropriate confidentiality release, and resolve any billing issues that might arise prior to launching the new SMA program.

Failing to Design Four Major Dimensions into Every SMA: Quality, Census, Economy, and Assessment

Another common beginners' mistake is to fail to carefully design four different critically important dimensions into each and every SMA that is launched: (1) build all possible quality into the design and flow of each and every group visit program; (2) ensure that targeted census is consistently met during each and every session; (3) keep overhead costs of the program down (while still trying to secure excellent promotional materials and personnel); and (4) measure all important outcomes from the SMA program on an ongoing basis.

Designing the DIGMA or PSMA to Be More Homogeneous than It Needs to Be

Yet another especially common mistake is for a physician to design the DIGMA or PSMA to be more homogeneous than it needs to be. This occurs as frequently as it does because physicians often initially feel more comfortable with a homogeneous grouping of patients, which at first seems to be a more intuitively appealing option. However, as a result, such physicians almost always end up designing a DIGMA or PSMA that is too homogeneous—with the ultimate result being that they have a hard time consistently filling the sessions and meeting targeted census requirements. They therefore end up designing a SMA program that is intuitively appealing, but at high risk for failure.

Do not make this common beginner's mistake of designing your PSMA or DIGMA around your interests or comfort level rather than around patient demand. Therefore, if you are a primary care physician and thinking about designing a DIGMA for diabetic patients in your practice, then I would strongly encourage you to instead make it a *Hyperlipodiabesity* DIGMA (or Endocrine Syndrome DIGMA) that includes almost all of the hypertensive, hyperlipidemia, diabetic, and obese patients in your practice—as there is much overlap in the issues that all of these patients face. By doing so, you will probably increase the percentage of patients in your practice qualified to attend the group visit from 15 or 20% in the case of diabetes to perhaps as many as 70–80% of your patients when you open the SMA up to those dealing with obesity, hypertension, hyperlipidemia, or diabetes—a consideration that holds as true for PSMAs as it does for any group visit program.

Failing to Consistently Meet Pre-established Census Requirements

By far, the most common reason for DIGMAs and PSMAs to fail is insufficient census. Always design your DIGMAs and PSMAs to increase your productivity during group time by at least 200–300% or more (i.e., compared to actual, not scheduled, productivity during individual office visits)—and try to have full sessions right from the start. You can learn to adapt to the full group size by debriefing after sessions with your team for the first 2 months, focusing upon how to make future sessions even better and more efficient. It is a common mistake to try to start with small groups and then gradually work up in size—an approach that seldom allows you to ever reach your targeted census level, as you will probably reach a group size you are comfortable with and then not try to increase census any further.

Also be careful to not let your census gradually drop off over time, which sometimes happens when we have an initial history of success and then become complacent. Do not settle for partial benefit from your DIGMA or PSMA program by rationalizing unfilled groups and telling yourself that they are allowing you to provide better care and

to have highly satisfied patients. Keep in mind that full sessions result not only in an economically viable program but also in more lively and interactive groups that are more likely to be optimally beneficial to your patients.

Not Promoting the DIGMA or PSMA Effectively to All Appropriate Patients

It is also a common beginners' mistake to not promote a DIGMA or PSMA program effectively to all appropriate patients. Effective promotion means that you do all of the following:

1. send an announcement letter out to all of your appropriate patients at the start of the program;
2. prominently display an appropriately sized, professional appearing framed poster on the walls of your lobby and exam rooms (with an flier holder next to it containing 100 or so graphically matching program description fliers for patients to take);
3. have your receptionist(s) give all appropriate patients an invitation letter (plus tell them some kind words about the program) on an ongoing basis when they register for regular office visits;
4. have your nurse/MA give patients a program description flier to read while waiting for the physician to enter in the exam room (plus say a few positive, personal remarks about the program) when rooming all suitable patients during normal office visits;
5. personally invite all your appropriate patients during normal office visits through a carefully worded script to attend your PSMA the next time they need a physical exam (this is *the most important single promotional step*);
6. train your scheduling staff to offer (and promote) your group visit to all suitable patients when they call for an appointment (i.e., regardless of whether they are calling for a physical examination, or whether they are calling for a follow-up visit but happen to be due for a physical), and to then offer them the choice of either a 90-minute PSMA appointment within 2–3 weeks or your first available individual physical examination appointment (which might be months away);
7. have a dedicated scheduler attached to your PSMA who can reach out to the patients you want to have invited by telephoning them and encouraging them to attend (i.e., for weeks where this service is needed due to low census for the upcoming session); and finally
8. inform patients about your new PSMA program through patient newsletter articles and positive coverage in the local mass media (TV, radio, newspapers, etc.);

9. Invite patients attending your PSMA to return when they next need another physical exam.

Assembling the Cheapest or Most Available PSMA Team, Rather than the Best and Most Appropriate One

Another common mistake is to assemble the cheapest or most available personnel for your DIGMA or PSMA team—i.e., rather than assembling the most appropriate team. Get the best team (i.e., a skilled, trained, and compatible team) for you and your practice, and do not short-change your program by trying to do without critical personnel. In larger systems, be certain to get help from, and to fully utilize the services of, the champion and program coordinator. Select a skilled and experienced behaviorist that you trust and feel you can work with—one with a complementary skill set that can effectively perform all the behaviorist's duties that are required in a well-run PSMA. If you are a physician who frequently finishes late in the clinic, be certain to select a behaviorist with good time management skills—who can at least pace the interactive group segment of the PSMA and ensure that it finishes on time.

Similarly, select one or two appropriate nursing personnel who are motivated and capable of expeditiously performing the expanded nursing duties that the PSMA involves—one of whom will typically be the physician's own nurse or MA. If at all possible, especially if you are on electronic medical records, try to secure a documenter for your SMA—and then see an additional patient during each PSMA session to cover the added overhead cost of having a documenter, which will almost certainly prove to be a wise choice.

Be certain to train your reception and scheduling staff regarding inviting and scheduling patients into your SMA—and be sure to also have them sit in on a session or two (one or two at a time) just as soon as possible after your PSMA is launched (particularly if they are of the same sex as the patients that the PSMA is designed for). This will help your reception and scheduling staff to later be able to explain and *sell* the program to patients thereafter. Finally, try to secure an appropriately skilled and trained dedicated scheduler for 2–4 hours per week on an as-needed basis to help you *top off* any unfilled sessions and ensure that PSMA sessions are consistently filled to targeted census levels. If the most appropriate resources do not happen to be available to you—i.e., so that you are unable to construct an *ideal PSMA*—then you might still want to set up the best PSMA that you are able to with the resources at your disposable (as a *good enough PSMA* is often better *than no PSMA* at all).

Physicians Not Fully Delegating to the Various SMA Team Members

Another frequently made mistake when starting a DIGMA or PSMA program is for the physician to not fully delegate as many duties and responsibilities as appropriate and possible to the various members of the SMA team. This is particularly important, as the ability to delegate is not always a physician's strong suit. Remember that one of the overarching principals of DIGMAs and PSMAs is to gain efficiency by delegating all that is possible and appropriate to less costly members of the PSMA team. This means that the physician must fully delegate to the champion and program coordinator in larger systems, as well as to the behaviorist and nursing personnel—who have greatly expanded roles and responsibilities in PSMAs. The physician must also delegate as much as possible to the documenter and the physician's own support staff—especially the scheduling staff, nurses, and receptionists.

However, the one exception here is to not delegate as much as possible to the dedicated scheduler, who is only there to *top off* the census for those sessions that the physician and support staff have failed to adequately fill. The dedicated scheduler is meant to strictly play a *backup* role in the PSMA, so that ideally the dedicated scheduler's efforts would never prove necessary. Because nobody else can be as effective and efficient in getting patients scheduled into the PSMA, the physician will always need to take a little time with all suitable patients seen during office visits to personally invite them in a positive manner to attend their PSMA—preferably through a carefully worded script that is warm, inviting, and effective. A successful strategy that some physicians employ is to try to invite enough patients seen during individual office visits each day to get at least 2 to accept this invitation and schedule their next physical exam appointment into the PSMA—or, in the case of a DIGMA, to get 3 patients each day to accept the invite and schedule their next return visit into the DIGMA. For full-time physicians working 5 days a week, this translates into ten patients scheduling future PSMA appointments every week, and/or 15 scheduling DIGMA visits on a weekly basis. Over time, this strategy will virtually guarantee the long-term success of their SMA program.

The Physician Not Staying Focused and Succinct Throughout the Entire PSMA Session

Another common beginners' mistake is for the physician not to stay focused and succinct throughout the entire

DIGMA or PSMA session. There are temptations and alluring potential inefficiencies at every turn, and it is very easy for the physician to lose focus, get into tangential discussions, or enter into unnecessarily lengthy explanations that are interesting but of minimal benefit to patients. Try not to leave the group room once the session has commenced—either to attend to clinic matters or to unnecessarily step out with patients individually in the mistaken belief that you are somehow providing them with better and more personalized care. If you do so, what you will likely be doing is entering into private and inefficient, one-on-one discussions that all of the other patients in the group will no longer be able to hear or benefit from.

Nonetheless, you will undoubtedly need to leave the PSMA setting on rare occasion, perhaps to deal with a clinic emergency or to handle a private matter with a patient. However, try to minimize this by only stepping out of the group room when it is truly necessary. Furthermore, when it is necessary for you to step out of the group room with a patient, try to make it towards the end of the interactive group segment (as this will be less disruptive to the flow of the group) and as brief as possible. Similarly, try to defer as much discussion as possible from the PSMA's inefficient exam room setting to the subsequent interactive group segment where all can listen and learn—and try to avoid unnecessary talk while actually conducting the private exams in order to conduct these exams thoroughly but efficiently. It is also a common mistake to take too much time with the first patient or two that you work with in the PSMA's private exam and interactive group settings. Therefore, along with your behaviorist, take every reasonable precaution to not make this common mistake—i.e., by limiting the amount of time spent on the first two patients accordingly. Then, once you have established an appropriate pace in the PSMA (one that will allow you to finish on time with all documentation completed), try to maintain that pace throughout both the private exam and interactive group segments of the session.

Failing to Encourage Any Group Interaction, or Fostering Too Much to Finish on Time

One final beginner's mistake that is frequently made is that, while it is very important to foster some group interaction during the interactive group segment of the PSMA, it is equally important to not foster too much interaction—as that will slow you down too much, and will make it impossible to finish on time. I usually recommend that the physician sit on a stationary chair, just like everyone else in the group room, rather than sitting on a stool or chair with wheels—which creates a temptation for the physician to fall into the old individual office visit habit of wheeling over to the patient and talking quietly and privately to that patient. Unfortunately, by doing so, the physician's back will be turned to the rest of the group and others will not be able to hear what is being said—thus preventing any meaningful group learning or interaction to occur. If the group cannot hear and learn from what the physician is saying, patients will quickly turn to others sitting next to them and begin distracting side conversations—which can cause the physician and behaviorist to rapidly lose control of the group.

Another tip would be for the physician to stay focused upon the patient that the physician is working with in the interactive PSMA group segment at that moment, and to keep any group interaction that is fostered focused upon what is helpful to that patient—such as in confronting any noncompliance by that patient with recommended treatment regimens. This also helps to keep the physician on track for running the PSMA like a series of individual office visits with observers. Simultaneously, it limits the amount of group interaction that can occur (which could otherwise quickly become too time-consuming) to that which is most helpful to the patient that the physician happens to be focusing upon at the moment. It is a common beginners' mistake to instead foster a type of group interaction that shifts almost randomly from one patient to another in the group until all focus is lost—thus allowing group interaction to bounce around like a pinball from one patient to another in the group room. It is helpful to remember that, if you have a documenter in the room and are using electronic medical records, the documenter has the chart note of the patient that the physician is working with at that time up on the computer screen—and is systematically working through that patient's chart note from start to finish. The documenter simply cannot keep up with such a rapidly changing focus in the group by quickly switching computer screens from one patient to another—and then quitting each patient's partially completed chart note in midstream—as the group interaction is allowed to jump indiscriminately from one patient to another.

One of the best ways to use a limited amount of group interaction is to use it to obtain help from the group when confronting a noncompliant patient's behavior—especially regarding the long-term consequences that such noncompliance is likely to ultimately have upon the patient. It is often better and more effective to have other patients in the group room, especially those who have already suffered such negative consequences by similarly being noncompliant to the physician's advice, confront the noncompliant patient on his/her behavior. I say this because they will likely be seen by the patient as being more credible due to having already gone through the same experience themselves. Such patients will therefore be much more likely to get through to the patient, and will probably be more successful than the physician in changing the noncompliant patient's behavior.

A Concluding Comment on the PSMA Model

I would like to conclude this chapter on the PSMA model with the following quotation which, I believe, captures the exciting potential of this remarkable—albeit counterintuitive—SMA model. Once they understand this innovative model and its multifarious benefits, some have referred to the PSMA as a "no brainer"—i.e., because of the remarkable efficiency, quality, service, and economic benefits that it can offer. While counterintuitive, this remarkably efficient model can be an exciting addition to any busy, backlogged physician's armamentarium for better managing high-volume patient demand for private physical examinations—and one that typically results in exceptional productivity, improved access, high-quality care, and satisfied patients and physicians.

A 2003 Managed Care article puts it this way: "Noffsinger developed PSMAs in response to access problems specifically for physical examinations in the private sector, in the armed services, and in the VA system. The actual physical exams are done in private and take only a few minutes. As in the other models, its the subsequent group dialogue where patients benefit and physicians gain tremendous efficiencies, seeing up to 3.7 times as many patients as they would otherwise in the same amount of time. PSMAs are segregated by sex and age. A typical group might be men over 50, where PSA tests would be on the agenda, or women over 45, who would be interested in issues such as hormone replacement therapy. 'I started with some apprehension,' says Palo Alto Medical Clinic family physician James Stringer, MD, whose patients are mostly men. He has been doing PSMAs for a year and a half and is starting weekly DIGMAs for follow-up visits. 'I thought you'd have to be an entertainer type person, but you just talk to patients as you do in the exam room. They enjoy it and I look forward to it' " (8).

"Mary Ann Sarda-Maduro, MD, an obstetrician-gynecologist at the Palo Alto Medical Clinic in Fremont, Calif., has been doing PSMAs with her obstetrics patients for two years, as have three of her OB-BYN colleagues. 'I love doing them,' she says. 'I have them on Thursday mornings, and if I have a great SMA, I feel great for the weekend.' These days, anything that elicits this kind of enthusiasm from physicians is worth looking into" (8).

References

1. Noffsinger EB. Physicals shared medical appointments: a revolutionary access solution. *Group Practice Journal* 2002;51(1): 16–18, 20–22, 24–26.
2. Noffsinger EB. Operational challenges to implementing a successful Physicals Shared Medical Appointment program. Part 1: choosing the right type of shared medical appointment. *Group Practice Journal* 2002; 51(2):24–26, 28–30, 32, 34.
3. Noffsinger EB. Operational challenges to implementing a successful Physicals Shared Medical Appointment Program. Part 2: maximizing efficiency. *Group Practice Journal* 2002;51(3):32, 34, 36, 38–40.
4. Noffsinger EB. Operational considerations for a successful Physicals Shared Medical Appointment program. Part 3: hints and guidelines. *Group Practice Journal* 2002;51(4):22, 24–26.
5. Kaidar-Person O, Swartz EW, Lefkowitz M, et al. Shared medical appointments: new concept for high-volume follow-up for bariatric patients. *Surgery for Obesity and Related Diseases* 2006;2(5):509–512.
6. Belfiglio G. Crowd Control: group office visits provide efficiencies, patient support. *Modern Physician* 2001;5(9):34–36.
7. Noffsinger EB. Working Smarter: group visits are proving to be a valuable antidote to harried physicians. Would a 200% increase in productivity make you feel better? *Physicians Practice* 2002;12(3):P22.
8. Carlson B. Shared appointments improve efficiency in the clinic. *Managed Care* 2003;12(5):46–48.

Chapter 6
Physician Buy-In: The Key to Successful SMA Programs

Substantial benefits also accrue to me from the group. I find the group to be a meaningful enhancement to the quality of my professional life, particularly because (a) it gives me the feeling that I am satisfying previously unmet needs of my patients, (b) I get to know my patients better, and (c) sometimes I get to know my patients in ways that would simply never come up one-on-one in the exam room. Furthermore, some office visits and phone calls are avoided through the use of the group. It is gratifying to feel more available to my patients. And the group is a pleasant and gratifying professional diversion—sort of like dessert—I look forward to with great relish.

Dr. Mason from Noffsinger EB, Mason JE Jr., Culberson CG, et al. Physicians evaluate the impact of Drop-In Group Medical Appointments (DIGMAs) on their practices. *Group Practice Journal* 1999; 48(6):22–33.

Physicians and Healthcare Organizations Recognize the Need to Change

Faced with the multiple pressures and harsh economic realities of today's highly competitive healthcare environment, which include rapid change, large practices, less time available per patient, and weakening bottom lines, physicians and healthcare organizations alike are grappling to meet these modern challenges through innovative new approaches to delivering accessible, high-quality, and high-value medical care. In this challenging environment, a rare combination of benefits makes the DIGMA and PSMA models exciting and unique: physicians see considerably more patients in the same amount of time; patients enjoy more time with their doctor and a more relaxed pace of care; access is improved through use of existing resources; greater attention is provided to patient education as well as psychosocial needs; patients and physician alike benefit from a multidisciplinary, team-based approach to care; the help and support of other patients is integrated into each patient's healthcare experience; the professional skills of a behaviorist are provided; patients and physicians are more satisfied; and the bottom line can be strengthened. It is this rare combination of benefits that has enabled DIGMAs and PSMAs to consistently work so well in a wide variety of applications in actual practice.

While the judicious use of individual medical appointments will always play a vital role in the delivery of quality medical care, highly efficient DIGMAs, CHCCs, and Physicals SMAs—as well as other group visit models still to be developed—are expected to play an increasingly important role in the appointment mix offered by physicians in primary care and the various medical subspecialties as we continue to move into the 21st century. These group visit models have broad applicability to integrated healthcare organizations (HMOs, PPOs, IPAs, VHA, DoD, community health, etc.) struggling with issues of quality of care, accessibility, service, adequacy of staffing levels, cost containment, and strengthening the bottom line.

Physician Acceptance Is Critical to Success

Properly run DIGMAs, CHCCs, and Physicals SMAs can offer major economic benefits to the organization as well as numerous benefits to patients. However, equally important to the benefits that well-run group visits can provide to the organization and to patients are the multiple benefits that they can also offer to the physicians who run them for their practices—benefits that physicians must understand if they are to be expected to embrace these relatively new shared medical appointment (SMA)

E.B. Noffsinger, *Running Group Visits in Your Practice*, DOI 10.1007/b106441_6, models. Many physicians will at first be reticent to initiate DIGMAs and PSMAs in their practices for a variety of reasons: they might have various concerns and resistances that have not been adequately addressed; they could be comfortable with the status quo; and they may cling to the mistaken belief that the individual treatment model in which they have been trained and practicing is simply the best form of providing medical care. Clearly, these issues must be thoughtfully addressed with physicians; however, they must also be properly balanced against the many real benefits that DIGMAs, CHCCs, and PSMAs can offer to physicians, patients, and the organization alike.

Physician buy-in hinges on two key factors: (1) all physician questions, concerns, and resistances need to first be promptly and fully addressed; and (2) physicians must clearly understand the multiple benefits that DIGMAs, CHCCs, and PSMAs can offer to them as well as their practices.

Extensive Experience Demonstrates that Physician Acceptance Is Achievable

Although I originally expected patients and healthcare organizations to like DIGMAs, I was not as certain that physicians would embrace them. In my experience to date with over 400 different providers and 20,000 patient visits in the DIGMA and PSMA models, I have found that physicians who choose to run them for their practices do in fact generally like them. This is true in both primary care and the numerous medical subspecialties in which these models have been applied—as well as in the different fee-for-service and capitated medical groups around the country (and most recently, internationally) that have launched such SMA programs. Even physicians initially reluctant or resistant to starting a DIGMA or PSMA, but willing to try one and give it their *best shot*, are often rapidly won over by the concept once their SMA has been implemented—as, almost always, physicians quickly grow to like their SMA once they have participated in it for a few sessions and have grown comfortable with it.

Generally speaking, I have found physician resistance to be greatest for the PSMA and heterogeneous DIGMA models, less for the homogeneous and mixed DIGMA models, and least for CHCCs. In other words, initial physician acceptance appears to hinge upon how intuitively appealing each of these models is, rather than upon the ultimate benefit and utility that each of these models offers to the physician's practice—e.g., to better managing both a busy, backlogged practice and chronic illnesses. In any case, extensive personal experience with

these models demonstrates that physician acceptance is nonetheless achievable with all of these SMA models, so long as all physician concerns are thoroughly addressed and physicians grow to understand how these various SMA models can be of benefit to them and their practice.

Physician Acceptance from Pilot Study to Full-Scale Implementation

The initial goal in starting a SMA program in mid-sized and larger healthcare organizations is typically to interest enough physicians in the concept to be able to start a pilot study. Once the SMA pilot study has been launched, evaluated, and demonstrated to be successful within the organization, the objective then typically immediately shifts to having the champion advance the SMA program toward full-scale implementation as rapidly and effectively as possible throughout the entire organization in order to fully capture its multiple benefits to patients, physicians, and the organization alike on the largest possible scale. Clearly, full-scale implementation requires widespread physician acceptance of these SMA models throughout the entire system—something that the champion and program coordinator can be most helpful in achieving.

Physician Buy-In Occurs at the Grassroots Level

Ultimately, successful large-scale implementation of a SMA program in an integrated healthcare delivery system will only be achieved through physicians hearing positive reports from their colleagues who are already running DIGMAs, CHCCs, and PSMAs for their practices with benefit. When coupled with the ongoing efforts of the champion and program coordinator in advancing the SMA program throughout the system, such positive reports encourage other physicians to try DIGMAs, CHCCs, and PSMAs for their own practices as well. Through this word-of-mouth process between peers, a critical mass of positive reports from colleagues can eventually begin to circulate within the organization—so that more and more physicians eventually become willing to give them a try. However, this will only happen if every effort is made to ensure that these initial DIGMAs and PSMAs are successful—which means that they must be carefully designed, appropriately resourced, well promoted, and properly run.

DIGMAs and PSMAs Provide Healthcare Organizations with a Golden Opportunity

In this manner, DIGMAs and PSMAs can provide healthcare organizations with a golden opportunity to initiate system reform toward leveraging existing resources, increasing productivity, containing costs, and enhancing service and quality from the ground up, instead of having to be dictated top-down to physicians by administrators (an approach that can be rife with problems). However, it is important to note that even when physician concerns and resistances are addressed, and when provider acceptance is ultimately achieved, successful DIGMAs, CHCCs, and PSMAs do not just happen. They require considerable effort and work for such innovative and dramatically different programs to succeed, particularly on the parts of the champion and program coordinator (in larger systems). Furthermore, because they represent such a major paradigm shift, there are steep learning curves for all involved. Successful DIGMAs, CHCCs, and PSMAs require administrative support, the best possible champion and program coordinator, detailed planning, appropriate facilities, a skilled and trained multidisciplinary team, effective promotion, buy-in from physician and support staff, constant attention to maintaining targeted census levels, and an ongoing effort to optimize and max-pack each and every SMA session—including the quantity and quality of medical care delivered.

Physicians Have Many Initial Concerns About the Group Model

Physicians have not been trained in these group visit models. For the most part, physicians have also not been trained in how to manage groups or how to deliver medical care in a group setting. As a result, they often have many initial concerns, worries, and anxieties about starting DIGMAs, CHCCs, and Physicals SMAs in their practices. Physicians worry and ask many questions. Will it work for me? Will it fit my personality and practice? What if somebody asks a question that I can't answer? Will I eventually become comfortable with this new modality of delivering care? What if I lose control of the group? How can I possibly get all of the chart notes done? Is this really better patient care, or is it just another way to squeeze more work out of already beleaguered physicians? Is this just another crazy idea that won't stand the test of time?

Interestingly, I have found that providers initially worry about innumerable relatively trivial, anxiety-

based concerns such as those just mentioned, concerns that will prove to be of little long-term significance once these physicians gain some experience and comfort in actually running their DIGMA, CHCC, or PSMA. However, this is certainly not to say that such worries as these could not keep physicians from ever trying one in the first place because this is, unfortunately, all too commonly the case—which, together with inadequate SMA designs and insufficient resources, has much to do with why more healthcare organizations are not already doing group visits on a much larger scale. Yet these same providers seldom, if ever; worry about the single most important issue (and the key to a successful DIGMA, CHCC, or PSMA program): consistently maintaining targeted census levels during all sessions. Nobody seems to initially ask the most critical question of all: "Am I design my DIGMA, CHCC, or PSMA in such a way that I can be certain of consistently filling all sessions over time?"

Most Physician Concerns Are Anxiety Rather than Reality Based

Many of these physician concerns are anxiety based and come from considering something as dramatically different from traditional office visits and unfamiliar as group visits are. Generally speaking, these are irrational fears that will quickly dissipate once the DIGMA or PSMA has been started—and once experience and comfort has been gained with these new paradigms of care delivery. Many of these concerns—such as possibly losing control of the group, being overwhelmed by nursing responsibilities, or being unable to complete documentation during the sessions—are solved by appropriately delegating as many duties as possible and appropriate to the skilled behaviorist, nurse/MA(s), and documenter that are provided in these SMA models. Additional concerns (such as worries about being able to finish on time with all documentation completed when so many patients are being seen) can be gradually overcome by debriefing with the team after sessions for the first couple of months—focusing upon how to make future sessions even better and more efficient.

Group Visits Do Have Their Own Requirements for Success

Some physicians nonetheless remain skeptical and unconvinced, despite the accumulating body of evidence regarding the remarkable potential that DIGMAs, CHCCs, and

PSMAs can hold for them, their patients, and the organization. However, it is anticipated that this evidence should continue to accumulate over time and gradually become evermore helpful in persuading such skeptical physicians to eventually try one for their practices (see Chapter 9). However, when such skeptical physicians ultimately do start a DIGMA, CHCC, or PSMA for their practice, they should not expect a cakewalk, although, on the other hand, running a group visit program is certainly not rocket science. This is because DIGMAs, CHCCs, and PSMAs introduce much change and do require considerable effort on the physician's part (especially with respect to personally inviting all appropriate patients) if they are to be fully successful—plus, they have their own specific design, training, personnel, facilities, budgetary, and promotional requirements.

Addressing the Most Common Physician Concerns and Resistances to SMAs

Some physician concerns are legitimate challenges that must be grappled with; however, most are the results of unrealistic fears—either misunderstandings that arise from trying something as new and different as DIGMAs, CHCCs, and PSMAs are from traditional office visits, or anxieties about delivering medical care in a large group setting. Furthermore, these anxieties and worries are not helped by the fact that shared medical appointments tend to be so counter-intuitive and require so much change. Additionally, other concerns are realistic, but solvable. However, it will be seen that there are also a couple of physician concerns that involve forces greater themselves (such as a substantially increased patient panel size being their reward for running a successful group visit in their practice) over which they have little or no control—concerns that administration must be very careful about addressing appropriately lest they undercut the success of their SMA program. Because they are so dramatically different from the traditional individual office visits in which physicians have been trained and practicing, DIGMAs, CHCCs, and PSMAs are often initially difficult for physicians to envision as being workable for their personalities and practices.

"I'm Too Busy to Start One at This Time"

I start with this concern because it is, by far, the most common worry voiced by those very busy, backlogged physicians who would most benefit from a well designed and run DIGMA or PSMA program. Physicians often report that they are simply too busy, too backlogged, too overworked, or already experiencing too much change to start a SMA for their practices at this time. They say that they have neither the necessary time nor the extra energy required to invest in starting something so new, unfamiliar, and different for their practice. They are already too pressured dealing with current heavy workload demands and hectic day-to-day professional responsibilities to consider adding something burdensome and new to their schedule at this time. Many physicians report that they have already been working for sometime to: cut back; reduce professional demands upon them; simplify their lives; not feel so overloaded; and enjoy more personal and family time. So why, they ask, should they add a SMA to their practice and complicate their lives further at a time like this?

Although it might be difficult to view from this perspective—especially in the light of ever-increasing change and practice demands—the answer to this question is that such a concern provides exactly the right reason for starting a DIGMA, CHCC, or PSMA at this time. For example, coping with excessive workloads, trying to better manage a large and backlogged practice, and attempting to increase efficiency and professional satisfaction are precisely what DIGMAs and PSMAs have been specifically designed to accomplish, i.e., along with increasing capacity, reducing demand, and matching supply and demand.

Clearly, the solution to busy practices, overwhelming workloads, and inexorable change requires a long-term perspective and strategy. It is understandable that physicians who are already overburdened by the extent of their current workload would find themselves too busy to step back for a moment and take a longer view toward more effective practice management.

In the more than 400 primary and specialty care DIGMAs and PSMAs that I have personally assisted in designing and implementing with different healthcare providers to date (i.e., in medical groups nationally and internationally), my experience has been that virtually all of the pilot physicians involved were already extremely busy and having some degree of this type of angst and concern. All were tempted to say: "I'm too busy to start a DIGMA or PSMA for my practice at this time." In fact, many initially did say this, but later recanted and, with my encouragement as champion, did start a SMA in the hopes of creating a long-term solution to their current excessive workload demands and access problems.

Once their SMAs were launched, these physicians typically rapidly became comfortable with their new programs. They found their DIGMA or PSMA to be interesting and helpful, and gradually learned how to use their

SMA program to best advantage. In the end, they eventually grew to like their SMAs and the many benefits they provided. After successfully running their SMAs for a while, these physicians simply did not want to go back to their pre-SMA days of: being unable to effectively manage their large and busy practices; facing access problems and numerous patient complaints regarding poor access; enduring all-too-many *work-ins* and *double bookings*; coping with high patient telephone call volume; and getting exhausted each day on the fast-paced treadmill of delivering medical care through inefficient individual office visits alone. In addition, they found that their DIGMAs and PSMAs introduced some enjoyment and fun into their otherwise hectic and draining workweeks—plus, they often left SMA sessions feeling energized rather than depleted (Fig. 6.1).

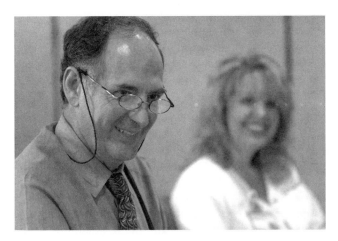

Fig. 6.1 SMAs are enjoyable to all in attendance, including the physician and behaviorist—which results in physician professional satisfaction being consistently high (courtesy of Dr. Patricio Aycinena, Diabetes DIGMA, Cleveland Clinic, Cleveland, OH)

"What if I Don't Know the Answer or Say Something Stupid in Front of 15 Patients At Once?"

This is one of those common anxieties that physicians often privately worry about prior to starting a DIGMA or PSMA for their practice, but one that quickly dissipates once the program actually starts and the physician has the opportunity to observe that this potential catastrophe seldom, if ever, occurs. Physicians must keep in mind that their patients have selected them to be their doctor for a variety of personal and professional reasons. All that their patients want is for the same doctor that they have grown to know and trust during individual office visits to show up for the SMA.

Physicians only need to be themselves in the SMA. They do not need to put on airs or suddenly become a genius, a scholar, a humorist, an entertainer, or anything different from what they normally are, just because they find themselves in a group setting. Physicians quickly come to realize that their patients are not out to get them in the SMA, nor are they likely to *jump* on them for making a mistake. Experience has shown that physicians are quite uniformly treated by their patients with kindness and respect in their DIGMAs and PSMAs—as patients appreciate having improved access, more time with their doctor, greater patient education, the professional skills of the behaviorist, an additional healthcare choice, and the opportunity to learn from (and be emotionally supported by) other patients in attendance.

Even if physicians were to say something they felt was foolish or incorrect in front of 15 of their patients at once, all that would need to happen is for them to say something like: "Oops, that wasn't what I meant to say. Let me try to answer that again." The patients would then likely briefly laugh with the physician, and the situation would quickly be corrected, with no harm done. If anything, you will appear to be all the more human to your patients. In fact, when this does happen, the patients often express that they now feel even closer to the physician than before, since their doctor now seems more human and approachable to them.

The same is true if you do not know the answer to a question. Simply acknowledge this, but add that you will try to find out the answer by the time the patient comes in for his/her next medical visit, unless, of course, it happens to be one of those important medical questions that nobody yet knows the answer to (in which case, just let the patient know that this is the case). Keep in mind that patients tend to be quite reasonable and supportive of their physicians in the group setting—so try to find some reassurance in this fact.

Nonetheless, the very fact that this fear happens to be unrealistically exaggerated in the physician's mind (in that it is extremely unlikely to actually occur in practice with anything close to a catastrophic consequence) certainly does not mean that it has not kept many physicians from ever trying a SMA for their practice in the first place. This is simply one of those many anxiety-based worries that physicians often have when initially considering a DIGMA or PSMA for their practice. I would encourage providers having such fears to simply trust me and put them aside for now, and try to proceed with starting a DIGMA, CHCC, or PSMA for their practice anyway—i.e., if that otherwise seems to be a wise choice for them. In other words: Just do it! You can always *fine-tune* the program later, and make adjustments as you go.

A contrary problem is the physician who has a false sense of security—i.e., the physician who thinks he/she knows more about running a DIGMA or PSMA than they in fact do, often because they have been associated with some type of group or class in the past. However, what is required for a successful DIGMA is often very different from that which is required for success in other types of group programs and classes. Worse yet, this false sense of confidence on the physician's part can lead to poorly designed, inadequately supported, hastily thrown together, and improperly run DIGMA and PSMA programs—as well as to many unnecessary beginners' mistakes. This could, in turn, frustrate the physician and ultimately foster the incorrect conclusion that SMAs will not work in their practice—when in fact they could, if only they had been properly designed, supported, and run.

"It Won't Work for My Personality and Practice"

Physicians sometimes state that, while DIGMAs and PSMAs might have worked well for others, their own personalities and practices are quite different for a variety of reasons, so that these SMAs would not work for them. For example, an internist or family practitioner might comment that while they can see how a DIGMA would work for the relatively homogeneous patient population of a specialist (such as a rheumatologist, cardiologist, nephrologist, neurologist, oncologist, obstetrician, or allergist), it would not work for them. Not uncommonly, primary care physicians will state that their patients are simply too heterogeneous for DIGMAs or PSMAs to work for them—adding that their patients often come in for one thing, but then also want a long laundry list of additional medical issues addressed.

One possible solution to the concern of heterogeneity could lie in selecting a mixed or homogeneous DIGMA or PSMA model rather than a heterogeneous one—so as to partition the physician's diverse practice into more homogeneous and compatible groupings of patients. For example, the mixed DIGMA model in primary care could be custom designed to the specific needs of the primary care physician's practice by focus upon: cardiopulmonary patients during the first week of the month; diabetes and obesity the second week; GI patients the third week (GERD, inflammatory bowel disease, irritable bowel, ulcers, etc.); and women's health issues on the fourth week. Other choices could include having chronic pain (headache, arthritis, fibromyalgia, musculoskeletal neck and back pain, etc.) on one of the weeks, and multi-morbid geriatric patients (or patients who are depressed, anxious, or having stress-related problems) on another week of the month. However, whenever you consider a mixed or homogeneous DIGMA for your practice, be certain to first ask yourself whether the patient groupings that you are designing the program around are sufficiently broad—and involve a large enough number of patients—to ensure that you will be consistently be able to fill all of your future DIGMA sessions.

Interestingly, extensive experience with primary care DIGMAs demonstrates that—even if the mixed or homogeneous model is initially used—it is not uncommon for the program to gradually evolve into a completely heterogeneous DIGMA over time. This is one of those observations about SMAs that is not intuitively obvious. But when one thinks about it, it does make sense. I say this because when patients come in for one reason that qualifies them for the session, but then bring up other unrelated issues on their *laundry list*, the physician will likely just deal with the entire list of medical issues brought up during the SMA. This not only keeps patients from needing to come back for these other issues (which would needlessly tie up an additional appointment), but also results in the mixed or homogeneous DIGMA gradually becoming more heterogeneous over time.

Unexpectedly, the heterogeneous DIGMA subtype is often the easiest to set up and run from an operational perspective—plus, it is typically the best subtype of the DIGMA model for better managing a large and back-logged practice. Because the follow-up visits of virtually all established patients qualify for inclusion, schedulers are more likely to schedule patients into a heterogeneous DIGMA—as they do not fear being reprimanded for putting the wrong patient into a session. Because of its operational advantages (plus the fact that it is easier to keep heterogeneous DIGMA sessions full, as the physician's entire practice qualifies to attend any given session), it is probably the most common DIGMA subtype used in primary care—despite being so counterintuitive. On the other hand, the homogeneous subtype is often the most common subtype used in chronic illness population management programs—i.e., where enough patients with a particular diagnosis are available to ensure that all homogeneous sessions can consistently be kept full. However, this would be much more difficult to accomplish if the homogeneous DIGMA was instead designed around the much smaller number of such patients that would be in an individual provider's practice.

Few heterogeneous DIGMAs have been more wide ranging and diverse than those that I experienced in neurology, where patients experiencing migraine and cluster headaches, younger patients with multiple sclerosis and seizure disorders, and older patients with stroke, dementia, and Parkinson's disease were all seen together during every sessions. Even here, this heterogeneous mix of patients worked out well. Patients were not only highly satisfied with these DIGMA visits but also found them to be very interesting and informative as well. Patients left the session realizing not only that they were not alone in dealing with a serious health problem but also that there were many others whom they felt were worse off.

Although the physician must have the necessary motivation to try a DIGMA or PSMA, experience has shown that physician personality otherwise appears to be a largely irrelevant factor to success. DIGMAs and PSMAs have worked for introverted, reserved physicians who feel painfully awkward and uncomfortable in groups—as well as for outgoing, gregarious physicians with exceptional interpersonal skills and no reservations whatsoever about delivering medical care in a group setting. DIGMAs and PSMAs have also worked with physicians who were initially highly resistant and skeptical to the concept, but were nonetheless willing to give a SMA a try despite their initial reluctance. They have also worked with providers who were initially so frightened by their SMA group experience that they actually broke out in full body hives, shook with nervous tremors, or spoke with a voice that kept cracking during their initial SMA sessions.

However, it must nonetheless be pointed out that DIGMAs are not for all physicians—especially physicians who are not willing to invest the necessary time and energy into making their SMA a success. This is particularly true for physicians who are not willing to personally invite—on an ongoing basis—all appropriate patients (i.e., through a carefully scripted and positively worded invitation) seen during regular office visits to have their next visit be in a DIGMA or PSMA. Nor are they likely to be as helpful to physicians with small practices, many unfilled appointment slots, and no access problems because of the difficulty that such physicians might have in filling their SMA sessions. Other than these few exceptions, the factor of physician personality appears to be largely irrelevant—an observation that initially came as a big surprise to me (as I felt in the beginning that DIGMAs would work best for physicians perceived either a technically brilliant or outwardly gregarious and entertaining), and which represents just one more factor about group visits that is highly counterintuitive.

"It Might Work for Others, but My Patients Are Different and Won't Want a Group"

I have heard this physician concern time and time again, in a variety of contexts, a few of which are mentioned here:

- "It won't work for my patients because they are highly educated managers and CEOs who are of too high a socioeconomic level to want a group."
- "It won't work for me because my patients are primarily the urban poor and of low socioeconomic levels."
- "It won't work for me because my practice is a rural one, and patients often know one another."
- It might work in America, but it won't work in our country because our patients are different."
- "It won't work for my military practice because of issues around rank and work proximity."
- "It won't work for my practice because I work in a public hospital with many homeless, poor, emotionally disturbed, and disenfranchised patients."
- "It won't work for me because I work in a prestigious academic setting, and my patients won't tolerate a group visit.
- "It won't work for my patients because I often work in nursing homes or domiciliaries."
- "It won't work for me because my patients are too complicated."
- "It won't work for my patients because they are too difficult, demanding, psychologically needy and require a lot of professional handholding."
- "It won't work for me because my patients are of tough Norwegian farming stock and tend to keep their problems to themselves rather than burdening family and friends."
- "I can see where it will work for the chronically ill, but it won't work for my patients because most of them have an acute health problem rather than a chronic one."
- "It might work for the elderly, but not for my practice because I primarily see younger patients who are still working."
- "It won't work for me because my patients won't be willing to stay for 1 ½ hours."
- "It won't work for me because my patients are used to having my undivided attention."

However, in all such cases where these suppositions have actually been put to the test, such initial concerns have ultimately proven to be unfounded—as DIGMAs and PSMAs have been shown to be robust SMA models that can work well in all of these situations. However, such concerns might translate into extra effort needing to be taken to ensure confidentiality or that the SMA is appropriately custom designed to a particular physician's practice. Whenever I heard such concerns, but was nonetheless able to persuade the physician to try a DIGMA or PSMA, we were able to custom design the program to the physician's particular needs, concerns, and patient panel—and the SMA was in fact almost always shown to work successfully in actual practice. It turns out that people are people, and they like the many patient benefits that well-run SMAs can offer—plus they like to talk about their health problems with others who can truly understand.

Although there will always be patients who prefer the individual office visits to which they have become accustomed, the point here is that when the SMA program is properly run and promoted to patients, there can still be a large enough number of patients willing to attend the group visit program to make it a success. In fact, I am still looking for applications where DIGMAs and PSMAs simply will not work—so, if you find any, please let me know at "TheDIGMAmodel@aol.com". Once we do know the limits of these robust SMA models, we will be better able to more accurately assess what types of patients and conditions will best be serviced by DIGMAs and PSMAs—and which types would best be seen in individual office visits.

"I'm Already So Busy that There Is No Way I Can See Three Times as Many Patients in a DIGMA or PSMA"

This is a frequently stated concern by physicians who are interested in trying a DIGMA or Physicals SMA in their practice, as it is with these particular SMA models that tripling a physician's productivity is a common goal. However, busy and harried physicians who are already overwhelmed by the demands of a large and busy practice frequently have a difficult time envisioning how they will be able to successfully address the needs of this added patient volume during the allotted 90 minutes of group time. This concern fails to take into consideration the substantial gains in efficiency that the physician can experience by delegating as much as possible and appropriate to the multidisciplinary SMA care delivery team—one that often includes a nurse/MA(s), behaviorist, documenter, and dedicated scheduler. It also fails to take into account the remarkable efficiency gains that can come from the group setting itself, where the physician can avoid repetition by only saying things once (but often going into greater detail) to the benefit of the entire group, and where sessions can be overbooked according to the expected number of no-shows and late-cancel—i.e.,

to avoid this burdensome source of waste and physician downtime.

The unfortunate fact is that, should physicians give in to this anxiety-based concern, they will probably make the common beginners' mistake of designing their SMA to be too small—and thus lose much of the economic and psychodynamic benefit that the program could in fact offer. If physicians start with a small census with the intention of then gradually making their group size larger over time (i.e., as they gain experience and comfort with the SMA), they are likely to find that this strategy will seldom work in actual practice. Instead, they will probably reach a group size with which they are comfortable, and then stop there—which will result in the physician never reaching the true productivity potential of the remarkable DIGMA and PSMA models.

What I recommend is that physician's adopt the opposite strategy. Start out with full groups having a target census that at least triples their actual productivity over individual office visits. The four exceptions to this rule (that I am currently aware of) would be for (1) prenatal visits in obstetrics; (2) well-baby checks and school, camp and sports physicals in pediatrics; (3) full body skin exams in dermatology; and (4) extremely productive primary care providers having only 10-minute office visits. Because of the very high initial productivity levels of these providers during traditional office visits, the DIGMA and PSMA models are frequently only able to double the productivity of such providers as these. This strategy of starting with full-sized groups from the outset will likely result in the physician soon learning to adapt to this higher census level, and soon becoming accustomed to running SMAs with these larger group sizes. Keep in mind that, with experience, some physicians have been able to successfully run DIGMAs with census levels considerably larger than the maximum of 16 patients that I typically recommend as an upper limit to DIGMA group size. When using this approach, accept the fact that you will likely finish late—plus possibly not have all of your chart notes completed—during your initial DIGMA and PSMA sessions. However, this is a temporary problem that you will quickly learn to overcome as experience and comfort is gained with these larger DIGMA and PSMA group sizes.

While finishing late without all documentation completed will likely happen at first (but not always, as some physicians are very efficient time managers from the very beginning), my recommendation for addressing this problem is to simply debrief with your behaviorist, nurse/MA(s), and documenter for 15–20 minutes after sessions for the first couple of months—focusing upon how to make future sessions even better and more efficient. By doing this, and then carrying the suggestions made forward into your next group sessions, you will likely soon become accustomed to this higher workload volume during your DIGMA or PSMA—and will gradually learn to pace the group so as to finish on time and with all charting done. By doing so, you will be able to achieve the optimal group size for your SMA from both psychodynamic and economic perspectives, and thereby derive its full benefit. Because of the increased efficiencies of the DIGMA and PSMA settings, this often translates into being able to see two, three, or more times as many patients (with three times being most common) in your SMA than you would be able to see individually during the same amount of time spent seeing patients individually in the clinic.

"I'm Not Comfortable Delivering Medical Care in a Group Setting"

Physicians differ as to how much medical care they are comfortable delivering (or are willing to provide) in the group setting, and often have strong feelings about this, which must be respected. Additionally, physicians sometimes worry about whether the group will demand more medical care than they can realistically provide. On the other hand, the delivery of medical care is the paramount feature of SMAs—which is why they are not support groups, health education classes, psychotherapy groups, or behavioral medicine programs. Over time, physicians generally appear to gradually gain comfort in delivering more and more medical care in the group setting—i.e., as they gain experience with their DIGMAs and PSMAs.

A common variant of this concern is that there will not be enough time during the SMA session for delivering quality medical care to all of the patients who are present—and to meeting all of their diverse medical needs. It can be argued that one of the major reasons that patients bring a long *laundry list* of medical issues to their appointments is, at least in part, a result of the inaccessibility and rushed nature of today's individual office visits. Because DIGMAs and PSMAs help to solve such accessibility and time problems, it could also be argued that such SMA programs can help these *laundry lists* of issues to be gradually worked through, so that single issue, focused visits ultimately become more achievable over time. This issue of enough time being available to deliver quality care to all attendees is addressed by requiring that the SMA census not be too large—i.e., that attendance remain within the recommended range for each SMA model.

Experience demonstrates that 10–16 patients plus 3–6 support persons is an ideal group size for most 90-minute DIGMAs in primary and specialty care. It is for this reason (plus the fact that physicians often find the pace of still larger groups to be exhausting) that I do not generally recommend groups larger than 16 patients in attendance for a 90-minute DIGMA. Nonetheless, DIGMA groups with as many as 22 or more patients have been successfully run in actual practice by physicians having years of experience in running DIGMAs in their practice—and with high levels of patient satisfaction. In fact, in one such group that was particularly large, there was even a spontaneous standing ovation by patients for the physician at the end of the session.

Ultimately, the amount of medical care delivered in the group setting will depend not only on the physician's goals in running the SMA for his/her practice but also on the physician's comfort level, practice style, and patient panel—and on the physician's level of experience in running the DIGMA or PSMA. Many physicians, especially those with busy practices and large backlogs, will want to deliver as much medical care as possible during their DIGMAs, so that as many appropriate patients as possible can attend in lieu of individual office visits in order to get their medical needs comprehensively addressed. On the other hand, there are certain physicians who have large numbers of patients with extensive informational and psychosocial needs. These physicians might therefore choose to have slightly smaller groups and to deliver some direct medical care in their DIGMAs—i.e., so as to focus upon meeting the extensive informational and psychosocial needs that these patients are experiencing. In either case, I have repeatedly observed that—as physicians become more experienced and comfortable with their SMAs—the amount of medical care they actually deliver during their DIGMAs and PSMAs typically tends to increase over time.

Although, at least in the case of DIGMAs almost all medical care is provided in the group setting, certain types of care are nonetheless provided by the physician in the privacy of the nearby exam room, typically toward the end of the session—e.g., brief private exams that require disrobing, brief discussions of a truly private nature, and some simple procedures (e.g., ear wax cleaning, liquid nitrogen freezes, trigger point injections, and brief hearing tests).

In addition, brief behavioral health evaluations, interventions, and referrals can also occur in the DIGMA setting. For example, information can be provided—with the assistance of the behaviorist—in the group setting (where all present can listen and learn) about: disease prevention and self-management; developing healthy eating and exercise habits; addressing anxiety, depression, and substance abuse; adopting healthy lifestyles and good sleeping habits; avoiding high-risk behaviors; available internal and external resources and treatment programs;

stress management techniques; and the importance of compliance and various self-help techniques.

"This Sounds Like More Managed Care Cost-Cutting, Not Increased Quality of Care"

When they first hear about DIGMAs and PSMAs, physicians sometimes express concern as to whether quality of care will really be increased or whether SMAs represent just another cost-cutting measure by managed care organizations in a dangerous trend toward justifying the overworking and understaffing of physicians. It is true that DIGMAs and PSMAs can leverage existing resources to dramatically increase physician productivity and efficiency—and thereby help to contain healthcare costs. However, this is a serendipitous concomitant of these group visit models—because the reason that I originally developed the DIGMA and PSMA models was to enhance the quality of care and healing experience that patients receive.

Although SMAs could be used in capitated settings to increase practice sizes, an issue which will be addressed shortly (see "Why should I run a SMA if my reward will just be a 200 patient increase in my panel size?"), my experience has been that well-run DIGMAs and PSMAs benefit physicians in a variety of ways (a topic discussed in detail during the second half of this chapter) and accomplish this while simultaneously enhancing service and quality of care to patients. SMAs provide medical care with a warm, personal touch, and allow physicians to interact with their patients in ways that short, rushed individual visits simply do not permit. In fact, some physicians have even commented that—through their DIGMA or PSMA—they are finally able to deliver to their patients the quality medical care that they originally envisioned being able to provide when they were in medical school.

DIGMAs offer a wide variety of quality of care benefits to patients. Patients are afforded *drop-in convenience* wherein they can spend 60, 90, 120, or more minutes (most typically 90 minutes) with their own doctor any week that they have a medical need and want to attend. Patients are amazed and appreciative about having this amount of time with their doctor—and this degree of prompt, barrier-free access to care. In addition to the increased patient education and broad range of medical services that DIGMAs and PSMAs offer, they also provide the additional benefits of: (1) the behaviorist (who can help the physician to diagnose depression, anxiety, substance abuse, and other psychiatric conditions that so often go under-diagnosed and under-treated in the primary care

setting); (2) an expanded nursing function; (3) a documenter (which enables to physician to look at the patient and more closely focus upon what the patient is saying); and (4) a supportive group of other patients from the physician's own practice who share similar issues, offer encouragement, give helpful advice, and can really understand.

Because DIGMAs can improve access to the physician's practice, patients requiring periodic monitoring and surveillance are able to be followed as closely as the physician deems appropriate—i.e., rather than being limited to the few individual appointments that might be available in the clinic, which might also be weeks or months away. For example, if the patient is started on a new medication or treatment regimen and the physician would like to see how the patient is doing the following week, then this is always possible with a weekly DIGMA—because all it means is that one more patient will be seen in the next week's group session. In other words, the patient will not have to wait for the next available individual appointment opening in the physician's schedule—which could be weeks or even months away.

Another quality of care benefit is that other patients in the DIGMA or PSMA session will often ask medically important questions that the patient never thought to ask, but would like to know the answer to. Similarly, other patients might describe significant medical symptoms they are having that the patient is also experiencing, but has neither recognized as medically important nor reported to the physician. This is of particular benefit with certain types of symptoms which patients are known to frequently deny, minimize, or underreport, such as cardiovascular symptoms. In addition, as the physician individually addresses each patient's medical concerns and answers their questions throughout the group session, everyone present is able to listen, learn, interact, and benefit. Patients report that they often find this information to be both interesting and helpful to themselves as well. Patients have described this experience as like being in a mini-medical school class taught by their very own doctor—and as being akin to *Dr. Welby care*.

DIGMAs provide patients with effective mind–body medical treatment in a relaxed setting—along with the information, encouragement, and support that they and their families need for better coping with and managing their health problems—and for living life as fully as possible, despite illness. The message is, "You might have an illness, but it doesn't have to have you." Others in the group might have the same condition as the patient, which can create patient bonding and provide a unique opportunity for the patient to ask questions and discuss important issues with someone else who is similarly afflicted. Others may have already undergone the treatment or procedure that is being recommended by the physician, but which the patient may be resisting (e.g., taking insulin, starting radiation or chemotherapy, beginning dialysis, undergoing a prostatectomy or mastectomy, or having a potentially disfiguring surgical procedure). The encouragement and support provided by other members of the group can improve not only the patient's mood but also the likelihood of compliance with the medical treatment regimens that are being recommended by the physician. Plus, SMAs are completely voluntary and provide patients with an additional treatment choice. In short, far from being managed care at its worst, there are many quality benefits that can be provided by a properly run SMA program (many of which we build in from the start, such as updated injections and health maintenance, Patient Packets, and appropriate handouts). This is not surprising given the fact that I originally developed two of today's three major group visit models as a disgruntled patient—i.e., because of what these group visit models could provide for our patients.

"What if I Lose Control of the Group?"

Another common concern that physicians express with DIGMAs and PSMAs is the loss of control they fear that they could experience in these group settings. After all, the reasoning goes, you can control a situation much better one-on-one than when you are facing a large group of your patients as a whole and are not certain about what will happen next.

In addition, there is the perceived loss of control that comes with delegating to others many responsibilities that you have traditionally conducted yourself. Interestingly, even though physicians not infrequently complain about all the workload responsibilities they carry, they often have considerable difficulty in letting go and delegating them to others. In SMAs, many such responsibilities are dispatched to a multidisciplinary care delivery team, although all team members (behaviorist, nursing personnel, and documenter) should have been specifically trained for these SMA responsibilities—and each should bring a helpful and complementary skill set to the group appointment.

When first contemplating a DIGMA or PSMA for their practice, physicians often initially envision a whole host of loss-of-control calamities that could occur to them if they should chose to proceed. They worry about losing control in the group, especially if there is an incessant talker who dominates the group and would not shut up or if there are many quiet patients who simply would not talk. They worry about receiving negative feedback from patients in the group, about the possibility of being confronted by angry patients, and about whether situations might develop that could spiral negatively out of control. These include the possibility of having an excessively demanding and difficult patient attend the SMA, of being embarrassed by patients asking questions in group that they are unable to answer, or of having a patient with such intensive and overwhelming medical and psychosocial needs that the physician does not know where to begin (or whether there will ever be any end to all of the medical needs that must then be addressed).

In part, the solution to many of these anxieties and concerns lies in the careful selection of a compatible, well-trained, and trusted behavioral health professional—such as a health psychologist or medical social worker—who is capable of handling many of the group dynamic and psychosocial issues that the physician might not be comfortable dealing with. The behaviorist should ideally possess a strong working knowledge of the DIGMA, CHCC, and PSMA models—plus be experienced in running large groups, working closely with physicians, and dealing with the emotional and psychosocial needs of medical patients. DIGMAs and PSMAs provide the physician with real and meaningful help from the behaviorist, nursing personnel, documenter, and dedicated scheduler, who assist the physician in running the group and in pacing the session to finish on time.

Because the physician and behaviorist function as a coordinated team, the behaviorist can take primary responsibility for handling the group dynamics and addressing behavioral health and psychosocial issues—which the physician may not be as skilled and comfortable in dealing with. The behaviorist can also run the group alone (focusing upon behavioral health and psychosocial issues) when the physician arrives late, provides a brief private discussion or exam, documents a chart note, or temporarily steps out of the group room to address an urgent clinic matter.

Dealing effectively with the emotional and psychosocial issues of difficult, angry, demanding, information-seeking, psychosocially needy, and high-utilizing patients is one of the great strengths of the DIGMA and PSMA models—and one upon which physicians actually running them frequently comment very favorably. Unlike individual office visits, where the physician frequently has little time and must deal with both medical and psychosocial issues alone, DIGMAs and PSMAs can actually provide more control by offering greater time plus the help of both the behaviorist and the group itself. Furthermore, other patients almost invariably support the physician's recommendations and often provide additional information that is helpful to the challenging patient. I have never found patients to be out to somehow get or embarrass their physician.

For this reason, the *in-your-face* angry patient, the distrustful patient, the anxious or depressed patient, the patient who is constantly bothering staff or telephoning the physician's office, the information-seeking patient (who refuses to leave until a long list of questions is answered), the lonely widow for whom her doctor's appointment is the high point of her entire week, the worried well, and the inappropriately high-utilizing patient with extensive psychosocial needs are all typically more effectively treated in SMAs than in relatively brief individual office visits. The overall net result of running DIGMAs and PSMAs for one's practice can actually be an *increase* in the amount of control that physicians have in better managing their practices—i.e., rather than the *loss of control* that physicians might initially fear.

"Group Programs Strip Away My Easy Patients, Leaving My Hard Ones for the Rest of the Week"

Physicians expressing this concern are saying that many group programs (such as some health education classes and behavioral medicine programs for hypertension, hyperlipidemia, early stage diabetes, and health and wellness) selectively remove some of the easiest patients that they normally see during their workweek. This can actually result in the physician experiencing an overall net increase in workload, because the patients that they are then left to see individually during the remainder of the week are the ones that are more difficult and time-consuming to deal with, i.e., those with more complex medical and psychosocial needs. The perception here is one of actually having to work harder as a result of establishing DIGMA and PSMA group programs, rather than finding some relief in workload through them.

The DIGMA and PSMA models address this issue because they have great flexibility, multiple parameters, and can be custom designed around the specific needs and requirements of the individual physician. Physicians considering a SMA for their practice must first ask themselves: "Specifically what do I want my DIGMA or Physicals SMA to accomplish for me and my practice?" Physicians who are capitation driven (i.e., who want their SMA designed so as to maximize productivity and efficiency in order to improve access, expeditiously manage their practice, and increase revenues) will opt for one type of SMA design—i.e., one that will maximally leverage their time and optimally increase their efficiency and productivity. On the other hand, physicians most wanting to preserve their easier patients (or patients whom they most enjoy working with) for their individual appointment slots will

instead want to design their SMAs to handle many of their more difficult, problematic, and demanding patients.

Although some physicians might be tempted to *cherry pick* their easy patients for their DIGMA or PSMA, I generally recommend against this. Why see your easy patients during a 1½-hour segment of your workweek, and then leave yourself with your most difficult, problematic and challenging patients for the entire remainder of your week? In other words, why not specifically target your most problematic, difficult, psychosocially needy, challenging, and information-seeking patients for your 90-minute DIGMA—and then leave many of your easier, more interesting, and pleasanter patients to enhance your professional satisfaction during the rest of your workweek? In addition, once you adopt such a strategy, you quickly come to realize that many of these patients that are so difficult and time-consuming to treat when you are seeing them one-on-one (e.g., fibromyalgia, chronic pain, headache, and irritable bowel) are often better and more easily handled in the DIGMA group setting, which is an additional, albeit counterintuitive, benefit of this group visit model.

Or else, why not adopt the strategy of trying to see all appropriate patients possible during your DIGMA—and reserve your individual office visits for those few patients who cannot be appropriately seen in your DIGMA. These can include such patients as those who: do not speak the language in which you are conducting the group; are too demented or hearing impaired to benefit; have highly contagious serious illnesses; refuse to maintain confidentiality; or are experiencing medical emergencies and rapidly evolving medical conditions. They can also include patients with urgent medical conditions, patients needing complex medical procedures, and patients who refuse to attend a group visit.

"I Will Still Need Individual Appointments"

My response to this frequently stated physician concern is that these SMA models were never meant to completely eliminate individual office visits, i.e., that DIGMAs, CHCCs, and Physicals SMAs are not designed to totally replace their individual appointments. Instead, these SMA models were designed to be compatible with individual office visits—and to complement and work together well with the judicious use of individual visits. This is not an *either–or* situation, but rather an additional healthcare choice that is available to patients. DIGMAs, CHCCs, and PSMAs provide physicians with an important tool to use in optimizing their management of time so that patients most appropriately seen in group medical appointments can be efficiently seen in that venue of care, thereby preserving more costly individual office visits for those patients truly needing them (or refusing to participate in a group visit).

In this way, patients and conditions best treated in the highly efficient and cost-effective DIGMA, CHCC, and PSMA settings can be seen in these group milieus, whereas patients best treated through individual office visits can then be seen in that venue of care. In fact, individual office visits should actually be more available to patients needing them as a result of the SMA program—i.e., because so many individual office visits are off-loaded onto the highly accessible DIGMA and PSMA group visits that individual visits should soon also become more available to patients needing or wanting them.

Each care model offers its own advantages. DIGMAs are often best for routine follow-up appointments and monitoring chronic illnesses because they offer the advantages of increased productivity and efficiency, improved access, a more relaxed pace of delivering care, closer follow-up care, and the support provided by the behaviorist and other patients in the group. PSMAs offer similar advantages, but for private physical examinations rather than follow-up visits. CHCCs are best for the follow-up appointments for the same group of 15–20 high-utilizing, multi-morbid geriatric patients. Individual office visits are often best for patients who are experiencing an urgent medical situation, having a serious acute infectious illness, needing a complex procedure, or refusing to attend a group visit. It is important to note that DIGMAs and PSMAs are meant to be voluntary to patients and physicians alike. In all of these SMA models, patients are to be told that they can still have individual office visits as before. However, if they prefer, they are also welcome to return to the DIGMA the next time they have a medical need—in which case, the follow-up visit can immediately be scheduled into the appropriate future DIGMA session.

Therefore, the challenge facing us now is to find that optimal mix of DIGMAs, PSMAs, CHCCs, and individual appointments to maximize benefit and value in the medical care that we are providing to our patients—i.e., while simultaneously providing quality care, excellent service, contained costs, and high levels of both patient and physician professional satisfaction.

"I'm Concerned About Confidentiality"

Physicians frequently express concerns about confidentiality, and whether patients might be unwilling to discuss (or have discussed) personal medical issues in a group setting.

One of the great counterintuitive surprises about SMAs is that patients are quite often unexpectedly open and candid in the group setting. Sometimes patients in the DIGMA will tell the physician that they did not feel comfortable bringing an issue up in their last individual visit, but that they feel safe with these nice people here—and then proceed to talk about topics that can be remarkably personal (erectile dysfunction; incontinence; diarrhea; vaginal discharge; sexual problems; mental health and substance abuse issues, etc.). In general, patients with concerns about confidentiality—as well as those who are unwilling to discuss their medical issues in a group setting—will typically opt not to attend a SMA in the first place.

Although physicians almost always worry about this issue of confidentiality when first contemplating a SMA, experience has shown that this issue has been surprisingly well handled in DIGMAs and PSMAs to date. This is accomplished in a conservative manner by: (1) having all promotional materials and scheduling personnel make clear to patients that this is a group visit and that other patients will also be in attendance; (2) having all patients and support persons sign an appropriate confidentiality release form prior to the start of every DIGMA and PSMA session; (3) having the behaviorist thoroughly address the entire issue of confidentiality in the introduction given at the beginning of each DIGMA and PSMA session; and (4) making private one-on-one time with the physician available to all patients wanting or needing it during every SMA session.

It is worth noting that, although they are typically willing to discuss the most personal of issues in a SMA, there are two things that patients are frequently unwilling to share with others in the group setting—i.e., their weight and age (unless it happens to be a weight management group). For this reason as well as others (e.g., it can be distracting to the group process when the patient and nurse/MA are talking and laughing together while vitals are being taken in a curtained off section of the group room), it is recommended that vital signs, injections, and other nursing duties be performed in a nearby exam room rather than in the group room itself. Also, when weight does need to be discussed (such as in a morbid obesity or weight loss DIGMA), the physician can always refer to Body Mass Index (BMI) and the amount of weight that has actually been lost since the patient joined the SMA rather than the patient's former or current weight—which is a much less sensitive issue for patients to have discussed in the group setting than their actual weight.

Experience demonstrates that, if the program is properly promoted, many patients will voluntarily attend a DIGMA or PSMA. Afterward, it is not uncommon for patients to state that they are willing to return, would recommend it to family and friends, or even that they prefer the group setting to individual office visits. One family practitioner, who had to cancel a DIGMA session at the last minute due to two deliveries she needed to perform, was surprised when one of her patients (who had driven 90 miles in a snowstorm in the middle of winter to attend her DIGMA) refused the physicians' offer to see the patient individually as soon as the deliveries were over. This patient said that he would "...rather be seen in the DIGMA"—which he did by returning the following week, again after another 90 mile drive in a snowstorm. Just as some patients will prefer traditional office visits, others will strongly prefer SMAs.

The entire issue of confidentiality has certainly not proven to be the overwhelming obstacle that physicians, upon first hearing about SMAs, often initially envision. Keep in mind that many successful group-based programs have been successfully running in psychiatry and behavioral medicine departments for decades. In fact, I am not aware of any cases where confidentiality has proven to be a problem with DIGMAs or PSMAs, which is undoubtedly due in large part to the conservative manner in which I recommend that confidentiality be handled.

"I Have Some Ethical Concerns"

Occasionally, a physician reports having an ethical concern about delivering medical care in a group setting. Such concerns certainly can play an important and healthy role in curbing any potential for abuse of group visits, either now or in the future. Although many of these ethical issues can be resolved (or avoided entirely) through careful planning and accrued experience, physicians must at all times stay well within their zone of comfort in the SMA, both medically and ethically. I strongly recommend this in each and every case. We must always remain cognizant that every SMA introduces practical and ethical concerns about quality of care and patient service issues: what should the targeted census level be for the group; what types of, and how much, medical care can be effectively delivered in the group setting; how is the program to be promoted to patients; which of the physician's patients can and cannot reasonably be anticipated to benefit; how will each session be designed and staffed so as to optimally meet both the patients' and physician's needs; etc. However, it has been my experience that physicians' ethical concerns regarding SMAs can be effectively addressed through appropriate sensitivity to such concerns, as well as careful planning and attention to detail.

"This Is 'Meat Market' Care"

The argument here is that SMAs represent managed care at its worst, *treating people like cattle* by *herding them* into a group instead of providing them with personalized, individual care—as the individual office visit has been considered by many to be the gold standard of care. When the idea of implementing a DIGMA or PSMA program for their practice is first presented, many physicians initially harbor some variant of this concern—a concern that is often exacerbated by pre-existing physician resentment over the amount of unwanted change that has already been imposed upon them and their practices from outside forces. Some physicians would like to maintain the status quo; however, they are also faced with many unwanted facts—that reimbursements have been reduced, patient panel sizes have increased, evermore patients need to be seen with less time per patient, and patients are frequently unable to obtain appointments to see them in a timely manner. Furthermore, the latest trend is for reimbursement to be increasingly tied—in any of a variety of ways—to meeting performance measures, to best practices, to demonstrated outcomes, and to patient satisfaction.

Based on extensive personal experience, I can comfortably state that carefully designed, adequately supported, well-promoted, and properly run DIGMAs and PSMAs are anything but *meat market* care. To the contrary, patients have remarkable accessibility, are able to spend considerably more time with their doctor, can attend any week that they have a medical need and want to be seen, have the convenience of max-packed visits, enjoy closer follow-up care, experience greater continuity of care with their own doctor, and report high levels of patient satisfaction. In addition, DIGMAs and PSMAs have the added benefit of the professional skills of a behaviorist to better address many patient behavioral health and psychosocial issues—which are known to drive a large percentage of all medical visits. Furthermore, these SMA models provide the added benefit of other patients with similar conditions who can provide the patient with encouragement, help, and support—which can enhance mood and increase compliance with recommended treatment regimens. In fact, the warm and enjoyable atmosphere of a SMA not uncommonly causes some patients to refer to DIGMAs and PSMAs as "Dr. Welby care."

Every possible effort needs to always be expended (through professional appearing marketing materials, distributing carefully thought out Patient Packets, providing healthy snacks, paying greater attention to patient education and psychosocial issues, etc.) to create the correct impression to patients that the physician, behaviorist, nurses, and support staff have all gone to a great deal of effort to ensure that patients receive an enjoyable and personalized form of high-quality healthcare in the DIGMA or PSMA. Compare this to the situation of the busy, backlogged physician who clings to the traditional individual office visit paradigm of care—where long waits for appointments are commonplace and where physicians are sometimes reluctant to schedule follow-up appointments for fear of further adding to their backlogs and wait-lists. I can only ask "Which of these two situations really results in better care?" Clearly, optimal quality, value, and service will only be achieved in today's highly competitive and fast-paced healthcare environment by providing that ideal blend of group and individual appointments based on patient needs and the individual physician's particular needs, practice style, and patient panel.

"What's In It for Me?"

This concern can easily be addressed by making it clear to physicians what the many provider benefits of properly designed and run SMAs really are—ranging from an opportunity to do something interesting and different to better physician management of busy, backlogged practices. Although the multitude of physician benefits that the various SMA models can provide are discussed in detail in the second half of this chapter, the important point here is that the many direct physician benefits that well-run SMAs can offer must be clearly communicated to all physicians.

"Why Should I Run a SMA If My Reward Will Only Be a 200 Patient Increase in My Panel Size?"

This concern is most frequently expressed by staff physicians in fully (or largely) capitated systems—particularly staff model HMOs. Of all the concerns expressed by physicians when they are initially considering starting a SMA for their practice, this is the most worrisome one in that this is the only physician concern that the DIGMA and PSMA models themselves cannot address and solve. The potential for long-term abuse here is real, as the organization could in theory strip away the entire physician benefit that the DIGMA or PSMA has been designed to provide by correspondingly increasing physicians' panel sizes. The organization could do this by simply increasing the physician's panel size commensurate with the expected efficiency gains

offered by the SMA program—i.e., typically an 8–9% gain in overall physician productivity for the entire week for each 90-minute weekly DIGMA or PSMA that successfully increases a full-time physician's productivity by 300%. Obviously, increasing the physician's panel size by 8–9% would completely absorb and nullify the entire efficiency gain that the DIGMA or PSMA provides the physician with. In effect, doing so would leave the physician with no net professional gain (at least in terms of improved productivity and access, and therefore in better managing a busy, backlogged practice) for having undergone the risk and change in practice style that running a SMA for their practice entails.

But if their potential gain in efficiency is completely offset by a corresponding increase in panel size, then physicians will likely resist DIGMAs and PSMAs. The physician's argument here would be "Why should I start a DIGMA or PSMA for my practice if the net result will only be a substantial increase in my panel size—i.e., one that completely nullifies any potential net gain in productivity and access that these models could otherwise provide for me and my practice?" Therefore, in a fully capitated system, a physician's panel size must be reasonably fixed before a physician will even consider the potential benefits of a group visit for his/her practice. If the reward for increased productivity is simply going to be more work through a larger panel size—and with no commensurate increase in reimbursement (time or dollars)—then the remarkable potential and multiple benefits that properly run DIGMAs and PSMAs can offer are doomed from the outset. Obviously, the situation in fee-for-service systems is quite different, especially in systems where reimbursement is 100% tied to the physician's productivity; however, even here, some physicians might not want such an increase in patient empanelment.

Clearly, this is an issue of fairness and trust, and ultimately involves the managed care organization's leadership objectives and long-term goals regarding access, productivity, and efficiency. Many physicians in managed care settings expect some modest future increase in panel size over time, but they hope that any such increase will be reasonable and manageable. Some feel that they are already being pushed to the outer limits of their ability to deliver adequate and effective care through traditional individual office visits alone. Many recognize the need for a practice management tool that will enable them to "Work smarter, not harder." However, they question how to accomplish this. Still others might recognize the multiple potential benefits that group visits could offer to them and their practices; however, they might choose to not do them—which is a decision that must be respected, as it has always been intended that SMAs be voluntary to patients and physicians alike.

For the DIGMA and Physicals SMA program to succeed, it must provide a *win–win–win* situation for patients, physicians, and healthcare organizations. In addition to the benefits that accrue to the patients and the organization, for DIGMA and PSMAs to be truly successful, physicians too must derive some substantial net benefit from the increased productivity and efficiency provided by their SMA program. From the physician's perspective, this is an issue of fairness and equitability. Therefore, integrated healthcare delivery systems wanting to fully capitalize on the multiple benefits that DIGMAs and PSMAs offer to patients, physicians, and the organization alike should adopt a long-term business plan that builds upon this trust—and provides meaningful benefits for all, including their physicians. Administration would therefore be wise to seek ways to equitably partition the overall gains provided by the SMA program in such a manner that they provide clear net gains to physicians as well as to the organization—which could include incentives based on money and time. By following this cautionary recommendation, managed care organizations could experience an acceptance of DIGMAs and PSMAs by practicing physicians at the *grassroots* level, so that SMAs are gradually and increasingly embraced from the *bottom-up*, instead of having to be dictated by administration *top-down* (which can lead to inefficiency and passive resistance).

The Multiple Benefits that Well-Run SMAs Offer to Physicians

The innovative DIGMA, CHCC, and PSMA models, which can provide efficient, cost-effective delivery of high-quality medical care while solving access problems with existing resources (the latter is for DIGMAs and PSMAs only), provide high-value care with a warm, personal touch. These models have broad applicability and can be especially helpful to health maintenance organizations (HMOs), independent practice associations (IPAs), preferred provider organizations (PPOs), and other profit and not-for-profit capitated, fee-for-service, and managed care organizations—i.e., for medical groups in the private, governmental, and public arenas that are struggling with issues of quality, service, accessibility, staffing levels, cost containment, and adequacy of staffing levels. Although the DIGMA and PSMA models offer clear advantages to managed care organizations (such as leveraging existing resources, reducing costs, improving quality and outcomes, increasing productivity and efficiency, and improving accessibility to care), the key to their long-term success ultimately lies in these SMA models being accepted by the physicians who will be running them in their practices.

However, this buy-in ultimately depends upon physicians clearly understanding the multitude of physician benefits that these SMA models can in fact provide—which is what the last half of this chapter is dedicated to.

Physician Professional Satisfaction with SMAs Is High

Among the more than 400 primary and specialty care providers that I have personally worked with to successfully launch DIGMA and PSMA programs, physician professional satisfaction has always been consistently high. Dr. John Scott has similarly found high levels of physician professional satisfaction with the various CHCCs that he has helped to launch over the years. The fact that these innovative models of healthcare delivery can increase physician professional satisfaction, and can therefore be embraced by physicians, is absolutely critical to the ultimate success of the DIGMA, PSMA, and CHCC models.

Physicians have found that they can relax a little, laugh with the group, interact in a positive manner with their patients, and enjoy themselves more than they otherwise could during a comparatively rushed individual office visit. Physicians often find that running a group visit for their practice can be both a positive experience and a welcome break from their normal, busy routine—and one which provides an *oasis* in their otherwise hectic workweek. One physician put it this way: "This is one of the things that I most look forward to every week." Another stated: "It's really interesting because I learn something new every week." Physicians also report: enjoying the collegial interaction they share with their behaviorist (who assists in meeting the emotional, psychosocial, and informational needs of patients and their families); appreciating the interesting learning experience that the group provides; and enjoying the intriguing opportunity to do something different and interesting—which also adds balance to the physician's busy medical practice and professional life.

Why do providers enjoy these group visit models so much? First of all, DIGMAs, CHCCs, and PSMAs are typically custom designed for the physician's own needs and practice. In addition, physicians benefit directly from well-run SMAs that help them to provide better care, leverage their time, get to know their patients better, and enhance their ability to manage busy, backlogged practices (Table 6.1).

Table 6.1 SMAs offer many benefits to physicians

- Customized to the needs of each physician
- The ability to deliver enhanced care
- A tool for working smarter, not harder
- An opportunity to do something new, interesting, different, and fun
- More time and a more relaxed pace of care
- A regular *oasis* in their workweek in which they are away from normal clinic duties and distractions—and are able to just focus on their patients
- SMAs are enjoyable, as most physicians like the group format
- Dramatically increased physician productivity and efficiency[a]
- Improved access[a]
- A means of better managing large, busy practices[a]
- Physicians enjoy the collegiality of the behaviorist[a] and SMA team
- A tool for better managing chronic illnesses
- Reduced telephone call volume, patient complaints, and double bookings[a]
- A tool for managing some of their most costly, high-utilizing patients
- Documentation support can be provided[a]
- SMAs can be used to help grow a practice[a]
- Providers can optimize their master schedule and appointment mix[a]
- Visits can be max-packed and defect rates can be decreased[a]
- The physician receives real, meaningful help from the SMA team
- Patients help patients and compliance can be increased
- Physicians can find out more information about their patients
- Reduced repetition of information
- An effective venue for difficult, demanding, noncompliant, information-seeking, angry, and inappropriately high-utilizing patients
- Increased patient education and attention to psychosocial issues
- Enhanced patient–physician relationships
- Enhanced continuity of care with patients' own physician
- The same group of 15–20 high-utilizing, multi-morbid geriatric patients is followed over time[b]
- Expensive downtime can be avoided by overbooking sessions according to the expected number of no-shows[a]
- High levels of patient and physician professional satisfaction
- A stronger bottom line can be achieved

[a]Primarily applies to the DIGMA and PSMA models
[b]Primarily applies to the CHCC model

When Properly Run, Group Visits Can Provide Better Care

Physicians' goals in running DIGMAs for their practices vary considerably. For many, the goal is to provide a higher, more satisfying level of care than they are able to provide during the rush of a brief individual office visit, especially when, as a result of access problems, such appointments are also limited and numerically inadequate for the large patient panels that many physicians currently have. Some physicians running DIGMAs and PSMAs have reported that, for the first time in years, they are able to adequately address both the psychosocial and medical needs of their patients during the amount of time allotted—and that this development represents "a quantum leap forward" in the care that they are able to provide.

Help from the Behaviorist as well as the Group Itself

Certainly, one of the great strengths of SMAs—due to the help and support of other patients as well as the professional skills of the behaviorist (at least in the case of DIGMAs and PSMAs) and multidisciplinary team—lies in their ability to better handle patients' behavioral health and psychosocial issues, which are known to drive a large percentage of all medical visits. To help maximize the physician's productivity in the DIGMA or PSMA, the behaviorist assists the physician throughout the entire session in every way possible (Fig. 6.2).

Mind and Body Needs Can Be Addressed

Because DIGMAs and PSMAs make available the professional skills of the behaviorist as well as the help and

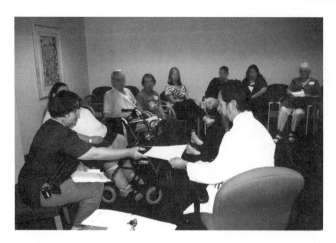

Fig. 6.2 Throughout the entire DIGMA or PSMA session, the behaviorist does everything possible to assist the physician in order to help maximize productivity (courtesy of Dr. Barry Eisenberg and behaviorist Gina Earle, LCSW, Internal Medicine DIGMA, Palo Alto Medical Foundation, Palo Alto, CA)

support of the patients themselves, they enable physicians to better meet the *mind* as well as *body* needs of their patients. This provides an important quality of care benefit in helping patients to successfully implement some of the lifestyle changes that the doctor is recommending (such as dietary changes, exercise regimens, and smoking cessation). Having a mental health behaviorist present in the group room can also help the physician to diagnose and treat such symptoms as anxiety, depression, and substance abuse—conditions that could otherwise go under-diagnosed and under-treated in the primary care setting.

Compliance Can Be Increased While Demand for Services Can Be Reduced

An additional benefit of having the help of a behavioral health professional as well as the group itself is that DIGMAs and PSMAs can increase compliance with treatment recommendations and do so while also better attending to the negative emotions and psychosocial needs that patients might have. It is not uncommon for other members in the group to gently confront and put pressure upon the noncompliant patient—encouraging them to adhere to the doctor's treatment recommendations. Also, because unmet behavioral health and psychosocial needs can result in a spate of otherwise unnecessary appointments, DIGMAs and PSMAs can thereby reduce patient demand on healthcare services, as well as increase supply, due to the exceptional productivity gains that well-run DIGMA and PSMA programs can provide. A 2003 article in *The Washington Times* by Christian Toto

quotes Dr. Kim McMillin (a family practitioner at Baylor Health Care System in Garland, TX, who had been running her group visit for almost a year at the time), who noted how many people watched the television show ER and how patients are attracted to SMAs because of their innate curiosity (1).

Physicians Get to Know Their Patients Better

Because physicians spend more time with their patients, get to know them better, and can monitor them more closely, they frequently report that their SMAs enhance their relationships with patients. Physicians not infrequently comment that properly supported SMAs also provide an *oasis* in their workweek in which they can get away from regular clinic distractions and just focus upon their patients. Also, patients often bring up different types of information in the group than they do in traditional office visits, especially when others first bring these issues up. Physicians frequently comment on how their DIGMAs allow them to discover things about patients that are medically important but were previously unknown to them—even with patients they have worked with and known for years.

William Peters, MD, discusses how his nephrology DIGMA has enabled him to get to know his patients better, and to thereby medically manage his patients in a more efficient manner that reduces both healthcare costs and the human toll of end-stage renal disease. "The group has more than fulfilled my original expectations. Personally, it has allowed me to grow and to develop my understanding and skill in treating end-stage renal disease and to recognize how this disease affects the lives of my patients and their families. It has provided an atmosphere in which I have been able to learn valuable skills from the behavioral medicine specialist...that I now use in other areas of my practice. I find the group to be a source of significant professional satisfaction for another reason. I communicate better with my patients as a result of knowing them better 'as people,' not just as patients with end-stage renal disease. Most important, the group has taught me firsthand by letting me hear from my patients what it is like to be 'on the other side,' an experience which has increased my awareness of the important human side to treatment of kidney disease. The group allows us to find out how kidney problems affect each person's lifestyle, psyche, and family life in a unique way that is not strictly tied to the medical point of view. My group has allowed me to observe how different individuals adapt to end-stage renal disease and has enabled me to learn from my patients in a way that I could not have learned from any other setting" (2).

Physicians Can Increase Productivity, Improve Access, and Better Manage Busy Practices

DIGMAs and PSMAs leverage physicians' time by enabling them to see a dramatically larger volume of patients in a given amount of time, to substantially increase productivity (which can then be applied toward working down backlogs and wait-lists), and to improve access to the physician's practice (Fig. 6.3). Moreover, this increased productivity is achieved with max-packed visits, quality care, and high levels of both patient and physician professional satisfaction. DIGMAs and PSMAs enable physicians to spend more time with their patients and to provide closer monitoring and surveillance. Also, because of the greater amount of time available, the pace of care feels more relaxed, and the physician–patient relationship can often be enhanced.

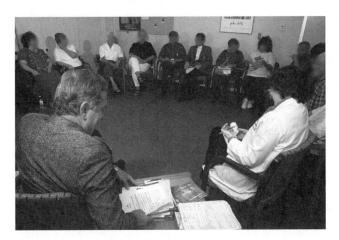

Fig. 6.3 Multidisciplinary team-based DIGMAs and PSMAs enable physicians to increase productivity by two to three times or more, and thereby help them to improve access and better manage busy, backlogged practices (courtesy of the American Group Medical Association and Dr. Lynn Dowdell, Kaiser Permanente San Jose Medical Center, San Jose, CA)

With regard to his weekly 90-minute DIGMA, neurologist C. Gregory Culberson, MD, said, "Considerable time savings are realized because patients need not be escorted individually to an exam room and because I need not return to my office before and after seeing each patient. During the one and a half hours that my DIGMA occupies, I am able to see three or more times the number of patients than I would ordinarily see individually during that interval, and I usually also feel less pressured. Patients perceive that I am less hurried and that we have enough time to discuss their current concerns—regardless of whether they are medical or psychological in nature.... The group experience has been positive for me as well: I look forward to it every week. In addition to the benefits mentioned, the group time has generally had a flow and cadence unmatched in the typical office day. It usually feels natural and unforced, and I generally feel better about what I've accomplished in that time. I can also be assured that I've increased my availability and service to my patients without spending more hours at the office and fewer with my family! My DIGMA truly enables me to "work smarter, not harder" (2).

Patients Have Not Abused the Excellent Access that DIGMAs and PSMAs Provide

Interestingly, experience has shown that the improved accessibility that DIGMAs and PSMAs provide is not abused by patients, and that this greater availability of appointments does not result in inappropriate high utilization, even when accessibility to appointments improves for an entire department (3). In other words, visits are replaced, not added. This is but one of the many surprising and counterintuitive findings regarding group visits. Nor does this improved access result, as some initially feared, in the same 10–16 patients returning week after week and clogging the DIGMA so that others cannot get in. By increasing productivity and by moving numerous individual return and physical examination appointments appropriately into highly efficient DIGMA and PSMA group visits, waiting lists can be rapidly diminished and individual appointments made more available for those patients truly needing or preferring them.

DIGMAs and PSMAs Enable Productivity to Be Dramatically Increased

It is through the inherent efficiencies of the group itself (where repetition can be avoided because all present can simultaneously listen and learn, and where sessions can be overbooked just like the airlines do)—as well as by allowing physicians to delegate as much as possible to less costly members of the SMA team—that DIGMAs and Physicals SMAs enable physicians to significantly increase productivity. To my knowledge, this increase in physician productivity has not been similarly demonstrated for CHCCs, which require a 2½-hour block of the physician's time (rather than 1½ hours like DIGMAs and PSMAs) and provide individual treatment to only approximately one-third of the patients in attendance. CHCCs also have patients return on a prescheduled basis, regardless of whether or not it is medically necessary (i.e., whether or not the patients happen to have a medical need to be seen at that time). However, the CHCC model has been shown to provide a different type of benefit (one that is realized *downstream*) by reducing the cost of the big ticket healthcare items for the 15–20 patients who attend on an ongoing basis—i.e., reduced ER visits, hospitalization stays, and nursing home costs (see Chapter 4 for a detailed discussion of the CHCC model).

One Weekly DIGMA Can Increase a Full-Time Physician's Productivity for the Entire Week by 8–10%:

Dramatically increased productivity, high-quality care, max-packed visits, improved access, better physician management of large practices, chronic illness treatment applications, and high levels of patient and physician professional satisfaction represent a virtual trademark combination of benefits for the DIGMA and Physicals SMA group visit models. In fact, it is this remarkable leveraging of existing resources (and resultant increased physician productivity) that enable properly run DIGMAs and PSMAs to improve access and enable physicians to better manage their busy practices. One 90-minute DIGMA or PSMA per week that increases the physician's productivity by 300% will improve a full-time physician's overall productivity for the entire week by 8, 9, or even 10% (depending on the exact number of patients in attendance and the number of clinic hours per week that physicians are expected to schedule in the system). It will also enable the physician to see the same number of patients during the 1½-hour DIGMA or PSMA as would normally require 4½ hours of clinic time to see individually through traditional office visits—providing the physician with a net gain in productivity of 3 hours per week. This benefit is equivalent to having an equally skilled and productive colleague help the physician 3 hours every week to better manage the physician's practice—and this benefit correspondingly increases with every DIGMA and PSMA that the physician runs per week.

Running Multiple SMAs per Week Increases the Physician's Productivity Correspondingly:

Of course, the physician could run more than one DIGMA or PSMAs per week (assuming that the physician has a busy enough practice to keep all sessions consistently filled), and thereby enjoy correspondingly greater benefits. There are physicians who run DIGMAs every day of the week—and who therefore can experience five times this amount of benefit. Running 2, 3, 4, or 5 90-minute DIGMAs per week (i.e., with each leveraging the physician's time by 300%) would, respectively, result in the equivalent gain of 6, 9, 12, or 15 hours of additional help

per week. And this increased help would effectively come from an equally productive and skilled colleague, because it is the physician's own time that is being leveraged.

The Increased Productivity of DIGMAs and PSMAs Can Be Used in Many Important Ways:

The physician can use the extra capacity generated by the efficiency gains of the DIGMA program in any number of ways: to increase RVUs (relative value units), revenues and income; to improve access and better manage a large practice; to convert some short individual office appointments on the physician's schedule into visits that are 5 or 10 minutes longer; to convert some individual patient contact time each week into nonclinic time (e.g., for administration, reading journals, research, training, or desktop medicine); or to simply work fewer hours in the clinic and go home earlier. However, if the physician elects to cut back productivity elsewhere on his/her schedule, the additional overhead costs of the group visit program must also be taken into account.

Improvements in Productivity, Access, and Patient Satisfaction Are Relatively Easy to Measure:

Certain economic benefits of DIGMAs and PSMAs can be relatively easily measured, such as evaluating the degree to which these SMA models leverage existing staffing, increase productivity, and solve access problems—i.e., without the need of hiring additional physician staffing. This is because it is relatively easy to measure decreases in backlogs and wait-lists, improvements in access, and how much DIGMAs and PSMAs are able to leverage physician time to create extra full-time equivalents (FTEs) for the system out of existing resources—i.e., by enabling providers to see dramatically more patients in the same amount of time. Recall the discussion of the economic benefit that comes from the DIGMA's (or PSMA's) increased productivity alone, which is analyzed at the end of Chapter 2 and can amount to millions of dollars over just a few years' time. Patient satisfaction is also a comparatively easy thing to measure, although an appropriate patient satisfaction form, a good experimental design, and both valid and reliable processes will need to be employed.

The Economic Benefits of Other DIGMA and PSMA Gains Can Be More Difficult to Measure:

There are also many other economic benefits other than improved productivity and access that can come from a well-run DIGMA or PSMA program (see Table 2.8). Although not impossible, it is often more difficult to measure the financial impact of many of these other benefits that well-run DIGMAs and PSMAs can offer. These can include economic gains potentially arising from such additional DIGMA and PSMA benefits as follows: enhanced quality of care; consistently bringing performance measures and routine health maintenance current; max-packed visits that provide patients with a one-stop shopping healthcare experience; increased patient education and disease self-management skills; building the help and support of other patients into each patient's healthcare experience; helping patients to comply with recommended treatment regimens; teaching patients how to more appropriately utilize medical services; reducing defect rates; reaching out to underserved high-risk patient populations; etc. There are additional potential downstream financial benefits as well. One further economic benefit not easily directly measured is the fact that DIGMAs and PSMAs can sometimes more effectively handle many of the behavioral health and psychosocial needs of patients—issues that are known to drive a large percentage of all office visits and to increase utilization.

For Every 12 DIGMAs and PSMAs Run per Week, an Extra Physician FTE Can Be Created:

Because each weekly 90-minute DIGMA or Physicals SMA that increases a physician's productivity by 300% on average enables the physician to see as many patients in the 1½-hour group as would normally require 4½ hours of clinic time to see through individual office visits alone, an average saving of 3 hours of physician time per week occurs for each such weekly DIGMA or PSMA that is run. In systems where 36 hours per week of direct patient contact time is the clinic standard for a full-time physician, this translates into one extra physician full-time equivalent (FTE) being created out of existing resources for every 12 such weekly 90-minute DIGMAs and PSMAs that are run. In turn, this translates into the need to hire one less physician in the future due to this increased capacity created by the DIGMA and PSMA programs.

However, the true savings to the system is probably closer to 1.5 times the number of physician FTEs created through the DIGMA and PSMA programs because these additional FTEs are created out of existing provider staff—i.e., without the need of actually hiring any additional physician staff. Therefore, these extra physician FTEs will not require any additional office space, exam rooms, durable medical equipment, support personnel (beyond that required for the SMA program itself), or

recruitment costs. This translates directly into the true savings from the DIGMA and PSMA programs (i.e., based on the reduced physician staffing ratios required to provide good service and quality care) being closer to 150% of the savings from that of the saved physicians' salaries alone. Of course, to determine the true net savings for the DIGMA and PSMA program, one would then need to deduct the additional overhead from the additional personnel, facilities, and promotional costs of the program (see illustrative financial analysis at the end of Chapter 2).

Reduced Telephone Call Volume, Patient Complaints, and Need for Double Bookings

Because of the increased productivity and improved accessibility that DIGMAs and Physicals SMAs provide, physicians often report a decrease in the volume of patient telephone calls, in patient complaints about poor access, and in the need for double bookings (i.e., forced bookings or work-ins). Because patients can attend a DIGMA any week that they have a medical need and want to be seen, patient complaints about poor access as well as patient telephone volume often decrease. Why call when you can simply come in?

Help in Getting Physicians Back on Schedule when Running Late in the Clinic

One less obvious physician benefit of DIGMAs is that—by acting as a shock absorber in the physician's fast-paced schedule—they can help physicians to get back on schedule by the end of the DIGMA session, even if they happen to enter the group a little late and behind schedule because they happen to be running late in the clinic. Although physicians are encouraged to not be more than 3–5 minutes late for their DIGMA (as the behaviorist will start the group on time with a 3- to 5-minute introduction, for which the physician does not have to be present), this is not always possible as physicians do in fact occasionally run late in the clinic.

Normally, when a physician falls behind schedule during regular clinic hours, the only way to get back on schedule is to: (1) cut the remaining visits during the day a little short; (2) miss lunch; (3) forego some desktop medicine or administration time later in the day; or (4) go home late. This is not true when the physician enters the DIGMA a little late, because the behaviorist can start the group on time and make good use of this extra time in a manner that is helpful to both patients and the physician. For example—after the introduction and while waiting for the physician to enter the group room—if there are some late arriving patients, the behaviorist can also write down on the flip chart their medical concerns which they want to discuss with the physician that day. If there is still more time available before the physician enters the group room, then the behaviorist can go over the contents of the Patient Packet that patients received upon registering for today's visit. The behaviorist could also continue fostering some group interaction and warming the group up, or else discuss community and organizational resources that are available to the patients (or address any relevant behavioral health and psychosocial issues of common interest to the patients in attendance).

In the rare circumstance that the physician arrives later still, the behaviorist can then go over some of the handouts that have been preselected by the physician, or else have the patients briefly introduce themselves to each other (which is something that I normally do not recommend, as this can take up too much valuable group time). What the behaviorist has discussed with the group can then be briefly related to the physician when she/he arrives—hopefully, with the physician not being more than a few minutes late. While attention to actual medical issues is postponed until the physician arrives, the intent here is to make the best possible use of the time that the behaviorist shares with the group until the physician does in fact arrive. The goal of each and every DIGMA or PSMA session is to make the entire SMA useful to patients from start to finish, and to complete all business (including the documentation of all chart notes) within the allotted amount of time. Upon arriving, the physician then begins promptly addressing in turn the unique medical needs of each patient individually (but at a slightly faster pace due to being late)—i.e., until the work is finished with each patient, which will hopefully be completed by the time that the group is scheduled to end. The physician then leaves the group room back on schedule, preferably without any unresolved group-related issues that might require attention later on. Nonetheless, whenever possible, I strongly recommend that the physician arrives in the group room no later than 3–5 minutes late for the session.

SMAs Are Customized to Each Physician's Particular Needs

It is important that physicians understand from the outset that their DIGMAs, CHCCs, and PSMAs are being customized around their own particular needs, goals, practice style, and patient panel constituency—and that every effort is being made to extract every possible physician benefit from their group visit program so as to optimally improve the physician's professional work-life. Individual physicians can select the specific benefits that they most want, and their DIGMA, CHCC, or PSMA can be customized accordingly. However, to optimize the benefits that SMAs can make available to physicians, the managed care organization must provide the necessary administrative support, personnel, promotional materials, and facilities required for success. The many ways that SMAs can be customized to the physician's specific needs are listed in Table 6.2.

Table 6.2 How SMAs can be customized to the physician's particular needs

- Whether to use the DIGMA, CHCC, or PSMA model
- Selection of the homogeneous, heterogeneous, mixed, or Specialty CHCC subtype
- The frequency and length of SMA sessions
- The weekday and time of day that sessions will be held
- Selection of particular SMA team members—nurse/MA(s), behaviorist, and documenter
- Specific expanded duties that the behaviorist and nursing personnel will perform
- What training will be provided, and to whom (including physician's support staff)
- The group and exam rooms to be used, and how they will be furnished
- What medical equipment, forms, etc., will be available in the group and exam rooms
- Marketing materials to be used, and how the SMA is to be promoted to patients
- Whether announcement letters will be sent to patients at the start of the SMA (how many, to whom, some each week or all at once, etc.)
- Whether a Patient Packet will be handed out, and specifically what it will contain
- The particular educational materials and handouts to be used
- Whether or not a documenter will be used
- Will a dedicated scheduler will be attached and, if so, how many hours per week
- The amount of medical care to be delivered during each group session
- What types of exams, procedures, and discussions will be provided in private
- The specific chart note template to be used
- The level of involvement by billing and compliance
- The particular physician benefits the SMA will be designed to primarily achieve

When custom designing a DIGMA or PSMA to the physician's needs, any of the three subtypes of these models can be used: (1) the *heterogeneous* subtype, in which each session is open to most or all patients in the physician's practice (regardless of diagnosis, age, sex, or condition); (2) the *homogeneous* subtype, in which each session is only open to patients with the same or similar diagnoses or conditions; or (3) the *mixed* subtype, an in-between concept that usually partitions the physician's entire practice into four major diagnosis or condition-related groups, one for each week of the month. However, the mixed subtype also allows patients who are not able to attend the session which best fits their particular condition that month to attend any other appropriate SMA session that happens to better fit their schedule (see Chapters 2 and 5 for more information on the subtypes of DIGMAs and PSMAs). Similarly, physicians can select either the CHCC model or the Specialty CHCC subtype when customizing their group visit program.

When custom designing a DIGMA or PSMA to accommodate the particular desires of the physician, careful consideration should be paid to preferred time, day of the week, length of the session (60–120 minutes, with 90 minutes being most common), and frequency of sessions (daily through monthly or quarterly, with weekly being most common, at least initially). As depicted in Table 6.2, DIGMAs have great flexibility, and can be customized to the physician's precise needs and practice along many different dimensions.

Individual physicians can select the benefits they most want, and their DIGMAs and PSMAs can be custom designed accordingly. To optimize the physician benefits of SMAs, it is strongly recommended that the organization provide: the necessary budget; the best possible champion and program coordinator; an appropriate behaviorist; one to two nursing personnel; a documenter; a dedicated scheduler for 2–4 hours per week; professional appearing marketing materials; appropriate group and exam rooms (if there is no group room space available, consider using the lobby during off-hours); the time required for training; and sufficient time dedicated to the program each week for each member of the team to fulfill their respective duties (including debriefing after sessions for the first 2 months). Also, it is advisable to have the physician's primary scheduling staff—and afterward, the reception staff—sit in on a session (or at least part of a session), one or two at a time, as soon as possible after the SMA is up and running.

Documentation Support Can Be Provided

One of the great physician benefits of a DIGMA or Physicals SMA is that documentation support can be provided to generate a superior chart note, i.e., one that is done in real time and is both comprehensive and contemporaneous, and can therefore optimize billing.

Efficiency Is Gained by the Physician Delegating to the Entire SMA Team

This is in line with one of the basic overarching principles of a well-run group visit program—i.e., that efficiency can be gained by having the physician delegate as many tasks and responsibilities as appropriate and possible to less costly members of the SMA team, which includes the documenter (Fig. 6.4). This approach also offers the additional advantage of more consistency in the actual performance of these duties—i.e., as theses duties that are delegated to the SMA team are then done on all patients per the protocol previously agreed upon with the physician. This is particularly true of the expanded nursing duties provided by the nursing personnel attached to the DIGMA or PSMA, as these are performed upon each patient in attendance by protocol—i.e., without the *hit and miss* approach of expecting this to be consistently done by the physician and nurse in the individual office visit setting.

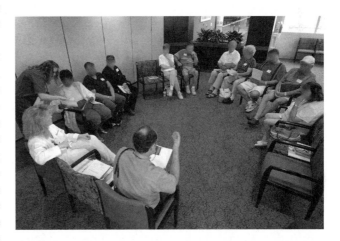

Fig. 6.4 To optimize productivity in DIGMAs and PSMAs, physicians delegate as much as possible and appropriate to the entire SMA team (behaviorist, nurse/MA(s), documenter, and dedicated scheduler)—from whom they get real and meaningful help (courtesy of Dr. Patricio Aycinena, Diabetes DIGMA, Cleveland Clinic, Cleveland, OH)

Having Documentation Support Provides a Strong Incentive for Physicians

Physicians view having a documenter in the room—who actually takes care of approximately 70–90% of the chart note responsibilities (as the physician does need to spend a little time reviewing, modifying, and signing off on each chart note immediately after working with that patient in the group setting)—as being a major benefit of running a

DIGMA or PSMA for their practices. This is especially true because the documenter has been specifically trained by the physician to draft the chart note exactly as the physician wants it done, and because the documenter is also trained to use the physician's own chart note template.

A Documenter Is Especially Helpful for Systems Using EMR

This benefit is particularly helpful for systems using electronic medical records (EMR) because, for systems using paper charts, it is relatively easy for the physician to use a chart note template that is largely in a preprinted, check-off form. Likewise, for physicians who use a microcassette recorder to dictate chart notes into, this is also relatively easily handled in the group setting by the physician (i.e., immediately after working in turn with each patient individually) saying something like, "OK, listen up everybody while I dictate the chart note for John, and let me know if I leave anything out." The physician then proceeds to dictate the chart note out loud (so that all can hear) immediately after completing the work with each patient individually, thereby using the dictation process as an additional teaching tool within the group setting.

However, there are two major problems with dictating in this manner. First, it means that all of the work, which includes the documentation of all chart notes, will not be completed by the time the SMA is over—i.e., because the physician will still have to read, modify, and sign off on all chart notes for the group after they are later completed by the medical transcriptionist and returned to the physician's office for signature. Second, this approach squeezes out the invaluable minute or two of time that the behaviorist would otherwise have to foster some group interaction and address psychosocial issues while the physician is briefly reviewing and completing the chart note on each patient—i.e., immediately after finishing the work with that patient.

Although EMR offers many benefits and can generate a very professional appearing chart note, this process does take a certain amount of time on average for each of the many patients in attendance. By multiplying this average amount of time per chart note by the number of patients in attendance, one quickly comes to realize that a great deal of the DIGMA or PSMA session could be occupied by the physician documenting chart notes on the computer. In addition, it also takes considerable expertise to completely utilize the potential of EMR, and to do so in a highly efficient manner—e.g., taking full advantage of the various shortcuts, smart phrases, smart texts, etc. for accessing and incorporating an assortment of *stock* or *standardized*

paragraphs and templates into the finalized chart notes (such as *dropping in* the hypertension, hyperlipidemia, or diabetes paragraphs). Because documenting chart notes is all that the documenter does (i.e., this is the documenter's sole job in the DIGMA or PSMA), and because of the specific training that the documenter has received, the documenter quickly develops a high degree of proficiency in working with EMR to full advantage—often soon becoming more efficient and capable of drafting high-quality chart notes than the physician.

DIGMAs and PSMAs Can Help to Grow a Physician's Practice

Because they can off-load many follow-up visits for established patients onto highly efficient DIGMA visits (or individual physical examinations for new and established patients onto cost-effective Physicals SMAs), DIGMAs and PSMAs can add sufficient capacity for physicians (especially those who are new to the system) to grow their practices. By doing so, many individual office visits on the physician's schedule can thereby be freed up—which can ultimately permit the physician's master schedule to be changed accordingly so as to add extra new patient intake appointments onto the schedule, and thus bring additional new patients into the practice. When this is done for DIGMAs, one change option is to reduce the number of short follow-up appointments offered by the physician each week—and then consolidate and convert the time thereby opened up on the physician's master schedule into additional new patient intake appointments. In addition, the physician's PSMA can itself include up to a certain number of new patients.

SMAs Enable the Physician's Master Schedule and Appointment Mix to Be Optimized

In addition, physicians can use DIGMAs and PSMAs to optimize the appointment mix they offer on their master schedules each week to best meet their professional goals and objectives. For example, physicians can reduce the number of individual return office visits or physical examination appointments that they offer each week, and then correspondingly increase the number of other types of appointments they offer on their master schedules. This could include additional new patient intakes or additional time set aside for administration, research, desktop medicine, phone calls, e-mails, consultations, teaching, etc. In other words, this equivalent of extra hours of help from an equally talented and productive colleague that is gained by leveraging the physician's time through a well-run DIGMA or PSMA each week can be spent in many ways—including optimizing the physician's master schedule—depending upon the needs and priorities of the individual physician.

Certain specialists and surgeons can use the additional time that DIGMAs and PSMAs provide to ratchet up income substantially, i.e., by off-loading lower compensated visits (such as intake appointments and follow-up visits) onto highly efficient DIGMAs and/or PSMAs, and then converting the time thereby freed up to providing more highly compensated appointment types, such as additional surgeries and procedures.

In addition, because of the increased productivity that properly run DIGMAs and PSMAs can provide, physician incomes should also be correspondingly increased due to the improved productivity of 200–300% or more—at least to the extent that physicians' salaries are determined by their productivity. However, a comprehensive cost–benefit analysis would need to be conducted in order to assess the true economic gain of the DIGMA or PSMA program, as full groups are critical and the overhead costs of the program would need to be appropriately factored in and, of course, deducted from the revenues generated in order to determine the actual net positive economic impact upon the physician's income and practice.

routine part of the care that is systematically delivered by protocol to all patients during their DIGMA or PSMA visit. Ultimately, this consistency in nursing duties performed on all patients should lead to fewer mistakes and oversights—and therefore, to decreased defect rates. When I visited one mid-sized medical group that I had consulted with and helped to start several DIGMAs and PSMAs a year earlier (i.e., with the intent of helping them to celebrate the 1-year anniversary of their SMA program), I asked them what their greatest surprise was about their DIGMA and PSMA program during the previous year. They told me that neither the high levels of patient satisfaction that they were documenting nor the high level of physician professional satisfaction they were experiencing was surprising to them. What surprised them most was that a very large percentage of all the patients attending their DIGMAs and PSMAs during the previous year had not had their tetanus shot updated during their last individual office visit, even though having this done was a clinic standard that had previously been established in the system for all individual office visits in primary care. Despite their best efforts during traditional office visits, they had a very large defect rate regarding tetanus shot updates. By making it part of the routine protocol for nursing duties in the DIGMAs and PSMAs, virtually all patients attending a DIGMA or PSMA had their tetanus shot checked and appropriately updated during the visit.

Visits Can Be Max-Packed and Defect Rates Can Be Reduced

Not only can visits be max-packed but also certain aspects of care can be systematically built into the DIGMA or PSMA in order to reduce defect rates. For example, due to the fast pace of individual office visit care, one dermatologist was very concerned about forgetting to give a full disclosure (or failing to fully document the fact that a full disclosure was given) to every patient for whom he was recommending cosmetic surgery. This concern has been greatly reduced in the DIGMA setting by appropriately designing the physician's full disclosure into every session—so that if the physician should happen to forget to provide a full disclosure to a patient for any reason, the behaviorist would then remind him/her to do so.

Similarly, by expanding the nursing role in the DIGMA or PSMA and by consistently including a wide variety of additional nursing duties that are performed on all patients in attendance, this becomes a

Physicians Receive Real, Meaningful Help from the Entire Multidisciplinary SMA Team

In addition to the enjoyable collegiality of the behaviorist and entire SMA team, DIGMAs and Physicals SMAs provide physicians with real and meaningful help from the entire SMA team. Physicians appreciate the help received from: the *champion* in designing and implementing the SMA program (with a minimum amount of time commitment on the physician's part), and in moving it forward throughout the organization; the *program coordinator* in training the team and in getting the program launched (as well as in later evaluating the SMA on an ongoing basis); the *dedicated scheduler* in keeping all sessions filled; the *documenter* in completing all chart notes during the allotted amount of group time, using the physician's own chart note template; and the one or two nursing personnel (MAs, RNs, LVNs, nursing techs, etc.) in performing the expanded nursing duties and bringing injections, vital signs, and routine health maintenance current. Even the physician's own *support staff* is trained to be helpful and involved, especially in informing appropriate patients about the PSMA, inviting them to attend, and scheduling them into the PSMA. Physicians also appreciate the information, encouragement, help, and support provided by *patients* themselves in the group setting.

Physician also value the friendship and help received from the *behaviorist* on an ongoing basis— i.e., by coming in early to *warm up* the group; giving the introduction; controlling and pacing the group to keep it running smoothly and on time; handling group dynamic and psychosocial issues; tactfully bringing depression and anxiety to the physician's attention; managing various difficult and challenging situations that might arise in the group setting; responding effectively to angry or demanding patients; temporarily taking over the group when the physician documents chart notes or steps out of the group room to conduct brief private discussions and exams; and staying late for a few minutes after sessions to address any last minute patient issues, clear the room, and quickly straighten up the group room.

For example, in an article centered upon how physicians evaluate the impact of DIGMAs on their practices, family practitioner Monica Donovan, MD, reported the following with regard to the help that she received from the author when serving as behaviorist in her Family Practice DIGMA of mixed design. "Of the four group sessions held during each month, my pain group is most difficult for me. It meets on the third Monday of each month and is open to all my pain patients, who have such conditions as neck and low back pain, arthritis, chronic pain, headache, and fibromyalgia. Because such patients are often difficult and sometimes show manipulative or drug-seeking behavior, I especially welcome the outside help and assistance that Dr. Noffsinger provides as a health psychologist, both in addressing the extensive emotional and behavioral issues of these patients and in guiding the direction and pace of the group. The participation of Dr. Noffsinger permits me to improve my ability to remain sympathetic to this patent population while minimizing my own negative feelings and thoughts about some of their behaviors" (2).

Dr. Donovan goes on to state: "I believe that attending the group sessions can help people to build on their strengths, to pay closer attention to the positive aspects of their lives, and to make their medical care a more pleasant experience. The group also gives patients the opportunity to spend more time with me, to see me interact with them and others, and to get to know me better. This enables my patients to feel more comfortable in expressing what they need to say in order to get their medical needs met" (2).

Patients Help Each Other, Which Makes the Physician's Job Easier

One of the great benefits of SMAs is that patients help each other in a variety of different ways—by supporting one another, by genuinely caring, by sharing important information, and by discussing their personal experiences (heartaches as well as successes). They share hard-earned coping strategies and disease self-management skills that they have learned through trial and error in dealing with their own health problems. By confronting noncompliant patients with the potential future consequences of not paying attention to what their doctor is telling them (and doing so in a manner that the patient is able to hear and understand), other patients assist the physician and help to increase the compliance of such patients with recommended treatment regimens.

Also, patients interact and ask questions from time to time throughout the SMA session, which keeps it interesting and enables other patients to benefit by getting answers to important medical questions that they might not have thought to ask. Patients also learn from each other when they bring up medical advice gleaned from friends, family, television, direct pharmaceutical ads, and the Internet, which gives the physician an opportunity to correct any misinformation or incorrect beliefs that patients might be espousing. They also share a myriad of helpful information with one another. All in all, when coupled with the prompt access and greater time with the physician that the SMA provides, it is the caring and support of other patients (as well as the multidisciplinary SMA team) that makes group visits so unique—and such a warm and rewarding experience for all.

When he was Chief of the Department of Neurology at the Kaiser Permanente Medical Center in San Jose, neurologist Rajan Bhandari, M.D., reported on the following case from his heterogeneous Neurology DIGMA, which clearly illustrated how patients help patients in the group visit setting. "An elderly man had Parkinson's disease for approximately 25 years and was having frequent falls and a poor response to most dopa agonists and replacement drugs. The disease progressed to Hoen and Yahr stage 4. The patient had been mostly confined to his bed until 18 months previously, when he had a pallidotomy; thereafter, he could ambulate using a walker, responded to both dopa replacement and dopa agonist medications, and had far fewer falls. He and his wife visited my Neurology DIGMA every three to four months and acknowledged that the group visits helped them by enabling them to interact with other patients and families struggling with severely limiting medical illnesses. Indeed, they greatly inspired my other patients with chronic debilitating neurologic conditions. He did not mind having his limb tone and motor function checked in group, nor did he mind performing motor tasks in the presence of others. Having the opportunity to watch him walk around the room and observe how he appeared was important for me as his physician. I have still seen him in individual appointments, but less frequently. Both the patient and his wife felt that they were getting more benefit from the group visits than from individual office visits" (2).

Because of the Multiple Benefits They Provide, Physicians Tend to "Own" Their SMAs

Because they provide a whole host of benefits to the physician, SMA programs tend to be *owned* by the physicians running them. As a result, there tends not to be any invisible or orphan DIGMA, CHCC, and PSMA programs without strong physician ownership, which could be the case with some types of group programs that provide fewer direct physician benefits, and to which the physician might not be as strongly identified or attached. Physicians typically grow very fond of their DIGMA, CHCC, and PSMA programs, and come to enjoy them very much—with many commenting that their SMA is one of the things that they most look forward to each week. One physician even told me that it was the only thing that he looked forward to each week. Interestingly, even for those DIGMAs and PSMAs that do ultimately fail (which is almost always due to insufficient census for economic viability of the program), the physicians are often very reluctant to stop their program, because they have grown to enjoy it and recognize the many benefits that it provides to both their patients and themselves.

Reduced Repetition of Information

Almost all physicians find that they have certain things that they keep saying over and over to different patients individually throughout the course of the workweek—which is a sure sign that they should start a DIGMA or PSMA for such patients, where such issues would only need to be discussed once. Furthermore, because more time is available, this information can often be covered in greater depth during the SMA session—and with less likelihood of forgetting to cover something important in the explanation.

Example 1: Hormone Replacement Therapy and Peri-menopausal Issues in Gynecology

One of the most dramatic examples of this physician benefit was offered by an experienced, middle-aged gynecologist whose busy practice consisted mostly of peri-menopausal women. She reported being "...bored out of my mind by repeating the same types of information over and over to different patients all week long." She went on to state that she had 20- and 40-minute appointments on her clinic schedule, but that such repetitive discussions with her patients completely filled the available time. She added that: "My sessions are so full that I don't want patients to talk or ask questions, because that takes too much time and ends up making me late for my next patient." Needless to say, her patient satisfaction scores with traditional office visits had not been very good.

By inviting all of her peri-menopausal and hormone replacement patients to attend her Peri-menopausal DIGMA any week they needed to be seen, she was able to have lively, interesting, and more comprehensive discussions regarding these issues with all such patients in attendance at once—but in the context of sequentially working with each patient individually. Interestingly, on the patient satisfaction form that was used to evaluate this system's DIGMA program (which consisted of a 5-point Likert scale for each of the seven satisfaction questions that patients were asked to respond to), this physician received the highest possible rating on all questionnaires turned in during the first 4 weeks that her DIGMA was held (which was the length of the pilot study to which I was attached)—something that I have never seen before or since. Her patient satisfaction scores had gone from mediocre to exceptional through her group visit program, and she grew to truly enjoy her group experience. It is dramatic result such as this that cause me to wonder if DIGMAs and PSMAs could not be used to actually raise patient satisfaction scores for those physicians whose scores are currently unsatisfactorily low, especially by pairing them off with a behaviorist who happens to have exceptional communication skills.

Example 2: Treating Headache in Neurology and Primary Care DIGMAs

As another example, consider how a physician can handle headache in a neurology or primary care DIGMA in which there happens to be many different headache patients in attendance. Here, common medical issues regarding headache can be addressed simultaneously with many similarly afflicted patients—issues that the neurologist would otherwise need to keep repeating over and over to numerous patients individually throughout the entire workweek. The various types of headaches (rebound, migraine, cluster, tension, etc.), treatment options, self-help techniques, and medication management issues (including typical side effects, addiction potential, scheduling, dosage, and alternative medications) could be discussed with the entire group at once while the physician is sequentially working with one headache patient after another in the DIGMA setting. By fostering group interaction, this discussion could simultaneously be helpful to all headache patients who are present—and could also lead to a stimulating and helpful group discussion.

In addition, when one patient then asks a follow-up question, the entire group has the opportunity to hear the answer, which might simultaneously apply to many other patients in the group as well. Even if the answer does not happen to relate directly to some of the other patients' current personal circumstance, it might in the future in the event that they started having headaches later on. Nonetheless, these other patients without headaches often state that they find the answers to such questions interesting— as they see how it might apply to others they know, and state that they now know what to do should the same type of thing happen to them in the future. In addition, because of the professional skills of a behaviorist and the gentle confrontation of other patients—both of which are potentially present throughout the entire session— limits can often more easily be put on drug-seeking headache patients that put considerable pressure on the neurologist to give them drugs that they want (but which are medically contraindicated).

DIGMAs Are Excellent for Difficult, Demanding, and Psychosocially Needy Patients

DIGMAs provide an excellent modality for treating some of the most difficult, demanding, time-consuming, and problematic patients in the physician's practice—patients who have extensive informational and psychosocial needs, are inappropriate high or low utilizers of health-care services, are angry and litigious, are distrusting and anxious, or are depressed and filing numerous complaints. Because of the greater amount of time available, the professional skills of the behaviorist, and the help and support provided by other patients, psychosocial issues such as these can often be much better addressed in DIGMAs and PSMAs than in traditional office visits.

Greater Patient Education Can Be Provided

In addition to providing greater attention to psychosocial issues, DIGMAs and PSMAs can also provide more patient education. Because the physician is able to efficiently provide information of common interest to many patients at once in the DIGMA group setting, questions can be answered and medical recommendations provided in a setting where all present are able to listen, interact, and learn. In addition, the patients themselves are also often able to help and support each other, which include the sharing of important information they have obtained as well as successful coping strategies.

The Doctor–Patient Relationship Can Be Improved

In the DIGMA, patients have the opportunity to spend a full 90 minutes with their doctor, the behaviorist, and the other patients. They can get their *mind* as well as *body* issues addressed, see their physician laugh and be more relaxed, and get to know their doctor better—all of which can lead to improved patient–physician relationships (which is something that patients attending DIGMAs and Physicals SMAs often report). Patients and physicians alike often leave the SMA setting reporting that they have gotten to know each other better, that their relationship has changed in a positive manner, and that they now feel more comfortable and able to work effectively together.

Psychosocial Issues Can Often Be Better Handled in SMAs

Although psychosocial issues are often difficult to address during a brief individual appointment, they can often be better handled during a DIGMA or Physicals SMA because of the combination of more time available plus the support and help of both the behaviorist and the group itself. After one DIGMA session, the physician commented: "This group is excellent for patients who are lonely, depressed, or lack the support of others— also for patients experiencing a great deal of life stress that we couldn't begin to address in a relatively brief individual appointment." Also, because of the added diagnostic skills that an experienced and skilled behaviorist can bring into the treatment setting, the behaviorist can help to diagnose clinical depression, anxiety, and substance abuse (and to tactfully point these out to the physician)—conditions that are known to often go under-diagnosed and under-treated in the primary care setting, and to drive many office visits.

Refer Some of Your Most Problematic and Demanding Patients into Your DIGMA

Physicians have not infrequently commented upon how valuable their DIGMA has been for handling and containing some of their most demanding, time-consuming, and draining patients. Any of the following types of patients could be included here: (1) information-seeking patients who, despite being 40 minutes into a 20-minute office visit, bring out a typewritten sheet filled with questions that they still want the physician to answer; (2) the patient who comes in with a folder containing several articles downloaded from the Internet that they want the physician to promptly read and comment upon; (3) the lonely widow who looks forward the entire week to her doctor's appointment; (4) the *doctor shopper*, who is repeatedly dissatisfied with medical care received; (5) the litigious and chronically unhappy patient who frequently files complaints both internally and externally; (6) the uncommunicative patient who frequently withholds information, gives only minimal responses, and fails to voluntarily let the physician know what her/his important healthcare issues are; (7) the patient with vague and ever-changing physical complaints who refuses to accept the possibility of contributory lifestyle factors or a psychogenic origin of symptoms; (8) the *frequent flier* who inappropriately overutilizes healthcare services, who constantly telephones the doctor's office, or keeps making unnecessary medical appointments; (9) the patient who interacts inappropriately with the healthcare system, and misuses or abuses the services offered; (10) the *worried well* with the multifarious and varied medical complaints that they so frequently present with; etc.

Negative Feelings Are Often Better Handled in SMAs

Although DIGMA and PSMA sessions largely have a positive and upbeat tone, anger and negative feelings are nonetheless expressed and responded to. Patients sometimes bring up, openly discuss, and favorably resolve their frustration and anger with the system—or with prior medical care. Such negative feelings can arise from any of a large variety of perceptions and misperceptions—that initial treatment or follow-up care was inadequate; that too little time was spent with their physician; that too much time elapsed between appointments; that the doctor or staff seemed disinterested; that their doctor was not reachable and did not return calls; that their diagnosis and treatment had been delayed; etc. In instances such as these, the improved access, drop-in convenience, and additional time that DIGMAs offer—coupled with the help and support of the behaviorist and other patients—can provide real and meaningful help to the physician, and invaluable assistance to the patient in resolving these negative feelings.

My Most Difficult Single DIGMA Experience as a Behaviorist

Because of my extensive experience in the DIGMA and PSMA settings, both as a behaviorist and as a champion, I am sometimes asked to describe the most difficult moment I ever had in a DIGMA session. The answer to this question provides an excellent example of the benefit that a skilled behaviorist—as well as the group itself—can provide to the physician and patient alike when challenging moments arise in the group. It occurred during a large oncology DIGMA session with approximately 18 attendees, a session that was particularly full of negative energy because two recently diagnosed cancer patients who were attending the group for the first time were extremely angry at their disease, their primary care doctor, and their healthcare plan. Their fury escalated even further as first one patient and then the other spoke loudly in an absolute rage. They loudly blamed their doctors, medical negligence, and the system for their plights. In addition, the oncologist (who was not used to being attacked and talked down to in such a negative, hostile manner) was becoming increasingly irritated and defensive as these two patients kept spewing their venom. To put it mildly, the group room immediately became very hot and tense with their vociferous accusations and seemingly insatiable fury.

As the behaviorist in this group, I waited for a couple of minutes (although it seemed like an eternity), listening intently to what these patients were saying before I said anything myself—trying to first get a handle on exactly what it was that these patients were so furious about. It seemed to me that these two patients were actually very fearful that, now that they were truly ill, the managed care organization would let them die or suffer needlessly rather than spend the necessary dollars to ensure that they received appropriate treatment and the care that they now so desperately wanted. When I asked them if this might not be the case, these patients seemed to stop dead in their tracks, and immediately became tearful as they acknowledged that this was indeed their greatest fear. They said that they had just that week read a national magazine article to this effect about managed care organizations—how they would let patients suffer needlessly and die, rather than spending the necessary money on them to ensure that they get appropriate care.

I was then able to immediately ask the physician whether or not this was a realistic concern on their part, which gave the oncologist an opportunity to intervene and reassure the patients—with heartfelt sincerity I might add—that this would definitely not happen regarding their treatment. He went on to say that neither he nor the healthcare system would stand for this, and that in his decades with the organization this had never happened with any of his patients—and that, if it ever did, he would promptly resign. The oncologist was then able to add that his facility was a test site in cancer research, and on the cutting edge with regard to the latest in cancer treatment studies. All of this went a long way toward reassuring these patients that they would in fact be receiving the care that they needed and toward greatly reducing their hostility.

It Is Unlikely This Positive Outcome Could Have Been Achieved as Quickly with Individual Office Visits

As a result of these interventions by the behaviorist and physician (together with other patients in the room acknowledging that what the oncologist was saying was certainly true in their case), the intense anger of these two patients was successfully resolved within 15–20 minutes. Afterward, both patients became very cooperative and compliant with the oncologist's recommended treatment regimens, and they both continued to appropriately attend future DIGMA sessions on an as-needed basis without further incidents or problems. During that trying session, an important positive shift had occurred in the therapeutic relationship that these two patients had with their oncologist—whom they now began to trust and listen to, and started viewing as an ally and partner in the treatment of their disease.

At the end of that singularly hot and heavy DIGMA session, which was initially so full of hostility and negativity, the oncologist commented on "what a good and helpful group it was today." He pointed out that the fierce rage that had been expressed by these two patients that day was much better handled in the DIGMA than he could possibly have dealt with it during individual appointments. He added that, "It would probably have taken several individual appointments to achieve a similar result, if it would have been possible at all."

Expensive Physician Downtime Can Be Avoided by Overbooking SMA Sessions

Another benefit that DIGMAs, CHCCs, and PSMAs offer physicians is that, by appropriately overbooking sessions, expensive physician downtime during the DIGMA can be avoided. With individual office visits— when patients fail to keep their appointment or cancel too late for the appointment to be refilled with another patient—the result is typically an expensive loss in physician productivity and revenues. With group visits, this costly problem can easily be avoided by simply overbooking sessions according to the expected number of no-shows and late cancels, a number that can readily be empirically determined with considerable accuracy for any given physician after only a few SMA sessions.

Some Concluding Comments

As we continue to expand and exploit the multiple benefits that DIGMAs, CHCCs, and PSMAs can offer (to improve quality and outcomes, to optimize productivity and efficiency, to increase the amount of medical care delivered, to increase patient education and disease self-management skills, and to solve real-life healthcare delivery problems such as improving access and containing costs), we must always remember that the foundation for this entire effort lies with the individual physician running a SMA for his/her practice. In the many medical groups where SMAs have been tried, physician professional satisfaction with the program has generally been very high.

Only with physician acceptance and buy-in can the remarkable benefits that DIGMAs, CHCCs, and PSMAs offer to patients, physicians, and the organization alike be fully realized. As we have seen in this chapter, there are two things that are absolutely critical to securing physician acceptance of any DIGMA, CHCC, or PSMA program: (1) one must promptly and thoroughly address the many concerns and resistances that physicians need to have resolved before they will be willing to try a SMA for their own practice; and (2) physicians need to clearly understand the many potential physician benefits that properly run and supported SMAs can offer to them and their practices.

References

1. Toto C. Group appointments mean more attention. *The Washington Times* 2003;18:B1, B4.
2. Noffsinger EB, Mason JE Jr., Culberson CG, et al. Physicians evaluate the impact of Drop-In Group Medical Appointments (DIGMAs) on their practices. *Group Practice Journal* 1999;48(6):22–23, 25–33.
3. Noffsinger EB. Solving departmental access problems with DIGMAs. *Group Practice Journal* 2001;50(10):26–28, 30–32, 34–36.

Chapter 7
A Comprehensive Chronic Illness Treatment Paradigm that Makes Full Use of Group Visits

Chronic conditions such as Type 2 diabetes and heart failure have become epidemic. This is not just a problem unique to the United States; it is a global problem. A contributing factor to the increase in many of the chronic conditions has been the epidemic of obesity. In the past 20 years, the rates of obesity have tripled in developing countries that have adopted a Western lifestyle involving decreased physical activity and overconsumption of inexpensive, high calorie foods. Today more than 1.1 billion adults and 1.7 billion children are overweight.[1] The impact of this problem has staggering numbers attached to it. In the US the combined costs for diabetes and heart failure exceed $200 billion per year.[2] Worldwide by 2030, there will be approximately 366 million people with Type 2 diabetes (Footnote 1). Our current models of providing care have not worked in addressing this problem. If we are to have a broad impact in reversing this trend we must find more effective ways in helping patients address the necessary health behavior changes. Group visits that help foster self-management support can have a substantial impact on the efficient use of resources necessary to reverse this trend. Not only can they impact the effects of conditions such as diabetes and heart failure, they have a broad applicability to a host of problems faced by an aging population.

Jim Nuovo, MD, personal communication, February 1, 2007

SMAs Offer Many Benefits to Chronic Illness Population Management Programs

In this chapter, we discuss a comprehensive chronic disease treatment program that I developed, implemented, and first published in the February 2008 issue of *Group Practice Journal*—one that takes full advantage of the multiple benefits that group visits offer and should work equally well for managing virtually any chronic illness (1). This paradigm represents a high quality, high volume, and cost-effective approach to chronic disease management that makes full use of the multiple quality, service, economic, and satisfaction benefits that well-run SMA programs can offer. As will be seen, of all the group visit models, the DIGMA model has many specific advantages that make it singularly well suited to chronic disease and lifestyle management programs—although the other group visit models can also be applied in certain unique ways. For illustrative purposes, diabetes is

used in this chapter as a specific application of the proposed chronic disease management paradigm. However, the reader should keep in mind that this is but a single example, and that this same paradigm could work equally well for any chronic illness treatment program (CHF, asthma, diabetes, hypertension, hyperlipidemia, stroke, Parkinson's disease, etc., provided that there are sufficient patients with that diagnosis to fill the SMA groups).

Delivery of Medical Care Is Central for All Group Visit Models

Recall that the central characteristic of a *group visit* (or shared medical appointment, group medical appointment, group appointment, etc.) is the efficient delivery of medical care in an informative and supportive group setting that includes other patients. Despite working long hours as hard and efficiently as possible, many physicians are nonetheless finding that access problems are worsening, that patient panels are becoming larger, and that these increasingly large practices are becoming more difficult to manage. In addition, patients are becoming

---

[1] Hossain P, Kawar B, El Nahas M. Obesity and diabetes in the developing world. A growing challenge. *New England Journal of Medicine* 2007;356:213–215.

[2] Nuovo J, editor. *Chronic Disease Management.* New York, Springer, 2007.

E.B. Noffsinger, *Running Group Visits in Your Practice*, DOI 10.1007/b106441_7,
© Springer Science+Business Media, LLC 2009

more informed and demanding; the patient population is aging; multiple chronic diseases are becoming commonplace; obesity is becoming an epidemic; and tens of millions of uninsured are likely to soon gain universal healthcare coverage. Furthermore, many providers are striving to move toward same-day access, but are finding that they need a tool such as group visits to increase their productivity and help them to achieve—and then maintain—this high level of accessibility to their practices. In addition to helping physicians better manage large and busy practices, group visits can also be used with an equally positive effect in better managing chronic illnesses and high-risk patients—a topic to which this chapter is dedicated.

Their Unique Combination of Benefits Makes Group Visits Ideal for Chronic Disease Management

Group medical appointments truly represent a glimpse into the future because of their unique ability to simultaneously cut costs, save time, enhance quality, update routine health maintenance, improve outcomes, and better meet the needs of patients and physicians alike. Typically involving the patient's own physician and a multidisciplinary treatment team, shared medical appointments (SMAs) have the flexibility to allow patients to bring one support person along with them (spouse, adult family member, caregiver, or friend)—at least this is the case for DIGMAs and some PSMAs, but not for CHCCs. Group visits also make full use of the complementary skill sets of all members of the SMA team—for example, the nurse/MA(s), who are pushed to do the maximum amount possible, but always stay at a level that is within their skill set and scope of practice. The goal here is to off-load as many responsibilities as possible from the shoulders of the physician to less costly (and often more specifically trained) members of the care delivery team. Because these shared medical appointments occur in a group setting (i.e., where all can simultaneously listen and learn), a broader scope of prevention and disease self-management information can be efficiently delivered—and this can be accomplished while greater attention is also paid to the psychosocial and educational needs of patients, which can drive so many office visits.

The Greatest Untapped Resource in Medicine Today—The Patients Themselves

I have always felt that perhaps the greatest untapped resource available to medical groups around the world

(and one that group visits fully tap into) is the patients themselves—not only in their own disease self-management but also in the altruistic sense of helping one another. Because they efficiently incorporate not only all the elements of the traditional individual office visit but also the help and support of other patients (as well as a multidisciplinary treatment team), group visits offer many advantages in the treatment of the chronically ill. Because shared medical appointments also have the potential to provide more time with the physician, unimpeded access to care, greater patient education, more attention to psychosocial needs, and closer follow-up care, they offer an ideal venue for treating both the chronically ill and the elderly.

SMAs Validate Patients as Legitimate Sources of Information and Help

As patients share helpful information, encourage each other, learn from one another, and provide an incentive to each other for improving their health, group visits validate patients as legitimate sources of information for other patients. It is amazing how much more effective an animated positive report from one patient proclaiming success with a particular dietary, exercise, smoking, or medication change can be in motivating others to also comply with recommended treatment regimens than can the advice or admonitions of the physician. Also, because of the warm, relaxing, and supportive nature of the group environment, patients often volunteer sensitive personal issues more readily than they would during regular individual visits with their physician. This social support can not only reduce the feelings of isolation, alienation, anxiety, and despair that chronically ill and geriatric patients so often experience, but also provide a healing balm that comforts and consoles—and accomplish all of this while validating patients as legitimate sources of information and help.

Patient Participation Is a Critical Ingredient to a Successful SMA Program

Because patients are the key underlying ingredient to the interactive educational and emotionally supportive processes that occur in the group visit milieu, patient participation is critical to the full success of any group visit program—which is something that patients need to be reminded of and valued for. It is important to recognize that, in addition to the physician actually providing medical care, patients are themselves primary caregivers in their own chronic disease management. They are the ones having the most first-hand experience in coping with their illness and in developing the requisite coping skills. It is the relationships between patients, as well as a healthy group dynamic, that are the keys to this interactive process—i.e., to enabling patients to help and support each other and to building the necessary self-efficacy skills. Although no patient is required to comment at any particular time during the SMA session, nonparticipation could negatively impact both effective group dynamics and the potential benefit that each patient receives. Therefore, it is critically important that patients be strongly encouraged to speak candidly and openly during every SMA session. As can be seen, it is essential that group interaction be fostered to the appropriate degree and that any contributions by patients are acknowledged as being worthwhile and valuable.

DIGMAs Offer Singular Benefits to Chronic Disease Management

DIGMAs were specifically designed to: (1) dramatically increase physician productivity (by 200–300% or more); (2) improve patients' access to medical care through use of existing resources; (3) provide more time with the patient's own physician, a more relaxed pace of care, and closer follow-up care; (4) integrate the help and support of others dealing with similar experiences into each patient's healthcare experience; (5) enhance quality, increase patient education, and better attend to patients' psychosocial needs; (6) reduce repetition, increase efficiency, and strengthen the bottom line (although cost-effectiveness requires consistently maintaining targeted census levels); (7) increase patient and physician satisfaction; (8) provide medical care from start to finish (i.e., as a series of individual office visits with observers); (9) provide only medically necessary visits (as patients only come in when they have an actual medical need); and (10) enable physicians to better manage both chronic illnesses and busy, backlogged practices.

In terms of a treatment paradigm for the population management of various types of chronically ill patients, DIGMAs offer certain advantages over CHCCs because: (1) they are open to virtually all patients having that particular chronic illness (i.e., rather than just the same 15–20 high utilizers being covered over time, as is the case for CHCCs); and (2) patients can come into any DIGMA session they wish, whenever they have a medical need and want to be seen (as opposed to coming into a prescheduled series of visits regardless of whether or not they happen to have a medical need, as with CHCCs and Specialty CHCCs). With DIGMAs, patients can typically be seen any week that they

happen to have a medical need (or any day, in the case of daily DIGMAs)—although sessions could be held more or less frequently.

An additional advantage of the DIGMA model is the fact that DIGMAs provide accessible care to all chronically ill patients who are willing to attend even a single session, no matter how weak their motivation might be—as, unlike CHCCs, they do not need to initially commit to coming on an ongoing basis. Finally, because DIGMAs permit patients to come in whenever they have a medical need, different patients typically attend each session—which is diametrically opposed to the CHCC model in which the same 15–20 patients are followed over time, with all patients needing to start at the same time. This means that every DIGMA session is open to all (or almost all) patients in the chronic illness population management program, and that they are welcome to come in any time that they happen to have a medical need. Therefore, DIGMAs are unique with regard to the exceptional access to care that they can provide within a chronic disease management program—even with patients only willing to commit to just coming once.

Also, because they focus upon delivery of medical care from start to finish (and because they can best be conceptualized as a series of individual office visits with observers attending to each patients unique medial needs individually), DIGMAs are never perceived as classes—which can be the case for CHCCs. Furthermore, DIGMAs are often billed by fee-for-service organizations through use of existing E&M codes according to the level of care delivered and documented (although they do not typically bill for either counseling time or the behaviorist's time). Finally, while DIGMAs are primarily used for return or follow-up visits, they can also be used to intake new patients into a chronic disease management program—unless the intake process requires a physical exam that must be completed in the privacy of the exam room (for example, because it involves disrobing), in which case the Physicals SMA model would instead be used for intakes.

For these same reasons, DIGMAs are ideal not only for chronic disease population management programs, but for lifestyle medicine as well—i.e., where the goal is for certain patient populations to make important and appropriate lifestyle changes (in such behaviors as diet, exercise, smoking, etc.). The same is true for geriatric patients, where the remarkable combination of benefits that DIGMAs (as well as CHCCs) offer can provide a remarkable level of care to these medically needy and often time-consuming patients—and do so while also bringing a certain degree of relief and joy back into the practice of medicine for the providers treating them.

DIGMAs Also Offer Some Disadvantages to Chronic Disease Management

On the other hand, while DIGMAs offer many advantages over CHCCs in chronic illness population management programs, they also suffer from a couple of disadvantages. For example, because different patients attend each session, DIGMAs have the disadvantage of requiring constant vigilance as to census—which is a less critical issue for CHCCs once the 15–20 committed, high-utilizing patients have initially been selected. In addition, although adequate, patient bonding is generally less for DIGMAs than for CHCCs—as patients in some CHCC groups have already been meeting together for over 10 years. In addition, while both require nursing personnel and a program coordinator, DIGMAs require certain additional personnel that CHCCs do not—the most obvious of which are the behaviorist, the documenter, and the dedicated scheduler.

Because different patients typically attend every DIGMA session, and sometimes include patients attending for the first time, another weakness lies in the importance of conservatively handling the entire issue of confidentiality. With DIGMAs, it is particularly important that patients know what to expect and understand that their medical issues will be discussed in front of others in the group setting. In addition, I always have every attendee (patients and their support persons) sign a confidentiality release prior to the start of every DIGMA and PSMA session, a release which makes clear that, by signing, patients are affirming that they will hold confidential anything that is said about other patients in the group setting—and to not disclose this information to anyone else after the group is over. This critically important issue of confidentiality is covered in the following quotation taken from Dorothy L. Pennachio's cover story entitled "Should you offer group visits?" in the August 8, 2003 issue of Medical Economics (which includes quotes from Steve Ingraham, an attorney with Harris Beach in Rochester, NY, and from D'Arcy Guerin Gue of Phoenix Health Systems in Montgomery Village, MD) (1):

> "HIPAA doesn't prevent people from voluntarily discussing personal health information with others. The intent is to protect patients' privacy," says Ingraham. "The focus of the privacy standards is on the doctor, whether he treats one-on-one or in a group. He has obligations under HIPAA with respect to permissible disclosures." This means a doctor can't reveal personal health information acquired from a patient during a group session for nontreatment purposes, such as research, publication, or promotion—any more than he can reveal information learned during a one-on-one visit, unless the patient authorizes him to do so. "Beyond that, there's nothing in HIPAA that precludes group appointments, provided the patients are willing and competent to participate," says Ingram. D'Arcy Guerin Gue of Phoenix Health Systems

in Montgomery Village, MD, advises caution, though: "HIPAA's read on group visits hasn't been tested, but I suggest erring on the side of conservatism. If tested, a decision by HHS would come down on the side of the patient"(2).

CHCCs Also Have Unique Advantages and Disadvantages

However, CHCCs do offer certain advantages. Because the care provided in a CHCC focuses upon the same 15–20 patients over time, the patient bonding and continuity of care—as well as the quality of care—can be exceptional for these patients. On the other hand, CHCCs also have several disadvantages because they fail to offer many of the advantages that DIGMAs do when it comes to managing the chronically ill. For example, CHCCs fail to offer the convenience of being able to drop in and require that patients only enter during prescheduled sessions—which might be held on a monthly basis or, in the case of the Specialty CHCC, sessions could be held according to a schedule recommended by best practices. Also, because CHCCs involve patients committing to attend a series of ongoing follow-up visits, they are used for follow-ups rather than new patient intakes—whereas DIGMAs can be used for both, so long as the exam does not require disrobing and can be completed in the group setting (or else the PSMA model would be used). Furthermore, with CHCCs, patients would be expected to come for each session—i.e., regardless of whether or not they happened to have a medical need at that time.

One of the major drawbacks of the CHCC model is that participation would likely be limited to a relatively small percentage of all the chronically ill patients in the program—perhaps to just 15–20 high-utilizing patients, because that is where the economic offset is. However, it is important to keep in mind that only approximately 40% of these high utilizers will make the necessary commitment to attend regularly. Therefore, the CHCC might not be so useful for the remaining 60% of high utilizers—as well as for the low and moderate utilizers in the program (which will likely be the vast majority of chronically ill patients in the program). Whereas CHCCs provide excellent and accessible care for the 15 or 20 high-utilizing chronically ill patients fortunate enough to attend regularly, they do little to either increase physician productivity or to solve access problems—nor do they provide ongoing care for the vast majority of patients in the disease management program who happen to have that particular chronic illness (i.e., all the other patients who are not a part of the 15–20 patients in the CHCC program, as it is not open to them). It is for reasons such as these that the DIGMA model provides the backbone of the proposed chronic disease population management program.

A Few Comparative Comments on Use of CHCCs and DIGMAs in Chronic Disease Management Programs

As can be seen, DIGMAs and CHCCs are both important and solid group visit models for the follow-up visits of established patients—models that can play important roles in chronic disease management programs. However, these models are also very different in design, accomplish different ends, have different strengths and weaknesses, are open to different groups of patients—and would appear to have different billing issues. However, because of these differences, CHCCs and DIGMAs provide complementary shared medical appointment models for follow-up visits. They can, and do, work very well together in actual practice. In addition, they also combine well with both individual office visits and Physicals SMAs (which is the preferred group visit model when the physical examinations involve disrobing and/or must be conducted in private).

In chronic disease management programs, the bulk of appointments will be for follow-up visits—which means that DIGMAs and CHCCs will be of paramount importance here. Although improved access to private physical exams can sometimes be important, it is clear that the CHCC and DIGMA models will play the major role in chronic illness population management programs because of their focus upon return or follow-up visits (although sometimes DIGMAs are also used for new patient intakes). With the same 15–20 patients returning on a monthly basis to all sessions, CHCCs tend to focus upon a small but costly subsegment of the chronic disease management program—i.e., high-utilizing, multi-morbid geriatric patients. Therefore, CHCCs would most likely be used in the individual case management component of a chronic illness population management paradigm (provided that the case manager had enough patients to fill a CHCC), although DIGMAs could be used for these very high risk patients as well.

With different patients typically attending every session (and all qualifying patients invited to attend whenever they have a medical need and want to be seen), DIGMAs are unlike CHCCs in that they typically cover most or all of the patients in the provider's practice or in the chronic illness program. In addition, patients can come into any DIGMA session they wish (i.e., whenever they have a medical need) rather than being expected to start at the same time and then return on a prescheduled monthly basis—i.e., regardless of whether or not they happen to have a medical need at that time, as is the case for the CHCC. An additional important

distinction is that DIGMAs leverage existing resources to dramatically increase productivity, improve access, and deliver medical care from start to finish. From the standpoint of chronic disease management programs, DIGMAs therefore offer many critically important and uniquely beneficial features.

Unlike CHCCs, which are typically held monthly, all patients within a diabetes program would be invited to come into DIGMAs any week that they had a medical need—i.e., assuming that the DIGMA is held weekly. Furthermore, unlike CHCCs, chronically ill patients within the diabetes program would be invited to attend DIGMAs regardless of whether they are high or low utilizers, compliant or noncompliant, motivated to attend on an ongoing basis or not, and irrespective of how long it has been since their last visit. Although the CHCC and DIGMA models can both offer high-quality care, improved outcomes, excellent patient education, the help and support of others, private time with the physician, and high levels of patient and physician professional satisfaction, it is important to keep the defining characteristics and benefits (as well as the weaknesses) of each model in mind when you are designing your chronic illness population management program and selecting which model to use.

A Comprehensive SMA Treatment Paradigm for Managing Chronic Illnesses

A comprehensive treatment paradigm that especially involves DIGMAs (but also CHCCs and PSMAs) for the population management of various chronic illnesses is depicted in Fig. 7.1. This chronic disease management paradigm, which fully utilizes group visits, consists of three basic

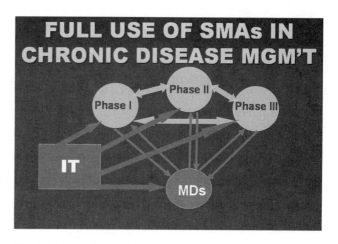

Fig. 7.1 A comprehensive treatment paradigm for all types of chronic illnesses that makes full use of group visits (as well as other types of group-based programs)

components. *First*, a system-wide capability (often an IT function) for identifying, assessing, tracking, and referring chronically ill patients into the appropriate form of care within the proposed chronic illness treatment program. However, direct referrals from providers throughout the entire system could also be made into the various components of the disease management program.

Second, there is a critically important 3-phase chronic illness treatment pathway for delivering the appropriate types of care to all of the patients in the program having this particular chronic illness. In the case of diabetes, these three phases would likely include: (1) a Phase 1 diabetes education class as an entry point into the program; then (2) a whole host of additional Phase 2 programs (most of which would be group based) for delivering additional care; and finally (3) a Phase 3 individual case management component for those patients at highest risk. *Third*, group visits would be used in the practices of virtually all of the providers attached to the chronic illness treatment program who are delivering medical care to these chronically ill patients. So as to leverage their time and maintain good access to their appointments.

An overarching principal of this proposed chronic illness treatment paradigm is that it be possible to expeditiously refer patients from any one component to any other within 1 week's time—i.e., that there be no bottlenecks at any point in the paradigm with regard to appropriately referring patients from any one element to another in a timely manner. Because of the large number of patients anticipated to be enrolled in any such disease management program, it is anticipated that—in order to leverage resources sufficiently to achieve this degree of accessibility throughout—it is likely that almost all of the care delivered in each component of the proposed paradigm would need to be provided in groups. Group visits would therefore be employed for the vast majority of medical care delivered, with individual office visits largely being reserved for applications where SMAs are not appropriate. In terms of the group visit models to be employed in the various components of this paradigm, it is the DIGMA model that would be the primary *workhorse* playing the major role, followed by the CHCC (which would likely be used to a considerably lesser extent) and then the PSMA—which would only be used in a limited way, as it would be reserved for those patients requiring a private physical examination.

First Component: A System for Identifying, Assessing, Tracking, and Placing All Diabetic Patients into the Program

The first step in the proposed population management program for diabetic patients (or for any other chronic illness) is

to establish a reliable, cost-effective IT system—including the necessary personnel, resources, computer systems, and processes—for identifying and tracking all diabetic patients within the healthcare organization, and for placing them into the appropriate care pathway within the chronic illness treatment program. In addition, direct referrals from physicians and other providers throughout the entire system could also be made into the chronic disease management program in a similar manner. The IT system must ensure that all diabetic patients are afforded ongoing monitoring and surveillance and that they are referred at proper times into the appropriate treatment modalities. This IT function needs to determine which patients within the system have a diagnosis of diabetes, and then ensure that they are referred into the appropriate level of treatment within the proposed diabetes disease management program—i.e., for their needs and stage of illness (with the most common entry point being placement into Phase 1 of the 3-phase care pathway).

Ideally, this should be a comprehensive, ongoing system for identifying, placing, and monitoring the progress of all diabetic patients—one that should play an important role throughout all stages in the treatment of diabetes to ensure that all affected patients are receiving appropriate care, and that no patients end up *slipping through the cracks*. Additionally, this system must be capable of tracking outcomes and performance measures. For most patients, regardless of whether they are referred into the program through the IT system or by direct physician referral, entry into this chronic disease management program will involve referral into Phase 1 of the proposed chronic illness treatment paradigm. In the example of diabetes that we are using in this chapter, Phase 1 would most likely be the diabetes education class.

Second Component: A 3-Phase Care Pathway

For this proposed chronic illness treatment paradigm, which is meant to make full use of group visits, the second component is a 3-phase care pathway.

Phase 1—The Diabetes Education Class

Phase 1 is the educational, self-help component of the proposed chronic illness treatment paradigm—i.e., the diabetes education class. Because patient education and the presentation of critically important information regarding the basics of diabetes and its treatment are the central focus of Phase 1, it is here that information about diet, exercise, medications, available treatments, insulin, and disease self-management skills are taught.

Allow Patients to Enter the Diabetes Education Class at Any Point

Phase 1 would normally consist of between one and five diabetes education class sessions, with one to three sessions being most typical. If the diabetes education class consists of more than one session, then I would strongly recommend that these sessions be designed in such a manner that patients are able to enter into the program during any of the sessions and then cycle through the entire sequence of sessions from that point forward in a manner that best fits their own schedule. This allows for best possible access to the program—i.e., for prompt placement of all patients into the program within 1 week's time.

It Is Here that the Basics About Diabetes and Its Treatment Are Taught

In Phase 1, patients are taught the basics about diabetes and its treatment—i.e., what diabetes is, its various forms and progressive nature, and the different types of treatments that are currently available. They also learn about the importance of: (1) making key lifestyle changes (such as diet, exercise, and smoking cessation); (2) complying with recommended medical regimens; (3) keeping blood glucose levels under tight control and within an acceptable range; and (4) understanding the potential long-term health consequences of this disease (hyperglycemia, hypoglycemia, hypertension, hyperlipidemia, neuropathy, retinopathy, nephropathy, cardiovascular complications, amputations, strokes, heart attacks, etc.). In addition, patients learn about the various healthcare services that are available to them (both internally and externally), how and when to access these services, how to make the best use of these services, the potential consequences of noncompliance, and the importance of appropriate and ongoing treatment—and of keeping all their appointments.

The Nutritional Aspects of Dealing with Diabetes Are Also Taught in Phase 1

It is in the diabetes education class (which constitutes Phase 1 of the proposed chronic illness treatment paradigm) that patients also learn about meal planning, the food pyramid, how to count carbohydrates, the importance of maintaining ideal body weight, and the critical role that proper nutrition can play in the effective self-management of diabetes. Patients also learn about resources available to them—e.g., the proposed diabetes program, smoking cessation classes, health education and exercise classes, mental health services, diabetes support groups in the community, weight control programs, etc.

The Importance of Exercise Is Also Taught During Phase 1

The need for proper exercise—particularly the need for aerobic exercise and improving one's body mass index (BMI)—is also explained to patients in Phase 1. It is here that patients learn about the different types of exercise they can undertake with benefit, the need to start slow and to build up gradually, the way to employ interval training, and the importance of involving their medical care team in decisions regarding exercise. It is here that the importance of selecting an appropriate form of exercise that one enjoys and can *stick with* over time is also emphasized.

The Different Medication Treatments Can Also Be Covered in Phase 1

Patients can also be taught about the different kinds of oral medications and insulin regimens currently available for treating diabetes, the potential side effects of these treatments, and when and how to take/inject these medications. The Phase 1 diabetes education class can also include discussions regarding injection site rotation and the possible use of pill boxes (i.e., with clearly labeled compartments for daily doses) so as to avoid patients forgetting about whether or not they have taken their pills. They can also be taught how to properly store their insulin and how to dispose of syringes and needles. In addition, the diabetes education class can teach patients about how to test their blood glucose levels—and the importance of regularly checking these levels each day according to the regimen their doctor has prescribed for them (but often before and after meals, as well as upon arising and at bedtime). They also learn about the importance of tracking their test results on an ongoing basis in a logbook or diary as well as the significance of having their glycosylated hemoglobin level checked at periodic intervals.

During Phase 1, Patients Also Meet, Support, and Learn from Each Other

It is in the Phase 1 diabetes education classes that patients have an opportunity to meet one another during group meetings, and to share with each other some helpful hints and successful coping strategies that they have learned. It is for this reason that I recommend that the Phase 1 diabetes education classes be somewhat interactive in nature—i.e., rather than just being a lecture-type class format—as patients will likely learn more and it will better hold their interest. Patients in attendance learn that the concern and support of others can help them to feel better, to cope more effectively with their disease, and possibly even to have better outcomes. In addition, patients learn that coping with diabetes can be stressful, can involve multiple losses, and will likely include significant lifestyle changes. They gain understanding about how stress can impact blood glucose levels and can even be taught specific stress management techniques that can be employed to help them deal more effectively with their disease.

Phase 1 Will Be Enough for Some Patients, but Not for Others

For many patients, Phase 1 of the 3-phase chronic illness care pathway that is being proposed here will provide them with enough information to understand and control their diabetes—at least at this point in time. For them, the diabetes education class will be sufficient to: motivate them to comply with recommended treatment regimens; help them to gain the skills necessary to self-manage their disease; and enable them to make the best use of their future medical appointments. Unfortunately, there will likely also be many other diabetic patients for whom Phase 1 will not be sufficient—i.e., Phase 1 will not provide these patients with enough information, support, and help for them to be able to appropriately self-manage and cope effectively with their disease. Such patients will therefore need more than Phase 1. In most cases, such patients will subsequently need to attend one or more of the various programs in Phase 2 (and in some cases, even Phase 3) of the proposed 3-phase care pathway for the treatment of diabetes. One of the goals of the proposed chronic illness treatment paradigm is, whenever possible, to keep patients from deteriorating to the point that they need Phase 3 (individualized case management) care; therefore, a whole host of Phase 2 programs must be employed to reduce this risk.

Phase 2—An Assortment of Relevant Group Programs

Phase 2 in this proposed chronic illness population management paradigm, which naturally is located between Phase 1 and Phase 3 of the 3-phase care pathway, is for those patients who do not yet qualify for Phase 3 (i.e., individual case management)—yet need more than the Phase 1 diabetes education class because their diabetes is still not sufficiently tightly controlled. Due to limited resources and the large number of chronically ill patients likely to be in a chronic illness population management program, the great majority of these Phase 2 programs are likely to be group programs in order to adequately handle the high anticipated patient volume. In Phase 2, we might have smoking cessation groups, chronic illness support groups, cognitive behavioral treatment programs for depression and anxiety, nutrition

classes, exercise groups, etc. These Phase 2 programs could include behavioral medicine group programs, psychiatry groups, health education classes, support groups, community programs, and any other types of lifestyle or disease-specific group programs that these patients might require.

These Phase 2 group programs are specifically designed for those chronically ill patients requiring additional help beyond Phase 1, as most of these patients will have already completed Phase 1. In our example of a diabetes population management program, the therapeutic goal of these Phase 2 programs would be to provide the additional medical care, information, emotional support, disease self-management skills, and resources required for these patients to get their diabetes under better and tighter control as quickly as possible. Clearly, the goal of these Phase 2 group programs is to give these patients what they need and to keep them from deteriorating to the point where they reach Phase 3—i.e., individual case management.

In Phase 2, Many Types of Group Programs (as well as SMAs) Can Be Utilized

It is in Phase 2 that the various types of group programs (including possibly some group visit programs) can play their greatest role. It is here, in Phase 2, that such group programs as weight management groups, smoking cessation classes, nutritional classes, exercise programs, hypertension and hyperlipidemia programs, cognitive behavioral treatment programs for depression and anxiety, chronic illness support groups, grief groups, and caregivers groups can all be offered. However, group visits such as DIGMAs and CHCCs can also be used not only in Phase 2 but also in Phase 3 as well as in the practices of all of the providers attached to the chronic illness program—which is where SMAs can play their greatest role. However, this is only true if these programs are promoted well enough to ensure that enough patients are willing and able to attend to keep all such group visit sessions filled to targeted census levels, so that census requirements for these SMA programs can be consistently met.

Mid-Level Providers Often Provide Most Phase 2 Care

In actual practice, it is often mid-level providers (nurses, diabetic nurse educators, social workers, psychologists, etc.) with a special interest in working with chronically ill patients (diabetic patients in the example being discussed here) who are involved with many of these Phase 2 group programs. However, group visits such as DIGMAs, CHCCs, and PSMAs will clearly need to involve a medical provider (physicians, nurse practitioners, physician assistants, etc.) attached to the chronic illness program.

The Precise Content of Phase 2 Programs Will Vary According to Need

The exact types of Phase 2 group programs offered, as well as the precise content of these programs, will vary according to the particular needs of the chronically ill patients attending the programs. Although some individualized care could also be made available to certain chronically ill patients on an as-needed basis, Phase 2 programs in the proposed paradigm would characteristically be group based—and built upon best practices whenever possible—so as to best serve the needs of the anticipated large volume of patients. These Phase 2 group programs could include educational, support, behavioral medicine, and mental health groups in addition to SMAs. In addition to being efficient and cost-effective, these reasonably large group programs would also provide the help and support of other patients dealing with similar issues—i.e., as well as a multidisciplinary care delivery team. Because of the helpful presence of other patients, these Phase 2 group programs could offer not only additional patient education and emotional support but also closer attention to such important psychosocial issues as patient noncompliance—and accomplish all this while expanding upon the medical and self-care information presented in Phase 1.

Phase 3—Individual Case Management

In the 3-phase care pathway of the proposed comprehensive chronic illness treatment paradigm making full use of group visits, Phase 3 represents the individualized case management of those patients who are at greatest risk because their disease is most out of control. In the example of diabetes being used here, Phase 3 would be the intensive, individualized case management stage of diabetes care for those diabetic patients whose illness is advancing most severely. Although each system will have its own particular cutoff point for patients to qualify for Phase 3, this criterion is often something like HbA1c levels over 10, 11, or 12. Phase 3 will often include patients having advanced disease, those whose disease is currently most out of control, those with compliance issues, and patients who are high utilizers of healthcare services.

While Phase 3 Is Primarily for Individualized Case Management, SMAs Can Also Be Used

It is in Phase 3 of the proposed population management paradigm for treating chronically illnesses that individualized case management is typically provided for these high-risk patients—often by mid-level providers such as nurses and medical social workers. The goal in Phase 3 is to provide individualized case management—i.e., to deliver close, appropriate, and ongoing monitoring and care to these high-risk and costly patients so that they can get their diabetes under better control as quickly as possible. The hope here is that this improved control will occur before further and irreversible medical damage is suffered by the patient, and before the healthcare system incurs the additional cost of a chronic illness unnecessarily turning into an acute medical emergency. However, this having been said, the DIGMA and CHCC models can still play an important role in Phase 3—provided that enough Phase 3 patients are willing and able to attend the group visit so that census requirements can be met and the program can be economically sustainable. By using group visits, the individual case manager's time can be leveraged and more patients reached with the care that they need. As an additional healthcare choice, the group visit format will actually turn out to be the preferred care delivery modality for many of these patients. The CHCC model would be used in Phase 3 when one desires to set up say monthly meetings with the same group of out-of-control diabetics over time, and where these same 10–20 patients would be expected to attend all periodically scheduled sessions. On the other hand, DIGMAs would typically be held on a weekly basis and could be attended by most if not all Phase 3 diabetic patients; however, different patients would typically attend each session as they would only attend DIGMA sessions when they had an actually medical need to be seen.

A Word of Caution Regarding Phase 3 SMAs

The one word of caution here is that—because Phase 3 DIGMAs consist solely of patients with HbA1c levels over some criterion level, say 10 or 11—they are often filled with noncompliant patients who minimize or deny their disease, and those who are living their lives in a singularly unhealthy manner. Therefore, the word of caution here is that these patients are often all-too-willing to support each other's noncompliant and unhealthy behaviors. In such DIGMAs, it is not uncommon to hear one patient say to another something like, "Yeah, I know exactly what you mean, Jim. Like you, I've also eaten red meat and cheese all my life—and I'm not about to change now either!" Or patients might say, "The doctor told me the same thing and actually expects me to quit smoking. It's easy for her to say, but I've also been smoking for over 40 years. I can't quit now, and I'm not about to. I understand exactly how you feel." Or else, a patient might say something like the following to another patient that is resisting the doctor's advice to start exercising: "I'm like you. I hate to exercise. I don't like getting all sweaty and tired out either. I just don't see the sense of it. I understand what you're saying."

Individual Case Managers Using Group Visits Must Be Ready to Promptly Handle Certain Challenges

Clearly, any provider running DIGMAs or CHCCs for Phase 3 patients will need to be aware of this, and will need to promptly confront such poor advice from other patients in the group whenever such comments and recommendations are put forth—i.e., by other patients whose HbA1c is also currently out of control. I have only found this tendency for patients to side with one another's noncompliance (i.e., rather than with the doctor's recommended medical advice) to occur in DIGMAs consisting almost solely of patients whose chronic illness is out of control. It is for this reason that I usually choose to not run DIGMAs solely for patients with out-of-control diabetic symptoms, and generally prefer to include patients with a wide range of HbA1c levels. This is because the patient whose HbA1c used to be over 10—but has worked very hard to gain tighter glucose control during the past year, and is now below 6—will often not be tolerant of such erroneous advice being offered by patients whose diabetes is still out of control. This patient will therefore likely strongly support the advice that the physician is giving to such patients in the group setting. This does not mean that Phase 3 DIGMAs cannot be run; it simply means that extra effort will need to be taken by both the physician and the behaviorist to remain ever-vigilant to this possibility, and to counter such counterproductive advice from other patients promptly just as soon as it occurs.

Third Component: SMAs in the Practices of All Providers Attached to the Chronic Illness Program

In the chronic illness treatment program depicted in Fig. 7.1 (which makes full use of the multiple benefits that group visits can offer, and covers all patients having a particular chronic illness within the system), the third critical component is to have all providers attached to the program—at least those providers willing to do so—run SMAs for the chronic disease management program (and possibly also in their own separate practices).

SMAs (Especially DIGMAs) Offer Many Potential Benefits to the Chronically Ill

Because of the high volume of patient visits that are anticipated, it is likely that the providers attached to the chronic illness program will quickly become overwhelmed by patient demand unless their capacity is somehow increased to the

point where it balances demand—i.e., so that access problems do not develop in this paradigm at the provider level. The solution here is for providers in the program to make optimum use of group visits. By being highly productive and efficient, these SMAs could be designed to improve patient access to care and to enhance quality within the program. DIGMAs, CHCCs, and Physicals SMAs (and their various subtypes) could be used with benefit both in the proposed chronic illness population management program's 3-phase care pathway (especially in Phase 2, but possibly also in Phase 3) and in the practices of all providers involved with the program.

In addition to the potential for improving access, productivity, and efficiency by leveraging existing resources that these SMA models can offer, they can also provide chronically ill patients multiple quality, service, education, support, and patient satisfaction benefits as well. In addition to chronic disease management, group visits can also be extremely helpful in both geriatric and lifestyle medicine—i.e., due not only to the help and support of other patients in the group setting but also to the professional skills of the behaviorist (at least, in the DIGMA and PSMA models).

The homogeneous subtype of the DIGMA model is especially helpful in chronic disease management because it can positively impact all chronically ill patients of that particular diagnosis—both in the population management program and in each physician's practice (Fig. 7.2). Furthermore, DIGMAs are also particularly well suited to population management programs because they: offer drop-in convenience; are held frequently; are open to all appropriate chronically ill patients within the program (high and low

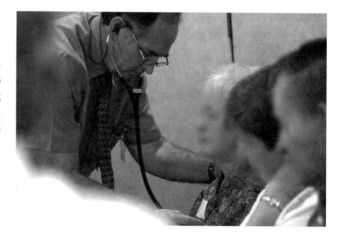

Fig. 7.2 To maximize efficiency while minimizing repetition, the proposed chronic disease management paradigm would have most or all providers attached to the program leveraging their time by running homogeneous DIGMAs in which follow-up care would be sequentially delivered to each patient individually—but in the group setting, whenever appropriate and possible. (Courtesy of Dr. Patricio Aycinena, Diabetes DIGMA, Cleveland Clinic, Cleveland, OH)

utilizers alike, as well as those not willing to commit to attending more than a single session); and deliver medical care from start to finish—i.e., in the group setting, where all present can listen, learn, ask questions, and interact.

In addition, patients can start attending the DIGMA any time that they have a medical need rather than only in a prescheduled series of appointments, like the CHCC. Therefore, all patients in the chronic illness treatment program can attend any DIGMA session they would like—i.e., rather than just the same group of 15–20 patients, who would need to start the CHCC at the same time, being followed as a group in a prescheduled series of appointments over time. However, CHCCs can play a helpful role in the treatment of the chronically ill, especially for treating the most costly and highest risk subset of patients in the program (especially in Phase 3). In other words, both CHCCs and, in some cases, PSMAs can play meaningful supportive roles in this chronic disease management paradigm, albeit a less important role than the homogeneous DIGMA model.

Access to the Chronic Illness Program Is Improved

By having all providers attached to the diabetes program run one or more homogeneous DIGMAs each week (and possibly a CHCC or Physicals SMA as well), the time of the providers attached to the program can be leveraged—hopefully, to the point where all diabetic patients within the program should be able to be seen in a timely manner whenever they have a medical need. Clearly, these DIGMAs can be a part of any provider's practice; however, they could also be specifically designed for the chronic illness treatment program as well. In the case of a diabetes program, the various internists, family practitioners, nurse practitioners, and endocrinologists attached to that program could have homogeneous or mixed DIGMAs specifically directed at diabetes, hypertension, hyperlipidemia, obesity, sleep apnea, etc.—or they could have a more heterogeneous "hyperlipodiabesity" DIGMA open to all endocrine syndrome patients in the event that pre-diabetic patients are also included in the disease management program.

In a similar manner, nephrologists attached to the diabetes population management program could run DIGMAs for hypertension, kidney disease, dialysis, predialysis, etc. Similarly, podiatrists could run Podiatry DIGMAs for diabetic foot care as well as for the various types of foot problems associated with diabetes. By offering group visits such as DIGMAs and PSMAs, all providers attached to your diabetes population management program would be able to dramatically increase their efficiency and productivity within the program—so that patients are always afforded prompt access into appropriate care. In addition, by offering CHCCs (which do not

increase physician productivity or improve access) to the most high-utilizing subsegment of the chronic illness population management program, these 15–20 patients could receive intensive care on a prescheduled basis—with the expected result being a reduction in ER, hospitalization, nursing home care, and referrals to specialists for this cohort of 15–20 high-risk patients.

In other words, by having all providers attached to the chronic disease management program offer DIGMAs on a weekly, twice-weekly, or even daily basis (while perhaps also offering them outside of their work within the program to better manage their own large, busy practices), access to these providers should be greatly improved (Fig. 7.3). The intent here is to improve access to these providers to the point where their appointments within the disease management program remain sufficiently open to referrals from all other components of the paradigm that any patients who are referred can be seen by these providers within a week. As depicted in Fig. 7.1, it permits patients to be promptly referred from any Phase 1, 2, or 3 program (or even from the IT function or other providers inside or outside of the program) in a timely manner into the DIGMA of the appropriate provider within the population management program.

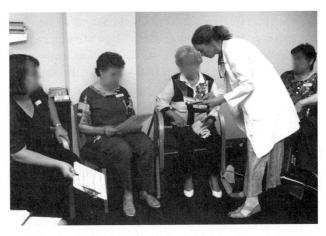

Fig. 7.3 Most follow-up visits within the proposed chronic illness population management program are seen in the highly efficient DIGMAs offered by providers attached to the program (rather than costly individual office visits), wherein most of the medical care (other than private matters) is delivered in the group setting. (Courtesy of Dr. Margaret Forsyth, Internal Medicine DIGMA, Palo Alto Medical Foundation, Palo Alto, CA)

In addition, although having homogeneous DIGMAs offered by most or all of the providers attached to the program would undoubtedly be best for the bulk of the patients within the population management program, also having a Specialty CHCC for the same group of 15–20 high-utilizing diabetic patients would enable the provider to follow this small but costly group of patients more closely over time.

This is also true in Phase 3 of the proposed paradigm, for those out-of-control diabetic patients at especially high risk to be high utilizers of healthcare services. Similarly, Physicals SMAs could also be used within the diabetes treatment program to efficiently provide any private physical examinations that might periodically be needed. However, because group visits are meant to be voluntary for patients and physicians alike, it goes without saying that for any patients who might refuse to attend a SMA, individual office visits should still be available to them as before.

Homogeneous DIGMAs Work in Chronic Disease Management Programs, but Less So in Providers' Own Practices

Please note that there are two major differences between the DIGMAs that are run by physicians involved with the chronic illness treatment paradigm under discussion and DIGMAs that are designed for these providers' own individual practices. *First* of all, DIGMAs that are a part of a chronic illness population management program are generally of a homogeneous design, so that the DIGMA focuses specifically upon patients with that particular illness or condition—and the various issues they must deal with. The homogeneous DIGMA design works well in this application because there are typically hundreds, thousands, or even tens of thousands of patients attached to a typical chronic illness population management program so that consistently filling all sessions of a homogeneous DIGMA is not that difficult.

Because so many patients having a particular diagnosis or condition are referred into the disease management program by IT and multiple providers throughout the system, the issue of keeping a homogeneous DIGMA filled to targeted census levels becomes less of an issue than it would be if it were only for the physician's own practice. This is because, even in primary care, the physician's own practice would typically include only 1–3 thousand patients in total—of which only a relatively small percentage would have that particular chronic illness (and most of these would not have a medical need to be seen at any given time). Homogeneous DIGMAs for physicians' own practices are typically more challenging to consistently fill because only a relatively small percentage of the physician's own practice (perhaps just 10–30%) would typically have any given chronic illness such as diabetes, CHF, or hypertension. Therefore, only a comparatively small number of patients from the physician's own practice would qualify to attend any particular session, so that homogeneous DIGMA sessions for the physician's own practice could be difficult to consistently fill.

A *second* difference is that chronic illness SMAs offered through a chronic disease management program lack continuity of care in that they are typically open to all patients with that disease who are interested in attending, and most of these patients will have been referred from other physicians practices throughout the system for that component of their care—although some of these patients might well come from the provider's own panel. By way of contrast, DIGMAs that are designed for better managing a providers' own busy, backlogged practices are typically open only to patients from that provider's own practice—so that continuity of care with the patient's own provider is ensured.

Group Visits Enable the Program's High Workload Demands to be Met

In this paradigm, enough providers must be involved with the chronic illness population management program to systematically meet the predicted high volume of demand for medical services that is expected to be generated by the large number of chronically ill patients with a particular diagnosis that are covered. In order to be able to productively meet the anticipated high level of demand generated by a chronic illness treatment program, DIGMAs (and to a lesser extent, CHCCs, Physicals SMAs, and other group visit models still to be developed) need to be frequently employed throughout. With DIGMAs and Physicals SMAs, the goal would typically be to triple the provider's productivity (i.e., vs. individual visits) during the same amount of time. This would not hold true for CHCCs, which have been demonstrated to provide other types of benefits—but not to substantially leverage the physician's time.

In effect, by tripling the provider's productivity during a 90-minute DIGMA, one would increase the number of patients that a full-time provider attached to the chronic illness program could see each week by approximately 8–10% (16–20% in the case of half-time providers). For full-time physicians running two, three, or even five successful DIGMAs per week for the program, these numbers would increase to 16–20%, 24–30%, and 40–50%, respectively—percentages that would be twice as large for half-time providers within the program. The latter is important because many of the providers attached to the chronic disease management program will only work part-time within the program; therefore, by leveraging this time through DIGMAs, they can experience a tremendous increase in their productivity within the program.

Simply put, such large increases in productivity are critical to the success of any chronic illness population management program due to the high volume of anticipated patient demand for medical services from such a large number of high-risk patients. For example, in the case of a diabetes population management program, the incidence of Type 2 diabetes in this country is currently reaching epidemic proportions—which places great workload demands upon the providers participating in the program. This high level of patient demand simply cannot be efficiently and cost-effectively addressed through traditional individual office visits alone; therefore, the multiple efficiency, economic, and quality benefits that well-run DIGMAs and other group visit models can offer are much needed in diabetes treatment programs.

In other words, without offering a sufficient number of DIGMAs (and perhaps some CHCCs and Physicals SMAs as well) each week to stay on top of this high level of patient demand, the practices within the program (i.e., of any providers attached to the chronic illness treatment paradigm) could quickly become overwhelmed, backlogged, and inaccessible. An additional advantage of DIGMAs is that sessions can be max-packed, so that optimal care can be systematically and consistently provided according to the needs of patients with that particular chronic illness. This ensures that all desired care is provided to patients during each and every visit, and that all relevant health maintenance, injections, and performance measures can consistently be addressed and updated.

The Chronic Illness Treatment Program Must Be Well Promoted

Because patients find SMAs to be a dramatic departure from the traditional individual office visits to which they have become accustomed—and because of the high volume of diabetic patients expected to participate—it is imperative that a diabetes population management program be well promoted to all appropriate patients in order to get patients to voluntarily attend the DIGMAs (as well as any CHCCs and PSMAs) that are being offered. Therefore, for these group visit programs to be optimally successful, it is very important that all diabetic patients be strongly encouraged by providers and staff alike—through high-quality promotional materials and carefully worded personal invitations—to attend the SMAs that have been specifically designed for the diabetes treatment program.

SMAs Are Appropriate for Most, but Not All Diabetic Patients

It is important that traditional individual office visits be reserved for those patients truly needing them, as well as for those few patients who refuse to attend a SMA despite being informed about the program and strongly encouraged to attend. Meant to be voluntary to patients and providers alike, SMAs will not be appropriate for all patients and health conditions (e.g., monolingual patients speaking another language, patients too demented or

hearing impaired to benefit, highly contagious acute infectious illnesses, medical emergencies, etc.).

Experience has shown that some patients will always refuse to attend DIGMAs, CHCCs, and Physicals SMAs—although the number of such patients has been observed to decline over time as patients gradually become more accepting of these models and aware of the multiple benefits that they can offer. This having been said, it is nonetheless important to mention that many of the components in Phases 1, 2, and 3 of the proposed chronic illness treatment paradigm will be available in a group format only, with no comparable individual offering being available to patients—for instance, the diabetes education class that constitutes Phase 1 as well as many of the group programs in Phase 2 (such as anxiety and depression groups, support groups, smoking cessation classes, exercise programs, substance abuse programs, and nutrition classes).

Try to Have Most of the Chronic Illness Program's Providers Offer SMAs

By leveraging existing resources and having most, if not all, providers associated with the chronic illness population management program run one or more DIGMAs a week, patients should always be able to be seen promptly whenever they have a medical need that requires medical attention (e.g., within a week in the next available DIGMA session). Furthermore, one would want to have any CHCCs and Physicals SMAs available through the program to also remain accessible to patients. However, for reasons already discussed (e.g., by being offered frequently, having max-packed visits, offering drop-in convenience, and being open to all patients with a chronic illness whenever they have a medical need), the DIGMA model offers many unique advantages vs. other types of group visit models for population management programs.

Patients can attend a DIGMA through physician, staff, or self-referral—either by prescheduling the visit (which the vast majority of patients typically do) or by simply dropping in whenever they have a medical need. However, if they do drop in, patients are requested to telephone the office at least a day beforehand so that: (1) census can be monitored; (2) they can check to ensure that the session will in fact be meeting; (3) appropriate preparations for their attendance can be made; and (4) they can be telephoned should the group later need to be canceled at the last minute due to a clinic emergency or the physician being ill.

On the other hand, the goal is for patients to be able to be referred that same week into any DIGMA from any other component of the proposed chronic disease management paradigm by: (1) the IT system that has been instituted for identifying, assessing, tracking, and appropriately referring all diabetic patients within the healthcare delivery system; (2) the health educators or diabetes nurse educators running the Phase 1 diabetes education class; (3) the mid-level providers running the various Phase 2 group programs (as well as any providers running Phase 2 SMAs); (4) the individual case managers employed in Phase 3; or (5) any other provider attached to the chronic illness population management program.

There Needs to be a Prompt, Ongoing Exchange of Referrals Between All Parts of This Paradigm

There needs to be an open, timely, and free flowing exchange (or cross-referral) of patients between all components of this chronic illness treatment paradigm that makes full use of group visits—a prompt and fluid exchange that is only made possible by taking full advantage of the quality, efficiency, productivity, and access benefits that properly run SMAs can offer.

Referrals into the Phase 1 Diabetes Education Class

For example, whenever physicians or other providers attached to any phase of the proposed program see patients who do not have important basic knowledge about their illness and how to better manage it, they can promptly refer them back into the next available session of the Phase 1 diabetes education class for a refresher course. For this reason, the diabetes education class should ideally be set up so that patients can enter any week that they are referred (either for the first time or for a refresher course), even if these classes should be held as a series of multiple sessions. In the case of larger population management programs, it would even be better if such referrals to the diabetes education class could be made within a day or two.

Prompt Referrals from Phase 1 into Phase 2 and 3 Programs

If patients have already attended the Phase 1 diabetes education class, but are continuing to have problems controlling their diabetes or need some type of additional help, then they can be referred from Phase 1 into the next appropriate Phase 2 group session. Therefore, whenever possible, Phase 2 groups should also be designed so that patients can be referred into them within a week, if not sooner. For example, if there is a 10-week Phase 2 cognitive behavioral treatment program for depression,

then it should ideally be set up in such a way that patients can enter at any point (i.e., during any of the 10 weekly sessions) and then cycle through all 10 sessions from that point onward. Similarly, if the patient's diabetes is completely out of control, then the patient should be able to be promptly referred by any Phase 1 or 2 provider (or by any physician attached to the program) into an appropriate Phase 3 program for individualized case management—preferably within a week.

Prompt Referrals from the Physician to Phase 1, 2, and 3 Programs

Whenever physicians attached to this diabetes treatment program see diabetic patients (during either group or individual visits) who are in need of additional diabetic education, who require some Phase 2 group program, or who have out-of-control blood glucose levels that require Phase 3 care, it is important that they be able to promptly refer such patients directly into the appropriate Phase 1, 2, or 3 program, respectively, in this 3-phase care pathway (plus, be able to have the patient start that program within a week or two at most).

Physician Referrals to Phase 1

For example, whenever physicians or other providers attached to the program see patients (i.e., either in SMAs or in individual office visits) who do not have important basic knowledge about their illness or about how to better manage their disease, they can promptly refer them into the next available session of the appropriate Phase 1 program—either for the first time or for a refresher course. Remember that Phase 1 programs should be set up so that patients can enter during any session of the diabetes education class and then rotate through all sessions in a manner that best fits their own schedule. This allows patients to start Phase 1 any week that they are referred—or perhaps even any day in the case of larger population management programs where daily Phase 1 programs might be offered.

Physician Referrals to Phase 2 Programs

If the patients being referred by the physician attached to the program have already attended the Phase 1 program, but are continuing to have problems controlling their diabetes or making the necessary changes in lifestyle, then they could appropriately be referred by the provider either (1) back to Phase 1 for a *refresher* course, where they would be able to build further upon the knowledge that they might have already gained when they previously attended; or (2) into the next available Phase 2 program that the provider deems most appropriate for the patient—which, in this chronic illness treatment program paradigm, should ideally be available to the patient within a week, if not sooner (i.e., regardless of whether it is a health education class, behavioral medicine program, psychiatry group, support group, etc.).

Physician Referrals to Phase 3 Case Management

Similarly, if the patient's diabetes is completely out of control (i.e., their HbA1c level exceeds some benchmark criterion such as 10, 11, or 12), then the physician might refer the patient into Phase 3 for individualized case management—i.e., in the form of individual or group visits. Again, the chronic illness program should be set up in such a way that Phase 3 is promptly accessible to all patient referrals—preferably within a week or less. DIGMAs and CHCCs could be most helpful in achieving and maintaining this degree of accessibility in Phase 3, provided that enough patients are under individual case management to ensure that Phase 3 DIGMA and/or CHCC sessions can be kept full.

Physicians Can Also Refer Patients into the Practices of Other Providers Attached to the Program

In the event that the provider attached to the program is seeing a patient that they feel could benefit from seeing another provider in the program (such as an endocrinologist referring patients into a podiatrist's diabetic foot care DIGMA or a nephrologist's end-stage kidney disease DIGMA), then it is important that such referrals can be made that week—and with a minimum amount of physician time investment being required in this referral process. The best way that I know to maintain this degree of accessibility between providers in a large chronic disease management program is for all providers attached to the program to offer at least one (and preferably several) DIGMAs per week in order to leverage their time, avoid bottlenecks and backlogs, and always have at least a group visit appointment available to patients who are being referred so that they can be seen that week.

Referrals by Providers Can Be Made so as to Build in Continuity of Care

When the physician or other provider attached to the chronic disease management program makes such referrals to any of the components of this population management paradigm (either directly from the provider's own practice or from the provider's work within the chronic illness program), an additional benefit of this paradigm is that these referrals can be made in such a manner that continuity of care is built in. That is, the physician can tell the patient that is being referred into an appropriate Phase 1, Phase 2, or Phase 3 program (or into another provider's DIGMA within the program) to be certain to return to the physician's DIGMA (or for an individual visit, if that is what the physician or patient prefers) in a month or two so that the physician can personally evaluate and keep abreast of how well the patient is doing. This approach signals to patients that the physician is not making the referral to get rid of them, which can be a concern to patients when they are referred to another provider's program without the physician simultaneously offering a personal follow-up appointment back into their own practice in the near future. This signals to the patient that the physician is interested in them and will remain involved in their care over time.

Referrals *to the Physician* from IT and Phase 1, 2, and 3 Programs

On the other hand, referrals must be freely made not only from physicians attached to the program into Phase 1, Phase 2, and Phase 3 programs, but also back into these physicians' DIGMAs from any other component of the proposed paradigm. For this reason, it would be preferable for all providers attached to the chronic illness program to offer a DIGMA that meets at least once a week so that patients could be seen by the physicians any week that they are referred from these Phase 1, 2, and 3 programs—or directly into the physician's care either from other providers in the healthcare system or the IT system that identifies and appropriately refers patients. Without question, making the physicians attached to the proposed chronic disease management program promptly accessible to referrals from all other components of this care pathway (which can be achieved by starting DIGMAs for their practices that meet at least weekly) provides an extremely important ingredient toward achieving prompt accessibility within the program, even when the workload demands are heavy.

Then, whenever staff (i.e., health educators, diabetes nurse educators, behavioral medicine or mental health personnel, case management workers, etc.) involved in Phase 1, 2, or 3 programs spot a diabetic patient in attendance whom they feel might benefit from a prompt medical appointment (i.e., with an endocrinologist, nephrologist, internist, family practitioner, podiatrist, or other provider attached to the diabetes program), they could simply refer the patient to the appropriate physician's DIGMA that week.

Referrals from Phase 1 Providers

For example, whenever the health educators or diabetes nurse educators leading a Phase 1 diabetes education class hear from a patient about a serious or new diabetic symptom (such as disconcerting hypoglycemic episodes, a new foot lesion, shortness of breath, severe fatigue, or any other significant deterioration in the patient's health status), it is important that they be able to promptly refer that patient back into the physician's next available DIGMA session. Preferably, such referrals within this chronic illness paradigm should be able to be made that week—without any barriers to care—for any of the physicians, nurse practitioners, podiatrists, etc., attached to the chronic illness program.

Referrals from Phase 2 Providers

There will be occasions when a mid-level provider running a Phase 2 group program (such as a smoking cessation class, a depression program, a provider-led support group, a health education class, or a behavioral medicine group program) will hear from a patient about symptoms which the provider feels might require prompt medical attention. When this does happen, it is important that the Phase 2 provider be able to schedule the patient with a medical appointment in an appropriate physician's DIGMA within a week—i.e., into the care of a suitable physician attached to this chronic disease management program. In other words, the Phase 2 provider needs to be able to schedule such patients directly into the appropriate physician's next available DIGMA session (or into an individual appointment)—preferably within a week or at most two. However, if the Phase 2 group program happens to be a DIGMA or CHCC, then the provider running it (physician, nurse practitioner, PA, osteopath, podiatrist, etc.) might be able to directly address such medical problem during the session—and, if not, could then refer the patient into the appropriate physician's DIGMA for treatment that week.

Referrals from Phase 3 Providers

The same is true for the case managers involved in Phase 3, as they must remain ever-vigilant as to any significant changes in the health status of the high-risk, out-of-control diabetic patients with whom they are working. Phase 3 case managers will sometimes need to refer these high-risk diabetic patients promptly to a physician attached to the program for medical care—e.g., for the prompt treatment of serious new diabetic complications just as soon as they become aware of them. This necessitates that any such referrals to physicians in the program be able to be made promptly—preferably within a week—which is a level of accessibility which DIGMAs

can help them to achieve and maintain. In addition, it would be beneficial to have a same-day referral service to providers within the program for any urgent medical issues that might arise with patients being seen in any component of this paradigm which need to be dealt with immediately.

Referrals from Other Providers Attached to the Program

Similarly, it is important that other providers attached to the programs also have prompt and unfettered access to making referrals that week into the physician's DIGMA. For example, the podiatrist running the diabetic foot care DIGMA (or the nephrologists running the hypertension DIGMA) might want to refer some of their patients into the endocrinologist's diabetes DIGMA. When that happens, it is important that they be able to make such referrals that week.

IT Referrals from the System Set Up to Detect, Monitor, and Refer All Chronically Ill Patients

In addition, this IT system should be able to refer suitable patients directly into the practice of an appropriate physician attached to the program. Whenever the IT system that has been put in place to identify, track, and appropriately refer all diabetic patients within the system detects a patient that requires evaluation, monitoring, or treatment by a physician attached to the program, this patient should then be able to be promptly referred into the physician's next available DIGMA session within the disease management program—or into an individual appointment, if that is preferred. Having DIGMAs in their practices can help physicians in the program to achieve and maintain this level of unfettered access.

Similarly, this identification and referral system should be set up in such a manner that it can also promptly refer patients appropriately into all other components of this proposed chronic disease management paradigm. For example, it should be able to refer appropriate patients into any suitable Phase 1, 2, or 3 program—although most such referrals will typically be into the Phase 1 diabetes education class, which usually serves as the entry point into the chronic disease management program. This IT system can also offer the advantage of monitoring the progress of patients on an ongoing basis to ensure that no diabetic patient ends up being overlooked or *falling between the cracks*. That is, processes need to be put in place to follow the progress of all diabetic patients over time (including noncompliant patients, inappropriate low utilizers, etc.) to ensure that they are followed up with and provided with appropriate care in a timely manner.

Referrals Back and Forth Between Phase 1, 2, and 3 Programs

In addition, the providers in the Phase 1, 2, and 3 programs (which, for the most part, are group programs) also need to refer patients back and forth between their own programs. For example, the group leaders in the Phase 1 program might feel that certain patients, upon completing the diabetes education class, still need more information, support, or care—in which case, they might refer them directly into an appropriate Phase 2 group program (preferably, one that is sufficiently accessible so that such follow-up can occur within a week or two). In a similar manner, the mid-level providers offering Phase 2 group programs might spot patients who still do not understand the basics about diabetes (what it is, its treatment, disease self-management, lifestyle issues, etc.) and want to encourage these patients to return to Phase 1 for a repeat or refresher course. When this happens, it is important that the Phase 2 provider be able to readily make any such referrals back into Phase 1 that week.

Likewise, leaders in either Phase 1 or 2 programs will occasionally identify patients whose diabetes appears to be completely out of control, in which case they should be able to promptly refer them directly into Phase 3 to be evaluated for individualized case management that week—or else be able to refer them back to a physician attached to the program that week with the recommendation that these patients be evaluated for Phase 3 care.

In an identical manner, Phase 3 case managers might have some patients who need more basic information about their disease, in which case they might refer them back into a Phase 1 class—perhaps for a repeat or *refresher* course. Or these Phase 3 case managers might have some patients who improve to the point where they no longer need individualized case management, but could nonetheless benefit from some additional information, support, or care—in which case they might refer such patients into an appropriate Phase 2 group program (such as a provider-led diabetes support group, a cognitive behavioral depression program, a smoking cessation class, a weight loss group, a nutrition class, or an exercise class, etc.). Or else, they could refer such patients back into the DIGMA of the appropriate physician attached to the program that week for follow-up care.

When Finished with the Program, Patients Can Be Referred Back to Their Own Providers

When patients have completed this chronic disease management program and are now appropriately self-managing their disease, they can then either be referred back to their own providers for their follow-up care or else put into some type of *holding pattern* within the program—perhaps by seeing their own provider within the program at regular intervals (such as every 3–6 months) or on an as-needed basis. In any case, the patients will continue to see their own providers outside of the chronic disease population management program for all other aspects of their care. The only question is whether, after finishing the program and achieving the desired level of control over their chronic illness, the patient is referred back to their own provider for that aspect of their care as well—or whether they continue to be followed over time within the chronic disease management program for that portion of their care (at least for a certain amount of time, such as until all are convinced that the patient is stable and doing well). In part, the answer here will lie with the wishes of the physicians who refer their patients into the program in the first place—although it also depends upon the design of the chronic illness treatment program, the wishes of the providers within it, the proposed treatment plan, and the amount of patient demand vs. supply of services available within the program.

PSMAs Also Offer Some Unique Benefits in This Paradigm

The Physicals SMA is unique among the various group visit models because it focuses upon delivery of private, individual physical examinations (with as much talk as possible being deferred from the inefficient exam room into the highly productive, interactive group setting)—i.e., rather than upon the follow-up care of established patients, which is the focus of DIGMAs and CHCCs. As such, the PSMA model can also play an important role—although typically a secondary rather than primary role—in the chronic illness population management paradigm that is being proposed here. If the physicians attached to the chronic illness program have one or more PSMAs (either as a part of the chronic illness program or for their own practice), then any chronically ill patient in the program needing a private physical exam can be promptly, efficiently, and cost-effectively provided with one.

Such patients can then be directly referred, with the physician's permission, into one of the physician's Physicals SMA sessions within 2 or 3 weeks. This includes patients referred for private physical examinations by the various providers attached to the program, by providers running Phase 1, 2, and 3 programs in the proposed paradigm, by providers outside of the chronic illness treatment program, and by the system set up for identifying, tracking, and monitoring chronically ill patients.

In addition, by off-loading many time-consuming physical examinations from the costly individual office visit setting to highly efficient PSMA visits, much time can be freed up on the participating physicians' schedules—time that can then be allocated to other purposes, such as teaching, research time, desktop medicine, seeing more individual follow-up visits, or running more DIGMAs and CHCCs in this diabetes care paradigm.

No Matter How Successful SMAs Become, Individual Care Will Always Be Important

I have always felt that, despite the almost certain growth of highly efficient and cost-effective SMA programs, there will always be a need (albeit a reduced need) for traditional individual office visit care in tomorrow's fully integrated healthcare delivery systems. This holds equally true for the chronic illness population management paradigm that I am proposing here, as some patients will undoubtedly either prefer or need individual appointments from time to time. In the future, our challenge will be how to best use group visits for patients who can be appropriately treated in them, while utilizing the limited supply of individual office visits for those patients needing or preferring them.

However, in order to optimally utilize the mix of group and individual appointments available in the chronic disease management paradigm making full use of group visits that is being discussed here, it is important to recognize the different applications of individual vs. group appointments. Traditional individual office visits are often preferred for serious acute infectious illnesses, rapidly evolving medical conditions, complex medical procedures, patients too demented or hearing impaired to benefit from a group visit, patients not speaking the language in which the SMA is being conducted, and patients refusing to voluntarily attend the group visit program. On the other hand, group visits excel for treating the relatively stable chronically ill; those needing routine follow-up care; patients with extensive informational and psychosocial needs; patients requiring simple procedures or physical examinations (PSMAs); the *worried well*; patients needing more physician contact and *professional hand holding*; and patients needing closer monitoring, surveillance, and follow-up care. The important point here is that much of the medical care that has heretofore been provided through traditional individual office visits can now be appropriately provided through the effective use of group visit programs.

DIGMAs, CHCCs, and PSMAs Work Well Together in the Proposed Paradigm

The intent of this chronic disease management paradigm is to efficiently provide high-quality, high-value, economical, and accessible medical care to all patients having a particular chronic illness—and to fully capture the multitude of benefits that SMAs offer by making full use of group visits (as well as other group-based programs). As it turns out, DIGMAs, CHCCs, and PSMAs work very well in this paradigm—both together and in conjunction with individual office visits.

When to Utilize the DIGMA Model

In chronic illness treatment programs, the homogeneous and mixed subtypes of the DIGMA model are most commonly employed. The chronic disease management program's SMA will be a DIGMA when: (1) the SMA is open to most or all diabetic patients, most commonly for follow-up visits; (2) different patients typically attend each session, coming only when they have a medical need; (3) sessions are held regularly and frequently, typically once a week for 90 minutes (although they are sometimes held more or less frequently, and can last from approximately 60 to 120 minutes); (4) drop-in convenience is sometimes offered; (5) most medical care and exams are performed with the patient's permission in the group setting (although private time with the physician is always made available for brief private discussions or exams, normally toward the end of the session); (6) virtually all patient education occurs in the context of the doctor sequentially working with each patient individually while others present are able to listen, learn, ask questions, and interact (i.e., there is usually no prepackaged *class* type of educational presentation to the group as a whole); (7) a behaviorist is present, and often a documenter to assist in the documentation process; (8) expanded roles are played by all members of the treatment team, especially by the nurse/MA(s) and behaviorist; and (9) the SMA is run like a series of individual office visits with other patients as observers (i.e., like a series of one doctor–one patient encounters addressing each patient's unique medical needs individually), while fostering some group interaction. In addition, DIGMAs have frequently been used with success in both fee-for-service (FFS) and capitated systems.

When to Utilize the PSMA Model

The Physicals SMA model is used when the focus is upon private physical examinations rather than follow-up visits—often because of the private nature of the exam, such as when disrobing is required. Here, in addition to the interactive group segment that typically follows (which is basically a small DIGMA), an individual physical examination is initially provided for each patient in attendance in the privacy of the exam room. The PSMA model can be used for routine or periodic physical exams, for inducting new patients into the chronic illness treatment program, for working down physical exam wait-lists and backlogs, and for a variety of other applications in this chronic disease management paradigm where a private physical examination is required rather than just a follow-up visit. Like DIGMAs, the PSMA model has been successfully employed in both FFS and capitated systems. PSMAs can be used either to better manage a provider's busy, backlogged practice or (especially in the case of the homogeneous and mixed subtypes) as a part of a chronic illness population management program such as that which is being discussed here—i.e., by providing private physical examinations efficiently and cost-effectively to patients with a particular diagnosis or condition.

When to Utilize the CHCC Model

On the other hand, the shared medical appointment program is a CHCC when it includes the same 15–20 high-utilizing patients during each session (typically prescheduled to be held monthly), when the session is typically approximately 2½ hours in duration, and when the session is structured into group and individualized treatment segments (and where the group segment is itself divided into warm-up, educational, working break/care delivery, question and answer, and planning for the next visit components). If the SMA is a CHCC: (1) medical care will typically not be provided in the group setting; (2) the program will generally focus upon high-utilizing, multi-morbid geriatric patients; (3) there will be a formal class-type educational presentation during the group segment; and (4) the SMA will usually have ongoing monthly sessions for the same group of 15–20 patients being followed over time. The benefits will be largely downstream in terms of reduced hospital, emergency department, and nursing home costs.

When to Utilize the Specialty CHCC Subtype of the CHCC Model

If the SMA is a Specialty CHCC, it will be similar to the traditional CHCC model in that: (1) the same 15–20 patients will normally attend each session; (2) the focus will often be upon high-utilizing patients, because that is where the economic cost offset can be maximized (but typically in the medical subspecialties rather than primary care); and (3) the same basic organization of a 90-minute group segment (structured into warm-up, educational, working break/care delivery, question and answer, and planning for the next visit segments) followed by an hour of individual care would be maintained. However, unlike ongoing monthly CHCC sessions for multi-morbid geriatric patients in primary care, the Specialty CHCC sessions would be irregularly spaced according to best practices and—rather than being for multi-morbid geriatric patients—they would typically be designed for 15–20 high utilizing patients having the particular chronic illness that this chronic illness management paradigm is designed to treat.

Start with One Group Visit Model and Later Try the Others as Well

It is likely that most healthcare organizations will start with one of these SMA models (typically the one that best suits their purposes), and not all three at the same time. Nonetheless, it is quite possible that they will eventually employ all three models in their chronic illness population management programs—as these SMA models are mutually enhancing and not mutually exclusive, with benefits that build one upon the other. Because the DIGMA, Physicals SMA, and CHCC models are complementary, they can work well together—and often have. In addition, these SMA models can also be used with any other components employed in your current chronic illness population management program—because they are compatible not only with each other, but also with individual office visits, health education classes, support groups, and both psychiatry and behavioral medicine programs.

Applying This 3-Phase Chronic Illness Treatment Paradigm in Actual Practice

The author has worked with several hundred different fee-for-service and capitated healthcare organizations—as well as numerous governmental (USAF, Army, Navy, VA) and public systems—to help them institute group visits both in provider's practices and in chronic illness treatment programs. The chronic illness population management paradigm discussed above, which is designed to fully utilize group visits, is proving to be a very robust model indeed—and to have a wide range of potential applications.

Some Systems Might Choose to Only Use Some Components of the Proposed Paradigm

Some healthcare organizations, especially smaller ones, might be interested in developing a more abbreviated version of this chronic illness treatment model for use in their system. For example, they might choose to only include a Phase 1 diabetes education class, DIGMAs in the practices of just one or two providers attached to the chronic illness program, and a system for identifying and referring appropriate patients. Being somewhat larger in size, some mid-sized systems might choose to institute a more comprehensive diabetes program—perhaps involving a couple of Phase 1 diabetes education classes, a few diabetes DIGMAs run by providers attached to the program, and Phase 3 individualized case management for their most out-of-control diabetics (along with a system for identifying, monitoring, and referring appropriate patients).

Still larger systems might want to implement all components of the proposed chronic illness treatment paradigm described above—i.e., in order to fully capture the multiple potential benefits that it can offer to the numerous chronically ill patients within their system having a particular diagnosis (such as diabetes, CHF, depression, and hypertension). It is important to note that abbreviated versions of the proposed paradigm can also be of great value to patients and physicians in larger organizations as well—i.e., as they progressively develop, on a step-by-step basis, what will ultimately be their comprehensive chronic illness population management program. The key here is to go slowly and carefully at first and to then develop this chronic disease management program within one's organization gradually—component by component—until the desired overall goal is ultimately achieved.

A Real-Life Example of This 3-Phase Chronic Illness Treatment Paradigm

I have successfully used the proposed 3-phase chronic illness treatment paradigm several times while consulting with various medical groups both nationally and internationally. One of the larger healthcare systems that I worked with had approximately 10,000 diabetic patients—and had previously set up a rudimentary chronic illness treatment program for better managing these patients. Unfortunately, it took patients approximately 18 months to get in, and even then the program was quite limited in scope.

The Problem

At the time I was called upon to consult with this integrated healthcare delivery system, their program was not only relatively rudimentary, but also completely *log-jammed* and overwhelmed—with waits of 18 months and longer just to enter the program being typical. Basically, their diabetes program consisted of three parts: (1) a means of identifying the diabetic patients within their system; (2) a diabetes education class consisting of two consecutive weekly 2-hour sessions that included just 10–12 patients; and (3) individual office visits with the providers attached part-time to the program (which included an endocrinologist, a nephrologist, a podiatrist, and a couple of nurse practitioners). Because the entry point into their program was a diabetes education class that permitted just 10–12 diabetic patients to be inducted into the diabetes program every 2 weeks, backlogs were clearly inevitable due to the fact that they had over 10,000 diabetics in their system at that time, yet could only enroll an average of 5–6 patients per week into their program.

The problems with this diabetes program were: (1) it had a very limited scope; (2) almost all care was being delivered through inefficient one-on-one office visits; (3) except for the diabetes education class, there was no opportunity for patients to help and support one another; and (4) it was severely impacted and backlogged. Once referred, it took a patient approximately 1½ years to get into the diabetes education class (which could never be repeated by patients needing a refresher course because of the high demand for this class)—and therefore into the program. Furthermore, once in the program, it often took months to get an appointment and actually be seen by a provider for a follow-up visit. It was a classical case of patient demand overwhelming the system's capacity to meet that demand.

Why Was This Problem Occurring?

In taking a close look at why this was happening, it became clear that a major roadblock was the two-session (with each session taking 2 hours) diabetes education class. Because the patients had waited so long just to get in, the two nurse practitioners running this class were delivering some medical care to patients during these sessions, which resulted in their only being able to see 10–12 patients during each class—which took two weekly sessions to complete. Clearly, the 5½ patients entering the diabetes program on average per week were only *a drop in the bucket* compared to the potential demand generated by the system's 10,000 plus diabetic patients—with the result being a hopelessly severe backlog of patients trying to get into the program.

The Solution

After analyzing the problem that they were facing, I initially recommended instituting a two-pronged attack on this problem. *First*, by using the chronic disease management paradigm being discussed in this chapter, we completely redesigned their diabetes program to better meet the high-volume medical needs of the system's approximately 10,000 diabetic patients. The diabetes education class was immediately retooled to become a single session, 3-hour class (i.e., rather than two weekly 2-hour classes). In addition, the actual delivery of medical care during these sessions was stripped away, so that it became a true diabetes education class. These changes enabled the diabetes education class to be redesigned to accommodate 35–40 patients per session—i.e., rather than the 10–12 patients that had previously been seen every 2 weeks. In addition, two diabetes education classes were offered per week, which enabled 70–80 patients to be inducted into the diabetes program every week.

Second, we needed to address how to efficiently handle this greatly expanded bolus of new patients entering the diabetes program each week—i.e., both initially and on an ongoing basis, through use of existing staffing. The answer to the question was to dramatically leverage existing resources, which was accomplished by leveraging providers' time via DIGMAs. Every provider attached to the diabetes program began running at least one 90-minute DIGMA per week for their work within the program. Ultimately, the goal was to develop enough highly accessible DIGMAs within this chronic care paradigm to efficiently handle their increased workload volume in a timely manner.

The Results

Over the first 6 months, a total of seven weekly 90-minute DIGMAs were instituted by the providers attached to this diabetes program—three diabetes DIGMAs (one run by the endocrinologist and two by the nurse practitioners associated with the program), two hypertension DIGMAs (run by the nephrologist attached to the diabetes program), a diabetic foot care DIGMA (run by the podiatrist in the program), and even a highly specialized sleep apnea DIGMA for this costly subset of the diabetes population. Over time, the number of DIGMAs offered in this program continues to expand. In all cases, the DIGMA census targets were set so as to at least triple the providers' actual productivity over individual office visits. As a result, the wait time to enter the program quickly went from 1½ years to a couple of months—

and then more gradually decreased to just a couple of weeks. Furthermore, as a result of their highly productive DIGMAs, all providers within the program became much more accessible to the patients in the diabetes program. This resulted in patients already in the diabetes program often being seen within a week or two for a routine follow-up visit—i.e., rather than having to wait for months, as was the case before.

Many Objectives Were Simultaneously Accomplished

Within a year of instituting the new design of their diabetes program, this healthcare system was able to accomplish all of the following goals: (1) patients were able to get into the diabetes program within a couple of weeks, rather than having to wait 18 months or longer; (2) patients already in the diabetes program were allowed to repeat the diabetes education class for a *refresher course* whenever one was needed or wanted; (3) patients were able to promptly see providers within the program, typically within a couple of weeks; and (4) the diabetes program rapidly expanded to better meet the medical needs of this system's plethora of diabetic patients (i.e., rather than just a select few).

Ongoing Developments and Future Goals

Through continuous process improvement, the development of this chronic illness paradigm—which was designed to fully utilize the multiple benefits that properly run group visits (and other types of group programs) can provide—is ongoing. In the case that we just discussed, the system is now looking toward gradually increasing the number and types of DIGMAs run by providers attached to their diabetes population management program—i.e., to better meet the steadily increasing patient demand as evermore patients are inducted into the program. They are also discussing additional plans to expand the program, which includes gradually instituting several Phase 2 group programs as needed—possibly including such new group programs as a smoking cessation class, a cognitive behavioral depression program, and exercise and nutrition classes. They are also looking toward instituting a Phase 3 individualized case management program for their most out-of-control diabetic patients, with the ultimate goal of including DIGMAs (and possibly CHCCs as well) for those Phase 3 patients willing to attend.

Concluding Remarks on Why You Should Institute Such a Chronic Illness Program

As can be seen, by developing high quality, efficient, and cost-effective chronic illness population management programs (particularly those that involve group visits), your patients can be better served—not only with the benefits of an additional and effective healthcare choice, but also with accessible, high-quality care targeted at specific diagnoses. This can result in greater patient education, enhanced disease self-management skills, better outcomes, and high levels of patient (and provider) satisfaction. Patients also enjoy a multitude of additional benefits from properly run chronic disease management programs that make full use of group visits, including the following: prompt access to care; more time with their doctor; a more relaxed pace of care; a multidisciplinary care team; greater patient education; closer attention to their mind as well as body needs; closer follow-up care; and the help and support of other patients having the same diagnosis integrated into their healing experience.

Physicians benefit by being able to do something new and different that gets them off the fast-paced treadmill of individual office visit care—a treadmill that somebody always seems to be tweaking so that it keeps going faster and faster, with evermore patients needing to be seen and ever-less time available per patient. Physicians also benefit from: the productivity and efficiency benefits that group visits offer; the quality benefits that chronic illness care pathways can provide; their enhanced ability to better manage chronic illnesses; the help of a multidisciplinary care team; and the added fun that group visits can bring into their workweek—as group visits are meant to be voluntary, energizing, and enjoyable for patients and providers alike.

Similarly, the organization benefits in numerous ways by having effective care pathways in place for efficiently treating various chronic illnesses: high-quality care and better outcomes for the chronically ill; more consistent attention to performance measures and routine health maintenance; cost containment that comes from lever-aging existing resources and increasing productivity; the competitive advantages that new chronic illness treatment programs can offer in the marketplace; and the increased levels of patient and physician professional satisfaction that can be achieved—as happy physicians and patients translate into retained physicians and patients. Similar benefits also accrue to third party insurers and corporate purchasers.

In this chapter, we have closely examined a broadly applicable chronic disease management paradigm originated by the author that makes full use of group visit for population management programs covering virtually any chronic illness—but using diabetes as an example. Because of the multifarious benefits that properly run group visits offer, the DIGMA, CHCC, and PSMA models—along with other SMA models that are currently less well known or are still to be developed in the future—are expected to play an increasingly important role in tomorrow's healthcare environment. They work well not only as stand-alone models, but also in conjunction with individual office visits, other SMA models, and many other types of group programs. These group visit models can be fully utilized in chronic disease management programs to provide a multitude of quality, efficiency, access, economic, and patient/provider satisfaction benefits—and accomplish all this while simultaneously improving outcomes for our chronically ill patients. However, to fully capture the multiple benefits that such chronic illness treatment programs making full use of group visits can offer to patients, physicians, and the organization alike, these programs must be carefully designed, adequately supported, fully promoted to patients, and properly run.

References

1. Noffsinger EB. Group visits for efficient, high-quality chronic disease management. *Group Practice Journal*. 2008; Feb 57(2): 23–40.
2. Pennachio D. Should you offer group visits? *Medical Economics*. 2003; 80:70–85.

Chapter 8
Do Not Abuse Group Visits

But even the staunchest supporters of group care worry there is a potential for abuse. Organizations could attempt to force patients to attend multipatient meetings rather than providing them with individual care. Penny-pinching medical offices could give physicians bigger patient loads and order them to hold most of their exams in these efficient group settings. Such fears, however, have not yet materialized during the few years since some centers have tried it.

The doctor is in for group visits. San Jose Mercury News, Tuesday October 10, 2000, pp. D5, D7

The Potential for Abuse of Group Visits Is Real

In today's highly competitive and challenging healthcare environment, as physicians and healthcare organizations alike try to leverage existing resources and do evermore with less, the potential for abuse of group visits looms very real. Healthcare organizations are struggling with the challenges of insufficient resources existing within the system to meet the quality, access, service, and patient satisfaction mandates—as well as the workload demands—facing them through traditional means alone (i.e., by hiring evermore physicians in a misguided attempt to meet these mandates and workload demands through individual appointments alone). They are increasingly recognizing that what is needed is a new tool for leveraging existing resources and better addressing all of these demands—which is something for which group visits are ideally suited. It is for this reason that, despite resistance to change and organizational inertia, group visit programs are gradually but progressively emerging—to enhance quality and service, to increase productivity, to leverage existing resources, to improve access and patient satisfaction, to strengthen the bottom line, and to better manage large, busy practices as well as chronic illnesses and high-risk patient populations.

Because of their proven ability to deliver better and more efficient care at reduced cost, and with high levels of patient and physician professional satisfaction, today's established group visit models can therefore be expected to play an increasingly important role in the future of healthcare services. Personally, I feel that as much as 60–80% of all that we do in the outpatient ambulatory care setting—and some of what we do in the inpatient, residential care, and urgent care settings as well—could ultimately be provided by carefully designed, properly run group visit programs. It is because of the many benefits that a well-run group visit program can offer to patients, physicians, and the organization alike that it is imperative to begin safeguarding against any potential for abuse now—i.e., before the reputation of group visits is any way sullied or tarnished.

Abuse Could Have an Enormous Negative Impact upon Group Visit Programs

Certainly, there is always the potential risk that healthcare systems could abuse group visits in a misguided attempt to extract even more benefit from SMAs than they were ever designed to achieve, which, if allowed to occur, could potentially undermine the very credibility of group visit programs. If they become concerned about abuse and fraud, payers will worry about opening the window to such healthcare innovations as group visits. Patients would likewise begin to balk at group visits if they were to get the impression that they are *mass medicine* and a means for doctors and healthcare organizations to gouge patients out of more money, spend more time out on the golf course, and improve their bottom lines.

This would be most unfortunate in view of the many legitimate benefits that properly run group visit programs

E.B. Noffsinger, *Running Group Visits in Your Practice*, DOI 10.1007/b106441_8,
© Springer Science+Business Media, LLC 2009

can in fact provide—e.g., greater time available with one's own physician and a more relaxed pace of care, improved productivity and better access to care, max-packed visits and the benefits of *one-stop healthcare shopping*, increased attention to the informational and psychosocial issues that are known to drive so many office visits, the potential for closer follow-up care and greater patient satisfaction, and the information and support provided by other patients being integrated into each patient's healthcare experience.

Preventing Abuse Will Require Safeguards and an Ongoing, Vigilant Effort

Therefore, it is imperative to safeguard against any such potential for abuse even at this early stage in the development of group visits and to start planning now so as to prevent any such possibility for abuse. In fact, early on Dr. John Scott and I were so sensitive to, and concerned about, this potential for abuse of that we published an article entitled "Preventing Potential Abuses of Group Visits" in AMGA's *Group Practice Journal* way back in May 2000. Many of the concerns that we discussed then are just as applicable today. In this chapter, I address many of the ways in which group visits can be abused—now or in the future—in the hopes that by understanding what these potential sources of abuse are, we can avoid making such mistakes in the future, and thus prevent the irreversible damage that could thereby be done to group visits.

Potential Abuse Could Take Either of Two Forms

While the potential for abuse of DIGMAs, CHCCs, PSMAs, and other forms of group visits yet to be developed is quite real and must therefore be strenuously guarded against, it is important to note that almost all such abuses will take one of the two basic forms: *First*, by attempting to extract even more benefits from a group visit program than these SMA models were ever designed to provide, i.e., beyond that which is commensurate with reasonable workload and quality care; and *second*, by not putting sufficient resources into the group visit program for these various SMA models to provide the full range of benefits that they were originally designed to deliver, i.e., by putting fewer personnel, facilities, promotional, and budgetary resources into them than properly supported and run group visit programs require.

It is important to always remember that today's major group visit models were designed to put patients first by emphasizing patient empowerment and self-care, and by providing them with what they most want—i.e., prompt access to quality medical care; more time with their doctor; greater attention to patient education and psychosocial issues; a more relaxed pace of care; and the help and support of both a multidisciplinary treatment team and others dealing with similar experiences. Anything that can potentially take away from this primary focus being upon patients, such as attempting to extract even more economic advantage from the SMA program than it was ever intended to deliver, would constitute an abuse of group visits.

First Form of Abuse: Attempting to Extract More than Group Visits Are Designed to Provide

The first major source of abuse is of particular concern because, as a group, this first source of abuse always boils down to trying to extract even more benefits from the SMA program than group visits were ever designed to provide. Almost all patient abuses (and most physician abuses) fall into this category, and these will therefore be discussed first. These abuses are especially unfortunate as they go *against the grain* of the overarching principal that both Dr. Scott and I have had from the outset in developing our models, which is to put patients first. Despite the multitude of legitimate patient care, service, productivity, and economic benefits that properly run group visit programs can and do in fact provide, there seems to always be a temptation in all of us to become even more greedy—so that we end up attempting to extract still more benefit than these group visit models were ever designed to provide. By examining the various ways that this can happen, my hope is that—by having this knowledge beforehand—we can promptly check any such greedy impulse that we might have, and thereby avoid all such potentially catastrophic sources of abuse.

Part One: Avoid Patient Abuses

Patient abuses of group visits must be avoided if we are to expect patients to trust group visits and fully participate in them. For patients to attend and wholly participate in SMA programs, we must understand that patients will need to trust the group visit experience—and that this trust can only be engendered and allowed to develop by scrupulously guarding against all types of potential patient abuses. Because patients are key to the interactive educational and emotionally supportive processes that occur in the group visit milieu, patient participation is critical to the full success of any group visit program. This is also true because, together with the physician providing medical care, patients are primary caregivers in their own disease self-management process because they have the most direct firsthand experience in dealing with their illness and in developing the requisite coping skills—something which patients need to be reminded of, and valued for.

Active Patient Participation Is Critical but Requires Trust

By sharing personal experiences, information, helpful tips, and hard-earned pearls regarding the disease self-management skills they have gradually learned over time with one another, patient participation makes the entire group visit experience a more beneficial one for everybody in attendance. Therefore, it is critically important that SMAs be conducted in such a way that the entire group visit environment is conducive to feelings of comfort, safety, and trust so that patients will be willing to speak up and participate—but this requires that any potential for patient abuse be meticulously safeguarded against.

In fact, patients need to be encouraged to speak up, candidly and openly. This is because patient participation is the key not only to the relationships that develop between patients in the group but also to the healthy group dynamics necessary for the building of self-efficacy skills and for enabling patients to help one another. Conversely, patient nonparticipation negatively impacts not only the SMA's group dynamic but also the amount of benefit that each patient can be reasonably expected to derive from the group visit experience itself.

Patient Abuse 1: Making Group Visits Mandatory Rather than Voluntary

Although DIGMAs, CHCCs, and PSMAs have the net effect of substantially off-loading numerous individual office visits onto highly efficient group visits, it is nonetheless important to ensure that access to traditional office visits not be restricted for patients needing or wanting them. If anything, group visits should increase—and not decrease—availability of individual office visits to those choosing or requiring them. It would certainly be a patient abuse of group visits if one were to use SMAs as a means of restricting patient access to individual office visits. It is important that all patients attending DIGMAs, CHCCs, and PSMAs be fully informed not only that participation in these SMA programs is totally voluntary, but also that they will still be able to have individual office visits just like before—and that SMAs are simply an additional healthcare choice that is now available to them.

Certainly, using group visits to largely or totally replace traditional office visits would violate this important tenet. Plus, restricting access to the appropriate use of individual office visits could have unintended consequences—as patients would almost certainly perceive this as an unwanted intrusion and an abuse of group visits, and thus grow to dislike and resist them. Using group visits to largely replace individual office visits and restrict patient access to them (as opposed to making the appropriate use of individual visits more accessible to patients) would cause patients, physicians, insurers, and corporate purchasers alike to grow distrustful of group visits and to lose confidence in them. The judicious use of individual office visits will always play an important role in the future of healthcare delivery. Both Dr. Scott and I have always intended that our group visit models be completely voluntary (i.e., for patients as well as for physicians and staff), and that they be designed to provide patients with improved care—as well as freedom of choice—by offering them an additional healthcare option.

In an article on group visits, the San Jose Mercury News addresses the importance of always offering voluntary choice to patients regarding group visits as follows: "This is what Richard Schelin considers superb medical care: driving several hours to see a physician. Being shepherded into a meeting room with a dozen other patients. Jockeying for a few minutes of attention as the doctor addresses everyone's individual concerns. And having to forget all about privacy as he discusses his medical condition *while everyone else in the room listens in.* 'It's well worth it,' says Schelin, 75, who along with his wife, Georgia, makes the long trek from the Gold Country to Stanford each month for a group doctor visit. 'We make it a point to be there.' No, Schelin does not suffer from dementia. And patients and physicians alike are emphasizing this is not an example of a managed-care system gone mad. 'This is the cutting edge of medicine,' says Edward B. Noffsinger, director of clinical access improvement at the Palo Alto Medical Foundation. 'It offers great benefits to patients, first and foremost' (1).

This article goes on to state: "Although it flies in the face of conventional wisdom, this new model of healthcare—the group doctor visit—is increasingly being embraced for its potential to increase patient access to physicians and its ability to better inform people how to cope with a chronic condition. Because patients are often placed in a group with others who suffer from the same medical problems, participants can receive practical tips, and emotional support from their peers...But clinics in San Jose, Palo Alto, Sacramento, Denver, Atlanta and Tampa, Fla., are among those that have unveiled their own group visit programs, convinced that the benefits far outweigh the drawbacks....Surprisingly, however, many patients have felt quite comfortable being examined in a room filled with strangers....Yet group visits aren't for every patient—or for every health problem....'If you said, 'You can come see the doctor with 20 other people and that's the only option you have,' I don't think that would fly,' says Margaret Wellington, coordinator of Stanford's Health Partners program, which holds group visits for anyone with a chronic disease" (1).

There are a couple of relevant points worth making at this time: (1) because DIGMAs and PSMAs are designed to off-load numerous individual office visits by appropriately converting them into group visits, individual visits should eventually also become more accessible to patients needing or wanting them; (2) as patients become more aware of group visit programs and begin to hear evermore positive comments from other patients about them, the number of patients refusing to attend a group visits is expected to gradually decline over time; and (3) the single most important component to winning patients over (i.e., and getting them to be willing to try something as different as a group visit for the first time) is effective promotion of the program.

Experience has shown that effective promotion of the SMA program especially requires that the physician take approximately 30 seconds during every regular office visit to personally invite, through a positive and carefully worded script, each and every suitable patient they see in the clinic to have their next visit be in a DIGMA or PSMA. In other words, the solution to patient buy-in to group visits does not lie in forcing or requiring patients to attend a group visit in lieu of an individual office visit (which would likely only engender patient resentment and resistance anyway), but rather in keeping group visits voluntary and instead actively promoting the SMA program to patients in a positive and effective manner.

Patient Abuse 2: Failing to Address Confidentiality and Concerns About Privacy

It is imperative that group visit programs address any patient concerns regarding confidentiality and privacy, and that time always be made available during each and every SMA session for patients to have brief private discussions as needed with their physician (or brief individual exams, whenever appropriate, in the privacy of an exam room). To my knowledge, issues around confidentiality have seldom if ever been brought up by patients as a result of DIGMA, CHCC, or PSMA visits. The rarity of such concerns is undoubtedly due in large part to these group visit models being designed and conducted with considerable sensitivity to the patients' needs for confidentiality and privacy. For example, because patients are often sensitive to having their weight and age discussed in public, these issues must be handled with tact in the group—e.g., by having the nurses take vitals in the privacy of the exam room and, in morbid obesity SMAs, by limiting discussions of weight to the amount of weight that the patient has lost since entering the program rather than discussing absolute values in the group setting (unless the patient decides to bring them up and discuss absolute values).

Also, patients have a right to feel that their medical issues and what they discuss in the group visit will not go outside of the group room. In order to keep the SMA a safe place for all, it is important that patients agree of their own free will to have their medical issues addressed in the group setting and to have all attendees agree not discuss the health issues of others—or to identify others in attendance—once the group is over. Therefore, at least in DIGMAs and PSMAs, all patients and support persons who attend are asked to sign a confidentiality waiver—which is written in understandable, patient friendly language—at the beginning of each and every session. This is a brief, concisely written full disclosure/informed consent document that describes all important points regarding privacy and confidentiality—including limits of confidentiality in the group visit format, and what is expected of all who attend—that all attendees are required to sign at the beginning of each SMA session. Also, all promotional materials used in these programs are to make clear that this is a shared medical appointment program and that it occurs largely in a group setting with others being present.

In addition, the behaviorist thoroughly discusses all aspects of confidentiality during the introduction given at the beginning of each and every DIGMA and PSMA session. This introduction by the behaviorist covers the facts that patients are still entitled to individual office visits just like before and that some one-on-one time will be made available to all requesting or wanting it—although it will typically be offered toward the end of the session so as to not interrupt the flow of the group. In the CHCC model, one-on-one time with the healthcare team is provided as needed during both the working break and the individual care segment that follows the group component of the session. Unlike DIGMAs and PSMAs, with CHCCs the actual delivery of medical care is typically done in private—and is generally not delivered in the group setting, where others can listen and learn. Also, because the same 15–20 patients typically attend all CHCC sessions (often for many years) and support persons are not invited to attend, the issue of confidentiality is somewhat different for CHCCs than for DIGMAs and PSMAs—so that confidentiality agreements could perhaps be signed say every 6 months in the CHCC rather than at the beginning of every session, as is required in DIGMAs and PSMAs (where different patients and support persons typically attend each and every session). However, this is something about the confidentiality agreement/release that the reader would have to discuss with their own medical risk department or corporate attorney in order to determine what would be recommended in their own particular circumstance and situation.

Patient Abuse 3: Billing for the Behaviorist's Time and Counseling Time (Which Could Also Constitute an Insurance Abuse)

As discussed elsewhere in this book, with DIGMAs and PSMAs, most fee-for-service (FFS) medical groups typically bill according to the level of care delivered and documented; however, they do not bill either for the behaviorist's time or for counseling time. This is because if they were to bill for the behaviorist's time, then patients would receive two bills—one from the physician and another from the behaviorist—involving two co-payments for the same medical visit, which would anger patients and turn them off to group visits. Therefore, the behaviorist's time is instead typically treated as an overhead expense to the SMA program, so that patients in fact only receive one bill (requiring one co-payment) for their group visit—and that bill is from their doctor.

Furthermore, billing several patients at once for the same block of counseling time because many patients happened to simultaneously benefit from this counseling would be egregious (if not outright fraudulent)—and would constitute an abuse of group visits that would almost certainly not be welcome by insurers. The fact that they are not generally being billed for either counseling time or the behaviorist's time certainly represents a substantial net gain for third-party insurers—which is fine by me as I believe that there is enough benefit in group visits so that some net gain should accrue to patients, physicians, healthcare organizations, insurers, and corporate purchasers alike.

Therefore, physicians typically bill DIGMAs and PSMAs according to history, exam, and medical decision-making—but not for counseling time. However, if the counseling specifically pertained only to a particular patient that the physician was actually working with in the group setting at that time (but not to other patients in the group who were observing and might also be benefitting), then it would seem that a case could probably be made for billing that one patient for the counseling provided. Nonetheless, to my knowledge, most FFS systems do not bill for counseling time, which represents one of the benefits that properly run DIGMAs and PSMAs can provide to insurers. Any gain that happens to accrue to the observers in the group room who are fortunate enough to be listening and benefiting, while fortunate for them, is not billed for.

Patient Abuse 4: Starting Sessions Late, Not Pacing the Group, and Not Finishing on Time

It is important that patients' time be respected during the SMA setting by having sessions start and end on time, with everyone's healthcare needs adequately addressed. It is important to keep in mind that many patients are *sick and tired* of waiting in the lobby for their physician to see them, and consequently of finishing late during regular individual office visits—so let us not make the same mistake with SMAs. This means that: (1) the nurse/MA(s) must arrive sufficiently early to conduct their duties during the allotted amount of time prior to, or during the early part of, the DIGMA or PSMA session; (2) the behaviorist needs to arrive sufficiently early to *warm up* the group, write down the medical issues that patients want to discuss with the doctor that day, and start the DIGMA or PSMA session on time with the introduction; and (3) that enough reception help be provided for the SMA to ensure that the requisite number of patients can be expeditiously received and registered prior to the session.

In addition, and most importantly, it means that the physician must arrive on time to begin the private physical exams in the PSMA, or be in the group room no later than 2–3 minutes after the start of the DIGMA—i.e., by the time that the behaviorist's introduction has been completed. By doing so, patients will not feel rushed as a consequence of the physician arriving late—plus, physicians should pace themselves so that there is enough time for each patient's unique medical needs to be adequately attended to during the DIGMA or PSMA session. This is especially important for physicians who are poor time managers, frequently finish late during normal clinic hours, and would be at high risk for entering the group room more than 3–5 minutes after the start of the DIGMA session. For those physicians having such time management problems, it is recommended that they consider holding their SMAs either first thing in the morning or immediately after lunch—i.e., at those times when they are most likely to be running on schedule.

Starting and finishing on time also means that the physician and behaviorist must pace the entire SMA session so that each patient gets the time they need in order to get their medical needs appropriately met. This translates into not taking too much time on the first couple of patients, not becoming entangled with dominating or talkative patients, remaining focused and succinct throughout, and pacing the SMA appropriately throughout the entire session. It also means that physicians be brutally honest regarding their own time management skills. If they are not good time managers and frequently run late in the clinic, it is imperative that they choose a behaviorist who has the complementary skill set of being a good time manager—i.e., who is capable of pacing the group and keeping it moving along in a timely manner.

Patient Abuse 5: Scheduling Too Many Patients (Which Is Also a Physician Abuse)

To fully realize the multiple benefits that properly run DIGMAs, CHCCs, and PSMAs can offer to patients, it is important that adequate time be scheduled for the number of patients attending—i.e., sufficient time for all attendees to receive quality care and to have their medical needs met. To avoid scheduling too many patients into your SMA, try to initially adhere to the guidelines provided in this book as to ideal census levels. Even though substantially larger DIGMAs have been successfully held by experienced physicians, it is recommended for most DIGMAs that the ideal census be between 10 and 16 patients for a 90-minute session (not including family members or caregivers)—and that this census typically be set so as to approximately triple the physician's productivity over individual office visits. In 2 ½ hour CHCCs, the ideal census is typically between 15 and 20 patients. In 90-minute PSMAs, the ideal census is typically between 6 and 8 female (or between 7 and 9 male) patients in primary care and 10–13 patients in most of the medical subspecialties.

These ideal census levels are provided as guidelines only, as larger groups than these have certainly been successfully run on occasion. However, it is recommended that any deviations from these suggested ideal census levels be carefully examined beforehand, and then only changed if the physician feels absolutely confident that this can be accomplished successfully without any loss on the patients' part. For group visit sessions that are of shorter or longer duration than the 90-minutes that is typical of DIGMAs and PSMAs (or than the 2 ½ hours that is typical of a CHCC or Specialty CHCC), simply prorate these ideal group sizes accordingly.

Failing to adhere to these recommendations as to ideal group sizes would likely constitute a patient abuse of group visits because including too many patients relative to the amount of time available would likely result in SMA sessions that feel rushed, decrease personalized care, diminish group interaction, reduce quality of care, decrease patient bonding, and decrease patient as well as physician professional satisfaction. Furthermore, if insufficient time exists to attend to each patient's unique medical needs individually, then there is the risk that patients might start to view the group visit as being *mass medicine* rather than quality care—or as being more of a class or support group than a shared medical appointment occurring in a supportive group setting. In addition, the physician can get tired out from the increased patient workload of SMAs that are too large. This goes against one of the fundamental precepts of group visits, which is to make it a more enjoyable healthcare experience—both for the patients who attend and for the physicians running them.

Part 2: Avoid Physician Abuses

Critical to the success of any group visit program is physician buy-in based on self-interest. After all, well-run SMAs can be used by interested physicians on a voluntary basis to enable such physicians to increase productivity and access, to provide better and more cost-effective care, and to better manage both busy, backlogged practices and high-risk patients with chronic illnesses. However, achieving these SMA benefits requires physician buy-in—which, as discussed in Chapter 6—requires that any physician resistances and concerns be thoroughly addressed, that physicians fully understand the many potential physician benefits that properly run group visits can offer, and that any potential for physician abuse be avoided at all cost.

Physician Abuse 1: Making Group Visits Mandatory for All Physicians

Neither Dr. Scott nor I ever intended for the group visit models we originated and developed to be mandatory to physicians—as forcing physicians to do something they do not want to do can only be a recipe for disaster by engendering distrust, resentment, and passive-aggressive resistance to group visit programs. We always envisioned that the participation of physicians would be entirely voluntary and secured at the grassroots level out of physician self-interest—so that physicians would eventually be won over *from the bottom up* through positive SMA reports from physician colleagues, instead of group visits being imposed upon physicians by executive leadership *from the top down*.

It is important that physicians, SMA team members, support staffs, and any invited guest speakers be volunteers and share in the enthusiasm and the positive perspective that are required for the group visit to be fully successful. Reluctant or hostile participants will undoubtedly communicate their resistance—even if only unconsciously through their body language—and thereby inhibit the salutary impact of the group process. Consider the more gradual approach of first instituting group visits on a pilot study basis at selected sites, with those physicians who are willing to voluntarily try running one for their practices. Then, if the pilot is successful, consider eventually expanding and disseminating the group visit program throughout the entire organization, but by allowing physician buy-in to develop voluntarily and progressively at the grassroots level.

goal), the main point here is that most patients are willing to accept group sizes that are even substantially larger than recommended. Nonetheless, I generally recommend against DIGMAs that are larger than 16 patients actually being in attendance because the physician tends to get tired out by the workload—and physician satisfaction must always remain a priority for group visit programs to be fully successful.

Of course, no DIGMA organizer can completely guarantee that this maximum group size will never be exceeded. This is because one must usually overbook sessions in order to compensate for no-shows and late-cancels, which could occasionally result in larger group attendances in the comparatively rare event that all patients do in fact show up for a particular session. Also, the DIGMA model itself cannot completely control for the number of patients that will drop-in to any given session, even though patients are asked to call a day ahead of time in order to let staff know that they are coming. Actually, these overbooking and drop-in numbers are usually far more predictable that one might at first believe.

Physician Abuse 2: Demanding that Group Sizes Be Excessively Large

As discussed previously, enhanced professional satisfaction is a primary goal for DIGMAs, CHCCs, and PSMAs, and physician buy-in is critical to the success of these group visit models. Therefore, demanding that the group size be excessively large (i.e., beyond the recommended ideal census levels for these SMA models) in an imprudent attempt to extract even greater physician productivity than these models were originally designed to achieve, would not only be self-defeating but also represent a physician abuse of these SMA models. It is essential that all aspects of the SMA program stay well within the physician's comfort zone—ethically, professionally, and in terms of group size.

Interestingly, it appears that physician professional satisfaction rather than patient satisfaction is the primary limiting factor in determining the upper limit to an SMA's group size. For 90-minute DIGMAs, physicians seldom like to have group sizes that exceed approximately 16 patients—even though many DIGMAs have been successfully conducted with substantially larger group sizes, and with reasonably satisfied patients. In one case that comes to mind, the endocrinologist actually received a standing ovation from the patients after successfully conducting a particularly large session with 20 patients in attendance. While I am sure that many of these patients would have preferred 90 minutes alone with their physician (which would, of course, likely be an unrealistic and unachievable

Physician Abuse 3: Increasing Panel Sizes to Extract All Benefit from the SMA Program, so that Physicians Are Left with No Net Long-Term Gain

I caution against (especially in systems that are largely or entirely capitated) stripping away most or all of the increased productivity benefit that the DIGMA or PSMA program provides the physician with through a correspondingly large increase in the physician's panel size. Physicians are by no means stupid, and they will strongly resist any type of group visit program that only leaves them with more work to do and no net long-term gain. Physicians often express this concern by asking such questions as "Why should I start a DIGMA or PSMA program if the net long-term effect will only be 200 more patients on my panel?"

With DIGMAs and PSMAs, Physicians Need to Know Practice Sizes Will Not Be Correspondingly Increased

Especially in capitated systems, full-time physicians worry that participation in a group visit program that leverages their time, increases their productivity, and enables them to better manage a large and busy practice will only have the net effect—in the long run—of administration substantially increasing their practice size by 8–10% (or 16–20% in the case of half-time physicians). This would leave them with no net long-term benefit whatsoever for having undertaken the group visit program in the first place—i.e., for taking the risk of establishing a SMA for their practice and learning to deliver medical care in the dramatically different milieu of a group visit. From the physicians' perspective, in the long term, such an increase in patient panel size would completely nullify any net productivity gain that the DIGMA or PSMA might have initially provided them with. Note that this is an issue for DIGMAs and PSMAs only. While CHCCs provide other types of gains, most of which are downstream (such a reduced ED, nursing home, and hospitalization costs for the 15–20 patients being followed in the CHCC), they do not dramatically increase physician productivity like DIGMAs and PSMAs are able to do.

Administration Needs to Reassure Physicians that They Will Retain a Substantial Net Gain

Therefore, any integrated healthcare delivery system seeking to achieve the many patient, physician, and organizational benefits that DIGMAs and PSMAs can offer must adopt long-term business policies that build upon physicians' trust in the SMA program. This, in turn, requires leaving physicians with some substantial net long-term gain for having undertaken the risk and change in practice style that group visits entail. Physicians in capitated as well as fee-for-service systems need reassurance from administrators that, should they choose to implement a DIGMA or PSMA in their practices, they will be left with some tangible and meaningful net long-term benefit for having done so.

Do Not Use SMAs as an Excuse to Cut Back Further on Physician Staffing Levels

One variant of this same theme would be to use the enhanced efficiency and productivity benefits that a well-run DIGMA or PSMA program can offer as an excuse to substantially reduce physician staffing levels—i.e., rather than using this added productivity to improve access, service, or quality of care. It is important to keep in mind that today's major group visit models have been designed as tools to enhance service and quality of care, to better manage both backlogged practices and chronic illnesses, and for improving outcomes as well as access to medical care. They were never meant to completely replace individual office visits or to give healthcare organizations an excuse to further reduce physician staffing levels in primary and specialty care, especially to the point where job doability becomes even further eroded.

While Some Increase in Practice Size Is Anticipated, It Needs to Be Reasonable

In today's hectic and fast paced healthcare environment, many physicians expect some future increase in panel size—but hope that any such increase will be reasonable and achievable. For physicians in a capitated healthcare environment (as well as physicians in other types of organizations where their income is not substantially determined by the number of patients seen), this translates into any such future increase in panel size being small enough so that physicians are nonetheless left with some meaningful net long-term gain for having started a DIGMA or PSMA in their practices. This certainly means that (at least in systems that are largely capitated, or where salaries are not appreciably determined by production) physicians must be assured that any future increase in panel size resulting from the increased productivity that the DIGMA or PSMA provides will be reasonable—so that the physician will be left with a substantial net gain for having undertaken risk and invested the time that running a group visit in their practice entails.

Physician Abuse 4: Not Rewarding Physicians with Either Time or Money

In an effort to maximally improve access and productivity, administrators might be tempted to allow physicians barely enough time to actually conduct the group visit (often with 10–16 difficult, high-intensity patients) and then expect them to rush back to immediately begin seeing more patients in the clinic just as soon as the group is over. Although this may work for some physicians in fee-for-service settings (in particular, those who might choose to do this in order to maximize productivity and revenues), this practice will provide little incentive to many other physicians and may even be a disincentive—especially for those in capitated systems.

To ask physicians to be doubly or triply efficient in a group visit by seeing dramatically more patients in that venue, but then only rewarding them with more work as soon as the DIGMA or PSMA is over, will almost certainly prove to be an unsuccessful strategy in the long run. In all likelihood, it will not help in recruiting physicians to start group visits either in their own practices (i.e., to improve productivity and access, and to better manage large, busy, and backlogged practices) or in chronic illness population management programs—i.e., to help care for the burgeoning population of chronically ill patients.

Why not instead consider providing physicians who participate in well-run group visit programs with a substantial and meaningful reward for doing so? This could include such powerful incentives as additional money or time—i.e., time that could be used for desktop medicine, phone calls, administration, research, teaching, or paperwork. For example, as SMA champion at Harvard Vanguard Medical Associates/Atrius Health, I am soon going to begin looking for a busy full-time physician or two who want to be the first to completely change their style of delivering medical care. That is, instead of primarily doing individual office visits and only secondarily working in a group visit or two each week, shifting to primarily running DIGMAs (e.g. at least one every day of the workweek) plus one or two PSMAs per week—and only secondarily seeing patients individually. I say DIGMAs and PSMAs because these are the group visit models that dramatically increase physician productivity and access (i.e. to follow-up visits and private physical examinations, respectively), and because this approach of daily DIGMAs and weekly PSMAs would enable patients to be seen any day that they happened to have a medical need.

Provided that such physicians would be willing to open their practices (i.e. in the event that they are closed) and increase panel sizes to create sufficient patient demand to keep all group sessions filled, this will directly translate into a 40–50% increase in their productivity each week—i.e. at the same time that they are feeling more energized, finishing on time, and enjoying their professional life more. The percentage increase in patient volume each week would be even greater in the event that the physician ran two DIGMAs on certain days (perhaps one in the morning and one in the afternoon) and/or one to two PSMAs per week—partly for the efficient delivery of annual physicals on established patients and partly to intake new patients into their practice (i.e. in the event that a private physical exam is necessary to intake a new patient).

In return, such physicians would not only be given a documenter for each SMA session they conduct, plus would also be given a full-time documenter for their individual office visits as well (or, if they prefer, given one less clinical hour per day during which they would need to see patients—i.e. using this hour instead to better manage their practice as they see best fit, such as to deal with e-mails, phone calls, teaching, paperwork, etc.). Although taking an hour per day for desktop medicine would reduce the overall weekly productivity gain of these providers from those stated in the previous paragraph, it would nonetheless leave them with a substantial net positive weekly gain—and much more enjoyment during the workweek. Such an approach would reveal the true potential that group visits can have as a practice management tool—i.e. for increasing quality, productivity, access,

patient empowerment, and patient as well as physician professional satisfaction. The key here is to provide physicians with some sort of potent incentive, a sizeable net long-term benefit, for having instituted a successful group visit program in their practices. By providing physicians with such a strong (but reasonable) incentive for running a group visit, administration will make it much more likely that the group visit program will rapidly expand at the grassroots level throughout the organization—a process that a SMA champion (particularly through the use of a documenter as a potent incentive to physicians) can be most helpful in achieving (at least in larger healthcare systems).

Physician Abuse 5: Forcing Physicians to Go Beyond Their Level of Comfort in the SMA

If the organization is to expect their group visit program to prosper and be fully successful, then it is important to not alienate physicians by forcing them to go beyond their level of comfort in the group setting. This could include such demands as forcing physicians to deliver more medical care than they are comfortable with providing in the group setting, to conduct examinations in the SMA setting that they prefer to provide individually, and generally pushing physicians outside of their comfort zone. The one exception here is that physicians will need to see sufficient patients during each and every SMA session to ensure that the program is economically viable—even if they are initially uncomfortable with doing so. Experience has shown time after time that when this is properly done and census targets are consistently met, physicians soon adapt to this increased patient volume and become comfortable with it—plus it makes for a more informative, interactive, interesting, and fast-paced group. Furthermore, without this baseline level of physician productivity within the SMA, the group visit program cannot succeed financially in the long run.

Second Form of Abuse: Not Putting the Necessary Resources into the SMA Program

The second form of abuse lies in not putting sufficient resources into the group visit program, i.e., for the various SMA models to be able to provide the full range of benefits that they were originally designed to deliver. This includes putting fewer personnel, facilities, promotional, and budgetary resources into the group visit program than properly supported and run DIGMAs, CHCCs, and PSMAs require.

Insufficient Resource Abuse 1: Expecting Physicians to Conduct the SMA Without the Appropriate Support Personnel

I cannot tell you how many times healthcare organizations have failed to provide the full complement of appropriate SMA team members required for a physician to efficiently and effectively conduct a SMA program. In fact, this is so common that I am listing it as "insufficient resource abuse number one." Demanding that the physician run the group visit either alone or without all of the SMA personnel that the group medical appointment program has been designed to operate with, would greatly reduce the physician's efficiency, productivity, satisfaction, and likelihood of success. In the case of DIGMAs and PSMAs, this means having the best possible SMA team—including the behaviorist, documenter, and nursing personnel required to correctly run the DIGMA or PSMA program. It also means having the dedicated scheduler assigned to the program to ensure completely full sessions, as well as the champion and program coordinator needed in larger systems to expeditiously move the program forward throughout the organization.

Do Not Try to Extract Even Greater Benefit from the SMA by Understaffing It

Insisting that the physicians run their DIGMA or PSMA without the full complement of recommended support personnel—behaviorist, nurses, documenter, and dedicated scheduler—in a misguided attempt to even further reduce costs and strengthen the bottom line beyond what these models were designed to provide would certainly represent a physician abuse of group visits. This is because any cost savings that might occur as a result of not providing required SMA personnel would likely be made at the physician's expense—as the physician would consequently have to work correspondingly harder due to the reduced efficiency and excessive physician workload that such an approach would involve. Furthermore, there is also a high probability that such an approach would also be self-defeating due to the likelihood that the physician would be correspondingly less efficient and productive during the SMA session, which would ultimately result in group census being reduced as a consequence of this understaffing of the SMA. In other words, by trying to *save a buck* by not providing the required less costly members of the SMA team, we end up undercutting the productivity of the most costly person—i.e., the physician—and consequently end up reducing the overall net financial gain that the SMA is capable of providing.

To Be Optimally Productive, Physicians Must Delegate Fully to All Members of the SMA Team

Keep in mind that although this might be a less important issue for the CHCC model, it is by off-loading, whenever appropriate, as many physician responsibilities as possible onto less costly support personnel associated with the DIGMA and PSMA that these group visit models are able to so dramatically leverage expensive physician time. Yes, some efficiency gains come from these group visit models simply due to the fact that they occur in a group setting (i.e., in which sessions can be overbooked to avoid expensive physician downtime, and where efficiency can be gained by avoiding repetition); however, most of the productivity gain in a well-run DIGMA or PSMA comes from the physician effectively delegating as much as possible to less expensive personnel in the SMA team. Ultimately, the goal is for the physician to only do that which the physician alone can do—and to delegate all other physician duties onto less costly members of the SMA team. This is accomplished by expanding the nursing, behaviorist, and documenter duties within the SMA to be all that they can be—which also enables DIGMAs and PSMAs to be max-packed, and for patients to be provided with an *one-stop healthcare shopping experience*.

Each Member of the SMA Team Dispatches Important Responsibilities

It is important to keep in mind that each and every member of the SMA team plays a critical role in its success, dispatches many important duties and responsibilities, and often has a complementary skill set that enables them to perform certain duties better than the physician could. For example, take the role of the behaviorist in the DIGMA and PSMA models, who often has complementary skills that augment those of the physician. By carefully selecting and training a behavioral health professional (health psychologist, social worker, marriage and family therapist, nurse, health educator, etc.) who is experienced in running large groups, handling group dynamics, pacing groups to finish on time, and addressing the psychosocial needs of medical patients, many duties that would otherwise fall onto the physician's shoulders can be off-loaded onto this less expensive person with special skills.

For example, the behaviorist: (1) enters the group room a few minutes early to warm the group up; (2) starts the SMA on time, even if the physician is late, with a 3–5 minute introduction; (3) paces the group to keep it running smoothly and on time; (4) handles group dynamic and psychosocial issues; (5) temporarily conducts the group alone whenever the physician documents a chart note, steps out of the group room to conduct a brief private exam or discussion, or (more rarely) to handle an unforeseen clinic emergency; (6) does everything possible to support the physician throughout the entire session; (7) and stays a few minutes late (after the physician has left) to address any last-minute patient questions and to quickly straighten up the group room after the patients depart.

Insufficient Resource Abuse 2: Not Providing the Physician and SMA Team with Adequate Time for Preparation and Training

For SMAs to be successful, physicians (along with their SMA team members and support staffs) must be provided with a small but reasonable amount of time for planning, designing, developing, and implementing their group visit program—much of which can be done outside of normal clinic hours and through use of existing templates already developed for the SMA program (many such templates are included in the DVD attached to this book).

Physicians Need Some Time for Training and to Prepare for Their SMA

In larger systems, the champion and program coordinator can handle much of this preparatory work—i.e., through use of the *pipeline* discussed in Chapter 11 and existing templates already developed for the SMA program (many such templates are included in the DVD attached to this book). In spite of this assistance, physicians still need some time in order to: draft the promotional materials for their group visit program (preferably from templates already developed for the program); develop a chart note template for their SMA; and select the appropriate handouts and patient education materials for their program. Physicians also need some planning and training time regarding how to both run a group visit and refer patients into it. Interested physicians will also need some additional time in order to meet at different times with the champion, program coordinator, SMA team members, and support staff—time that should, whenever possible, occur outside of normal clinic hours.

Support Staff and All SMA Team Members Also Need Time for Training and Preparation

In addition, adequate staff preparation time and training must be provided for the group visit program to be successful. For example, DIGMAs and PSMAs require that physicians not only understand these models and their role in them, but also learn how to effectively and efficiently refer patients into these group visit programs during normal office visits. Furthermore, the various members of the physician's SMA team—including nurse/MA(s), behaviorist, documenter (if any), and dedicated scheduler—must be appropriately trained with regard to their respective duties and responsibilities. In addition, the physician's office manager and entire support staff (especially the physician's schedulers, receptionists, and nurses/MAs—as well as their supervisors) need to be provided with adequate meeting time to address their concerns, discuss their roles in the program, and provide proper training for a successful SMA program. Without adequate training, the physician, SMA team, and support staff are likely to experience unnecessary stress and frustration with the program—and the SMA itself will be at significantly greater risk for failure.

Insufficient Resource Abuse 3: Not Providing the Appropriate Group and Exam Rooms

As discussed below, all three of today's major group visit models have their own respective facilities requirements.

An Appropriate Group Room Is Required

The necessary facilities for a DIGMA and CHCC typically include a properly equipped group room of sufficient size which is adequately ventilated—preferably one which is wheelchair accessible, nicely decorated, and with bathrooms nearby. The group room needs to be well lighted, clean, stocked with two working computers and a printer, and equipped with enough comfortable chairs to accommodate all attendees—patients, support persons, physician, and members of the SMA team. In addition, the group room must be large enough (perhaps containing 18–25 comfortable chairs) to also accommodate any observers. A few pictures and an artificial tree or two will go a long way towards *warming up* what would otherwise be a rather sterile appearing group room. In addition, a well-stocked exam room should be located nearby that contains a computer, all necessary forms, and the required medical equipment. On the other hand, the Physicals SMA model requires a group room that can be considerably smaller than that required for a DIGMA; however, PSMAs also typically require 2–5 examination rooms—although they can be located in the physician's own office area rather than adjacent to the group room. If no appropriate group room space is available, be creative by using: (1) any available conference rooms; (2) unused storage or staff lunchroom space that could be converted into a group room; (3) the lobby during off-hours; or (4) in the absence of any appropriate group room space whatsoever, consider taking the SMA offsite to a nearby building (or even into the community).

Appropriate Examination Rooms Are Also Required

If there is no examination room located in the vicinity of the group room (i.e., for a DIGMA), then consider converting any available nearby space into one—such as an office, small storage room, vending area, or staff break room. Only if no other space is available should you consider improvising an exam room by curtaining off a corner of the group room, as the constant noise and chatter emanating from this area throughout much of the session could prove to be an annoying distraction for the physician as well as group members. Such an arrangement could also prove problematic in terms of confidentiality—because many patients will likely not want to have the entire group within hearing range when their vitals are taken (especially when their weight and age are discussed).

Use Existing Facilities for the Pilot Study, but Recognize that More Appropriate Facilities Will Eventually Be Needed

It is critically important that the necessary, appropriately furnished group and exam room facilities be provided to ensure that: (1) the SMA can be held successfully with a full cohort of patients; (2) patients are kept comfortable throughout the entire session; and (3) the privacy needs of the patients are adequately addressed. Although physicians and the organization can often make do with whatever group and exam room facilities might happen to be available during the initial pilot study phase (i.e., so that the success of the pilot SMA program can be evaluated within that system), this is at best a temporary solution. One suggested long-term solution—i.e., when later moving toward full-scale, organization-wide implementation—would be to reinvest a portion of the savings created by the group visit program back into retooling the physical plant in such a manner that the necessary group and examination room space can ultimately be provided.

Insufficient Resource Abuse 4: Not Providing the Required High-Quality Promotional Materials

Historically speaking, healthcare organizations have all too often failed to provide the high-quality promotional materials that SMA programs require in order to help fill all sessions. We must always remain cognizant of the fact that patients have a lifetime of experience in expecting an individual office visit with their physician. This means that professional appearing promotional materials are needed in order to both reflect the high-quality care that patients can expect to receive in the SMA and help persuade patients to attend something as different from traditional individual office visits as group visits are.

Use High-Quality, Coordinated, and Eye-Appealing Promotional Materials

If we want to adequately inform patients of the new SMA program (and expect them to consider attending in lieu of a traditional office visit the next time they need to be seen), then we must use high-quality, coordinated, and eye-appealing promotional materials that accurately represent the high-quality care and multiple benefits that patients can in fact expect to receive. The framed wall poster, which should be prominently displayed on the physician's lobby and exam room walls, can be used as a template to establish a particular trademark look for all promotional materials developed within the organization for the SMA program. Such marketing materials include the program description flier, the announcement letter, the invitation to attend, any educational handouts, and the Patient Packet that might be used.

Not Providing Appropriate Marketing Materials Could Undermine the SMA

Do not attempt to avoid spending the necessary funds on quality promotional materials. Such an approach would neither inform patients adequately about the many patient care benefits that the new SMA program provides nor help persuade them to attend. The inevitable result would likely be to undermine the success of the entire SMA program, which would be unfair to the many patients who might otherwise be willing to attend—i.e., if they only understood the new program and its many potential patient benefits. The use of cheap appearing, sloppy, or inappropriate promotional materials will likely result in poor attendance and a lack of patient buy-in— which could sabotage and undermine the success of the entire SMA program. This is not the time to hastily run off a few Xerox copies of a poorly drafted poster and quickly scotch tape it onto the lobby walls in the hopes that it will somehow persuade uninformed patients to attend something as dramatically different as a SMA.

Many Organizations Fail to Provide the Needed Promotional Materials

The lack of any marketing materials whatsoever would likely even be worse, and it would almost certainly undermine the success of the SMA program. The goal of all of these SMA marketing materials is to persuade patients to attend for the first time (and for it to take less time later for the physician to personally invite patients and get them to attend)—after which, experience has shown that patients will almost always be willing to return to the SMA setting in the future. And remember that the key to a successful SMA program is group sessions that are consistently filled to targeted census levels. Despite this harsh warning, abundant personal experience to date as a consultant in the area of group medical visits has made it clear that numerous healthcare organizations frequently fail to develop the appropriate promotional materials for their SMA program—and that, as a result, group census during SMA sessions is all-too-often subpar.

Insufficient Resource Abuse 5: Failure to Evaluate the SMA Program on an Ongoing Basis

Another potential source of abuse is not providing the ongoing evaluation that is needed for a successful SMA program.

Ongoing Evaluation of the SMA Program Is Critically Important for Many Reasons.

It is critically important that the quality, outcomes, service, productivity, access, utilization, economic, patient and physician satisfaction, etc. benefits of the SMA program be accurately evaluated on an ongoing basis. Only then can we correctly assess whether patients, physicians, and the organization alike are receiving the desired level of demonstrable benefit from their group visit program. The great importance of this ongoing evaluation effort is emphasized here because it is only through such measurements and data analyses that the organization will be able

to track the effectiveness of their SMA program—and determine whether it is achieving the expected results. Furthermore, it is only through such ongoing evaluations that we can hope to ultimately improve the SMA program because, as it is often said, "If we keep doing what we are doing, then we will keep getting what we've got."

Innovations such as group visits must be data driven and provable in order to convince physicians and healthcare organizations to adopt them—and to demonstrate their validity and economic value to payers and corporate purchasers so that they support them. For example, without such data analyses and evaluations of the effectiveness of their group visit programs, the various studies reported in the outcomes chapter of this book would not have been possible. Also, patients need to be convinced of the benefits that group medical appointments can offer to them and come to believe that SMAs provide improved care and a better way. For insurers and healthcare bureaucrats to take full notice, it will ultimately take hard evidence in the form of data-based research and publications from reputable universities and healthcare systems that are beyond reproach demonstrating that group visits can in fact yield better results, provide more affordable medical care, and make doctors and patients happier.

As can be seen in Chapter 9, this process is now beginning to occur—and should continue to increase exponentially into the foreseeable future as evermore SMA programs are launched in healthcare systems both nationally and internationally. Although community support groups and psychiatry therapy groups have been widespread for decades (and a 1907 JAMA article discussed how some tuberculosis patients treated in groups did better) (2), the group visit concept did not really take off in primary care until the emergence of the CHCC, DIGMA, and PSMA models during the past decade and a half—a trend that should continue in primary and specialty care, but only as long as data demonstrating the effectiveness of SMAs continues to be collected and published (and as long as potential abuses as well as substantial billing problems do not emerge).

While Important to Long-Term Growth, Many Systems Are Not Evaluating SMA Programs

It is often stated that "If we fail to plan, we plan to fail." The importance of this ongoing evaluation process (i.e., of continuously gathering and analyzing all relevant data) is key to the ultimate success of any group visit program. If we are to expect group visits to continue to grow and receive appropriate reimbursements, ongoing documentation must be generated to demonstrate the effectiveness and consistency of these SMA models in achieving their stated objectives—i.e., in terms of quality, service, outcomes, productivity, and economy. Despite such recommendations, experience has all too frequently demonstrated that healthcare organizations are often reticent to make this commitment to measurement and analysis—and to evaluating the success of their SMA program on an ongoing basis.

Caution: Do Not Evaluate a SMA Program Without First Ensuring It Is Being Properly Run

The only word of caution that I would make here is to first be certain that you are running your SMA program relatively correctly before undertaking this time-consuming and somewhat laborious evaluation process. Otherwise, all that you will be measuring is that which is currently not being done correctly—i.e., rather than anything meaningful or significant as regards the true potential and capabilities of group visits within your organization. Before measuring and analyzing your SMA program, be certain that the basics are first correctly put in place. For example, we know that consistently maintaining targeted census levels (which is most frequently set to be a 300% increase in physician productivity over individual office visits) during all sessions is critical to the success of any DIGMA or PSMA program—especially in terms of achieving their potential productivity, access, and economic benefits. As a consequence, it is hardly worth the effort to generate a 20–40 page report on your DIGMA program if you only have five or six patients on average attending sessions—because such a program is, even on its surface, clearly insufficiently attended and therefore not economically viable(3).

Should such poor patient attendance be occurring during your DIGMA and PSMA sessions (recall that almost all problems in a SMA program ultimately result in reduced census), I would recommend that you instead put your energy into first correcting this problem—i.e., before going through an extensive data analysis on a program that is clearly neither economical nor correctly run. There is a wide variety of such factors that could be underlying the poor attendance of your SMA program—such as inadequate promotional materials, lack of appropriate physician and staff involvement in the referral process, hostility toward the SMA program by some on the physician's reception or scheduling staff, SMAs being too homogeneous and narrowly defined to ensure full groups, running SMAs at times that will likely result in low attendance (e.g., holidays, after dark with elderly patients, during heavy snow storms), patients not being informed about the SMA and invited to attend, etc. Should you instead proceed to evaluate a SMA program that has insufficient attendance, you will likely incorrectly conclude that DIGMAs and PSMAs do not work in your system—i.e., when they in fact very well could, if only the problem underlying such poor patient attendance was first ferreted out and solved.

Insufficient Resource Abuse 6: Physicians Must Avoid Misusing Their Group Visit Program

In addition to physicians being abused with regards to their group visit program, it is important to note that SMAs can also be misused and abused by the physicians themselves.

No Matter How Much Others Do, Some Physician Time Involvement Is Nonetheless Required

For example, even though the champion, program coordinator, and other support personnel are trained to assist the physician in many ways in planning, designing, implementing, and conducting the group visit program, some modicum of physician involvement during each phase is nonetheless required. It is not realistic for physicians to expect that their SMA program will be designed and implemented solely through the efforts of others—and that it will be successful without any personal investment of their own time and energy.

Physicians Cannot Avoid Personally Inviting Patients into Their DIGMA or PSMA

Also, it is imperative that physicians be willing to play an active role on an ongoing basis in inviting all appropriate patients during regular office visits to attend the SMA for their next follow-up visit (DIGMA) or physical examination (PSMA). Having the physician personally invite all appropriate patients as they are seen in the clinic (through a positive and carefully worded script) is the single most important key to successful SMA—as it is the critical ingredient to consistently achieving full group sessions. While others on the physician's support staff (receptionists, nurses, schedulers, etc.) can help, only the physician can perform this vital function so effectively and efficiently. Yet, one problem in this regard is that personally inviting patients is somewhat of a foreign concept for many physicians (which makes it easy for this critically important SMA function to be overlooked)—especially for those physicians who are busy and backlogged. For these physicians, all they normally have to do with regards to having full schedules each day is to show up at work in the morning. I say this because at least for these busy physicians, patient demand exceeds their capacity to meet that demand. As a result, when they arrive in the morning, they will naturally find that their individual office visit schedule for the day is already completely full. Despite the best of intentions, some physicians fail to follow-through on inviting all appropriate patients during normal clinic hours—with the result all too often being that their SMA fails because it does not consistently maintain the desired level of group census.

Physicians Must Not Arrive More than 5 Minutes Late, or Leave Sessions Unnecessarily

Another way that physicians can misuse group visits is to constantly arrive late to their group sessions—especially when they arrive quite late. Physicians must keep in mind that by consistently arriving more than a few minutes late, they are missing more than just the behaviorist's introduction—which is OK to miss, but only takes 3–5 minutes. Arriving later than this will likely result in the session feeling rushed and in finishing late—and ultimately, possibly even in being able to see fewer patients in the SMA. Some physicians also sometimes leave the group inappropriately to make a telephone call or attend to a non-urgent personal or clinic matter—all of which can take time away from the group setting and could communicate to the patients that they are not that important. Arriving late to sessions (or unnecessarily missing time during the group) will in all likelihood ultimately translate into insufficient time remaining in the session to adequately address the medical needs of all patients in attendance.

Physicians Need to Keep the SMA Team and Support Staff Appraised as to How Well They Are Doing

Yet another responsibility that physicians must be willing to shoulder with regards to their group visit is to keep all personnel associated with their program appraised of how satisfied the physician is with what they are or are not doing satisfactorily. This includes SMA team members as well as the physician's scheduling and reception staff, and it also covers what improvements need to be made and what changes still need to occur for the desired results to be achieved. Nobody else can do this because only the physician knows how satisfied they are or are not with each person's performance. Should the physician not do this, the SMA program will likely be negatively affected.

For example, if the documenter is not generating the type of chart notes that the physician wants, then the physician needs to talk to the documenter about this, giving constructive suggestions as to what is wanted or what additional training might be helpful. If the physician's scheduling staff is not filling sessions sufficiently, then the physician needs to discuss this with them and explain exactly what is expected. The same holds for the reception staff handing out invitations, and the nurse/MA distributing fliers to all appropriate patients as they are roomed—plus saying a few kind words about the program. In addition, the physician needs to give constant, ongoing feedback to the behaviorist as to what they are or are not doing correctly from the physician's perspective.

Patients, Physicians, Organizations, Insurers, and Purchasers Alike Should Benefit

One final point regarding the possible abuse of group visits by physicians needs to be made which is perhaps a little less obvious. I have always felt that group visits offer enough benefits to provide a "win-win" situation for patients, physicians, healthcare organizations, insurers, and purchasers alike—so that each gains some long-term net benefit from the SMA program.

No single entity should extract all the benefit at the expense of the others. To do so would constitute an abuse of group visits. For example, the physician could take the entire benefit for themselves by reducing his or her workweek by 3 hours (or by increasing their salary by 8–9% in fee-for-service systems that are 100% productivity based) for every weekly, 90-min DIGMA or PSMA that is run which increases productivity by 300%. Or capitated healthcare organizations could take the full benefit of full-time physicians running such a weekly DIGMA or PSMA in their practices by increasing physicians' patient panel sizes by 8–9%. Similarly, the insurer could extract the entire benefit by reducing reimbursements by 8–9%, or the corporate purchaser could reduce what they are willing to pay by 8–9%. Instead, I believe that some sort of intermediate compromise be struck that provides some sort of substantial and meaningful net benefit to accrue to each of these entities.

Organizational Abuse

As we have been discussing, there are numerous ways that healthcare organizations can abuse group visits. For example, they can make group visits mandatory to physicians, bill for the behaviorist's time as well as for counseling time, or demand that group sizes be excessively large. In addition, they can force providers to go beyond their level of comfort, fail to put the necessary resources into the SMA (personnel, facilities, promotional materials, budgetary, etc.), or fail to provide adequate time for preparation and training—i.e., to the physician, SMA team, and support staff. Furthermore, healthcare organizations could expect physicians to conduct SMAs without the appropriate support personnel, make group visits mandatory rather than voluntary to patients, fail to evaluate the SMA program on an ongoing basis, or fail to reward physicians with either time or money.

Finally, healthcare organizations could also attempt to extract the entire benefit of the SMA program for themselves (i.e., to the exclusion of all others), which could include increasing panel sizes to the point that physicians are left with no net long-term gain for running a SMA program. We have already discussed this issue with regards to capitated healthcare organizations, in the context of the system extracting the entire benefit of the program for themselves by correspondingly increasing full-time physician's panel sizes by 8–9% (or half-time physicians by 16–18%), which would not leave physicians with any net long-term gain for running a group visit in their practice. Fee-for-service systems could similarly extract the entire benefit of the SMA by correspondingly reducing the financial reimbursement that passes through to full-time physicians by 8–9%.

Physician Abuse

What is less obvious is that physicians can (and, on occasion, have) take the total net productivity gain of the SMA program for themselves. They have done this in managed care organizations by cutting back their workweek in a manner that is directly equivalent to the productivity gain that the DIGMA or PSMA provides in their capitated or fee-for-service system (in the latter case, where the physician prefers extra free time to additional money). For example, in the case of a 90-minute weekly DIGMA or PSMA that leverages the physician's time by 300%, the increased productivity of the SMA would translate into the physician seeing as many patients in the 1½ hour SMA as would normally require 4½ hours to see in the clinic—or a total net gain of 3 hours per week for every such weekly DIGMA or PSMA that the physician runs.

If such a physician were to reduce his or her workweek by 3 hours (which would certainly be all right for a solo practitioner, but not for a physician in a managed care

organization), then they would extract the entire net efficiency benefit of the program for themselves—and thereby leave no net economic gain from this increased productivity for the organization, which would also be faced with covering the overhead cost of the DIGMA or PSMA program. Of course, even here, the SMA program could also provide other economic benefits to the organization (such those that might accrue from improved compliance, performance measures, health maintenance, outcomes, etc.); however, for the sake of this discussion, let us just focus upon the benefits of the improved productivity that the DIGMA or PSMA offers.

Instead, why not compromise and share the benefit? Perhaps a wiser approach would be for the physician and organization to split this efficiency benefit up in some reasonable way, such as the physician being able to take 1 hour each week and convert it into time for desktop medicine, administration, phone calls, etc.—or else, perhaps, to work 1 hour less per week (or enjoy a 1–3% raise in salary in fee-for-service systems where salaries are 100% productivity based) for every such DIGMA or PSMA that the physician runs each week which leverages the physician's time by 300% or more. The remainder of this benefit could then be used by the organization to cover overhead and increase capacity—which could, in turn, result over time in improved access to care.

Insurance Abuse

Just as is the case with organizational and physician abuses, we must likewise prevent any potential for the abuse of group visits by insurers—which could possibly take the form of insurers being overly intrusive by either underincentivizing or overincentivizing SMAs.

Avoid Unwarranted Insurance Intrusions into Group Visits

Unwarranted organizational and insurance intrusions into group visit programs could prove to be very problematic and could even constitute an abuse of group visits. For example, organizations that force unmotivated providers to offer group visits (or so highly incentivize them that even reluctant physicians are eventually forced to offer them) would constitute an abuse, as SMAs were always meant to be voluntary to patients and physicians alike. Furthermore, if you want to have a group visit program of poor quality, I can think of no better way of doing so than by forcing providers who do not want to run them to do so despite their personal reluctance.

Similarly, if insurers should deny reimbursement for group visits unless patients are taken outside of the group room, one by one and treated individually, this would certainly undermine and dramatically undercut the value that a well-run group visit program can offer to patients. I say this because, by forcing physicians to comply with such an unfortunate requirement, other patients in the group room would thereby be denied the benefit of learning from the physician while treating each patient individually outside of the group room—i.e., so that other attendees could no longer listen, learn, interact, and benefit. What would the rationale for such a requirement be? It certainly represents a *throw-back* to the same old way of doing things—i.e., by forcing patients to be seen individually.

If there is no difference in the care that is actually being delivered (which would, of course, not be the case for discussions of a truly private nature or for physical examinations that are inappropriate for the group setting), then why not provide that medical care in the group room—i.e., where all can listen and learn, and so that patients can feel that they are spending 90 minutes with their doctor? Although PSMAs would be largely unaffected (since the actual physical examinations are already being conducted on all patients individually in the privacy of the exam room, with only the subsequent interactive group segment occurring in the group room), DIGMAs and CHCCs could definitely be deleteriously impacted by such an unfortunate and intrusive requirement by insurers. In the majority of cases (i.e., as for DIGMAs, where all the medical care that can appropriately be delivered in the group is in fact provided in the highly efficient group room setting), such a requirement would dramatically undercut the benefit that a well-run group visit program could offer to all patients in attendance.

CHCCs might be less impacted than DIGMAs by such a requirement since approximately one-third of the patients in attendance are already being seen individually during the individual visit segment that follows the CHCC group. However, it could dramatically and negatively impact the CHCC group experience for the other two-thirds of patients if they need to be sequentially shuttled out of the group room—i.e., just in order to be seen individually for insurance billing purposes, even if this happens to not be medically necessary. I am particularly concerned about this as a result of hearing that some physicians are actually taking patients out of their group room setting solely for reimbursement purposes—i.e., one at a time in order to treat them individually, which is what they understand they must do in order to get reimbursed. Clearly, this would undercut not only much of the efficiency benefit but also the patient education, support, and interaction benefits

that properly run SMAs can offer. What an unfortunate waste that would be.

What if Insurers Underincentivize SMAs?

It is clear that should insurers underincentivize SMAs, the likely result would be to undermine all group visit programs—and preclude their widespread use. This would be most unfortunate as it would be a terrible loss for patients, physicians, and healthcare organizations alike, as it would effectively kill the multiple benefits that a well run group visit program can provide to all—and basically leave us with the same old broken individual office visit health care system that we currently have. I am often asked by physicians, medical group administrators, and executive leaders what would happen to group visits if Medicare were to ultimately rule somewhat along the following lines: "We will pay you $100 for this medical service if you treat the patient through a traditional individual office visit, but will only pay $40 if you provide that exact same service through a group visit." To me, this scenario would not make much sense because precisely the same medical service is being provided, but at two different rates—with the only substantive differences being the number of observers present and the setting in which the care is being delivered (i.e., an exam room versus a group room). However, it is my understanding that neither of these differences is addressed by existing E&M billing codes. It is not that this situation could not occur; however, I fail to see how such a scenario would benefit Medicare.

In other words, it would seem that Medicare would have little to gain through such a scenario, which would leave them with exactly the same situation that they have had all along (i.e., until the recent advent of highly efficient group visits)—traditional individual office visits alone and an inefficient and inaccessible healthcare system that is already is stretched to the max. Obviously, the likely end result of such a decision would be devastating to group visits. As a result, patients, physicians, and Medicare alike would lose out on the many potential benefits that properly run group visits can offer. Despite the fact that this possibility represents a common fear amongst physicians and healthcare executives alike, it seems that all it would accomplish is to completely undermine and destroy group visits—along with the multitude of benefits that they provide. In other words, it would just leave Medicare with the same old broken system of individual office visits alone—which is something that they already have, but which is not working. Because it would seem that Medicare has as much to gain as anybody from a well-run group visit program, I have never worried a great deal about this scenario actually occurring in practice—which is certainly not to say that it could not happen.

Not being overly worried about the possibility of insurers underincentivizing group visits does not mean that I have not had a realistic concern in this regard. Certainly, if insurers and integrated healthcare delivery systems fail to adequately incentivize group visits through the appropriate levels of reimbursement and support, then there would be no meaningful financial incentive for physicians to significantly alter their style of practice to include group visits, rather than providing traditional individual office visits alone. My concern in this regard is apparent in the following quotation that appeared in the November 10, 2003 article on group visits in Time Magazine. "Doctors conducting one-on-one exams followed by a group discussion (AU: as in a PSMA) can bill for individual visits, but Noffsinger, for one, is concerned that insurers could reduce those payments once they realize doctors can triple the number of patients they see. 'The insurers have more to gain than anybody,' he insists. 'Their patients are serviced faster and better'" (4).

Insurers' Overincentivizing Group Visits Could Likewise Be Problematic:

There is another concern that I have had for a long time, which is quite different from the one discussed above. Clearly, if insurers and healthcare organizations underincentivize SMAs, the results could be devastating to group visits; however, there is another, less obvious concern as well. What if insurers should instead overincentivize group visits relative to traditional individual office visits? In other words, what if the above discussed scenario alternatively took the following form, wherein Medicare instead ultimately ruled along the following lines: "We currently pay you $100 for delivering this particular medical service. From now on, we will instead pay you $90 for providing that service; however, you can provide it either through traditional individual office visits or through group visits, the choice is yours." This could force reluctant physicians to run SMAs in their practices just to survive economically. This could be a particular problem for DIGMAs and PSMAs, as they are best viewed as a series of individual visits with observers occurring in a supportive group setting.

Unlike the previously discussed scenario, this one would provide clear economic benefit to Medicare—and might therefore be an approach they could consider. I have always had a concern that once insurers and managed care organizations gained a clear understanding of the multiple, substantial economic and patient care benefits that

properly run group visits can offer, they could overincentivize them relative to individual visits—perhaps by reducing compensation for individual visits, or else by offering a disproportionate reimbursement for group visits(5).

Should this happen, these excessive incentives for SMAs could end up reducing freedom of choice for patients and physicians alike—i.e., as physicians who do not want to run group visits might be forced to do them in order to survive economically. Similarly, if healthcare administrators were to overincentivize group visits with regards to physicians' future salaries in the organization, physicians who otherwise might not want to run a group visit could then feel compelled to do so. Not only would group visits no longer be voluntary to physicians under such a scenario, but also the likelihood of having many second-rate SMA programs would increase exponentially as evermore physicians not wanting to run group visits were forced to do them just to compete financially. This presents a surefire recipe for numerous low-quality group visits, a risk for failure of the entire SMA program, and a possible public relations nightmare for group visits in the making.

It Is Critically Important that Group Visits Be Appropriately Reimbursed

In our article on preventing potential abuses of group visits, Dr. Scott and I point out that—while no group visit billing codes currently exist—we strongly recommend against such practices as underincentivizing or overincentivizing group visits. This is because we always intended for group visits to be strictly voluntary to physicians and patients alike—i.e., so that physicians who choose to run a SMA do so on a strictly voluntary basis. To do otherwise could create physician resistance to the entire group visit program—plus result in many poor quality SMA programs because the providers doing them would be resentful about being forced to run one despite not wanting to (5).

As group visits continue to grow and play an increasing role in the delivery of high-quality, accessible, and cost-effective medical care in the progressive healthcare delivery systems of the future, there will nonetheless always be an important role for individual office visits to also play. It has always been intended that rather than completely replacing them, SMAs would work well in conjunction with the judicious use of individual office visits—i.e., so that patients who can appropriately be seen in cost-effective group visits are able to receive medical care in that highly efficient venue, whereas traditional office visits will always be available to those patients requiring or preferring them. In fact, because numerous individual visits could thereby be off-loaded onto highly productive group visits, it is anticipated that traditional office visits would eventually become more available to those patients wanting or needing them. However, for a proper future balance to be struck between individual and group visits, it is essential that both be appropriately reimbursed—both individually and with respect to each another.

A Concluding Comment on Potential Abuses of Group Visits

Barring some catastrophic public relations nightmare due to abuse—or some disastrous ruling with regards to billing—it is expected that despite all of the previously discussed concerns surrounding their potential for abuse, group visits will undoubtedly continue to grow and expand in their influence upon healthcare delivery during upcoming decades. Therefore, in terms of preventing any potential for abuse, now is the time to act. History has certainly shown that individual office visits can be abused, and the same is clearly true for group visits—which can also be abused. In spite of the numerous quality, service, efficiency, and economic benefits that properly supported

and run group visit programs can offer, the potential for abuse nonetheless looms very real. The various types of potential abuses must therefore be clearly recognized and scrupulously safeguarded against in order to preserve both the future credibility of SMAs and the numerous quality, access, service, economic, educational, support, and patient care benefits that properly run group visit programs can provide.

References

1. Stevens-Lyons J. The doctor is in for group visits. San Jose Mercury News. Tuesday October 10, 2000;D5, D7.
2. Pratt JH. The class method of treating consumption in the homes of the poor. *Journal of the American Medical Association* 1907;49:755–9.
3. Christianson JB, Louise H, Warrick LH. The business case for Drop-In Group Medical Appointments: a case study of Luther Midelfort Mayo System. Institute for Healthcare Improvement, field report. April 2003.
4. Brower A. The semiprivate checkup: tired of waiting two hours to see the doctor for 10 minutes? Try making your appointments en masse. *Time*. November 10, 2003: 71.
5. Noffsinger EB, Scott JC. Preventing potential abuses of group visits. *Group Practice Journal* 2000;48(5):37–38, 40–42, 44–46.

Chapter 9
Reports, Case Studies, and Outcomes Data

"Do more with less—that's what we all must learn. In the physician's office, when patients share their doctor's time, everyone benefits ... Shared medical appointments improve patient access, enhance patient and physician satisfaction, and increase practice productivity, all without adding more hours to a physician's work week. There is even evidence that they promote better outcomes and lower overall costs of care."

Bob Carlson, Contributing Editor, "Shared Appointments Improve Efficiency in the Clinic," Managed Care, 2003 May; 12 (5):46–83

Why Group Visits?

In this chapter, we look at several recent reports, case studies, and outcomes data regarding group visits from many different healthcare organizations. Although these data are still quite preliminary, certain trends are already becoming clear and much of the information is quite compelling. Because group visits are a relatively recent healthcare innovation, the outcomes studies are just now beginning to emerge—especially for the DIGMA and PSMA models, which were first published in 1999 and 2002, respectively. Undoubtedly, additional reports, case studies, outcomes data, and even more sophisticated randomized control studies will eventually be emerging in the not too distant future.

As the pressure increases for doctors and healthcare organizations to improve care and lower costs, innovations to the delivery of care become evermore important—innovations such as group visits have emerged during the past decade and a half as a means of enhancing care, reducing spending, and providing a "win-win" solution for doctors, patients, and healthcare organizations alike. With properly designed and run shared medical appointment programs such as DIGMAs and PSMAs: (1) quality and outcomes can be enhanced; (2) doctors' time is used more efficiently and access to care is improved; (3) patients enjoy more time with their doctor, plus a more relaxed pace of care; (4) patients help one another and benefit from the group experience; (5) psychosocial and informational issues are better addressed while the doctor–patient relationship is improved; (6) patient education and disease self-management skills can be enhanced; (7) closer follow-up care, surveillance, and monitoring can be efficiently provided; (8) costs can be contained; and (9) individual office visits can be allocated to those who can benefit from them most. Simply put, group visits offer a high quality, accessible, efficient, and cost-effective healing experience to our patients—plus, an additional healthcare choice.

Outcomes Studies Are Just Beginning to Emerge

Group visits provide an effective additional tool in the doctor's *black bag*—one that is voluntary for doctors and patients alike—for better managing both chronic illnesses and busy, backlogged practices. Although this innovative approach to care delivery is still quite new and outcomes data are just now beginning to emerge, the reader will see from the studies discussed in this section that the initial results from these early, preliminary studies are nonetheless quite exciting and persuasive. Because data related to the CHCC model have already been addressed in Chapter 4, this chapter is primarily dedicated to examining some of the important early studies related to today's other two major group visit models—DIGMAs and PSMAs (although one section, which has not yet been published, does deal with the CHCC model). As will be seen, the early data related to these two SMA models are already convincingly illustrating some of the important benefits that these two shared medical appointment models can

E.B. Noffsinger, *Running Group Visits in Your Practice*, DOI 10.1007/b106441_9,
© Springer Science+Business Media, LLC 2009

offer to patients, physicians, and healthcare organizations alike. Before proceeding with the actual outcomes data that we will be discussing in this chapter, I would like to first briefly review a couple of critically important issues regarding the DIGMA and PSMA models.

DIGMAs and PSMAs Are Widely Used in Both Fee-For-Service and Capitated Systems

DIGMAs and PSMAs are the two group visit models that are in widespread use today in both fee-for-service and capitated healthcare environments. Primarily, this is because these two SMA models can best be viewed as a series of individual office visits that happen to occur with observers in a supportive group setting—i.e., with the exact same types of care being delivered as during traditional office visits, and often more. From start to finish, these two SMA models are run like a series of one doctor–one patient encounters addressing the unique medical needs of each patient individually. DIGMAs (primarily designed for efficient, high-quality, and high-value follow-up visits) and PSMAs (primarily designed for the efficient, high quality, cost-effective delivery of private physical examinations) are unique in that they are the only group visit models that are run throughout just like a series of individual office visits with observers. When coupled with the fact that current CPT coding does not address either the setting in which the care is delivered (i.e., exam room, group room, or the *doc-in-the-box* at the local warehouse retailer) or the number of observers that you can have, this is the reason that many fee-for-service systems are currently offering DIGMAs and PSMAs and billing according to the level of care delivered and documented—but not for either the counseling time or the behaviorist's time.

Although billing for DIGMAs and PSMAs through use of existing billing codes according to the level of medical care delivered and documented might therefore seem reasonable, one must keep in mind that the issue of billing for group visits has not yet been completely resolved (i.e., either for group visits in general or for the different types of group visit models)—and it is complicated by the lack of specific billing codes for group visits. On the other hand, at least for DIGMAs and PSMAs, many question whether there is any need for separate billing codes as these two group visit models are run just like a series of individual office visits and deliver the exact same types of care throughout (and often, even more care). It is therefore recommended that, before starting any type of group visit program (at least until the billing

issue for group visits is fully clarified), each healthcare organization addresses for itself how it intends to bill for group visits—i.e., while still meeting all internal and external requirements and regulations.

Outcome Studies at the Level of the Individual Physician

DIGMA pilot studies at the individual physician level should prove to be relevant and helpful to the reader who is contemplating a group visit program for his or her practice. With properly designed and run DIGMAs and PSMAs, increased physician productivity is built in by first determining the *target* and *minimum* census levels, based upon both medical economics and effective group dynamics, and then subsequently ensuring that this predetermined group size is consistently met over time—which requires an organized and disciplined team approach to inviting patients and filling all group sessions. In DIGMAs and PSMAs, the predetermined census level is usually set so as to increase provider productivity over traditional individual office visits by 200–400% (and most commonly by 300%).

DIGMAs And PSMAs Are Unique in Their Ability to Solve Access Problems

The DIGMA and PSMA models are unique among all group visit models because of their ability to dramatically increase productivity and solve access problems through use of existing resources. This is because: (1) DIGMAs and PSMAs cover much—or most—of the individual provider's practice, rather than just a relatively small but costly subset of their patient panel (such as high-utilizing, multi-morbid geriatric patients, as is the case for the CHCC); (2) different patients attend each session, and they only come in when they have an actual medical need (i.e., rather than according to some predetermined schedule); (3) DIGMAs and PSMAs deliver medical care from start to finish, and all patient education is provided in the context of the physician working with each patient individually (i.e., there are no separate formal warm-up, educational presentation, break, question and answer, and planning for the next visit segments, as there are for CHCCs); (4) these two SMA models seem to work equally well in fee-for-service and capitated healthcare environments; and (5) they are able to dramatically increase physician productivity (by 200–300%, or more). Importantly, it is this increased capacity created by the enhanced productivity of the DIGMA and PSMA models that essentially creates additional physician FTEs out of existing resources.

Caution: Always Stay Focused On Providing Patients With a High Quality Healing Experience

One word of caution before we proceed: Always keep high-quality patient care as your primary focus. While we will be talking a great deal about gains in access and productivity in this chapter, it is important to keep in mind that properly run DIGMAs and PSMAs also offer a multitude of other benefits to patients as well (see Chapters 2 and 3)—including numerous potential quality and psychosocial benefits. In fact, it is for reasons of enhanced patient care that I first developed the DIGMA model. Remember that I originally developed DIGMAs as a patient, one who was disgruntled with the broken system of traditional care—and this despite having the best physicians that I could have hoped to have had. As it turns out, the productivity, access, and economic benefits that these SMA models offer were simply fortuitous and serendipitous concomitants. Always remain cognizant that it is the enhanced care benefits that these models are intended to deliver to our patients that are most important about DIGMAs and PSMAs—i.e., despite the economic, productivity, and access motivations they might engender.

Study 1: DIGMAs at the Erie, PA, Veteran Affairs Medical Center

The following is a personal case study of a provider who went from initial outright refusal to a willingness to try, to great anxiety during the initial launch, and to ultimate clinical success with her group visit—and who eventually came to enjoy her DIGMA so much that she soon wanted to do DIGMAs full time. Her story is one that many other providers will be able to identify and be sympathetic with. It underscores how any provider, even those who are initially very reluctant and scared to try one, can ultimately be successful in running a group visit for their own practice—if only they have the courage and tenacity to give it a try and put the effort into it. Group visits are not nearly as dependent upon physician personality and personal assurance as they are upon having the courage and willingness to try one and give it one's best effort. As is so frequently the case, the clinical outcomes data for her work with DIGMAs are now being collected and

analyzed—but, while on the horizon, is not yet quite ready for publication. Nonetheless, the preliminary clinical outcomes data are very encouraging and are expected to be available for publication within a year or so.

Background

My name is Stacey Lutz-McCain. As a Certified Registered Nurse Practitioner (CRNP) my story with group medical visits started in the spring of 2003. I became a nurse practitioner in May of 1998 and, after many trials, felt that I was a seasoned CRNP in the VA system by spring 2003. I finally felt comfortable in my role after 5 years, by which time I had a panel of about 1000 patients that I managed solely—and I could finally sleep throughout the night without waking up wondering if I killed someone or seriously hurt them.

Initially, I Rejected the DIGMA Concept

Then there was that fateful day in April 2003 when Dr. Adelman, Chief of Staff at that time, called a meeting of the medical center providers. He gathered all of the nurse practitioners and physicians together because he had a new idea that he found in his readings—i.e., group clinics. None of us had heard of this concept, and Dr. Adelman spent the next hour talking about how effective and efficient they could be and how we were going to love doing them. I still did not understand but was certainly glad that I did not have to do one. Then, the ball dropped. Dr. Adelman announced to everyone that he thought I should try it out. I did not see this one coming. All I could think of was how hard I had worked the past 5 years to establish my panel of patients and how I finally no longer felt like a *deer in the headlights*—and now it seemed as if he was going to take all of that away from me. I thought I had drawn the short straw since I was the youngest of the nurse practitioners. He then asked me what I thought about his idea. In all of my 29-year-old ignorance and immaturity I said "I think your idea sucks." That was the end of the conversation and we were all dismissed.

I Soon Had a Change of Heart

The next day my team leader sought me out to tell me how horrible Dr. Adelman felt and that I should just think about his idea—which I did, but chose not to follow through on at the time. Four months later, I was in Albuquerque, New Mexico, for a Preventive Medicine Conference—and there was a nurse practitioner from Georgia talking about group medical appointments and how efficient and effective they were. I flew back to Erie, PA, on a Sunday night, and first thing on Monday morning, I was in Dr. Adelman's office. I apologized for my behavior 4 months prior and offered my services for group clinics.

My Initial DIGMA Session

Shortly thereafter, Dr. Noffsinger came out to train us and show us how to do DIGMAs properly. In January 2004, we held our first DIGMA. I had a pharmacist and dietician (both of whom were certified diabetic educators), a nurse, and a secretary help me with the group clinic. In my first DIGMA session (which focused upon diabetes, hyperlipidemia, hypertension, and obesity), we had 10 of my patients in attendance. I made countless trips to the bathroom that morning and cannot believe I did not have to take a bathroom break during the group. As I walked into the room, I still had no idea how it would go but, boy oh boy, was I ever nervous. It went better than my wildest dreams could ever have anticipated. It took us almost 3 hours, but the patients loved it. I ended up with full-blown body hives and diarrhea.

I Am Now Very Comfortable in Running My DIGMA

We are now 3 ½ years into group visits and the hives and gastrointestinal distress have long since left. I now can sleep through the night again and eat my breakfast prior to group. With much help and support from Dr. Adelman (our current medical center director) and others in executive leadership, our group clinic for chronic disease has advanced a great deal over time. We are getting new referrals daily. I see 10–15 patients and their spouses in 2 hours. A secretary helps me enter my orders. I document my chart notes right there, during group time. The pharmacist counsels patients on meds and functions as the behaviorist, although the dietician serves as the behaviorist while helping patients with diet therapy and exercise.

The reason that the dietician and pharmacist both serve as behaviorists is that when the groups started to grow, I needed to divide them up to get behaviorist coverage during all sessions. We have even added a guest speaker for 5–10 minutes during each group who discusses various topics—such as advanced directives, living wills, depression, stress, exercise. We have networked with optometry and can get diabetic eye exams done on

DIGMA patients the same day, if needed. In addition to taking vital signs and providing injections, the nurse does diabetic foot exams, insulin teaching, glucometer training, and home blood pressure monitoring. It is a very effective and efficient group.

DIGMAs Provide Many Benefits—to Me as Well as My Patients

Whereas I have 30-minute individual return appointments (with some no-shows) during regular clinic time, I am now able to provide comprehensive mind–body care to 10 patients at once in my 2-hour DIGMA—and with greater patient education and training in disease self-management skills. But best of all, I am happy—I have finally found my niche in life. I truly enjoy the group setting and find it very effective. I run my DIGMA two–three times a week and manage a panel of 600+ patients outside of group. I also follow up on all of the patients from group with their sugars, cholesterol, and blood pressures in between group visits. Patients generally return to group every 3–6 months. I grew to like my DIGMA group so much that after 1 year, I asked if I could do DIGMAs full time, which was a remarkable turnaround from how I felt just a year earlier! We are up to 12 groups a month now, and I am also taking the DIGMA concept into our community clinics (CBOCs). In addition, I received my CDE in October 2006 and am now working on ADA certification for our program.

Preliminary Clinical Outcomes and Performance Measures Are All Positive

As a result of my DIGMA, my patients' scores for HbA1cs, HDLs, LDLs, triglycerides, hypertension, and urine protein have all improved—as have diabetic eye exams, foot exams, and weight loss. The patients truly love it. They look forward to their group visit, the friends they will meet, and the knowledge they will gain and share. Although formal outcomes data are not yet available, the preliminary data for our DIGMAs are quite positive. Data have been collected for our groups over the past 3 years. Although this data collection and analysis is still in the preliminary stages, results so far point to significant improvement in LDL values, triglyceride levels, HbA1c readings, and blood pressure readings. Results from patient satisfaction surveys are very positive, with most patients preferring group appointments to individual appointments for their chronic care. Official data will be published later.

Study 2: DIGMAs Work Well, but Only When They Are Properly Supported

This case study illustrates the point that DIGMAs (and PSMAs) work well in accomplishing the objectives for which they were originally designed, but only if they are appropriately supported. I have always found this to be one of the saddest DIGMA stories of all. In this section, we see how one extremely busy and backlogged physician's successful DIGMA program, which was accomplishing exactly what it was supposed to by leveraging her time, adding substantially to her supply of follow-up appointments, matching supply to demand, reducing her backlog over time, and providing high levels of patient and physician professional satisfaction, was ultimately undermined by a system that failed to appropriately support her program over time.

This longitudinal study, which was initially reported in the February–March 2001 issue of Hippocrates, demonstrates the dramatic positive impact that the DIGMA model was able to have on one of the most backlogged physicians that I have ever encountered, and how that benefit was subsequently undercut when the system later withdrew the critically important supports that were necessary for success. (1)

The Problem

This study was conducted by the author from September 1997 through June 1999 at a large staff model HMO serving more than 200,000 patient members and having approximately 85 physicians who reported to the department of medicine. One of these physicians, who was board certified in both internal medicine and endocrinology, decided to start a DIGMA in order to improve access to care—as she recognized the singular inaccessibility of her practice to patients. Whereas the other 84 physicians in the department had an average of 14 patients *past due* for a return appointment at the start of this study, this particular physician had 273 patients past due when she launched her first DIGMA session in January of 1998. Because of this severe backlog of patients past due their follow-up appointment, there was no opening left to schedule these patients into because her schedule for the next 3 months (i.e., which was as far out as the computer was able to schedule) was already completely filled. Because of her severe access problems, this physician was confronted daily with drop-ins, numerous patient telephone calls, complaints about lack of access, and double bookings—and her professional satisfaction was deteriorating.

Study Design

When she first began her DIGMA program, this physician chose an endocrinology DIGMA of mixed design in which (1) type 1 diabetes was the focus the first week of the month; (2) type 2 diabetes was the focus during the second and fourth weeks; (3) other endocrine disorders were the focus on the third week of each month (primarily thyroid, but all other endocrine problems as well—such as adrenal, parathyroid); and (4) the fifth weekly session (for those couple of months each year having five sessions) was open to all of her patients, regardless of diagnosis. Furthermore, as is typical of the mixed DIGMA model, patients were allowed to attend any other appropriate session that might happen to better fit their schedule (i.e., regardless of the focus of that particular session) in the event that the most suitable session for their particular diagnosis proved inconvenient for her endocrinology patients to attend that month.

Although each of her DIGMA sessions focused upon a specific endocrinology diagnosis during each week of the month, all of her primary care patients were also invited to attend any week they wanted—i.e., because her practice was so severely backlogged and because she wanted to provide more accessible care to all of her patients (primary care as well as endocrine patients). As a result of this (plus the fact that patients often brought in a *laundry list* of diverse issues and could attend any session that best fit their schedule), her mixed endocrinology DIGMA gradually became more heterogeneous over time—and had evolved into a completely heterogeneous design before the end of the first year of operations (i.e., in which all of her patients, regardless of diagnosis, were invited to attend any week that they happened to have a medical need and wanted to be seen).

Four Distinct Phases of the Study

Figure 9.1 shows the dramatic impact that this endocrinology and primary care DIGMA had on patient access to this endocrinologist's practice. This figure, which focuses on the number of backlogged patients on this physician's wait list over time (in particular, the number of patients *past due* for a return appointment), is broken into four distinct timeframes or phases.

Phase 1:

Phase 1, which covers the time period prior to starting her DIGMA program, extends from September 1997 through

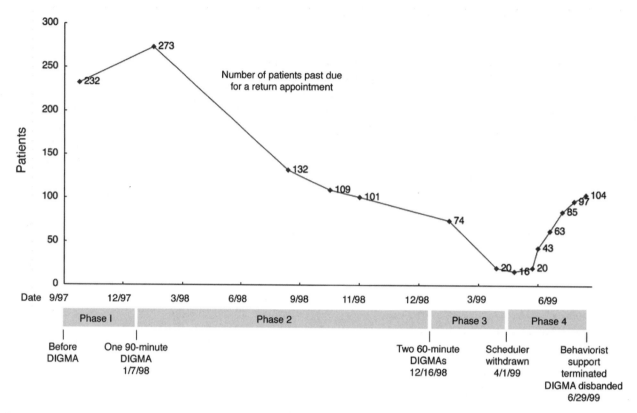

Fig. 9.1 The dramatic impact that this endocrinology and primary care DIGMA had upon patient access to this endocrinologist's practice is shown. Backlogged patients on this physician's wait list over time (in particular, the number of patients past due for a return appointment) is broken into four distinct timeframes or phases

January 7, 1998, which was when this physician launched her first DIGMA. The purpose of Phase 1 was not only to assess the severity of the backlog of patients *past due* at any given point in time but also to measure how rapidly this backlog was deteriorating over time. By *past due,* it is meant that the patient was told to return in say 3 months during their previous appointment (which, let us assume was 6 months ago), yet—even though this patient is already 3 months overdue for her/his follow-up appointment—there is still no place to put them on the endocrinologist's schedule for the next 3 months (which was as far out as the computer would allow appointments to be scheduled at that time). Thus the designation "past due" is used. Therefore, the *past due* portion of the waitlist is the most severe and problematic part. Phase 1 clearly reveals how severe this physician's access problems already were, and the fact that this alarming situation was further deteriorating at the rapid rate of an additional 10 or so patients per month. In two more years, it was projected that her backlog would likely be over 500 patients past due for a return appointments, which would certainly make for an almost impossible workload and professional life.

Phase 2:

Phase 2, which covers the 11-month timeframe extending from the launch of this physician's DIGMA on January 7 through December 16, 1998, during which time she conducted one 90-minute DIGMA per week at the same time and place (except when absent from the clinic due to vacation, illness, meetings, etc.). This weekly DIGMA program not only immediately reversed this trend of declining accessibility but also dramatically and continuously reduced the backlog of patients *past due* over time throughout Phase 2. There was a reduction in the number of patients past due for a return appointment throughout Phase 2—with the number of backlogged patients dropping from a high of 273 patients at the beginning of the DIGMA program to just 101 patients past due in November of 1998—at which time the rate of decline appeared to be tapering off and plateauing.

Because of this plateau in the curve that was beginning to form (which effectively represented a law of diminishing returns), the decision was made on December 16, 1998 by the physician and myself to start two back-to-back 60-minute DIGMAs per week instead of the single 90-minute DIGMA that she had been running during Phase 2.

Although doing so only took 30 additional minutes of the physician's time per week, she was thereby able to see considerably more patients in these two shorter DIGMAs combined than she was during the single weekly DIGMA of longer duration. By increasing her capacity through this change, she was able to again resume rapidly decreasing her backlog of patients past due—in fact, the rate of decline was even greater in Phase 3 than it was for the single, longer DIGMA during Phase 2.

Phase 3:

Phase 3 depicts the period extending from December 16, 1998 to April 1, 1999, during which time two properly supported, back-to-back 60-minute endocrinology DIGMAs were conducted per week. An important result of this change to two shorter DIGMAs per week was that the rapid decline in backlog resumed once more—in fact, as can be seen in the graph, at an even greater rate. The positive result of this DIGMA program was that by the end of Phase 3 on April 1, 1999, the endocrinology DIGMA program had continuously reduced this physician's backlog of patients *past due* for a follow-up visit from 273 to just 16. Furthermore, Phases 2 and 3 of this DIGMA program had, in combination, completely reversed the trend prior to the start of this study—i.e., during which the backlog of patients past due was increasing at the rate of approximately 10 additional patients per month.

Furthermore, this lengthy initial wait list of patients past due had been brought virtually current in just 15 months' time by this endocrinology DIGMA program—i.e., through use of existing resources alone and no other changes in this physician's practice. In just another couple additional weeks of operations, it was felt that her backlog of 16 patients past due could easily have been brought completely current (i.e., from 16 patients down to zero)—at which time the severe access problems to her practice would have been completely eliminated by the use of just the DIGMA model and existing resources. However, as will be seen, the system instead made two unfortunate decisions—both of which involved withdrawing critically important supports, decisions that completely undermined this heretofore highly successful DIGMA program.

Phase 4:

The first decision resulted from the misperception that once this endocrinologist's backlog had been reduced to just 16 patients past due, access to her practice had become essentially the same as access to any other physician in the department of medicine—as all 85 physicians in the department of medicine, which included this endocrinologist, now had roughly the same average number of patients past due (i.e., approximately 14–16 such patients past due). This extremely pressured, busy, and heretofore severely backlogged endocrinologist was now seen as facing essentially the same pressures in her practice as the other 84 physicians within the department. However, this perception was clearly mistaken as this physician had unique and enormous patient demands upon her practice—pressures that were only being relieved by the additional capacity created by two well-functioning efficiency engines in her practice (i.e., two appropriately supported DIGMAs).

Mistake 1, the withdrawal of critically important dedicated scheduling support: The result of this mistaken perception was that due to a lack of resources and competing demands upon the dedicated scheduler's time, the dedicated scheduling support for this DIGMA program was completely withdrawn. This scheduler, who had been dedicating a couple of hours per week on average throughout this program to the critically important function of telephoning patients from the wait list and inviting them to attend an upcoming DIGMA session, was thus removed from this responsibility. The natural result was that—because patients on the wait list were no longer being notified about this highly accessible alternative venue for being seen (nor were they being invited to attend by the scheduler)—the waitlisted patients no longer knew to come into the DIGMA. Therefore, this physician's backlog immediately began to grow quite rapidly. In other words, her practice promptly began to implode. The number of patients *past due* in this endocrinologist's practice immediately increased almost exponentially from just 16 return patients past due in April 1999 to 104 patients past due just a few weeks later (i.e., by the end of June 1999). The perception that her practice was somehow the same as everybody else's in the department of medicine once her backlog decreased to just 16 patients past due was clearly a misperception. In actuality, she had enormous pressure upon her practice due to heavy patient demand coupled with insufficient capacity to deliver accessible care—a degree of pressure that other practices simply did not have, as witnessed by the size of her backlog compared to others at the start of this study.

Mistake 2, the withdrawal of critically important support from the behaviorist: The second devastating decision, which occurred on June 29, 1999, was to discontinue support for a behavioral health professional to assist in the running of this physician's two 1-hour DIGMAs per week. Although I had been her behaviorist throughout her DIGMA program, I had made the decision to accept an early retirement package some 18 months earlier;

however, no replacement behaviorist was made available to take over after I had left the organization. Unable to run her DIGMA without a behaviorist, this endocrinologist discontinued her program as of that date—after which, her practice was quite different and reduced in scope. She later advised me that she no longer accepted new primary care patients, followed fewer patients overall, and frequently served as an endocrinology consultant to other physicians in the system regarding how to best manage their endocrine patients. She later told me that she missed her groups and that her patients did as well. She pointed out that her patients still occasionally asked her about the group and wondered if she would ever start it up again, saying that she really enjoyed her DIGMAs and the care that she was able to deliver (as well as the improved access that she was able to enjoy during this study).

DIGMAs Do Not Increase Utilization

When the data from this longitudinal case study were reviewed, it clearly demonstrated that the improved access provided by DIGMAs does not increase utilization of medical services—they do not simply provide a value-added service that drives up utilization (i.e., in which patients are coming in for additional visits). If this had been the case, the rapid and consistent reduction in backlog observed in this study simply would not have occurred. To the contrary, what was found was that patients were attending DIGMAs largely in lieu of traditional individual office visits, at least in Phases 2 and 3 (although not in Phase 4, where backlogged patients were neither informed about nor invited to attend upcoming DIGMA sessions in lieu of individual office visits). It is certainly the case that one of the important goals of a well-run DIGMA program is to have suitable patients attend highly efficient and cost-effective DIGMAs in lieu of traditional individual office visits whenever appropriate and possible.

Patients Did Not Keep Coming in Simply Because DIGMA Visits Were Now Available

Furthermore, initial concerns to the effect that patients might keep returning week after week for unnecessary DIGMA visits simply because they were now available to them, did not prove to be justified. Nor was it observed that the same group of patients kept coming back session after session, thereby effectively blocking availability of the group to other patients who might have greater medical need. In fact, patients attending DIGMAs during Phases 2 and 3 averaged only two group visits throughout these 18 months. The conclusion to be drawn from this study is that once patients have their medical needs properly met, they seem to have better things to do with their time than to simply go back to their doctor for additional visits—no matter how accessible those appointments might happen to be.

Why Was This DIGMA Program So Able to Reduce the Backlog and Improve Access?

One might wonder why this DIGMA program was so effective in reducing the backlog and in solving this physician's access problem. Because she had previously reduced her clinic hours from 0.9 to 0.7 full-time equivalents (FTEs) and had many other scheduling commitments, this endocrinologist had only 27 non-urgent return appointment slots on her weekly schedule during Phase 1—i.e., prior to the start of this DIGMA program. During Phase 2, when she ran a single 90-minute DIGMA per week, she was able to see an average of 9.94 patients per session—not counting support persons such as spouses, friends, and caregivers. This represented a 36.8% increase in the number of return patients that she was able to see each week.

Furthermore, during Phases 3 and 4 (i.e., when two back-to-back 60-minute DIGMAs were conducted per week), she saw an average of 12.84 patients in her groups each week—which represented a 47.6% increase in her productivity with regard to the number of return visits provided each week as a result of this DIGMA program. However, it is important to note that this 47.6% number would have undoubtedly been substantially larger had the needed scheduling support for the program not been discontinued throughout Phase 4—as the low attendance during phase 4 dramatically reduced the number of *past-due* return patients that were being seen on average from the number seen during Phase 3. Clearly, the number of attendees was greatly reduced when the dedicated scheduling support was withdrawn—as only 6.26 patients were seen on average during these two weekly Phase 4 DIGMAs combined during the last month of this study (which makes clear the degree to which the decision to discontinue scheduling support had completely undermined this DIGMA program).

Conclusion: DIGMAs Work Well, but They Need to be Appropriately Supported

The reason that the DIGMA program was so able to reduce the backlog and improve access to care was that this program dramatically leveraged the endocrinologist's time, increased her productivity for follow-up visits, and enabled her to substantially increase the number of non-urgent return appointments that she was able to offer patients each week. However, once the necessary scheduling support was removed by the system in Phase 4, the effectiveness of the DIGMA program with regards to increasing capacity, reducing backlog, and improving access was completely undercut. Furthermore, the final nail in the coffin of the DIGMA program was the fact that behaviorist support was eventually also withdrawn—despite the remarkable achievement of this DIGMA program—with the physician being expected to somehow run the DIGMA alone (something which she recognized she could not do, which resulted in her discontinuing the entire program despite its success).

I have often thought back upon just how unfortunate these two decisions to withdraw critical supports actually were. Not only was an effective and highly successful DIGMA program thereby lost but a remarkable resource in form of a well-liked, busy, capable, and highly efficient endocrinologist was thereby considerably reduced—and all of this loss in a futile attempt to save the few extra dollars that it would have cost to provide the appropriate support personnel for the program (a couple hours of time each week for both a scheduler and a behaviorist to assist this physician in running the DIGMA). It is for this reason that I often say that DIGMAs and PSMAs work very well, but only if they are carefully designed, appropriately supported, fully promoted, and properly run.

Study 3: Typical First Session of a Well-Run DIGMA Program

This study clearly demonstrates just how dramatic an impact DIGMAs (and PSMAs) can have upon provider productivity from the beginning (indeed, even during the first session)—and how that increased efficiency can be achieved with high levels of patient satisfaction. As a healthcare consultant specializing in group visits, I am often brought out to help integrated healthcare delivery systems launch their initial group visit sessions—typically just 3–5 days prior to their launch in order to help design the program and train all personnel associated with the DIGMA and/or PSMA. As a result, all that I am often able to witness and measure during these brief pilot studies is the increased physician productivity and patient satisfaction (and sometimes, the improved access) that these pilot DIGMA and PSMA programs can provide

to the physician and organization from the very beginning. This is one of innumerable such pilot studies that I have run. It is typical in every way except one—i.e., that this provider had 30-minute follow-up appointments in the clinic (whereas most providers today have 15 or 20 minute individual appointments), which resulted in a correspondingly larger increase in physician productivity—i.e., 520% in this case vs. the 200–400% (and, most commonly, 300%) increase that is more typically achieved in such pilot studies.

How I Typically Set Up the Initial DIGMA Session

In general, when setting up an initial DIGMA session with an interested provider (i.e., as a consultant), I typically spend 3 days (or 5 days if there are two providers launching DIGMAs and/or PSMAs that week): (1) securing the necessary high-level executive leadership and administrative support that is required for success; (2) custom designing the program to the provider's specific needs and practice; (3) developing the necessary promotional materials and forms (typically in template form); (4) selecting the required personnel for this multidisciplinary team-based approach to care; (5) securing the necessary group and exam room space; (6) training the team members regarding their respective roles and responsibilities in making the DIGMA a success; (7) actually running a mock DIGMA at the end of the last training session prior to the *go-live* session on the following day; and (8) meeting with, and giving presentations to, executive leadership within the organization and key administrative leaders in all of the departments that will be involved with the DIGMA program (billing and compliance, marketing, charting, IT, scheduling, reception, nursing, behavioral medicine, etc.). All of these issues are thoroughly addressed elsewhere in this book. In addition, I typically sit in the initial DIGMA or PSMA session when it is launched at the end of this 3–5 day period, as well as the team debriefing that usually follows.

Focus Carefully on the Size of Your DIGMA

In every case, I strive to set the DIGMA up so that it can be successful in the long run—which means in such a manner that full groups can be consistently achieved, patients and physicians will be satisfied, and the physician's goals for the program can be met. In order to have a DIGMA that is economically viable as well as lively, interesting, and highly interactive in terms of group dynamics, the goal is typically to set the group census such that the DIGMA: (1) approximately triples the provider's actual productivity in the clinic with individual office visits; and (2) is in the ideal range of between 10 and 16 patients for any primary or specialty care DIGMA (or 7–9 patients for a primary care PSMA for men, 6–8 patients for a primary care PSMA for women, or 10–13 patients for most PSMAs in the medical subspecialties).

The Design of This Study

As can be seen in Fig. 9.2, the physician was an internist in primary care who happened to select the heterogeneous DIGMA subtype. Although this initial 90-minute DIGMA pilot session happened to be held by an internist in primary care, it could equally well have been held by a family practitioner, nurse practitioner, osteopath, PA, etc. in primary care—or by a provider in virtually any of the medical or surgical subspecialties as well. Furthermore, although this DIGMA happened to be of a heterogeneous design, it could equally have been of a homogeneous or mixed design—i.e., so long as the same group census levels could have been achieved. Because this primary care physician worked with complex and multimorbid geriatric patients, individual return appointments on the clinic schedule were 30 minutes in length (note that it is not uncommon for certain medical and surgical subspecialists to have 30-minute return appointments as well). A patient satisfaction questionnaire very similar to those found on the DVD attached to this book (which employed several questions and a 5-point Likert scale) was used for this DIGMA session. This questionnaire focused upon how satisfied patients were with the DIGMA, the access they had to care, the amount of time they had, the information they received, the group interaction, and the quality of care they received. It was given to patients to complete anonymously at the end of the session.

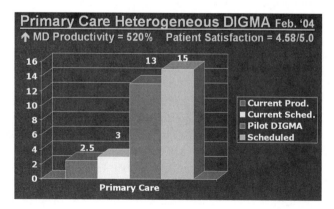

Fig. 9.2 Data from the first session of a well-run heterogeneous internal medicine DIGMA

First Determine the Provider's Actual Productivity During Normal Clinic Hours

We first determined this physician's pre-DIGMA productivity during traditional individual office visits in the clinic for the 6 months prior to this pilot—which turned out to be 2.5 patients per 90-minutes of clinic time. Although this physician had 30-minute follow-up appointments and could therefore have theoretically scheduled and seen three patients in traditional office visits during 90 minutes of clinic time, the number actually seen—i.e., 2.5 patients—was somewhat less because of no-shows, late-cancels, unfilled appointments, and some downtime on the physician's schedule. In this physician's case, the total amount of lost productivity from all of these causes combined happened to be 0.5 patients (3.0–2.5 = 0.5) on average per 90 minutes of clinic time—which is fairly typical for physicians having 30-minute office visits.

The Result: A 520% Increase in Physician Productivity, Plus Satisfied Patients

This particular physician targeted to have a group census of 13 patients in the DIGMA. However, with group visits we always try to overbook sessions just like the airlines do in order to make ourselves immune to the vexing and costly problem of no-shows. Because we wanted to overbook this physician's DIGMA sessions according to the expected number of no-shows and late-cancels (which we anticipated would total approximately 2.0 patients on average, which is often the case for 90-minute DIGMAs of this size), we actually scheduled 15 patients into this initial DIGMA session. As can be seen, of these 15 scheduled patients, 13 patients did attend this first session—as we did in fact experience the two *no-shows* that we had anticipated. By taking the ratio of the 13 patients actually seen in this initial DIGMA session divided by the 2.5 patients that would have actually been seen on average during 90 minutes of clinic through traditional individual follow-up office visits alone, we can see that this pilot DIGMA increased the physician's productivity by 520.0% right from the start—i.e., even during the first session.

In addition to this remarkable 520.0% increase in physician productivity, the level of patient satisfaction with the initial DIGMA session was also determined to be very high—i.e., with the average score reported on the patient satisfaction questionnaire being 4.58 out of 5 (which is typical, as patient satisfaction scores for DIGMAs and PSMAs typically range between 4.4 and 4.8 on a 5-point Likert scale). In addition, brief structured interviews with patients immediately after the session also revealed the high degree of satisfaction—and even enthusiasm—that the patients had with regards to this new DIGMA program.

Study 4: Development of the PSMA Model and How It Increased One Physician's Productivity Over 300%

The following study has historical significance because it reveals the development of the PSMA from what was initially an unworkable conceptualization to what eventually became a workable and successful model. Due to the lengthy backlogs for private physical examinations that existed in many healthcare systems during 2001, I recognized that there was a need for a better and more efficient way of delivering private physical examinations in both primary care and many medical and surgical subspecialties. I say private physical exams because the DIGMA model would accommodate non-private physicals that do not require disrobing and could be conducted in a group setting—for example, exams for carpal tunnel, tennis elbow, thyroid, gait disorders, sore throats, sprained ankles, facial lesions, swollen ankles, and earaches.

What makes this study important is that it nicely captures the transitional moment during which the correct version of the PSMA was developed. In addition, this study also clearly depicts that when it comes to group visits, that which seems to be intuitively obvious is often the incorrect approach to take. Despite all of my personal experience with group visits, I nonetheless made a common beginner's mistake by doing what I felt was intuitively obvious when originally conceiving of the PSMA model. Had I stopped there, that would have been most unfortunate as a remarkably effective model was just one step away from that which was initially conceived. As it turned out, going with what I found to be intuitively appealing proved to be a colossal mistake that frustrated three physicians no end, caused two of them to quit their PSMAs, and almost completely undercut the development of the entire PSMA model.

The Original Flawed Model

The model that I originally conceived involved registering patients 2–3 weeks ahead of the PSMA session, sending them a Patient Packet that contained several items—a welcome letter from the physician explaining the SMA, any handouts that the physician wanted included, and (most importantly) both the lab tests needing to be done prior to the visit and a detailed health history form needing to be completed by the patient and returned to the office a couple of days prior to the visit. Someone on the physician's staff would follow-up with pre-registered patients to ensure that they completed all lab tests in a timely manner prior to the visit, and that the completed health history form was returned to the office by patients at least a couple of days prior to the session.

In this manner, the nurse could carry lab test results over onto a erasable whiteboard wall chart with horizontal and vertical grid lines on it (or a flipchart) in the group room prior to the visit—and the relevant updated material from the detailed health history form could be carried forward prior to the group into each patient's chart note for the session by a member of the physician's staff. On the day of the PSMA session, patients would be registered at the front desk as they arrived for the session and asked to sign a confidentiality release. So far, so good. The flaw in this model, as I originally conceived of it, appeared during the next step.

It seemed intuitively appealing to me to have the initial segment of the actual SMA visit be the interactive group segment of the PSMA session—i.e., with almost all the talking occurring in this highly efficient and interactive group setting, which would basically be a small DIGMA. Once the interactive group segment was completed—which is where virtually all discussion was to occur, except for truly private matters and that which needed to be discussed in order to complete the physical exams—it would be followed by the second half of the session, the private physical examination segment of the PSMA visit. The PSMA promotional materials, as well as both the behaviorist and physician at the start of each session, would advise patients that almost all discussion was to occur in the initial interactive group segment of the visit—and not during the physical examinations that followed. Therefore, they should be certain to ask all of their questions during the group—i.e., during the first half of the session. Thus, the physical examinations that followed would be conducted with a minimum amount of talk and discussion.

After the first half of the PSMA session (i.e., the interactive group segment, or small DIGMA) was over, four patients would then be taken out of the group room by two nurses or MAs and roomed into four separate exam rooms. Each nurse/MA would be responsible for rooming patients, one at a time, into two of these exam rooms—and then taking vital signs, providing injections, and conducting any special nursing duties requested by the physician. When these nursing and exam room resources were available, I envisioned using two nurses/MAs and four exam rooms whenever possible so that the provider would be able to rapidly conduct physical examinations (and go quickly from one exam room to another) without ever catching up with the nurses/MAs and being left waiting in the hallway for the next patient to be roomed and prepared.

The physician would then leave the group room and start efficiently delivering private physical examinations, one at a time, upon all patients roomed in the exam rooms—i.e., with a minimum amount of discussion and social chit-chat. The physician would go in turn from one exam room to the next, until all patients were finished—i.e., providing thorough, but fairly rapid, physical examinations with a minimum amount of talk and discussion. After the physician finished with the private physical examination upon each patient in turn, then that patient would get dressed, leave the exam room, and be free to either leave the clinic or join the small group of unroomed patients being led by the behaviorist. The behaviorist would be addressing relevant behavioral health issues with this dwindling, small group of unroomed patients during the remainder of the PSMA session—i.e., while the next patients were being escorted by the nurse from the group room to the exam room. This process would continue until the private physical exams and nursing functions had been completed upon all patients and the session was over.

The Problem

Simply put, the problem with this model, as it was originally conceived, was that no matter how many times the physician and behaviorist told the patients at the start of the session that virtually all of the talk needed to occur during the initial interactive group segment of the session, patients always ended up saving some of their questions so that—when they later got the physician alone in the exam room—they almost always still had a few more questions to ask. The physician was therefore forced to answer these questions one-on-one in the inefficient exam room setting—i.e., just as is the case for the inefficient individual office visit model of care. Unfortunately, because answering all these questions individually is a very inefficient, time-consuming, and often repetitive process, these early PSMA sessions always ended up finishing late—and often very late.

By giving a flawed PSMA model to the first three physicians willing to give it a try, the end result was that the first two internists to ever try it promptly quit out of frustration—while the third, a family practitioner who was very seriously backlogged for private physical examinations, was also ready to quit. It was then that revelation struck—and I realized that we had *the cart and the horse* in the reverse order.

The Updated PSMA Model

After four frustrating sessions of finishing very late with the third physician mentioned above, it occurred to me that we were doing things the opposite of what we should—i.e., that if we would conduct the private physical examinations first, but without much discussion, then we would easily be able to defer most patient questions from the exam room into the subsequent interactive group segment. This could be accomplished by simply saying something like "That is a good question. Why not bring that up in the group that follows so that everyone can benefit from the answer?" That simple alteration in the PSMA model—i.e., from how it was originally conceived—was the solution to a successful PSMA model that could handle large group sizes and still finish on time. Upon realizing this, I called the family practitioner up at 10:30 pm that night and told him about my thoughts and recommendation. He immediately agreed to make this modification and to try it out during our very next PSMA session.

The Data

The results of the first 10 PSMA sessions with this family practitioner are depicted in Fig. 9.3. As can be seen, we were only able to see an average of 5.0 patients during the first four sessions of this family practitioner's 90-minute PSMA using the flawed original model—and were also finishing very late. Although this physician had both 30- and 40-minute physical examinations on his individual office visit schedule, when we went back and actually counted the number of patients that he saw on average during 90 minutes of clinic time dedicated to individual physical examinations, we found that he was only seeing an average of 2.2 patients—i.e., due to some late-cancels, no-shows, and downtime on the schedule. Clearly, by only seeing 5.0 patients during the original four 90-minute PSMA sessions, this physician was not experiencing any meaningful productivity or efficiency gain through the flawed version of the PSMA as it was originally structured—especially when all of the extra overhead and staffing for the model were factored in, along with the fact that these sessions were also finishing quite late.

As depicted in Fig. 9.3, these original four PSMA sessions were followed by four transitional PSMA sessions (i.e., session 5–8), during which this physician shifted to the revised and updated PSMA model and was able to see an average of almost seven patients per session. During these transitional sessions, the group sizes were increasing because the physician was gaining confidence and not having to waste time answering questions one-on-one in the inefficient exam room setting—

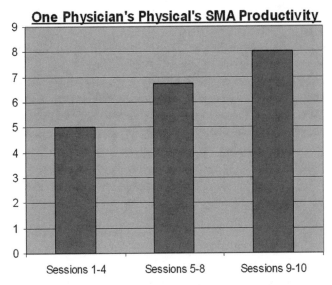

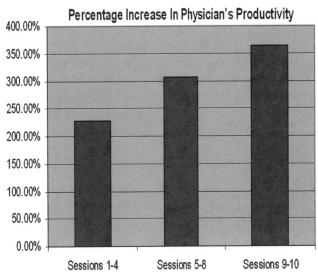

Fig. 9.3 How the PSMA model increased one physician's productivity as it evolved from its original flawed design to its final form. (From Noffsinger EB.[2], with permission from *Group Practice J.*)

Fig. 9.4 The percentage increase in productivity over traditional individual physical examinations as the PSMA model evolved to its current form and allowed for larger group sizes. (From Noffsinger EB.[2], with permission from *Group Practice J.*)

questions that were being better and more efficiently addressed during what was now the subsequent interactive group segment of the PSMA session—and was no longer finishing late. This data was discussed in the original series of four articles published on the PSMA model in AMGA's Group Practice Journal (2–5).

Finally, from weeks 9 and 10 onward, the newly redesigned (and now functional) heterogeneous PSMA model for male physicals enabled this physician to see full groups of 8.0 patients on average—and to finish on time. As it turns out, finishing on time with full census levels is a process that is typically only gradually acquired over time as experience and comfort are acquired with the PSMA and DIGMA models. As depicted in Fig. 9.4, by seeing 8.0 patients on average rather than the 2.2 patients that he would have been able to see on average during 90 minutes of clinic time using the old one-on-one office visit model, this physician was able to increase his productivity in delivering private physical examinations by more than 350%—which more than meets the goal that most DIGMAs and PSMAs have of tripling physician productivity. Not only was this family practitioner able to achieve this high level of productivity within just a few weeks of working with the new PSMA model, but also he was also able to consistently sustain that level of productivity during subsequent sessions as well.

The PSMA model has continued to demonstrate its many clear benefits over time and is now gaining widespread interest. However, the development of this model stands as a clear warning to all who would venture into the world of group visits on their own by doing what seems to be *intuitively obvious*—i.e., rather than starting

off with established models that have been proven successful in numerous applications.

Pilot Studies Involving Multiple Physicians

Let us now turn our attention to some rather typical DIGMA pilot studies that involve multiple providers, which will be of special interest to larger and mid-sized integrated healthcare delivery systems; however, the lessons learned should also prove interesting to smaller group practices and solo practitioners as well.

Study 5: DIGMAs Can Have an Immediate Impact upon Access—for Group and Individual Visits

In this section, we examine the improved access results that can reasonably be expected even at the earliest stages of a properly run DIGMA (or PSMA) program in primary or specialty care. Such results are due to the fact that these two types of SMA models dramatically leverage existing resources to increase provider productivity and enhance the supply of available appointments—with the net result typically ultimately being a substantial reduction in wait lists and backlogs. This study demonstrates how immediate and dramatic those reductions in backlogs from the DIGMA or PSMA program can sometimes be. The reason that this particular study was selected was because it so clearly demonstrates just how immediate the impact of a well-run DIGMA or PSMA program can be upon reducing backlogs and increasing appointment availability—i.e., with dramatic reductions sometimes becoming clearly evident even after just the first session of a newly established, ongoing DIGMA (or PSMA) program.

Two Months Prior to Launch, Substantial Access Problems Existed in All 3 Pilot Physicians' Practices

In this single session pilot study (which I conducted in a mid-sized medical group that was partially fee-for-service and partially capitated), three physicians were initially selected—a dual board certified internist and endocrinologist (Dr. A), a family practitioner (Dr. B), and a podiatrist (Dr. C)—all of whom worked full time and had established practices with substantial access problems, and all of whom decided to offer weekly 90-minute DIGMAs in their practices. As can be seen in Table 9.1, Doctors A, B, and C were initially quite backlogged prior to the start of this pilot study and had wait times for their second available return appointments (this organization happened to measure the wait times for the second available, rather than the more typical third available, upcoming return appointments) of 35, 39, and 103 days, respectively.

Right After the Launch of This DIGMA Pilot, Access to All Three Practices Had Already Improved Substantially

As seen in Table 9.1, from the very beginning, this DIGMA pilot immediately increased capacity and improved access to the practices of all three participating providers. This is because patients were being scheduled

Table 9.1 Improved access of three pilot physicians in a mid-sized medical group

Pilot physicians	Number of days until second available return		
	August 4, 2000(8 weeks prior to launch)	September 28, 2000(1 day after launch)	Percent decrease in wait time
Dr. A (internal medicine/ endocrinology)	35	16	54.3
Dr. B (family practice)	39	14	64.1
Dr. C (podiatry)	103	68	34.0
Average no. of days wait for second available return appointment	59.0	32.7	44.6

into not only the first DIGMA session but also the subsequent DIGMA sessions as well—all of which caused a dramatic reduction in these pilot physicians' backlogs. As a result, when the access to the second available return appointment was again determined for these three physicians' practices just 1 day after the launch of their new DIGMA program (for which all three pilot physicians selected a weekly 90-minute format), considerable improvement in access was already noted. This is because, right from the start, so many individual return office visits were instead being off-loaded and scheduled into highly productive future DIGMA sessions.

For example, Dr. A went from 35 to 16 days for the second available individual office visit (although the next available DIGMA visit was typically less than a week away), which represented a 54.3% decrease in wait time for his second available individual follow-up visit. Similarly, Dr. B went from 39 to 14 days, which represented a 64.1% decrease in wait time for the second available individual follow-up visit in the clinic. Finally, the most heavily backlogged provider of all, Dr. C had already gone from 103 to 68 days for his second available return, which represented a 34% decrease in wait time. These improvements in access were due to: (1) the increased capacity that DIGMAs provide each week (now and into the future as far out as the computer was able to schedule appointments); and (2) the fact that these providers' new schedules (which now included weekly 90-minute DIGMAs into which numerous follow-up appointments could be scheduled) were opened up for scheduling patients into. Overall, after just a single DIGMA session had been held, the decrease in wait time for the second available individual appointment for all three pilot providers had already decreased by an amazing amount—i.e., by an average of 44.6% after only the first DIGMA session had been held.

This Improvement in Access Is Typical, and Should Continue to Get Better Over Time

These results are actually not uncommon. They clearly demonstrate the improved access benefits that a properly designed, supported, promoted, and run DIGMA and/or PSMA program can offer—both to the physician's practice and to the organization—right from the very start. It is important to note that all of this improvement in access had occurred from the very beginning of the DIGMA program due to the extra capacity that a weekly DIGMA (or PSMA) adds to the physician's schedule every week into the indefinite future—i.e., by the time that just one DIGMA session had been held! Furthermore, patient satisfaction with the program was again found to be very high. Significantly, with the passage of time (i.e., as more and more DIGMA sessions are held and as evermore individual office visits are off-loaded onto highly efficient DIGMA visits), these benefits with regard to increased accessibility of individual office visits should continue to improve over time. However, the important point here is that—with DIGMAs and PSMAs alike—substantial improvements in access for both SMA and individual office visits can occur right from the very outset of the program (and with high levels of patient and physician professional satisfaction), a finding that I have been able to replicate time and time again.

Study 6: Improving Access to Care in the Face of Limited Physician Resources

The following study was submitted by Karen E. Jones, MD, FACP, who is both the physician champion for SMAs and the physician champion for chronic care initiatives at Well-Span Health and serves as an attending for the Medical Resident Service at York Hospital, Department of Medicine, York, PA. She was assisted in this effort by Meagan Renninger VanScyoc, PA-C, MBA, who was the SMA Project Manager and is currently the Medical Director for Employee Health at York Hospital. This write-up is interesting both because of the specialized applications of the PSMA model that it entails (i.e., pre-operative gastric bypass pulmonary consultations and sleep apnea consultations) and because it clearly demonstrates the robustness of this group visit model. That is, even when the SMA group census is considerably below the recommended level of tripling provider productivity whenever possible, the PSMA model is still so productive and efficient that it is nonetheless capable of solving access problems—and of doing so with high levels of patient and provider satisfaction.

Preoperative Gastric Bypass Pulmonary Consultations

WellSpan Health is a not-for-profit health system that provides more than $18 million each year in uncompensated medical and outreach services, supplies, and physician care to residents of York and Adams counties, which are located in south central Pennsylvania. It is an integrated delivery system comprised of two hospitals, a physician medical group providing more than 800,000 patient visits per year, a home healthcare organization, two managed care plans, and more.

WellSpan also collaborates with other healthcare professionals in the area to provide needed services to the community. An example of this collaboration is the bariatric program, which provides the full spectrum of needs for obese patients—including a medical weight loss program, bariatric surgery, and the many consultations required prior to surgery (which includes pre-operative gastric bypass pulmonary evaluations). Lung, sleep, and critical care consultants is the group of pulmonologists who serve this need. Due to tremendous demand for pulmonary and sleep services, this group experienced a large and growing access problem. Prior to starting the group visits program, there was a 6-month backlog for all non-urgent pulmonary consultations. As a result, there was a bottleneck in the pre-operative process that led to delays in bariatric surgery.

The pulmonologists joined forces with WellSpan's SMA physician champion, Karen E. Jones, and SMA project coordinator, Meagan Renninger VanScyoc. Dr. Ed Noffsinger was brought in as a consultant in July 2004 to help launch WellSpan's SMA program and to begin work on the pulmonary SMA.

The Physicals SMA (PSMA) model was selected for this project because of its ability to improve access, max-pack visits, and provide for a private physical examination to be performed upon each patient in attendance toward the beginning of each session. In addition to trying to improve access to care, the PSMA team also designed the program to make the appointment more convenient and comprehensive for patients—e.g., by incorporating any necessary Pulmonary Function Testing (PFTs) into the SMA instead of rescheduling the patient for a separate PFT appointment. The patient is simply escorted into the PFT lab after their private exam—i.e., before joining the group in the group room. Respiratory therapists serve as the pulmonary PSMA behaviorists and provide pulmonary education to the group while the doctor performs private examinations.

Sleep Apnea Consultations

Given the success of the pre-operative gastric bypass pulmonary evaluation PSMA program, the pulmonologists initiated a different type of PSMA in January 2005 for another backlogged consultative service—i.e., new evaluations for sleep apnea. The added benefit for patients in the sleep apnea SMA is that they get to see how an actual CPAP machine works and are exposed to a variety of CPAP masks during the appointment.

The Outcomes

From March 2005 through January 2006, the pulmonologists hosted 30 SMAs for pre-operative gastric by pass pulmonary evaluations in which they consulted on 159 patients—for an average group size of 5.3 patients. In that same time period, they hosted 141 SMAs for sleep apnea evaluations, consulting on 564 patients, for an average group size of 4.0 patients per sleep apnea session. One reason contributing to the low census of these PSMAs is the fact that all of these patients were consults—and therefore, had never been seen by the doctors and had never been to the practice before this visit. In combination, the 159 pre-operative gastric bypass pulmonary evaluations and 564 sleep apnea evaluations during this time period totaled 723 new patient consults. To compare the number of patients seen in the SMAs to the number of patients that would have been seen through usual individual appointments during that same time period, one must consider that individual consultation appointments are scheduled for 40 minutes—i.e., compared to SMA appointments that typically last about 2 hours and consist of 5–8 patients (with the greater time permitting much greater patient education and development of improved disease self-management skills). Had they seen only individual consultations during those 10 months instead of doing SMAs, the pulmonologists would have only seen 513 patients—i.e., assuming that every patient showed up for their individual appointment, which is of course not true and would have further reduced the number of patients seen individually.

In actuality, the pulmonologists saw a total of 723 patients during these 10 months of doing SMAs, a difference of 210 more new patient evaluations (assuming 100% attendance for individual appointments)—a number that would undoubtedly have been larger if the number of no-shows and late-cancels for individual office visits had been taken into account. This equates to 21 more patients per month, which is equal to approximately 3.8 more patients per week. Given 40-minute individual appointments, this equates to gaining an extra 3.25 hours per week of clinical time without adding any new hours to the schedule or new providers to the payroll. Within 6 months of initiating these SMAs, the pulmonary group's backlog for non-urgent consultations had dropped from 6 months down to 2 weeks.

Benefits of Improved Access to Care:

Several benefits and changes were noted from the improved access to care provided by these two PSMA programs:

1. By improving access, the pre-operative gastric bypass pulmonary SMAs substantially decreased the overall amount of time that patients had to wait before receiving bariatric surgery.

2. Increased access to care via sleep apnea SMA consultations got patients in for their appointment much sooner, but unexpectedly created the need for two additional beds in the sleep lab in order to accommodate the increased volume of sleep studies.

3. Providing PSMAs for these two types of pulmonary consultations opened up additional time in the pulmonologists' schedules, which helped to improve access for patients with other types of pulmonary conditions as well.

Patient Satisfaction:

In addition to the pulmonary SMAs described previously, WellSpan Health supports many other types of SMAs—including SMAs for diabetes, multiple sclerosis, pre-natal visits, and medical weight loss. Every patient receives a satisfaction survey at each SMA which they complete anonymously at the conclusion of the visit. A random compilation of 520 surveys from over 10 different SMA providers in York shows that patients are overwhelmingly satisfied with their SMA experience. Specifically, 94% of patients surveyed thought that the group interaction and peer support were helpful, 98% reported that they had a chance to ask questions about their medical condition and treatment, 98% were satisfied overall with their appointment, and 92% agreed that they would participate in a future SMA (Figs. 9.5–9.8).

Study 7: A typical DIGMA Pilot Study Involving Multiple Primary and Specialty Care Providers

The 6-session pilot project at Sutter Medical Foundation reported in this section represents a fairly typical pilot study involving multiple physicians over time in primary and specialty care. This pilot, which involved four physicians at two sites, was published as a 3-article series in the March, April, and May 2001 issues of AMGA's Group Practice Journal—a series of articles that I co-authored with Dr. Thomas N. Atkins who, at that time, was Chief Medical Officer at the Sutter Medical Foundation in Sacramento, California (6–8).

Overview of This Pilot Study

As the originator of the Drop-In Group Medical Appointment (DIGMA) model, I was brought in as a consultant to develop this DIGMA pilot project—which was to be conducted at two different Sutter Medical Foundation medical center sites (one urban and the other rural). A large multispecialty healthcare organization in northern California, Sutter is partially fee-for-service and partially capitated in nature.

Fig. 9.5 The percentage of patients reporting on their patient satisfaction survey that the group interaction and peer support of the SMA were helpful to them (N = 520 patient responses) at WellSpan Health

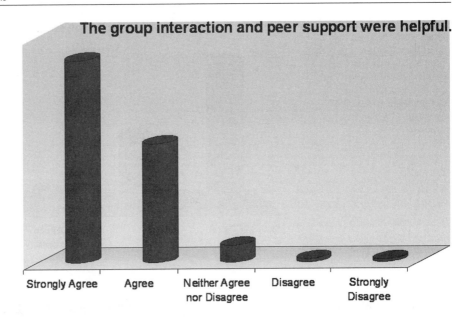

Fig. 9.6 The percentage of patients reporting on their patient satisfaction survey that they had a chance to ask questions about their medical illness and treatment during their SMA visit (N = 520 patient responses) at WellSpan Health

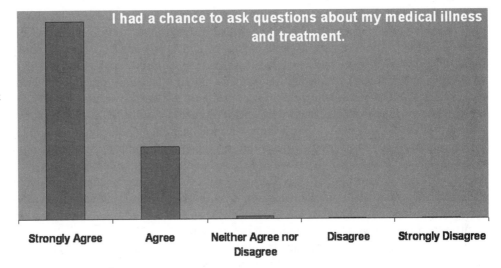

Fig. 9.7 The percentage of patients reporting on their patient satisfaction survey that overall, they were satisfied with today's SMA appointment at WellSpan Health. Note 98% patient satisfaction. (N = 520 patient responses)

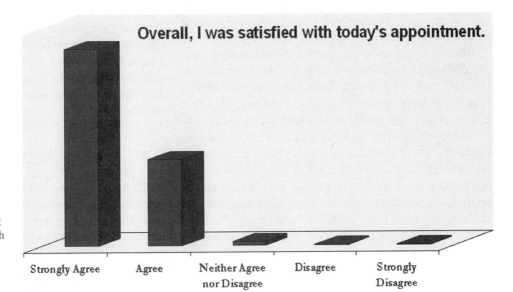

Fig. 9.8 The percentage of patients reporting on their patient satisfaction survey that they would participate in another shared medical appointment in the future at WellSpan Health. Note 92% agreed. (*N* = 520 patient responses)

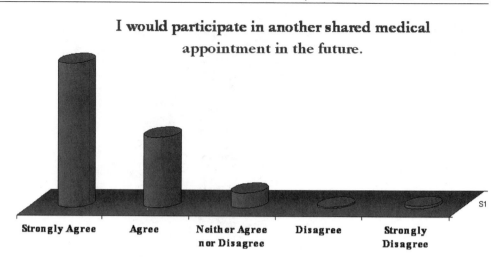

Reasons for This Pilot

Sutter Medical Group became interested in a DIGMA pilot because some members of the group felt that this shared medical appointment model might provide both a different way to practice and a means for working smarter rather than harder. It was noted that many of the group's physicians were becoming tired of the production pace required to achieve their income expectations—and that many physicians lacked satisfaction with their day-to-day practices even when their production goals were met. An additional negative contributor to this environment was the fact that financially supporting the additional capacity required to achieve access priorities through traditional means was also becoming more difficult. Moreover, patients were reportedly feeling disenfranchised and less satisfied with the depth of personal interactions with their providers—although basic medical needs were being met, it was becoming more difficult to introduce compassion into the process.

Reasons such as these caused administrators and clinicians alike to consider a different means of delivering care, one that would both better meet patients' needs and be more professionally satisfying. In other words, a tool was needed that would increase capacity by leveraging existing resources and increasing physician productivity—yet enhance patient as well as physician professional satisfaction. The DIGMA model was chosen for this study because it: (1) had been demonstrated to improve access through use of existing resources by dramatically increasing physician productivity (by 200–300% or more); (2) can be used to enhance quality of care as well as both patient and physician professional satisfaction; and (3) was being successfully employed in fee-for-service settings.

The Original Plan Envisioned for This Pilot Study

The original plan for this Sutter Medical Group DIGMA pilot study involved selecting three motivated physician volunteers (a medical subspecialist and two primary care physicians) who were highly respected by their peers and had busy practices and access problems. It was felt that such physicians would not only maximally benefit from a DIGMA for their practice but also be most influential in persuading colleagues to try a DIGMA for their practices as well. In turn, this would help to expand the DIGMA pilot to organization-wide implementation once the necessary administrative approval was secured based upon the results of this pilot. The following time line was originally proposed for this pilot study.

Preliminary Work (Mid- to Late–September, 1999):

Introductory phase in which I was to give a 3-day DIGMA presentation to Sutter administrative and physician staffs. Upon completion of these initial presentations to administration and interested physicians in primary and specialty care, the original pilot project plan called for the following three specific action steps to be taken during the time periods indicated.

Phase 1 (October 1–November 14, 1999):

Selection and training phase in which the three pilot physicians (as well as the necessary staffing to support their DIGMA programs) were to be chosen and trained. In addition, I was to act as DIGMA champion for this pilot study by meeting with each of three pilot physicians selected—i.e., in order to determine their particular goals, and then to custom design their DIGMAs accordingly so as to best meet their needs, practice style, and patient panel constituency. In addition, I also helped to get all marketing materials to be used in Sutter's DIGMA program designed and produced: the framed wall poster to be prominently displayed in physician's lobby and exam rooms; the program description flier (100 or more of which were to be mounted in a dispenser secured adjacent to the wall poster); the announcement letter to be mailed to each of the pilot physicians' 500 highest utilizing appropriate patients; an invitation letter to be given by receptionists to every appropriate patient registering for a regular office visit; and a "Dear Valued Patient" follow-up letter to be mailed by the scheduler to interested patients after telephoning those patients that the physicians wanted invited each week. Please note that examples of all of these promotional materials are included in the DVD attached to this book.

I also helped each pilot physician develop a list of appropriate patients to be invited to the DIGMA—especially high utilizers (except for those patients that the physicians felt were inappropriate). In addition, I assisted each physician in drafting the paper DIGMA progress note template that was to be used in the pilot. This was to be largely preprinted and in check-off form in order to optimize the efficiency of the charting process during group time (as no documenter was used in this pilot study), with completed chart notes then being entered into each DIGMA patient's medical chart after the session was over.

I also trained the pilot physicians' schedulers regarding how to best invite patients into the DIGMA—providing them with a scripted message plus talking points to be used when telephoning patients (see the sample scheduling scripts included in the DVD attached to this book). Schedulers were taught how to respond to commonly asked questions about DIGMAs as well as how to send follow-up letters to interested patients (again, see the DVD attached to this book for examples of commonly asked patient questions and how to respond to them). In addition, I trained the physicians' medical assistants regarding their expanded DIGMA responsibilities—such as taking vital signs, updating injections, and performing other special nursing duties. Finally, appropriate group and exam rooms were selected and reserved, the physicians' and medical assistants' schedules were cleared for all 90-minute pilot DIGMA sessions, and the various operational issues associated with the pilot were properly addressed.

Phase 2 (November 15–January 14, 1999):

Launching phase in which I would personally serve as both DIGMA champion and behaviorist for all three pilot DIGMAs. The ultimate goal here was to get all three pilot physicians comfortable with their groups prior to bringing a behavioral health replacement trainee in to eventually take over the behaviorist role in their DIGMAs. As is typical of DIGMAs, the behaviorist was to fulfill multiple duties, such as: giving the introduction at the beginning of each session; handling group dynamic and psychosocial issues; making behavioral health evaluations and interventions; pacing the group to keep it running smoothly and on time; taking over the group while the physician was documenting chart notes or stepping out to handle any private exams or discussions; staying late to address any last minute questions that patients might have before departing; and then quickly straightening up the group room after the session is over. By January 14, 2000, it was anticipated that all three pilot DIGMAs would be running smoothly, that any bugs in the system would have been worked out, and that all three pilot physicians would be relatively comfortable in running their DIGMAs.

Phase 3 (January 15–March 14, 2000):

Transitional phase in which the behavioral health replacement was to be increasingly trained in the group setting to gradually assume evermore responsibilities until ultimately being able to completely take over the pilot DIGMAs—at which time the consultant was to gradually transition out of the pilot DIGMAs. It was during Phase 3 that I was to begin training the behavioral health replacement for all three DIGMAs, and to have this replacement take over progressively more duties until able to ultimately act independently as the behaviorist in all three DIGMAs. By March 15, 2000, it was anticipated that: all three pilot physicians would be quite comfortable in running their DIGMAs; the behavioral health replacement would be well trained and established in co-facilitating these groups; all schedulers and medical assistants would be well trained in performing their respective DIGMA duties; and patients would be becoming increasingly informed about, and satisfied with, the DIGMA program.

Exiting Phase (March 15, 2000):

Behavioral health replacement to take over all three pilot DIGMAs while Dr. Noffsinger (who had been acting as consultant, DIGMA champion, and behaviorist) was to exit and evaluate the pilot study.

The Actual Plan That Was Utilized in This Pilot Study

As so often happens, the pilot study that was actually implemented at Sutter differed in many ways from the pilot as it was originally planned. Here we discuss the pilot study as it was actually implemented, what occurred along the way that caused it to deviate from the original plan, and the various challenges that needed to be addressed.

Pre-implementation Planning:

The initial phase of this pilot program, which included DIGMA presentations to administration as well as to primary and specialty care physicians who had indicated that they might be interested in running a DIGMA for their practices, generated a relatively large pool of interested DIGMA candidates. From this pool of potentially interested providers, three physicians were selected from two sites (Sutter Fort, an urban location in Sacramento, and Laguna, a rural site in northern California located approximately 15 miles away). Using the selection criteria previously established for this pilot program, three pilot physicians were chosen: (1) Dr. A, a full-time internist at Sutter Fort; (2) Dr. B, a full-time rheumatologist at Sutter Fort; and (3) Dr. C, a half-time family practitioner at Laguna.

As the consultant acting as temporary DIGMA champion and behaviorist for this pilot study, I held several initial meetings with each of these physicians and their support staffs—along with the social worker that had just been hired in a half-time capacity as the behavioral health replacement for this DIGMA pilot project. There were three primary goals for these initial meetings that were held with each of the three selected pilot physicians and their support staffs: (1) to custom design each of the three pilot DIGMAs around the specific goals, practice styles, and patient panel constituencies of the selected physicians; (2) to train the three pilot physicians (as well as their schedulers, medical assistants, and support staffs) regarding their respective DIGMA duties; and (3) to develop, in template form, all of the marketing materials (wall poster, fliers, announcements, invitation letters, and follow-up letters) and forms necessary for the DIGMA program—such as the DIGMA progress note, the confidentiality release, and the patient satisfaction form that was to be completed by patients anonymously at the end of each DIGMA session.

I therefore arranged several meetings with Sutter's Marketing Department to design and develop the wall poster (which is included in the DVD attached to this book) and the matching program fliers—and to develop a *trademark look* for their SMA program. All promotional materials were designed to be mutually compatible, professional appearing, and coordinated so as to work together and make lobby and exam room wall displays that would be pleasing to the eye. These marketing materials, which established the desired corporate look for the program, needed to meet Sutter's particular organizational requirements—plus have a warm and inviting look that would both help to recruit patients and accurately reflect the high-quality care that patients could expect to receive from the DIGMA program.

The confidentiality release (which was to be signed by each patient during every session, as well as by any support persons accompanying them) was printed on the back side of the DIGMA progress note, with space above it for the patient to write down the reason for today's visit—an approach that both conserved paper and made clear which DIGMA session the confidentiality release actually applied to. A group chart was also developed for each DIGMA pilot, which required that still other forms be developed for the program (such as attendance sheets and logs, which are included in the attached DVD). In addition, a computer code needed to be developed for this new visit type that could be entered into the computerized scheduling system so that patients could be pre-registered into DIGMA sessions months in advance—and so that reminder notices could be sent to pre-registered patients shortly before their DIGMA appointment.

Departures from the Original Pilot Study and the Reasons for the Changes:

During one of the early planning meetings, I became aware that Sutter had one of the most productive primary care doctors that I have ever encountered. He had only 10-minute return appointments—with no 15-, 20-, or 30-minute return appointments on his schedule whatsoever. As it turned out, Dr. D (a full-time family practitioner at the Laguna site) also had an extremely busy practice and a heavy workload, and was therefore also interested in running a pilot DIGMA for his practice. Although the DIGMA model had been shown time and time again to increase physician productivity by 300% or more, I knew that this could not be accomplished with such a highly productive physician. Nevertheless, I did feel that his productivity could be doubled through use of a carefully designed and run DIGMA, which was something that Dr. D initially doubted and took serious issue with—as he felt that he had already done everything possible to make his practice as efficient and productive as possible. In any case, we both felt that it would be a remarkable accomplishment if the DIGMA model was able to double the productivity of such a highly efficient physician.

As a result, the decision was made to establish four pilot DIGMAs rather than the three called for in the original plan. It was also felt that by having two busy, backlogged, and productive physicians attached to the DIGMA pilot from a relatively small facility like Laguna, a special opportunity would be provided for Sutter Medical Foundation to evaluate—in a microcosm—the potential impact that DIGMAs could have upon the organization. In addition, there were other meaningful departures from the original plan. For example, due to limited start-up funding being available, it was unfortunately the case that only 150 announcement letters could be sent out to patients per pilot DIGMA. In other words, we were no longer able to mail announcements to the 500 highest utilizing patients of each pilot physician, as was called for in the original pilot project plan (the intention of which was to *jump start* the pilot and produce high group census levels from the very beginning). It was felt that this mailing limitation would likely translate into reduced group census for this pilot study, and therefore into less than ideal increases in physician productivity (i.e., less than what might otherwise have been achievable through the DIGMA model and this pilot study).

Issues That Needed to Be Addressed

As we progressed toward the implementation phase of this pilot study, we found that there were many issues that needed to be addressed.

Training the Behavioral Health Replacement:

In another significant deviation from the original pilot study plan, the training of the behavioral health replacement was accelerated in order to (1) reduce the overall cost of the implementation process and (2) ultimately decrease the need for the author's direct involvement in the pilot study as an outside consultant—i.e., from the originally projected 4 months after actual launch to just 6 weeks. This meant that the behavioral health replacement would need to attend all four DIGMA pilots from their inception and immediately start taking over progressively more duties (i.e., from initially just sitting in and observing to gradually taking over more and more of the behaviorist's role), rather than waiting until 2 months after the pilots were launched as was originally planned. In addition, this behavioral health replacement was also to be groomed and trained from early on in this pilot to ultimately take over as the organization's DIGMA champion (and, as a result, attended all subsequent meetings that I had with administration, pilot physicians, and

support staffs)—i.e., so as to be able to ultimately assume responsibility for implementing all future DIGMA programs throughout Sutter.

As this training progressed, the behavioral health replacement gradually took over progressively more responsibilities in co-facilitating the pilot groups as the weeks went by. In addition, for all four pilot physicians, each of the initial six pilot DIGMA sessions that I was involved in was followed by a debriefing and training meeting. These debriefings were attended by the provider and the behaviorist replacement as well as myself, and focused upon improving and fine-tuning the DIGMA so as to make future sessions even better and more productive. In order to provide this replacement behaviorist and champion-in-training with the opportunity to experience running the pilot DIGMAs alone for a couple of weeks, the author attended the pilot DIGMAs for the first five consecutive sessions—and then took 2 weeks off before returning on the eighth week for the final session of this pilot study that he participated in (with all six of these pilot study DIGMA sessions being followed by debriefing meetings). During the two intervening sessions preceding the sixth session in which I did not participate, the replacement behaviorist acted alone as the behaviorist throughout.

Training the Support Staffs:

Before actually launching the pilot DIGMAs, several meetings were conducted with the pilot physicians and their staffs at both Sutter sites in order to familiarize all support staff members associated with the pilot with regards to the DIGMA concept, its intended benefits to patients and physicians alike, and their expected roles and duties in supporting the program. Additional presentations were also made to the support staffs and their managers in order to gain their full support for this effort—and to familiarize everyone with their respective roles and responsibilities. Schedulers were trained by providing them with scripts and talking points for telephoning and inviting patients into the pilot DIGMAs, and by then role playing various scenarios that could possibly occur. Receptionists were trained regarding both how to register patients into the pilot DIGMAs and how to handle incoming phone calls in the clinic—i.e., so as to inform patients about the pilot program and, when appropriate, to invite them to attend the group in lieu of an individual office visit.

Additionally, medical assistants and nurses were trained regarding their expanded DIGMA nursing duties—i.e., in taking vital signs, in giving injections, and in providing any special duties that the physician wanted to have performed. Unfortunately, the centralized telephone answering and scheduling service posed an ongoing challenge to this pilot study. This was the result of so many personnel being involved with handling incoming calls that accountability regarding the scheduling of patients into the pilot DIGMAs was all-too-often lacking within the call center. This made it difficult to fill all DIGMA sessions to capacity, and therefore to consistently achieve peak performance and optimal productivity.

Billing for DIGMA Services:

Another issue that needed to be dealt with was that of billing for group visits. DIGMA group patient appointments had not been specifically addressed in the most recent manual for billing and coding(6). Because it is the setting and the number of observers present rather than the content of the visit that differentiates individual office visits from DIGMAs, it was decided that any billing disputes with patients or insurers would be handled in the same manner as those arising from traditional medical services. It is important to note that DIGMAs provide—through a series of one doctor–one patient encounters with observers—complete medical visits with history, assessment, medical decision-making, physical exam (when appropriate), counseling, risk assessment and reduction, and treatment plan being provided according to the specific and unique needs of each individual patient. Medical charts are reviewed and an individual chart note is documented during group time for inclusion in each patient's chart.

All medical services provided in the DIGMA setting were subjected to the same evaluative and billing process as any other medical services. History, exam, assessment, medical decision-making, and treatment plans occurring in the DIGMA setting were documented through individual chart notes in each patient's medical chart and coded according to existing criteria—with the service being billed via standard procedures required by payers. Patients, along with the support person (spouse, adult child, caregiver, friend, etc.) whom they invited at no extra charge, signed a confidentiality waiver at the start of each DIGMA session. Research at Sutter confirmed that these billing procedures were in compliance with applicable regulations and contractual requirements; however, it was nonetheless recommended that other healthcare organizations interested in establishing DIGMA programs involve their own reimbursement analysts and compliance experts to develop their own billing procedures. It is further recommended that they document DIGMA visits carefully and thoroughly,

and that they adhere completely to billing procedures that fully comply with all applicable regulations, contractual requirements, and community standards.

The Custom Design Utilized in Each of the Four Pilot DIGMAs

Three of the four pilot DIGMAs were held weekly for 90 minutes; however, the fourth (that of the highly productive physician with only 10 minute office visits) was held weekly for 60 minutes—as it was felt that his patients, because they were accustomed to very rapid and short visits, would not be able to tolerate a 90-minute group visit. The design of each of these pilot DIGMAs differed from all the others as a result of being custom designed around the specific needs, goals, and practice of each individual physician.

Dr. A's Internal Medicine DIGMA:

Dr. A, a busy and backlogged full-time internist, selected a DIGMA of mixed design. Here, diabetes and obesity were the focus during the first week of the month; heart disease, hypertension, and hyperlipidemia were the focus during the second weekly session each month; allergy, asthma, and chronic respiratory problems were the focus of the third monthly session; gastrointestinal difficulties (GERD, diverticulitis, irritable bowel, ulcers, etc.) and chronic pain (headache, arthritis, fibromyalgia, musculoskeletal pain, etc.) were the focus during the fourth week each month; and general health issues were the focus of the fifth week—during which virtually all of the internist's patients were invited to attend, regardless of diagnosis or condition (i.e., for those couple of months each year having five sessions). However, as is typical of the mixed design, patients who were unable to attend the monthly session that best addressed their particular health problem were then invited to attend any other appropriate session that happened to better fit their schedule.

This internist was helped by a medical assistant assigned to his DIGMA and by receptionists from his office who both registered patients for his DIGMA and acted as DIGMA schedulers—i.e., whenever they had the time and were able to do so (which was not often enough, and therefore resulted in the census of group sessions often being less than ideal). By averaging his productivity data during normal clinic hours over the entire month preceding his pilot DIGMA, Dr. A's pre-DIGMA production rate for individual return appointments during 90 minutes of clinic time was determined to be 4.5 patients per 90 minutes. It was observed that he had 15-minute return appointments on his schedule (so that six return patients could theoretically be scheduled into 90 minutes of clinic time) and a moderate no-show rate. Therefore, in order to triple actual productivity during his 90-minute weekly DIGMA, he would need to see 13.5 (i.e., $3 \times 4.5 = 13.5$) patients on average in his group sessions. Because he wanted to at least triple his productivity for return visits during his DIGMA, this internist therefore set his minimum census level to be 13.5 patients—and his target census level to be 15 patients.

Dr. B's Rheumatology DIGMA:

Dr. B, a full-time rheumatologist, decided to utilize the heterogeneous DIGMA model for her pilot program. She made this decision because of her relatively small panel size (especially of rheumatology patients having intense medical needs), and due to concerns that her group census would be too small if a homogeneous or mixed DIGMA design was selected. She felt that a heterogeneous design would be best because it would permit all of her rheumatology patients to be invited to attend any given session, irrespective of diagnosis or condition. She was assisted by a medical assistant assigned to her pilot DIGMA and by receptionists from her office who both registered DIGMA patients and fulfilled the role of DIGMA schedulers (i.e., again, when they had the time and inclination, which was problematic). Because this rheumatologist's pre-DIGMA production rate for return appointments was determined to be 2.9 patients per 90 minutes of clinic time (as she had 30-minute return appointments and a very low no-show rate), her minimum census level was set at 8.7 patients—as she wanted to increase productivity during her DIGMA by 300%. However, with the hope of ideally increasing her productivity even more, she set her target census at 12 patients.

Dr. C's Family Practice DIGMA:

Dr. C, a busy halftime family practitioner, initially wanted to implement a mixed DIGMA design. It was structured to focus upon diabetes, obesity, hypertension, and hyperlipidemia on the first week of the month; pain management (headache, neck and back pain, fibromyalgia, and arthritis) on the second week; gastrointestinal problems (GERD, colitis, irritable bowel, diverticulitis, etc.) on the third; women's health issues (for women of all ages) on the fourth week of each month; and be open to all of her patients on the fifth week (i.e., for those couple of

months each year having five sessions). Unfortunately, her half-time practice proved to be too small to support this mixed DIGMA design during the first couple of pilot sessions, which, as a result, failed to achieve the group census levels required to make this a viable option for her. Because this mixed DIGMA design produced a group census that was too low during Dr. C's first three pilot sessions, it was promptly dropped at that time in favor of a heterogeneous DIGMA design—i.e., in which all of her patients were invited to attend any week that they happened to have a medical need and wanted to be seen, regardless of diagnosis or condition.

This family practitioner was assisted by a medical assistant assigned to her pilot DIGMA and by her own receptionists, who not only registered DIGMA patients but also occasionally acted as DIGMA schedulers for her program. As it turned out, scheduling support for the DIGMA pilots ultimately proved to be particularly problematic at the Laguna facility, which, as a result, negatively impacted group census for the two pilot DIGMAs held at that site. Because Dr. C's pre-DIGMA productivity rate for individual follow-up appointments was determined to be 4.2 patients per 90-minutes of clinic time dedicated to seeing return appointments (as she had 15-minute returns and a fairly high no-show rate), her minimum census level was set at 12.6 patients in order to triple her productivity during DIGMA sessions. In the hopes of ideally increasing her DIGMA productivity even further, she set her target census level at 15 patients; however, she was prevented from achieving this number for two reasons—initially as a result of selecting a mixed DIGMA design, and then as a result of the significant scheduling problems that she experienced at her facility on an ongoing basis.

Dr. D's Family Practice DIGMA:

Dr. D was an extremely busy and productive fulltime family practitioner with a very busy and fast-paced practice. Because he wanted operational simplicity and to have as many of his patients as possible qualify to attend all of his DIGMA sessions, he selected the heterogeneous design—as this model enabled all of his patients to attend any session they wished, regardless of diagnosis. He was also assisted by a medical assistant and occasionally by his scheduling staff, although DIGMA scheduling support (especially at the Laguna site) remained a significant and ongoing problem throughout this pilot study—which resulted in less than ideal census levels being achieved in many of Dr. C's and Dr. D's DIGMA sessions during this pilot study. Although this fast-paced family practitioner had only 10-minute individual return appointments on his schedule and could theoretically schedule six individual follow-up visits during 60 minutes of clinic time, his pre-DIGMA return appointment productivity rate during normal clinic hours was actually determined to be 4.7 patients per hour—which, although amazingly high, was considerably smaller than the six patients per hour theoretically possible (i.e., due to having some no-shows and late-cancels). This exceptional initial productivity rate would clearly place high demands upon any model, including the DIGMA model, which attempted to further increase the remarkable productivity of this extremely efficient physician.

Because only a relatively small group room was available at the Laguna site, and because his patients were used to a very rapid pace of care delivery, we decided to employ a weekly 60-minute DIGMA format—i.e., rather than the more typical 90-minute weekly DIGMA venue, as we felt that would simply be too long for this family practitioner's patients. Therefore, in order to increase his productivity by 200% during 60-minute DIGMA sessions, the minimum census for his pilot was set at 9.4 (i.e., $2 \times 4.7 = 9.4$) patients. Furthermore, his ideal target census was set somewhat higher at 13 patients for two reasons: (1) because it was the largest group size that the relatively small group room could possibly handle; and (2) because the DIGMA model was already being pushed close to its limits and, as a result, it was doubtful that more than 13 patients could realistically be provided with quality care during just an hour's time, no matter how efficient the physician might happen to be.

Results of Sutter's Pilot DIGMA Project

The data reported here were collected on the four pilot DIGMAs during the six sessions that I participated in as a consultant. Although I initially acted as the DIGMA champion and behaviorist (i.e., prior to and during the first 3 weekly sessions of each pilot DIGMA), I thereafter progressively delegated evermore of these responsibilities to the behavioral health replacement whom I was training to take over these roles.

The Data That Were Collected During This Pilot Study:

The data collected during the 6 weeks of the pilot study that I participated in are presented in Table 9.2, which depicts the following aggregate data for all four pilot physicians combined during each weekly session that I participated in: (1) the number of patients who were pre-registered into each session; (2) the number of pre-registered patients who actually attended each session; (3) the number of patients who simply dropped into each session without pre-registering; and (4) the number of support persons (spouses, adult children, caregivers, friends, etc.) who accompanied the patients. It needs to be noted that Dr. C was on vacation and did not hold her DIGMA on the second week of this pilot—i.e., the second session—which is the only pilot DIGMA session that was not actually held.

Overbook Sessions to Compensate for "No-Shows":

As can be seen from the numbers in Table 9.2, a total of 81.2% of all patients who pre-registered for sessions actually attended—whereas 18.8% failed to keep their appointments. Therefore, if one were to do as the airlines do and overbook sessions according to the expected number of *no-shows*, then these two Sutter medical center sites would need to overbook their DIGMA sessions correspondingly (i.e., by approximately two patients per session, less the number of patients who drop-in) in order to compensate for these no-shows—and to thereby make their DIGMAs immune to this vexing problem that can result in so much costly physician downtime with traditional individual office visits. However, when planning to ensure that targeted census levels are consistently met, one must take into account not only the number of no-shows that are expected but also the average number of *drop-ins* attending each session without pre-registering (in this case, approximately one drop-in per DIGMA session, on average)—which must be subtracted from the expected number of no-shows.

Table 9.2 Totals for all pilot DIGMAs combined

Pilot sessions	# Pre-registered Patients	# Pre-registered attendees	# Drop-ins	# Support Persons
First session	46	35	0	3
Second session	41	27	4	5
Third session	40	32	4	4
Fourth session	41	36	5	9
Fifth session	36	28	5	4
Sixth session	57	54	11	4

Overall average number of DIGMA patients seen per week in 4 pilot DIGMAs = <u>41.8</u> (i.e., during those DIGMA sessions that were actually held)

When Overbooking for "No-Shows," also Take the Number of "Drop-ins" into Account:

In the case of this 6-week pilot study, there was an average of 1.3 drop-ins per DIGMA session—although the number of drop-ins tended to be larger during the latter sessions, i.e., after patients had begun to find out about the DIGMA program and its drop-in feature. As is always the case with DIGMAs, the number of drop-ins was expected to gradually increase over time—i.e., as evermore patients in the physician's practice become familiar with this new program, give it a try with success, and are willing to return to it in the future. However, even after a DIGMA has been running for years, the number of drop-ins seldom exceeds 15–20% or so. With regards to the size of the group room that was necessary to accommodate all attendees into these DIGMA groups, it is important to also note that an average of 1.3 support persons typically attended each session during this pilot study. Therefore, based upon the data gathered so far, the data would indicate the wisdom in this case of roughly overbooking all sessions by 1 patient (i.e., the two that failed to show on average, less approximately one drop-in).

Physician Productivity Was Increased 256.4% During This DIGMA Pilot Study

Table 9.3 consolidates the individualized data depicted in Table 9.2 into a simpler format, showing the total number of patients attending each of the four pilot physicians' DIGMAs during each of the six sessions that I attended (i.e., regardless of whether the patients that attended pre-registered or dropped-in). Unlike Table 9.2, Table 9.3 does not show the number of patients who pre-registered or dropped-in, nor does it depict the number of support persons who attended sessions on average. As can be seen in this consolidated table, the average number of patients seen per session in each of the pilot physicians' DIGMAs ranged from a low of 8.7 to a high of 14.0 patients. Furthermore, when added up and aggregated for all four pilot physicians in combination, the average weekly total for all four pilot DIGMAs combined was 41.8 patients. In total, the four pilot DIGMAs combined consumed only 5.5 hours of physician time per week (i.e., in running three 90-minute DIGMAs plus one 60-minute DIGMA per week), although they did require additional facilities and support personnel (other than the behaviorist) in order to be properly run.

For each of the four pilot physicians, Table 9.3 also compares productivity data gathered during the four pilot DIGMAs with the pre-DIGMA productivity data that these same physicians had for traditional individual return visits. For the entire month prior to the start of the pilot study, the four pilot physicians saw an average of between 2.9 individual return patients per 90 minutes of clinic time (Dr. B) and 4.7 patients per hour (Dr. D). This table compares physician productivity between individual office visits and DIGMA group visits during the

Table 9.3 Increased physician productivity at the sutter medical foundation

	Week 1 (12/6/99) No. patients/ week	Week 2 (12/13/99) No. patients/ week	Week 3 (1/3/00) No. patients/ week	Week 4 (1/10/00) No. patients/ week	Week 5 (1/17/00) No. patients/ week	Week 6 (2/7/00) No. patients/ week	Average No. patients/ week	Percent increased productivity per physician
Dr. A, internal medicine; initial no. patients per 90 minutes = 4.5 (minimum group census 13.5)	12	12	14	16	5	25	14.0	311.1
Dr. B, rheumatology, initial no. patients per 90 minutes = 2.9 (minimum group census 8.7)	5	6	9	8	7	17	8.7	300.0
Dr. C, family practice, initial no. patients per 90 minutes = 4.2 (minimum group census 12.6)	8	Cancelled (illness)	7	11	8	14	9.6	228.6
Dr. D, family practice, initial no. patients per 90 minutes = 4.7 (minimum group census 9.4)	10	13	6	6	13	9	9.5	202.1
Total	35/4	31/3	36/4	41/4	33/4	65/4	41.8	256.4

length of time that the DIGMA occupied (i.e., 90 minutes in all cases but one, which was 60 minutes). With regards to individual return visits, these four pilot physicians would—in combination—have only been able to see an average of 16.3 (4.5 + 2.9 + 4.2 + 4.7 = 16.3) patients individually in the clinic during the 5.5 hours of physician time that the four pilot DIGMAs occupied each week.

Let us now compare this level of productivity for individual return visits to the 41.8 patients actually seen on average during a comparable amount of time spent during the initial sessions of the DIGMA pilot. For all four pilot physicians combined, this represents, on average, *a 256.4% increase* (41.8/16.3 × 100% = 256.4%) in physician productivity during the time spent running their DIGMAs. Instead of seeing 4.5 return patients on average during 90 minutes of clinic time, Dr. A was able to see an average of 14.0 in his 90-minute DIGMA, which translated into a 311.1% increase in his productivity. Instead of seeing 2.9 patients individually on average, Dr. B instead saw an average of 8.7 return patients during her 90-minute DIGMA—which corresponded to a 300% increase in her productivity. Similarly, Dr. C saw 9.6 return patients on average per week in her 90-minute DIGMA vs. the 4.2 patients she saw on average individually during that amount of time—which represented a 228.6% increase in her productivity. Finally, Dr. D increased his productivity by 202.1% by seeing 9.5 patients on average during his 60-minute DIGMA instead of the 4.7 return patients that he was seeing individually during the same amount of time.

A Few Teaching Points and Comments About This 256.4% Increase in Physician Productivity

As we have just seen, a 256.4% increase in physician productivity was demonstrated in this DIGMA pilot study during six of its initial weeks of operations, even though we knew from the start that one of the physicians would only be able to achieve a 200% increase in his productivity. Although all four pilot DIGMAs were still at a very early stage of implementation, we found that three out of four pilot physicians were able to meet the increased level of productivity that they originally had hoped for. In addition, Dr. C's case proved to be particularly informative—and it certainly warrants a closer inspection. All four pilot DIGMAs provided important teaching points.

The Internist Proved to be Especially Adept at Inviting His Patients to Attend:

Dr. A quickly mastered the process of referring patients into his DIGMA, and consequently quickly proved especially adept at filling his group sessions. He recommended his DIGMA in a persuasive and positively worded manner to all appropriate patients that he saw each day for a regular office visit—being careful to always invite them to attend his DIGMA whenever they might have a future medical need or require a follow-up visit. In addition, all of his office support staff (receptionists, schedulers, nursing personnel, etc.) were also quite enthused, well trained, and supportive of his new DIGMA program—and were certain to always inform all suitable patients of the new program and to encourage them to attend. When appropriate, patients telephoning the office to schedule an appointment or to talk to the doctor were always told about the DIGMA program and invited to attend that week. Because of these highly successful patient recruitment efforts from the very beginning (i.e., by both the physician and his support staff), he was able to see an average of 14 patients per session in his DIGMA during the six sessions of this pilot. This increased his productivity over individual office visits by 311% and met his original productivity goal for the program. By scheduling numerous patients into the DIGMA program, Dr. A and his staff were able to off-load many traditional follow-up visits onto the highly efficient DIGMA program—which freed up numerous individual office visits for those patients needing or preferring them and, as a result, improved access to individual visits as well.

The Rheumatologist, a Medical Subspecialist with Longer Appointments, Tripled Her Productivity:

Even during the early, pilot phase of her program, Dr. B's rheumatology DIGMA had already increased her productivity during group sessions by 300%, which was her targeted goal. However, she should be able to eventually increase her productivity by at lease 400% in the future—which, in her case, would only require an average group attendance of 11.6 patients, which is well within the recommended group size for a DIGMA of 10–16 patients. This is because, as more time passes, she will likely become even more comfortable in running her DIGMA program and capable of efficiently handling a group of that size—plus evermore patients will gradually find out about and experience the benefits of her DIGMA, and will therefore be willing to attend the group and return. Actually, I have set up many larger rheumatology DIGMAs (i.e., with several different rheumatologists in various fee-for-service and capitated systems around the country) that have often had groups with 15, 16, or more patients in attendance—i.e., group sizes that were much larger than those of Dr. B, yet were nonetheless highly successful.

Close Examination of Dr. C's Data Is Quite Revealing for Part-Time Physicians:

While Dr. C's overall 228.6% gain in productivity fell considerably short of the 300% increase that she had originally hoped for, a closer examination of the data reveals something quite different. Although the mixed DIGMA model that she employed during her first two DIGMA sessions did not prove to be viable (as she only saw an average of 7.5 patients during her first two sessions, which corresponded to an increase of only 179.6% in her productivity), the results of her following 3 sessions—during which she utilized a heterogeneous DIGMA model—stood in dramatic contrast to this finding. During the last three sessions of this pilot study, Dr. C was able to see an average of 11.0 patients per DIGMA session by using the heterogeneous model—which translated to a 261.9% increase in her productivity. Because her pilot DIGMA program was still quite new, it was anticipated that the small additional increase in her census (i.e., an average of just 1.6 more patients per session) that would be required to increase her gain in productivity to 300% could reasonably be expected to occur over time—although she would need to overcome the scheduling problems previously noted at the Laguna facility in order to optimize the efficiency benefits of her DIGMA program.

Because Dr. C worked only half-time, she had a correspondingly smaller pool of patients in her practice from which to draw attendees for her DIGMA. However, once she employed the heterogeneous design, virtually all of her patients qualified to attend every one of her DIGMA sessions—which contrasts sharply with the mixed and homogeneous subtypes, wherein only a considerably smaller subset of patients in a provider's practice qualify to attend any given session. While consistently having full groups certainly is possible, achieving targeted DIGMA census levels simply requires a greater effort from half-time providers—even if they do use the heterogeneous design. Because their patient panel is considerably smaller, consistently meeting group census requirements means that half-time providers must take particular care to adequately market their DIGMA program to all of their patients—and they must be certain to consistently invite, through a carefully worded and positive script, all appropriate patients seen during regular office visits to have their next visit be a DIGMA visit (plus be certain to invite all appropriate patients seen during DIGMA sessions to have their next follow-up visit back in a future DIGMA session). I say the latter because there is simply no *richer ore vein* in the universe for populating future sessions than that provided by the DIGMA groups themselves as, once patients do in fact attend, they are almost always willing to return—i.e., if only they are invited to do so.

The lesson to be learned here is that half-time physicians can run successful DIGMA programs for their practices. However, to achieve the increased levels of productivity that they desire, part-time physicians might need to employ the more all-inclusive heterogeneous model in order to attain the requisite census levels during sessions—i.e., rather than the more limited homogeneous and mixed DIGMA subtypes. This would not be the case, however, for large chronic illness population management programs where homogeneous DIGMAs could be kept full with relative ease, even for physicians who only work part time in such programs, because of the large number of patients having a particular chronic illness that are covered by that program. In addition, half-time providers must be certain to personally invite all appropriate patients seen in the clinic (or in a DIGMA) to have their next visit in the DIGMA, plus make certain that all schedulers and support staff are also recommending the program and inviting all suitable patients to attend. This process can sometimes be accelerated by having all support staff (especially the entire scheduling staff) sit in on a DIGMA session or two shortly after the DIGMA has been launched so that they can personally witness what a beneficial program it is—and so that their buy-in can be achieved (and so that they can later SELL it to patients).

Implications for Extremely Productive Physicians:

In addition, the results for Dr. D are also quite informative and have implications for all extremely productive physicians. This is because such a highly productive physicians (Dr. D's baseline productivity rate for individual return appointments during 1 hour of clinic time was 6.0 patients scheduled and 4.7 patients actually seen on average) place an inordinate burden—and a singularly difficult challenge—upon any model that attempts to even further enhance such exceptionally high efficiency. Certainly, it is quite unlikely that he would be able to further increase his productivity in any meaningful way through traditional individual appointments alone—i.e., by simply attempting to see even more patients than he already does by using the same model and delivering care at an even faster rate. Simply put, the time pie for such highly productive physicians is already cut about as thin as can realistically be achieved in the context of delivering quality care. Since Dr. D was already close to the efficiency limit of traditional individual office visits, what he needed was a tool that would enable him to "work smarter, not harder" and dramatically leverage his remarkable productivity even further, which is precisely what a properly run DIGMA should be able to provide.

Because the group room at Laguna was relatively small (with a maximum capacity of 15, should patients, staff, and support persons be willing to truly squeeze in), it severely limited the size of DIGMA groups and necessitated that Dr. D's sessions be limited to just 60 minutes in duration. This is because correspondingly fewer patients needed to be seen during 60-minute DIGMA sessions in order to double Dr. D's productivity—i.e., as compared to 90-minute sessions, which it is doubtful that Dr. D's patients would have been able to tolerate anyway. As it turned out, a remarkable accomplishment of this pilot study was that—despite these limitations and challenges with regard to scheduling and group room size at the Laguna site—his DIGMA was nevertheless able to further increase his already remarkable productivity by 202.1% during group sessions.

There Was a High Level of Patient Satisfaction with This Pilot DIGMA Program

From its earliest beginnings, high levels of patient and physician professional satisfaction have been goals of primary importance to the DIGMA model—and goals that have consistently been achieved in study after study. The data from this study demonstrated that patient satisfaction with the DIGMA program was once again very high, which is completely consistent with the results of numerous other DIGMA programs that have been implemented elsewhere (i.e., for studies that have been properly designed, supported, and run).

At the end of every pilot session in this pilot study at Sutter, all patients attending the DIGMA were asked to anonymously complete a 7-question Patient Satisfaction Survey, shown in Table 9.4, rating their level of satisfaction with the DIGMA visit.

Table 9.4 Patient satisfaction with DIGMAs on the 5-point Likert scale

1. The length of time I had to wait between making an appointment and seeing the doctor today was _____
2. The length of time I had to wait at the office to see the doctor was _____
3. I felt today's visit with the doctor was _____
4. I felt the explanations of medical procedures, tests, and drugs were _____
5. I felt the amount of time I had with the doctor and staff during today's visit was _____
6. I felt the personal interest in myself and my medical problems by the doctor and staff was _____
7. Overall, I felt the quality of care and services I received today were _____

Excellent (5), very good (4), good (3), fair (2), and poor (1).

Table 9.5 shows, for each of the pilot physicians, the range of average patient satisfaction scores on the seven questions over the various sessions of this study—i.e., during the six sessions that I participated in as a consultant (i.e., the first 5 weeks, which was then followed by the eighth weekly session). The overall average patient satisfaction score for the entire pilot project (i.e., for all seven survey questions, for all patients in attendance, and gathered over all 4 pilot physicians) was a remarkably high 4.67 out of 5—which, as it turns out, is fairly typical of the level of patient satisfaction demonstrated in other DIGMA studies as well (i.e., which, as it turns out, is almost always in the 4.4 to 4.7 out of 5 range).

Table 9.5 Patient satisfaction data for four pilot DIGMAs at the Sutter Medical Foundation

Physician	Average Patient satisfaction score(range of average scores by physician for all 7questions)
Dr. A (75 surveys)	4.3–4.7
Dr. B (42 surveys)	4.7–4.9
Dr. C (33 surveys)	4.5–4.8
Dr. D (62 surveys)	4.4–4.8
Overall average score (for all physicians)	**4.67/5**

Although it was not measured in this pilot study, it would also have been interesting to compare these patient satisfaction scores for DIGMA visits with similar scores (i.e., using the same patient satisfaction measurement instrument) gathered prior to the start of this study for traditional individual office visits for the same four pilot physicians—i.e., before the DIGMA program had begun to solve the serious access problems to these physicians' practices. Had this been done, it is almost certain that the level of patient satisfaction would have been significantly lower for individual office visits than for DIGMA visits (a finding that would be consistent with similar findings from other DIGMA studies—for example, see Study 10 in this chapter) as all four of these pilot physicians initially had busy practices and serious access problems. Not only would patients be expected to get frustrated (and thus rate their overall level of satisfaction as lower for individual office visits) when they are not readily able to get in and be seen in a timely manner, but they would also score lower on this patient satisfaction questionnaire as the first question specifically addresses the amount of time that the patient had to wait before being seen.

How the Pilot Physicians Evaluated Their DIGMAs

Upon completion of this pilot project, a structured telephone interview was conducted with each of the pilot physicians, who were asked to evaluate their level of satisfaction with their DIGMAs. I have included some representative physician comments from these telephone interviews in the paragraphs that follow (7). It is important to note that throughout these structured telephone interviews, all four pilot physicians made it abundantly clear that they were highly satisfied with their DIGMA programs. Thus, the results of this pilot study demonstrate not only dramatically increased physician productivity, but also high levels of both patient and physician professional satisfaction.

Dr. A, Internal Medicine:

"Drop-In Group Medical Appointments or DIGMAs are a unique way to deliver healthcare and provide an interaction between physician and patient that would not ordinarily occur. My DIGMA has primarily provided three things to my practice of internal medicine. It has allowed my patients greater access. It has allowed me to spend more time with my patients in an appointment setting where a wide range of issues can be discussed. My patients are given the opportunity to share their health issues in a group setting and receive information that may come from experiences of others sharing in the appointment. The Drop In-Group Medical Appointment allows me to educate my patients, identify and address their psychosocial issues, and provide support in a group setting. Thus far, my patients have enjoyed this appointment setting. The majority seem to like the easier access to my practice afforded by the DIGMA, and the opportunity to spend 90 minutes with their physician (7)."

> Professionally, the DIGMA has created more time in my schedule. It has increased the number of longer appointments available in my schedule where I can do physical exams or consultations. This has been made possible because I can schedule shorter appointments such as routine follow-up appointments, medication refills, blood pressure checkups, and straightforward medical issues into the DIGMA. Personally, this approach to delivering healthcare has relieved some of the burdens of juggling time between a busy internal medicine practice and time spent with my most cherished possession, my family. Drop-In Group Medical Appointments are not for everyone. The concept may sound interesting but be vague to both physician and patient. Some patients and physicians may prefer individual, one-on-one type appointments. DIGMAs don't take away this opportunity. They are not meant to be a substitute, but an alternative.

> My initial skepticism about DIGMAs dissipated quickly when I reviewed the high patient satisfaction scores obtained and the impact it has made on patient access in my practice. I now feel that I have a greater command over my time and schedule in my practice. I no longer feel under the gun to see 25–30 patients a day in order to be productive and meet my compensation standards. I feel that this appointment format allows me to deliver the highest quality healthcare while improving patient satisfaction and enhancing my efficiency.

As we move into the next century, healthcare systems must explore a variety of health delivery mechanisms that will foster quality, efficiency, and patient satisfaction. The Drop-In Group Medical Appointment is one way that this has been accomplished in my practice (7).

Dr. B, Rheumatology:

"There are some definite advantages and some disadvantages to the group. For chronic illnesses, for patients with rheumatoid arthritis or fibromyalgia, and for chronic pain and disability issues it works very well. It does not work as well for acutely ill or sicker patients because I'm afraid that I'll miss or overlook something important for patients who drop-in but actually require a thorough examination and an individual visit. I still have to learn how to best use my group and individual visits: How to have patients who need to be seen individually not drop into group and patients who can best be seen in group not be seen individually. Overall, the experience has been a very good one for me, and the patients absolutely love it. It seems like every day I have patients who have seen the poster or have heard about the group who tell me that it is a good idea and that they would like to attend. Over time, this should help keep the group filled with less effort on my part. In general, I would say that I like it, that patients really like it, and that what I need now is to learn how to best use it (7)."

Dr. C, Family Practice:

"My overall feeling is that it has expanded my horizons about my interactions with patients and different ways that I can interact with them. I've also gotten a lot out of the group dynamics that I've liked. It is heartwarming to see patients open up, share, and help each other. It warms my heart to see that. I also like the fact that I do not have to do any notes afterward—that I can get them all done during the group. I do not feel that I've gotten far enough off the ground yet to see as much from my group as I'm sure it will eventually provide, mostly because I only work half-time. Even if I only broke even as a result of having the group, it would still be worth doing the group because it is so enjoyable, different, and helpful to patients. I expect to see even more benefit with time as my patients and I get more used to using it. As schedulers and patients become more familiar with the group, and as I see and invite more patients, I expect that it will succeed exponentially—which is the key to increasing census. The biggest challenges to me are: (1) getting the census up; (2) learning how to best manage my time in the group; and (3) figuring out how to best do it as it is so different from what I am used to. I do not know of any negatives that have occurred as a result of the program. One thing I can say is that I did not anticipate how draining it would be to see such a large number of patients at once in the group. On the other hand, the group concept takes advantage of one of the greatest untapped resources we have—i.e., the patients themselves, both in managing their own disease and in helping each other. Also, I've appreciated all the help that I've received in group from the behaviorist (7)."

Dr. D, Family Practice:

"Challenges for me: Let the behaviorist be more active in it. Give up some control. As physicians, we have a long history of always having to be in control, so this is new to me. Use it more for follow-up—that is where it will be most valuable to me. Also, it is a good place to put follow-up care—to save time and improve quality of care. Many patients' issues only take two or three minutes of appropriate care, so why give them a 15-minute appointment if it can be handled better in just a couple of minutes in group? This will free up my office visits so that I can have more time available for patients who need them. Also, it reduces the need for my having to repeat the same information over and over, because I can say it one time in the group to many patients at once. Plus, patients are more likely to follow a lot more of the advice because other people in the group agree with what I'm saying. Also, I can spend more time in the group on lifestyle and non-compliance issues (like weight loss, stopping smoking, and better diabetes control) and get a better result. People will listen to and learn more from other people than from me (7)."

> I'm glad that I'm doing it, although it still causes me some anxiety because it's still a new thing and I'm not quite used to it. It's an effort to invite people and that's the key to success—I simply have to do a better job at making that effort. I think the schedulers are starting to get more enthused about the program, which should help. I think that it's a good idea to have them sit in on the group to see what it's like. Although it's hard to free them up from other duties in the clinic, perhaps we could have them each come in one time for 15 or 30 minutes. Do I enjoy it? Absolutely! I really like the fact that I get almost all of my notes written there so that when the group is over, it's over. Plus it's better for the patients too because there are things that happen there that are better care. We can follow some things closer and there's less chance of missing something or having it fall through the cracks because we can watch for it each time they come in (7).

Some Concluding Comments

Although the original plan for Sutter's DIGMA pilot study was carefully conceived and the result of much initial planning, for the reasons previously discussed, the pilot that was actually launched differed in many respects from the original plan. Nonetheless, the desired productivity—as well as patient and physician professional satisfaction goals—were in fact achieved during this pilot study.

DIGMA Programs Must Be Flexible:

Because each DIGMA is custom designed around the specific goals, practice style, and patient panel constituency of the individual provider—and because these needs are constantly changing over time—DIGMA programs must be flexible. This pilot makes it clear that, if DIGMAs are to be fully successful in the long run, they must be able to flexibly adapt to: (1) ever changing and evolving provider and practice needs; (2) new circumstances as they occur, and a rapidly changing healthcare environment; (3) organizational and budgetary constraints, and (4) unexpected operational challenges that can rapidly occur along the way.

Because DIGMAs Can Stress the System, Operational Challenges Must Be Promptly Resolved:

Healthcare organizations considering DIGMAs as a means of helping them to solve access, service, quality, productivity, and patient satisfaction issues will likely find that group visits tend to magnify any pre-existing problems within the system. This is because DIGMAs (as well as Physicals SMAs) so dramatically leverage existing resources and increase physician productivity that they can stress the entire system and exacerbate any pre-existing organizational problems and inefficiencies. Whereas such inefficiencies might not have proved particularly problematic when one patient was being processed through the system at a time for individual office visits, such difficulties are compound when 10–16 patients are going through the system at once for a group visit. And we must always remember that the key to a successful DIGMA (both economically and psychodynamically) lies in consistently meeting predetermined census levels for the program.

Unless addressed, all such inefficiencies and operational problems in the system tend to have the same common effect upon DIGMAs: They ultimately reduce group census and therefore the degree to which the physician's productivity can be increased through the DIGMA program. When operational problems such as promotional, scheduling, personnel, facilities, or budgetary challenges begin to emerge—problems that can substantially and negatively impact the entire DIGMA program—then it is imperative that these issues be promptly addressed and resolved in order for the DIGMA program to be fully successful over time. Otherwise, all such operational challenges can eventually result in the same ultimate difficulty—i.e., decreased attendance, and therefore reduced productivity and efficiency for the DIGMA and PSMA program.

For example, the scheduling problems—especially at the Laguna site, which represents a work in progress—certainly reduced the census of these DIGMA pilot study groups below what it otherwise could have been (and this in turn reduced the increased physician productivity that we were able to achieve below that which otherwise might have been attained). The size of the group room at the Laguna site also put limits on group size, and consequently the degree to which we were able to increase physician productivity. In addition, frustrations over such problems can also tend to decrease both patient and physician satisfaction with the DIGMA program. However, once such operational problems are successfully addressed (challenges that often arise either as a result of the increased productivity of the DIGMA program or because of its additional personnel, promotional, scheduling, and facilities requirements), these improvements can prove beneficial not only to the DIGMA program but also to individual office visits throughout the remainder of the workweek as well.

DIGMAs Have Specific Requirements for Success, and These Often Evolve Over Time:

Because DIGMAs deliver medical care in a manner that is dramatically different from traditional individual office visits, they must be carefully planned, adequately supported, well promoted, and properly run in order to be fully successful. They truly represent a major paradigm shift and a significant departure from traditional individual office visit care. Since DIGMAs are so different—and because they represent a multidisciplinary team-based approach to care—they require professional appearing marketing materials, specially designed forms, appropriate and well-trained team members, custom designed programs, and appropriate group and exam room facilities. In other words, there are numerous specific requirements that must be met in order for DIGMAs to achieve full success—i.e., to completely capture the multiple benefits (increased productivity and access, enhanced quality and service, and high levels of patient and physician professional satisfaction) that they were originally designed to achieve. In addition, as this pilot study at Sutter Medical Foundation has revealed, DIGMAs require considerable flexibility in the implementation plan. In the end, despite much initial planning, this Sutter Medical

Foundation pilot study experience reveals that medical groups implementing DIGMA programs should not be at all surprised if the program that they actually end up launching differs in many respects from that which they originally envisioned.

The Important Teaching Points Learned from This Pilot Project:

Results of this pilot study make it clear that part-time physicians (who have correspondingly smaller practice sizes from which to draw patients for their DIGMAs) will often be more successful in achieving targeted group census levels—and therefore in having a successful DIGMA—if they choose the all-inclusive heterogeneous subtype rather than the more restrictive mixed or homogeneous DIGMA designs. This is because the heterogeneous DIGMA design enables most or all patients in a part-time physician's practice to qualify to attend all sessions—and to therefore attend a DIGMA session whenever they have a medical need and wish to come in. This is particularly true for part-time physicians who happen to work half-time or less, as their patient panel sizes will likely be smallest.

Another teaching point from this study is that DIGMAs are potentially better able to leverage existing resources and dramatically increase productivity for those physicians that have either busy, backlogged practices or relatively lengthy return appointments, and consequently a relatively low level of productivity during normal clinic hours (such as 20–30 minute return appointments rather than 10–15 minute appointments). As an example of this, consider how much easier it was to triple provider productivity (and how much smaller the DIGMA group size needed to be) for Dr. B vs. Dr. D in this pilot study. Physicians who are extraordinarily productive—i.e., who have the shortest individual office visits during regular clinic hours—present the greatest challenge to any model, including the DIGMA model, which strives to further increase physician productivity.

Nevertheless, the DIGMA model can still be of great benefit to such highly productive providers—as was the case for Dr. D in this study—because it can still double productivity and efficiency. However, as was the case in this study, the DIGMA model typically cannot triple or quadruple the productivity of physicians who are initially so productive. There are four types of highly productive physicians where I have found this to be true in actual practice: (1) for pediatricians conducting physical examinations through a Physicals SMA (e.g., well-baby checks or school, camp, and sports physicals); (2) for obstetricians conducting prenatal exams through PSMAs; (3) for dermatologists doing full-body skin exams; and (4) for extremely productive primary care physicians running DIGMAs who have only 10 minute office visits available to their patients for return appointments (such as Dr. D in this pilot study). The reason for this is that all three of these groups of physicians often already have such high levels of initial productivity prior to launching their DIGMA or PSMA that it is very difficult for these SMA models to triple their productivity.

Specialized Applications for DIGMAS and PSMAS

In both primary care and various medical and surgical subspecialties, there are myriad specialized applications for all types of group visit models. In this section, we focus upon a couple of specialized applications of the DIGMA and PSMA models; however, we must keep in mind that there are innumerable such applications—the numbers and types of which are constantly expanding over time and only limited by our imaginations. The reader is invited to read and learn from these studies, and then to contemplate how to take these applications and results and best apply them to their own particular practices, needs, and circumstances.

Study 8: DIGMAs and PSMAs at the Memphis Tennessee VA Medical Center

The following contribution was written by Dr. Keith W. Novak, who is the Associate Chief of Staff for Ambulatory Care at the Memphis Tennessee VA Medical Center (VAMC). Dr. Novak discusses some of the experiences that he has had over the years in using the DIGMA and PSMA models. In addition to working with Dr. Novak in custom designing DIGMAs and PSMAs for his own practice, it was also an honor to help him design and launch the first ever Physicals SMA for Combat Veterans returning from Iraq and Afghanistan. Dr. Novak has been instrumental not only in moving group visits forward within the Memphis VAMC, but also in establishing the highly recognized Combat Veterans Physicals SMA, which he discusses in the following write-up.

This section will also be of interest to some readers because it discusses a minor variant of the DIGMA model which omits the drop-in component—a variant that is referred to herein as a "SIGMA" (Scheduled-In Group Medical Appointment). I (Dr. Noffsinger) have always referred to this as a minor variation of the traditional DIGMA format (and by no means an essential departure from the model) because, when first starting a DIGMA,

there are typically no drop-ins anyway—i.e., because patients are not yet familiar with the program or its drop-in feature. Furthermore, even after DIGMAs have been running for years and are well established, only 10–20% or so of the patients will typically drop-in (and having fewer than 20% of attendees be drop-ins is certainly the norm). Furthermore, since the inception of the DIGMA model, there have always been some physicians who preferred to not employ the drop-in component of the model (i.e., despite the fact that I generally recommend it) which we would then omit—considering it as just one more of the variables that can be used when custom designing the DIGMA to the specific interests, goals, and practice of the individual physician (see Table 2.2).

Going back to the early days of DIGMAs, I have not infrequently utilized this variant with providers who were anxious about, fearful of, or concerned over the drop-in component of this model. Nonetheless, I continue to prefer to hold to the original intent of the DIGMA model as it is optimally patient friendly in that it allows patients to come for a session whenever they happen to have a medical need and want to be seen—even if it is at the last minute and there is not time to call in and schedule the appointment. The original DIGMA design also allows the physician and healthcare organization to capture such patients (i.e., those who are willing to attend) in the highly efficient and cost-effective DIGMA venue whenever possible—i.e., even if it is at the last minute and the only option is to drop-in rather than having such patients occupy a less efficient and more costly individual office visit. In any case, I have never viewed the drop-in feature as critical to the DIGMA model.

The Combat Veterans Physicals Shared Medical Appointment (PSMA) Program

I (Dr. Novak) would like to start my piece by discussing the Combat Veterans PSMA that we have been running at the Memphis VAMC for our combat veterans who are returning from Iraq and Afghanistan. The PSMA for Operation Iraqi Freedom/Operation Enduring Freedom (OIF/OEF) combat veterans was launched in May 2004 to ensure a seamless transition from DoD to VHA care for our returning combat veterans. This SMA was designed to provide a multitude of services in one place at one time for returning combat veterans. These veterans have unique needs, both emotional and physical, that are addressed in the same forum. By treating both mental and physical concerns concurrently, we have been able to help *de-stigmatize* mental health and ensure that treatment for mental health conditions is received. I say this because our workload data show that when a primary care provider refs a patient to Mental Health clinic, only 1/3 of those patients keep the appointment. We also realize that treatment outcomes for mental health conditions are improved when treatment is received early in the course of the disorder, rather than years later as was the case with some Vietnam veterans who suffered with PTSD for 20 years before presenting for treatment. Because of these benefits in addressing mental health and medical problems during the same SMA visit, SMAs have helped de-stigmatize mental health. The OIF/OEF Combat Veterans PSMA has been found to be an "organizational strength" for Memphis VAMC.

General

The OIF/OEF Combat Veteran PSMA is a distinctive type of the Physicals Shared Medical Appointment (PSMA) model. Normally, six to eight patients participate in the PSMA. All participants must agree to receive their medical care in a group setting, to share information about themselves, and to keep group discussions confidential by signing a Confidentiality Release—i.e., which each patient and significant other must sign at the time of check-in for the appointment. Key staff assigned to this clinic includes an internal medicine physician, psychiatrist, psychologist, combat veteran case manager, and a licensed practical nurse. Other participants in the clinic include the Vet Center counselor, nutritionist, Veteran's Service Officer, and business office representative. Each veteran receives a private full physical exam in an exam room. After physicals are performed, patients present to the group room where all history is obtained, treatment plans are developed, education is given, labs are ordered, follow-up appointments are made, referrals are made, and prescriptions are written.

Advantages

The Combat Veterans PSMA offers several distinct benefits, including the following.

Efficiency, Access, and Overbooking Benefits:

PSMAs benefit patients by providing prompt access to healthcare with shorter waiting times. Efficiency can increase 300% or more by seeing six—eight patients in 120 minutes, instead of just the three patients (or considerably less, if our approximately 30% no-show rate is taken into account) normally seen in those three

40-minute slots. After taking the no-show rate into consideration, it becomes apparent that in 120 minutes we typically only see 2.1–2.4 patients (not three patients). PSMAs are more efficient because no-shows and late patients do not have the same negative impact on appointment availability when patients are seen in a group. This is especially true when groups are over-booked by the expected number of no-shows and late-cancels.

Patient Benefits:

PSMAs offer patients access to high-quality medical care. Activity is "max-packed" into the appointments to increase quality and service. Preventive health maintenance and performance measures are satisfied, vaccines given, screening labs obtained, and education provided. The OIF/OEF post-deployment screening, traumatic brain injury screening, posttraumatic stress disorder screening, depression screening, and substance abuse screening are routinely accomplished in the OIF/OEF Combat Veteran PSMA. In addition, patients have the opportunity to enjoy more time with their provider. Although the time is shared, patients see their provider for more than 60 minutes rather than the typical 15–30 minutes of face-to-face time. An additional great benefit is that the patients have the opportunity to enjoy the interaction with, and support from, other combat veterans who are dealing with similar issues. Combat veterans particularly benefit from this type of interaction as many are having a difficult time adjusting to civilian life after having been deployed with their units for the past 12–15 months. If a patient forgets to ask about a health concern, which happens frequently at individual appointments, it is not uncommon for someone else in the group to bring up the concern and everyone will learn from the discussion. Exiting patient satisfaction survey results have been dramatically positive.

Provider Benefits:

PSMAs benefit providers by improving access and productivity, providing an opportunity to practice medicine in an innovative way, allowing more time to educate patients without repetition, and fostering a team approach to care. Questions about eligibility and benefits, which hinder the physician's ability to deliver care during a typical appointment, can be addressed during the orientation segment of the Combat Veterans PSMA. Repetition is lessened by delivering education regarding sleep hygiene, diabetes, or substance abuse to the many patients attending the PSMA simultaneously, rather than eight separate times during individual appointments. In addition, including a clinical pharmacist on the PSMA team is helpful in making appropriate formulary substitutions for a new patient's non-VA medications.

Administration Benefits:

DIGMAs and PSMAs afford advantages to administration by being billable, being a great deal more efficient, leveraging existing staffing, decreasing waiting times, and providing high levels of patient and provider satisfaction.

Flow in Our OIF/OEF Combat Veterans PSMA

1. Patients check in at front desk
2. Patients and significant others sign confidentiality release
3. Vitals obtained, performance measures updated, and routine health maintenance provided
4. OIF/OEF data triggers reminders unique to OIF/OEF veterans (i.e., post-deployment screen, PTSD screen, depression screen, substance abuse screen, and TBI screen)
5. Each patient sequentially receives private physical exam (four exam rooms and two nurses used)
6. Un-roomed patients meet with behaviorist in group room during first part of session, while private physical exams are being conducted
7. Behaviorist/facilitator welcomes patients and reviews confidentiality with group
8. Facilitator documents each patient's complaints on the board in the group room
9. Patients assemble together in the group room immediately after all private physicals are completed for interactive group segment of the session
10. Provider arrives in group room once all private exams are done to start interactive group segment
11. Individual visits conducted in group room, with other patients present as observers (basically this is a small DIGMA)
12. Each patient's chart note is documented immediately after physician has finished working with that patient
13. Provider leaves after last patient's treatment plan is documented
14. Facilitator remains behind to clear and straighten up group room

15. Short break
16. Orientation session begins
17. Session is over

Memphis VAMC Data on OIF/OEF Combat Veterans PSMA

We have seen 693 patients in the OIF/OEF PSMA since it was launched in May 2004 (Fig. 9.9). Efficiency has increased 333% through utilization of the OIF/OEF PSMA. This is based on seeing an average of 7 patients compared to 2.1 patients in 120 minutes—as there is a historic 30% no-show rate for new patients.

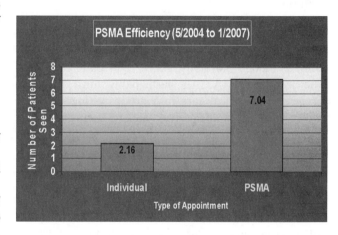

Fig. 9.9 Efficiency from May 2004 to January 2007 in the Memphis VAMC Combat Veterans PSMA

The OIF/OEF post-deployment screen is completed at rate of 97%—i.e., compared to 82% when patients are seen at regular appointments in one of the other Primary Care Clinics. Data from Patient Satisfaction Surveys indicate that patients prefer the OIF/OEF Combat Veterans PSMA to traditional individual appointments (80% reported "strongly agree" and 20% reported "somewhat agree"). In addition, 82% of participating patients "strongly agree" that the group interaction and peer support was helpful and 15% "somewhat agree" (Table 9.6). Furthermore, 89% of PSMA participants "strongly agree" that they got as much information about their health as needed and 11% "somewhat agree." Also, 91% "strongly agree" that they got understandable answers to their questions, and 7% "somewhat agreed." Finally, 91% "strongly agree" that all of their medical needs were addressed, and 9% "somewhat agree." Interestingly, there were no negative "somewhat disagree" or "strongly disagree" reports on any of the patient satisfaction questions from any of the attendees. As can be seen from this data, our veterans are extremely satisfied with this new modality of care delivery.

Table 9.6 Operation Iraqi freedom/operation enduring freedom post-deployment screen for combat veterans PSMA

Statement	Strongly agree	Somewhat agree	Neither agree nor disagree	Somewhat disagree	Strongly disagree
All my medical needs were addressed.	91%	9%			
I understand the answers that I got to my questions.	91%	7%	2%		
I got as much information about my health as I needed.	89%	11%			
The group interaction and peer support was helpful to my care.	82%	15%	3%		
I would recommend a shared medical appointment to others.	80%	20%			
How would you rate the quality of today's visit? (please circle)					
	Poor = 0%	Fair = 0%	Good = 9%	Very good = 36%	Excellent = 55%

Memphis VAMC Has Been Offering Four Separate Types of DIGMAs and PSMAs.

We have been offering four different types of DIGMAs and PSMAs at the Memphis VAMC—two of which are DIGMAs (heterogeneous and disease specific) and two are PSMAs (one for new patients and another exclusively for returning combat veterans). We find that these SMAs are great tools for improving access for the entire practice group. SMAs are able to better match supply and demand, which is one of the 10 key change concepts in Advanced Clinic Access (ACA). Although we use the DIGMA model for two of these, we prefer to use the term "Scheduled-In Group Medical Appointment" (or SIGMA) as we do not use the drop-in component of this model.

Scheduled-In Group Medical Appointment (SIGMA) of the Heterogeneous Subtype:

This type of DIGMA most resembles the customary individual visit that patients are familiar with. They are ideal for routine follow-up care, relatively stable chronically ill patients, those needing increased support and education, low maintenance patients needing intermittent follow-up, patients normally scheduled to nurse clinics, and patients needing to be seen before their normally scheduled follow-up appointment. SIGMAs are not appropriate for the demented, hard of hearing patients, or for those patients that refuse to attend or exhibit disruptive behavior. During the heterogeneous SIGMA, as in any general clinic appointment, the provider examines each patient and develops an individual treatment plan. However, the heterogeneous SIGMA offers the added benefit of other patients in the group being able to benefit by listening, interacting, and learning about various illnesses and treatments while the provider is speaking.

The medical provider sequentially speaks to each patient individually in the group and may do a focused exam in front of the group—or briefly take the patient to an exam room for a more private exam. An individual treatment plan is developed for each patient, preventive health maintenance records are updated, education is provided, prescriptions are written, a chart note is documented, and follow-up care is scheduled as needed. The ancillary assistant obtains vitals, administers vaccines (flu, Pneumovax, etc.), offers written patient education information, collects blood samples for lab tests, and completes preventive medicine reminders. What makes a SIGMA different, and what patients seem to prefer, is that patients get to share how they are feeling alongside comrades who may be experiencing similar medical problems. Patients also prefer the relaxing environment of a 90-minute appointment compared to the rushed feeling of a regular 15- to 20-minute appointment. A social worker or psychologist assists during this session.

The flow of the heterogeneous SIGMA (basically a heterogeneous DIGMA, but without the drop-in component) is as follows. The patient checks in at the Central Check-In Station and signs a confidentiality release. The family member, if attending the visit, must also sign the release. The behaviorist/facilitator collects the patients and brings them to the group room where he/she discusses confidentiality issues, provides an overview of the SIGMA, discusses what to expect during today's session, and addresses housekeeping issues (bathrooms, snacks, etc). The ancillary assistant performs the nursing functions by obtaining patients' vitals and updating health maintenance, and then the provider arrives and begins the SIGMA. During the session, patients may be intermittently pulled out of the group room to have vitals taken, blood drawn, or vaccines given. The provider addresses each individual patient's concerns and develops a treatment plan. The facilitator fosters interaction to ensure that the SMA is beneficial to all participants and may also elaborate on topics discussed (such as tobacco use, exercise). The provider also sometimes needs to examine a patient privately, or to discuss the assessment and plan with the documenter—during which time the behaviorist temporarily takes over the group. Patients and staff are encouraged to volunteer questions and advice. If necessary, patients may leave prior to the end of the session once all medical concerns are addressed.

Scheduled-In Group Medical Appointment (SIGMA) of the Homogeneous subtype:

The SIGMA homogeneous subtype is different from the heterogeneous subtype in that each group is disease specific. We have group clinics specifically designed for patients with diabetes, ischemic heart disease, hypertension, etc. The flow and support staff duties are similar to the heterogeneous subtype. These clinics evolved as a way to both improve patient outcomes as well as efficiently meet VHA performance measures, but without putting all the responsibility on the primary care provider (as is the case during traditional individual patient appointments)—i.e., as the multidisciplinary team, as well as the support of other patients, are most helpful in handling much of this responsibility. We created registries for ischemic heart disease, hypertension, and diabetes—and scheduled these patients into the respective homogeneous SIGMA. We have bundled all applicable disease specific performance measures and systematically addressed them during these SMA sessions.

New Patients' Intake Physical Shared Medical Appointment (Intake PSMA):

This type of SMA, which was specifically designed to efficiently intake new patients awaiting VA Primary Care, was developed by Dr. Noffsinger as a way to intake new patients awaiting VA Primary Care. This type of appointment is similar to a SIGMA (i.e., a no drop-in DIGMA) except that patients receive a full detailed physical examination in private (plus an Orientation to Primary Care and VA benefits). Also, since new patients tend to have many questions, fewer patients (about six—eight) meet during this group session. The flow of the PSMA differs from the SIGMA. Since patients receive full physicals, three to four exam rooms are needed near the PSMA group room. Half of the patients have vitals taken and are roomed in the exam rooms for private physicals. The remaining patients are taken to the PSMA group room and meet with the behaviorist/facilitator.

What makes the PSMA so efficient is that very little discussion takes place privately between the provider and the patient while completing the physical exam. Patients have completed health questionnaires prior to the visit, and the provider briefly reviews these to determine if a more disease or body system focused physical is needed in addition to the general physical exam. Most of the dialogue between physician and patient takes place afterwards in the group room, where all the other participants in the PSMA can benefit and where repetition can be avoided. In this way, each physical can be completed in three to five minutes. As each patient's physical is concluded, he/she is taken to the PSMA group room and another patient is escorted from the group room to be roomed in the exam room for the private physical examination—and to have vitals taken and other nursing duties performed. The role of the behaviorist/facilitator in the PSMA is more comprehensive than in the SIGMA. While the provider is completing the physicals, the facilitator is acquiring each patient's concerns and complaints and writing them on the board in the PSMA room. We suggest using a nurse in the PSMA facilitator role because he/she can sometimes address some of the patient's problems before the provider arrives in the PSMA room after completing the physicals. This practice further increases efficiency during the PSMA clinic. Typically, a clinical pharmacist is present to review the patient's medication list and make formulary substitutions, address polypharmacy issues, educate patients on side effects and pharmaceutical interactions, and instruct patients on refilling prescriptions.

Once all the physicals are concluded (usually, about halfway into the session) and the various patient complaints have been obtained in the group room by the facilitator, the provider joins all the patients that have now regrouped in the PSMA group room. From here on, the flow is very similar to the SIGMA. Each patient is spoken to individually and efficiently in the presence of a group of observers—i.e., while some group interaction is fostered. After all the patients are seen, the provider leaves the room to review the notes that were entered by the documenter, and edits or adds appropriately—or else the provider can review and modify the chart note drafted on each patient in the group room immediately after finishing working with that patient during the group (i.e., while the behaviorist temporarily takes over running the group). Lastly, once the interactive group segment is over, the orientation to primary care and other presentations on VA benefits are provided afterwards to the patients as they are new to the system.

Combat Veteran Physicals Shared Medical Appointment:

This special type of PSMA was specifically established to meet the unique medical needs of combat veterans returning from OIF/OEF while ensuring a "seamless transition" from DoD to VHA care. This appointment shares all the features of the New Patients' Intake PSMA except that these veterans are also screened for problems sometimes associated with combat, such as depression, posttraumatic stress disorder (PTSD), some infectious diseases, and other chronic symptoms. The use of a psychologist as the facilitator in this type of PSMA is recommended because these combat veterans tend to have more psychological and readjustment issues—i.e., as compared to non-combat veterans. The combat veterans seem to benefit most from the support of their peers with similar concerns. We also feel it is important to address both medical problems and psychological problems in the same context. Another goal of this program is to destigmatize mental health issues and to commence treatment plans for PTSD and depression as early as possible. The session includes an overview of veterans' eligibility and benefits. A Veterans Service Officer (VSO) is present to assist with filing benefits claims. A social worker and a Vet Center counselor are also available to handle combat-related, readjustment issues.

What Others Are Saying

To date, our SMA program—especially our Combat Physicals SMA program—has received some very positive press.

Newspaper Coverage:

In a May 9, 2004 article in the local Memphis, Tennessee newspaper, *The Commercial Appeal*, our SMAs were described as follows (9):

Instead of waiting for their doctor in individual exam rooms, the men sat on folding chairs arranged in a circle in a meeting room at the Memphis Veterans Medical Center's South Clinic. They wore street clothes and name tags. All pledged not to discuss anything heard in the group outside the gathering. Their chief health complaints—back and knee pain, lung disease, insomnia, ringing in the ears, stroke, a rapid heart rate—were listed on an erasable board. In one corner, foam cups were stacked next to the pot of freshly brewed coffee. Then Dr. Keith Novak arrived and the appointment began. In an era when patients typically spend more time watching the waiting room television than talking to their doctor, shared medical appointments are attracting interest as a way to boost efficiency, improve care and increase patient satisfaction.

...At the recent VA appointment, Novak, an internal medicine specialist, counseled one patient about heartburn and then asked who wanted additional information. Nearly every hand went up. Everyone raised his hands when Novak asked who had been exposed to potentially toxic smoke while serving in Iraq or Afghanistan. He recommended environmental screening for everyone...Nationally, the demand for VA health services has nearly doubled since 1996. That means

veterans now often face long waits for care...The Memphis VA now offers seven different shared appointments, including the nation's first such appointment for combat veterans. It is planning at least two more, said Novak, acting associate chief of staff for ambulatory care. They include appointments for returning combat veterans, new patients and those with diabetes, depression and heart disease (9).

Another local newspaper article by Daniel Connolly on April 28, 2007 entitled "Combat vets reach out to each other in VA appointments" on pages C1 and C2 in *The Commercial Appeal* features the Memphis VAMC's Combat veterans group and states the following (10):

On a recent Tuesday, Dr. Keith Novak performed physical examinations on former military men in a clinic in Whitehaven, then brought them all to a conference room to discuss their problems, which ranged from erectile dysfunction to depression. It was part of the combat veteran shared medical appointment program, which introduces people returning from Iraq and other recent conflicts to the federal Veterans Affairs healthcare system. Participants sign waivers allowing doctors to discuss their conditions in front of others. Novak said he got the idea from a professional conference and began using it for groups of recent veterans in 2004. "It's better for peer support, for one thing," he said. "And one of the things that the guys miss a lot and one reason why they have trouble adjusting when they come back is that they're not with their comrades (10)."

Now, Novak and colleagues plan to hire four more people to administer an expanded version of the program. They hope it will help veterans get the mental and physical treatment they need and guide them through a sometimes confusing VA system. The planned expansion demonstrates how the VA in Memphis is devoting more resources to deal with a stream of combat veterans returning from the wars in Iraq and Afghanistan (10).

Congressional Legislation:

In July 2004, Congressman Harold E. Ford, Jr., who represented the Ninth District of Tennessee, introduced legislation in the U.S. House of Representatives titled Enhancement of Veterans Mental Health Services Act. This legislation was intended to help combat service members and veterans better cope with posttraumatic stress disorder. The Ford legislation had four components, one of which specifically referred to our OIF/OEF Combat Veterans PSMA in Memphis VAMC. The bill directed the VA to use group visits because of their success in helping veterans. The bill is still in committee as of this writing (11).

Polytrauma SMA for OIF/OEF Combat Veterans with Traumatic Brain Injury

In addition to the types of DIGMAs and PSMAs discussed previously, we launched a Polytrauma SMA for OIF/OEF combat veterans with traumatic brain injury

(TBI). This clinic includes a multidisciplinary team (internal medicine, psychology, social work, physical therapy, occupational therapy, recreational therapy, and speech therapy) to evaluate patients. As OIF/OEF veterans screen positive for TBI in primary care, they are referred to the Polytrauma Clinic Support Team and scheduled into the Polytrauma SMA for further evaluation. We are responsible for completing the 22-question Neurobehavioral Symptom Inventory on these patients and for developing the multidisciplinary treatment plan.

Our first SMA session in this new program went very well. Although we only invited two patients to this first session in order to *test the waters* (one of them gave his left leg and the other gave his right arm and right hip to us in support of OIF—Operation Iraqi Freedom), I think the patients learned from each other and appreciated this experience.

Additional SMAs on the Horizon

Next month I am heading up a SMA for Homeless Veterans. The goal of this SMA is to enroll veterans into the Memphis VAMC Healthcare for Homeless Veterans Program. We will use the clinic to perform intake physicals. As we grow, I plan to expand it to run a heterogeneous DIGMA at the same time as the PSMA so that some patients can come to the group rather than present to ER for non-emergent conditions. I collaborated with Hampton VAMC, whom Dr. Noffsinger has helped to develop the VA's Homeless Veterans' SMA. The Homeless Veteran Social Worker will facilitate the SMA.

We have expanded our Diabetes SMAs to include management of diabetes mellitus, hypertension, and hyperlipidemia and we have renamed them Metabolic Syndrome SMAs. We now have these homogeneous SIGMAs running at all primary care locations, both at the Medical Center and our Community-Based Outpatient Clinics (CBOCs). These SMAs are headed up by Nurse Practitioners with help from endocrinology.

We have found that these SMAs have improved clinical outcomes. For example, we have found an increase in the number of patients with HbA1c<9%, BP<140/90, and LDL<100 performance measures through utilization of these SIGMA clinics. Success rates for these measures range from 70–90% in these SMAs compared to 55–75% with traditional care—i.e., when utilizing these Metabolic Syndrome SMAs compared to each individual primary care provider (PCP) addressing these performance measures during traditional individual office visits held in their own clinic. The PCPs can refer any of their uncontrolled patients into this SMA.

In addition, we have launched an Anticoagulation (Coumadin) SMA. The PharmD sees about eight patients at a time for PT/INR check ups (PT/INR is Prothrombin Time, International Normalized Ratio). This clinic is particularly efficient as we utilize point of care PT/INR testing in the SMA. We also have a "MOVE! SMA" which stands for "Managing Overweight Veterans Everywhere." The MOVE! SMA can be considered a hybrid between the DIGMA and CHHC models, as it is mostly an education and support group (rather than the pure delivery of medical care, as is the case for DIGMAs and PSMAs). Like CHCCs, the MOVE! SMA sessions do have different presenters attend on different weeks to speak—some of whom are providers.

Study 9: Using PSMAs in Dartmouth's Bone Marrow Transplantation Clinic

The following is another specialized application of the PSMA model. In a recent article Dr. Kenneth Meehan et al reported that, in their use of the PSMA model in their bone marrow transplantation unit, they found Transplant PSMAs to be satisfying to patients and provider, as well as to the caregivers accompanying the patients (12).

Positive Early Data for Dartmouth's Transplant PSMA

For the Transplant PSMAs held at Dartmouth, they found that: (1) more than 88% of patients reported that they would attend a future PSMA; (2) 94% reported getting the information about their disease and treatment options that they wanted; (3) each patient rated the medical care they received in the PSMA as "very good" to "excellent"; and (4) all patients felt that they benefited from the presence of other patients sharing similar issues and concerns. They went on to state that "The three care providers (two physicians and a nurse practitioner) and the transplantation nurse coordinator (who acted as the 'behaviorist' in this model) enjoyed the PSMA and recommended that the PSMA be continued on a regular basis as an adjunct to regular office visits. For the medical team, this type of visit broke the routine of an office visit and also provided a unique opportunity to spend a significant amount of time focusing on patient teaching and education" (12).

Increased Productivity and Efficiency, Plus a Program That Is Liked by the Entire Team

The authors point out that this new type of PSMA appointment has increased productivity and efficiency while simultaneously increasing patient, caregiver, physician, and staff satisfaction. They then go on to point out that the physician is able to see dramatically more patients during the same amount of time in the group visit setting. Before the Transplant PSMA was initiated, patients who had received transplants were usually scheduled for 1 hour appointments with a care provider (typically a transplantation physician) for a physical examination and review of lab results—the majority of which time was spent on discussions and Q&A, talk that was quite similar for the various transplant patients. However, in the Transplant PSMA, 10 patients could be seen and provided with the same types of care during just 2 hours time—something that would previously have taken 10 hours through traditional individual physical examination appointments. The authors' state (12) "Our results indicate that this specialized form of office visit for patients after autologous stem cell transplantation provides quality care in a setting that is preferred by medical care providers and patients who have received transplantations, a finding confirmed by others in the nontransplantation setting" (9,13).

The authors continue "In addition, we have discovered a high level of satisfaction and enhanced team-building among the transplantation care providers. This type of appointment is a team-based approach to care, with each member of our bone marrow transplantation team playing an important role in the overall success of the program. This led to not only increased efficiency and team rapport but also a mutual appreciation for the helpful role that each team member plays in the process. The PSMA used existing resources to increase productivity by supplementing and possibly enhancing the routine office visit." The authors go on to point out that their Transplant PSMA helps meet the six goals for patient care recommended by the Society for General Internal Medicine (i.e., safety, effectiveness, patient-centeredness, timeliness, efficiency, and equitability) and report that the Dartmouth Transplant PSMA model provides innovative care and fulfills these goals while improving provider and patient satisfaction (12).

Conclusion

Dr. Meehan's article finishes with the following conclusion: "The stem cell transplantation patient population is ideal for a tertiary-care PSMA. These patients are highly motivated individuals, with issues discussed during the group meeting being pertinent to the majority of autologous transplantation recipients, regardless of diagnosis, age, or sex. The PSMA allows patients to spend a considerable amount of time with their care providers while providing the care providers an opportunity to discuss general health questions pertinent to all transplantation patients in 1 appointment. With the rapid growth of our transplantation program and the outstanding success of the group appointments, our PSMA efforts are expanding into the pretransplantation (autologous) and posttransplantation allogeneic stem cell patient populations. Our ongoing goal is to provide the highest quality of care while improving access to care providers and better addressing patients' psychosocial, emotional, and education needs. This model could offer potential benefits to other specialized and unique patient populations" (12).

Follow-Up and Update

Upon reviewing and approving the foregoing write-up, Dr. Meehan added the following: "At the current time, we are continuing with our group visit program, although it is temporarily on hold due to minor personnel issues (medical leave of absences, etc.). Since these appointments have been placed on hold, a number of my patients have asked whether they could attend another group meeting and when the next meeting is planned. I believe this only emphasizes the quotes within the article—that is, both the transplant physicians and their patients really look forward to the Transplant PSMA group sessions. Of course, I always ask my patients why they would like to attend another group appointment. To my surprise, their answers differ. For some patients, it is the group rapport and camaraderie that provides the patient with a sense of 'belonging' and not being isolated in the world. These patients report that, through the group, they can hear and see other patients who have been through what they are now going through.

Another one of my patients would like to attend so he can teach. He describes a great sense of self-worth by sharing his experiences with other patients. He also feels that this 'sharing' helps him to emotionally deal with the fact that he is a cancer survivor. Finally, another patient stated she prefers to sit and learn at the group meeting, rather than spending a lot of time answering medical questions (such as naming her medications, addressing her performance status)—i.e., the types of questions that we typically ask patients to answer at traditional office visits. This patient felt she got more out of sitting and listening to others with similar issues at the group appointment then she did out of discussing her own problems with medical staff. What I find especially interesting is the fact that the vast majority of patients do *not* find it a problem that patients with different diseases are included within the group sessions. All of the patients seem to realize that they are dealing with (sometimes struggling with) similar issues that are not limited to disease, gender, age, etc."

Outcome Studies from Ongoing DIGMA and PSMA Programs

In this section, we discuss various outcomes studies from ongoing DIGMA and PSMA programs at some of our nation's larger and mid-sized integrated healthcare delivery systems—studies that demonstrate the multiple quality, access, productivity, psychosocial, service, and patient and provider satisfaction benefits that properly run DIGMA and PSMA programs can offer.

Study 10: Access and Satisfaction Results from Cleveland Clinic's DIGMA and PSMA Program

The following contribution came from Dr. Richard Maxwell, a pediatrician at the Cleveland Clinic Wooster Family Health Center, who has been the shared medical appointment champion for Cleveland Clinic since its inception several years ago. In this section, he writes about the DIGMA and PSMA program at Cleveland Clinic, its history and current status, and the access and patient satisfaction benefits that they are experiencing. This section of the chapter also addresses the background and current status of Cleveland Clinic's SMA program, why they selected the DIGMA and PSMA models, how they bill for these visits, and how their program is evolving. He also discusses lessons learned, hurdles that needed to be overcome, how their program is currently evolving, and specific recommendations to other medical groups interested in launching a SMA program of their own.

Background on Cleveland Clinic's SMA Program

In June 2002, Dr. David Bronson, Chairman of Regional Medical Practice, invited Dr. Ed Noffsinger to the Cleveland Clinic for a presentation to 50 key physicians and administrators. The decision was made to develop a shared medical appointment (SMA) program

throughout the various regional medical centers at Cleveland Clinic, and to bring Dr. Noffsinger out for 3 days on a monthly basis for a year (and on an *as needed* basis thereafter) to assist in the design, development, and implementation process. Dr. Bronson then appointed Dr. Richard Maxwell as physician coordinator and Bill Atkinson as project administrator—i.e., to act as physician champion and project coordinator, respectively, for the SMA Program.

Why We Selected the DIGMA and PSMA Models

We made the decision to use Dr. Noffsinger's two shared medical appointment models—his Drop-In Group Medical Appointment (DIGMA) model for return visits and his Physicals Shared Medical Appointment (Physicals SMA or PSMA) model for physical examinations. We had two specific reasons for selecting the DIGMA and PSMA models: (1) because, from start to finish, these are the two SMA models that are run just like a series of individual office visits with observers (and are therefore the two SMA models widely used in fee-for-service systems); and (2) because, in addition to providing the many quality and educational benefits that SMAs are known for, the DIGMA and PSMA models have also been repeatedly shown to substantially improve both physician productivity and access.

Dr. Bronson and I stated the reasons underlying this decision to move forward with a DIGMA and PSMA program in our article in the May 2004 issue of the Cleveland Clinic Journal of Medicine. "Shared medical visits are a new concept in patient care. Doctors perform a series of one-on-one patient encounters in a group setting during a 90-minute visit and manage and advise each patient in front of the others. Patients benefit from improved access to their physician and significantly increased education, while providers can boost their access and productivity without increasing hours. Such group visits are voluntary and for established patients only (14)."

Once the Decision Was made, the Next Steps Needed to Be Taken

The next step was to involve the Cleveland Clinic Legal Department for preparation of a HIPPA compliant confidentiality statement, a confidentiality release that all SMA attendees would need to sign at the beginning of every DIGMA and PSMA session. During these initial planning stages, we also involved a Cleveland Clinic coding and reimbursement specialist, the scheduling department, and our marketing department to assist in the development of all of the promotional materials for the SMA program. Two sites in CCF (Cleveland Clinic Foundation) Regional Medical Practice were chosen, and pilot programs were prepared at each using both the physicals (PSMA) model and follow-up (DIGMA) model. Providers and behaviorists were trained, rooms were prepared, patient service representatives were oriented to the model, and the marketing plan was developed.

Due to Success of Initial Groups, Many Other SMAs Have Been Launched

It was during a 2-week period in September/October 2002 that the first physicals shared medical appointment, the first heterogeneous DIGMA, and the first diabetes DIGMA went live. These initial groups performed smoothly, and the patients were vocal in their appreciation of this new model of care delivery. Subsequently, Dr. Maxwell and Bill Atkinson did presentations to departments throughout Cleveland Clinic to inform and attract new providers to the model. By January 2006, over 10,000 patients had been seen in 1300 different DIGMA and PSMA sessions. At that time, 35 physicians had been trained and had actually launched DIGMAs and PSMAs in their practices—of which 28 physicians continue to run them on a regular basis. On average, we run approximately 40 SMAs per month, and have over 300 patients in attendance.

Inadequate Census Has Caused Some SMAs to Fail

Those providers lost to the model were largely a result of their inability to consistently achieve desired census levels in their groups. At this time, eleven physicians conduct physical shared medical appointments on a weekly or biweekly basis. The remainder are conducting follow-up shared medical appointments (homogeneous DIGMAs) for diabetes, gastric bypass, gynecology follow-ups, asthma, panic disorder, depression, metabolic syndrome, medical weight loss, Parkinson's disease, women's health issues, arthritis, osteoporosis, headache, elevated PSA (prostate-specific antigen), OB visits, and hypertension. We have had challenges getting physician buy-in to the heterogeneous DIGMA model, as it is less intuitively obvious than the disease- or condition-specific homogeneous model. As the project matures, wide application throughout numerous disease states in our various medical and surgical departments is being realized (with inflammatory bowel disease, low back pain, uterine fibroids, insomnia, prostate cancer, open heart surgery, and congestive heart failure currently being considered).

As Planned, Access Was Dramatically Improved

It is important to note that Cleveland Clinic began the shared medical appointment project in order to improve access to our busiest services (especially for new patients)—and to decrease wait times for both follow-up visits and physical examinations. We also wanted to leverage our resources to boost physician productivity. After the first year of the SMA project, the data already showed that access to third available individual appointments had improved by 40 days on average for the various physicians that had initiated a shared medical appointment for their practices (as shown in Fig. 9.10), from an average of 73 days to 33 days for individual office visits, and to only 10 days on average for the DIGMAs and PSMAs themselves! Over the subsequent 4 years, this data regarding improved access to the practices of SMA physicians has consistently remained just as positive.

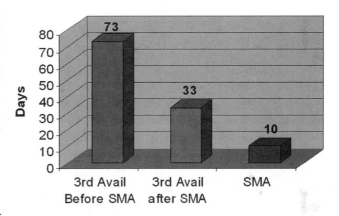

Fig. 9.10 Impact of the SMA program on access to individual and group appointments at Cleveland Clinic

Clearly, patients can get in to see their physician much sooner by agreeing to attend a SMA rather than waiting for an individual appointment. What is less obvious is that, by running a DIGMA or PSMA for their practice, the provider's individual appointments also steadily become more available to their patients. It is worth noting just how dramatically the DIGMA and PSMA models were able to improve access to some of our most backlogged physician's practices. For example, one of our physicians had a 5-month backlog for physical examinations in his practice, and this was despite providing 14 individual physical examinations per week. Within 3 months of starting his Physicals SMA, he had reduced his third available individual physical examination appointment from 150 to 66 days—plus, patients could get a PSMA physical exam appointment within a week.

For another physician, the third available appointment quickly went from 105 to 30 days out—plus, patients could be seen in the group within 1 ½ weeks. Although this physician had an eight-week backlog upon beginning the SMA in October, this backlog was gone by Christmas.

Patient Satisfaction Is Also High

In addition to remarkably improved access, the SMA program also provided yet another big plus—we quickly found that patients and providers alike really liked their SMA experience.

Most Patients Attending a SMA Choose to Return for their Next Visit:

For example, as shown in Fig. 9.11, we found early on that among those patients attending a SMA, 85% had their next follow-up visit back in a future DIGMA session rather than in an individual office visit. This indicated a very high level of patient satisfaction with the SMA program. We found this high rate of return into future DIGMAs to be surprising because this was often the first time that these patients ever attended a shared medical appointment, a paradigm of care delivery that differs dramatically from the traditional individual office visits that patients had come to expect.

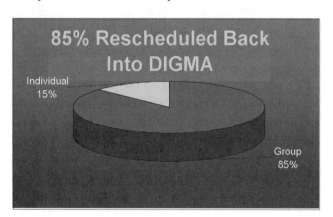

Fig. 9.11 The percentage of patients attending a DIGMA who reschedule their next visit back into a future DIGMA session at Cleveland Clinic

Substantially More SMA than Individual Visits Are Rated as "excellent:"

For the first 2 years of the SMA project, Cleveland Clinic utilized the American Medical Group Association's patient satisfaction survey. Although normed patient satisfaction surveys like AMGAs have the advantage of being excellent research tools, the items contained in the survey are typically much more appropriate to traditional

office visits than to SMAs. However, the AMGA's patient satisfaction tool did contain one important item that applied equally well to individual and group visits—and that was "How would you rate today's visit overall?" Because our focus at Cleveland Clinic is upon excellence, what interested us was the percentage of patients that would rate their care experience as "excellent"—i.e., for SMAs as well as traditional individual office visits.

In order to make this determination, the AMGA patient satisfaction survey was used for all Cleveland Clinic providers in the region in order to determine the percentage of patients that would rate their overall care experience as "excellent." Then we specifically looked at those providers running DIGMAs and/or PSMAs in their practices, and evaluated the percentage of patients that rated their care experience as "excellent"—i.e., for those patients seen individually as well as for those patients seen in SMAs by the same providers, and then comparing these two numbers. Let us now look at the level of patient satisfaction (i.e., as evaluated by using AMGA's questionnaire) with individual office visits vs. SMA visits for those providers who offered both types of appointments.

What we found was that, for physicians conducting shared medical appointments and for those patients that were seen individually through traditional office visits, patients rated their overall care experience as "excellent" 59.12% of the time—which, indeed, was a very respectable number. However, for those patients seen in SMAs by these same providers, 74.67% rated their overall care experience as "excellent"—representing a 15.55 percentile improvement in the percentage of "excellent" ratings for SMAs than for individual office visits (i.e., which actually represents a 26.30% increase over the baseline rate of 59.12% for traditional individual visits) (Fig. 9.12). In other words, the percentage of patients reporting their overall level of satisfaction with the visit as "excellent"

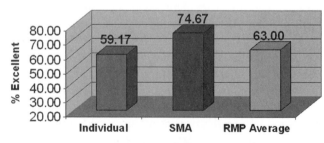

Fig. 9.12 The percentage of patients rating their overall satisfaction with the visit as "excellent" was much higher for SMAs (74.67%) than for either individual office visits with the same providers (59.17%) or for Cleveland Clinic Regional Medical Practice providers on average

went from 59.12% for patients seen individually to 74.67% for patients seen in a SMA by the same provider—a differential quite remarkable in its magnitude. Interestingly, by receiving an "excellent" rating from SMA patients 74.67% of the time (i.e., regarding their overall care experience), these providers were placed in the top 5% of providers around the country using this survey—i.e., but only for those patients seen in their SMAs (and not for patients seen individually).

Recent Results Using Our Own Patient Satisfaction Survey:

Since that time, we have used un-normed patient satisfaction surveys that we specifically designed for our SMA program. Throughout the Cleveland Clinic System, these patient satisfaction survey results have been remarkably consistent. Patients virtually always rate their experience with shared medical appointments as being either "very good" or "excellent." For all SMA providers (and for all of the various items in the questionnaire), the average score consistently ranges between 4.2 and 4.9 on a 5-point Likert scale. These findings are very consistent with the average patient satisfaction scores that Dr. Noffsinger has reported for DIGMAs and PSMAs that he has been involved with, which typically range between 4.4 and 4.7 on a 5-point Likert scale.

This patient satisfaction survey has specifically demonstrated excellent satisfaction with privacy and confidentiality, with patients having their medical needs and questions addressed, and satisfaction with the providers and support staff involved with the DIGMAs and PSMAs.

Providers Also Enjoy the SMA Setting

In the Cleveland Clinic Journal of Medicine article that I co-authored with Dr. David Bronson, we made note of the high level of provider satisfaction with our DIGMA and PSMA program as follows: "Physicians who run groups have typically reported that they are a great 'break' in their day: It is a very different, effective, and enjoyable form of patient care" (14). Overall, we have found that provider satisfaction is quite high with our DIGMA and PSMA program.

The Next Step Will Be to Demonstrate Improvements in Clinical Outcomes

The next step in the Cleveland Clinic Shared Medical Appointment Project is to produce genuine clinical outcomes improvement data. Patient and providers are

consistent in their opinion that these models are superior not only for annual physical examinations but also for follow-ups on chronic medical conditions. The lack of clearly identifiable markers for many medical conditions could make objective outcomes data difficult to produce; however, in the meantime, those involved with the SMA project are subjectively convinced that this is a superior model of care delivery. However, HbA1c is certainly a well-accepted marker for diabetes, and this type of outcomes data can certainly be obtained. Actually, the literature already contains numerous examples of significant improvement in hemoglobin A1c for diabetics seen in the group settings vs. traditional individual office visits—and this experience is also being echoed at the Cleveland Clinic.

Trento, Passera, et al. report on a 4-year randomized controlled study involving 112 patients with type 2 diabetes (not treated with insulin), and compared outcomes for those patients treated in shared medical appointments vs. those receiving usual care. Their findings revealed a weight decrease of 2.6 kg vs. only 0.9 kg—and a change in HbA1c level (which was 7.4% at baseline) that decreased to 7.0% vs. an increase to 8.6%—for the shared medical visit cohort vs. the control group (i.e., usual care through individual office visits) (15). Another study was a 24-month trial that randomly assigned 707 patients with type two diabetes (who were taking either insulin or oral medications) to either shared visits or usual care. The authors found that the shared visit cohort had fewer emergency room visits and disability days, plus better general health status than the control group; however, there was no difference in glucose control between these two groups as measured by HbA1c (16).

Start by Using the DIGMA and PSMA Models as Recommended

One word of caution: Be sure to design, support, and run DIGMAs and PSMAs exactly as Dr. Noffsinger recommends—as it seems that almost every time we have gone "off model," we ended up creating problems for ourselves. Therefore, be sure to develop professional appearing promotional materials; use appropriate group and exam rooms; staff your DIGMAs and PSMAs appropriately with behaviorists, nursing personnel, and documenters (although we have few documenters); assign a dedicated scheduler to each SMA that you launch; have both a champion and a program coordinator for your SMA program (at least in larger systems); and pay close attention to census at all times, ensuring that all group sessions are consistently filled to targeted levels.

The Cleveland Clinic introduced the shared appointment models with careful attention to the principles set down by Dr. Noffsinger. We are convinced that, in larger systems like our own, having both a physician champion and a project administrator are essential—i.e., both in initiating, and then in monitoring the progress of, a wide variety of DIGMA and PSMA groups. Introduction of a SMA into a practice can be used as a quality improvement tool; however, it also exposes the constraints in that system. Obviously booking appointments is a major constraint in ours. Dr. Noffsinger recommends having a dedicated scheduler attached to each SMA, and with enough hours available to the program each week to ensure adequate census for all group sessions. Cleveland Clinic did not utilized centralized scheduling for its SMA program, instead intensively training and orienting each department's patient service representatives to the task. Over the life of the project, our single greatest challenge has been maintaining consistent census in all group sessions—which might potentially be validating the need for a centralized dedicated scheduler. In addition, by having a busy physician champion with limited time available to dedicate to the SMA program, the speed with which SMAs can be moved forward throughout our large system has probably been affected—at least once the program achieved a certain size. Another challenge lies in finding a suitable replacement for our capable program coordinator upon his leaving the system.

Billing

Third party recognition of these models is in its infancy. After we had significant experience with the DIGMA and PSMA models and had produced videos to illustrate their use, we obtained a face-to-face interview with the medical directors of our regional Medicare (CMS) intermediary. After viewing the video and reviewing the data listed above, they enthusiastically approved of the Shared Medical Appointments and validated the use of individual Evaluation and Management codes. DIGMAs and PSMAs are unique among all group visit models because they alone are run, from start to finish, just like a series of individual office visits with observers. With these two models, there is no separate educational presentation as all patient education comes in the context of the physician working with each patient individually. Therefore, DIGMA and PSMA visits (although this very well might not be applicable to other types of group visits—i.e., because they are not run throughout as a series of one doctor-one patient encounters with observers) are billed just like individual appointments and are coded according to level of care delivered; however, the appropriate level of care must be both provided and documented. It is important to note that we do not bill either for counseling time or for the behaviorist's time (which are benefits to third party payors)—instead treating time spent by the behaviorist as an overhead expense to the program. Hopefully, as these models become widespread and their superior clinical efficacy recognized, CMS and other third party payors nationwide will welcome and promote these models.

Study 11: Group Medical Visits when Access Is Not an Issue

The following contribution, which regards their diabetes program and is largely based on the CHCC model, was made by Louis A. Kazal, Jr., M.D., Associate Professor and Chief Clinical Officer, Department of Community and Family Medicine, Dartmouth Medical School, Hanover, New Hampshire. Dr. Kazal is also Chief, Section of Family Medicine, Dartmouth–Hitchcock Medical Center, Lebanon, New Hampshire. He was assisted in this project and write-up by Gillian C. Jackson, Quality Improvement Coordinator, Dartmouth–Hitchcock Community Health Center, Lebanon, New Hampshire. I believe that the reader will find this material of interest because I am often asked how SMAs will work when access is not a problem. Furthermore, these results are important because they show that group medical visits—when applied to patients with diabetes in a setting where access was not a problem—not only increased the frequency of obtaining recommended diabetes tests and preventive medicine measures, but also resulted in very high levels of patient satisfaction.

It shows that when asked "If you were offered the choice of a group or individual appointment for the same reason you were seen today, which type of appointment would you prefer?"— patients strongly preferred a group visit to a traditional office visit. It also reveals that when asked "Please rate how well you like the experience of sharing with and learning from others in the group"— patients very much appreciated the opportunity to interact, share, and help one another. The results of this work at Dartmouth provide a compelling argument for integrating shared medical appointments into both chronic disease management programs and outpatient clinical practice settings—i.e., regardless of whether or not access happens to be a problem.

Background and Rationale

At the Dartmouth–Hitchcock Community Health Center, access to care for patients with diabetes was not a problem. Additionally, patients were not reporting that they did not have enough time with their physician, so why try group medical visits? At the encouragement of the support staff, one of the physicians decided to make such a model available by choice to his patients. The physician was attracted to the possibility of batching care and resources around a chronic illness and taking advantage of the potential benefits of group dynamics in helping people manage their disease. If nothing else, it would allow for more face-to-face time with his patients.

The first CHCC-type group medical visit was in 2005. What the patients have taught us during the intervening year and a half has been quite surprising. At the end of the first visit, the majority of the group wanted to meet again in 3 months, instead of their usual individual physician visit, and over time a core group of patients routinely attended most of the group medical visits along with a mix of new patients. They also decided to select a topic for the next group medical visit, which became a routine practice. Dates were set on a rotation of every 3 months on the same day of the week at the same time. Themes have been the pathophysiology of diabetes (patients' family physician), pharmacological management of diabetes (pharmacologist), nutritional aspects of diabetes (dietician), ophthalmologic manifestations of diabetes (optometrist), and prevention and complications of foot problems (podiatrist).

Design of the Program

The anatomy of the group medical visit program was as follows: Eight weeks prior to the visit, invitations were sent to the clinician's patients with type 2 diabetes. Patients were asked to call and confirm their attendance. Four weeks prior to the visit, the support team huddled to review room reservation, multimedia needs, supplies, patient needs, and the patient flow process. The clinician contributed input, but the majority of the pre-work and planning was completed by the support team. Once patients confirmed their attendance, a licensed practical nurse reviewed their medical records and noted the needs for laboratory tests and any preventive care measures. Patients were scheduled in advance for tests so results would be available at the time of the visit (although HbA1c levels were obtained real time).

On the day of the group medical visit, patients were registered 30 minutes before the planned start of the visit, a licensed nursing assistant obtained vital signs, and a licensed practical nurse gave any immunizations that were needed. At the start of the visit the clinician welcomed the patients, and the guest speaker typically presented for about 40 minutes and answered questions for another 20 minutes. In the remaining 30 minutes, the physician spent time putting the information in context for the patients, answered questions, and helped facilitate the group discussion. Prior to ending the visit, an exit survey was completed and afterward a group visit team huddle was done—i.e., for a debriefing and a "plan-do-study-act" (PDSA) cycle.

Overall, the Results of This Pilot Have Been Very Positive

We have found our preliminary results regarding our diabetes shared medical appointment program to be very positive and encouraging. Thus far, there have been five group medical visits with an average of nine patients (some accompanied by their spouses) per visit.

Patients Attending Our Diabetes SMA Decreased Their Frequency of Routine Diabetes Visits:

Those patients commonly attending the group medical visits have decreased the frequency of their routine diabetes visits. Although this program is still quite new and the results are of a preliminary nature, the early findings have been quite dramatic.

The Recommended Frequency of Diabetes Tests and Preventive Care Measures Were Better Achieved:

There was an increase in achieving the recommended frequency of diabetes tests and preventive care measures, including: HbA1C testing every 6 months; LDL testing and microalbumin every year; foot and eye exams every year; flu vaccine each year; and Pneumovax (Fig. 9.13). This improvement was most likely attributable to two factors: First, compliance for testing for each of the indicators of good diabetes care was assessed prior to the group medical visit, and second, group medical visits provided a captive audience with the opportunity to obtain the necessary tests or give the indicated vaccines. It is worth noting that, whereas some of the success may have been contaminated by other initiatives to improve diabetes care in general at the clinic, most of this group's care was in the group visit setting.

Diabetes Testing Outcomes-Group Visit Care

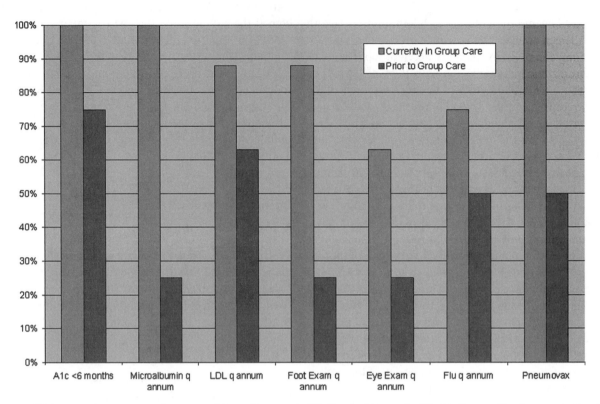

Fig. 9.13 Diabetes testing outcomes for group visits at Dartmouth–Hitchcock Community Health Center. The frequency of patients obtaining recommended tests and preventative care increased with the group visits

Patient Satisfaction with the Diabetes SMA Program Is High:

Patient satisfaction has remained high throughout the entire year and one-half of this diabetes group medical visit program. At the conclusion of each group medical visit, patients were asked to complete a satisfaction survey. When they were offered the choice of a group medical visit or individual appointment for their diabetes care, 71% preferred a group medical visit (Fig. 9.14). 96% rated their experience as "very good" or "excellent" (Fig. 9.15). There was not a statistically significant difference in A1C levels or LDL measurements.

Conclusion

In conclusion, Dartmouth–Hitchcock Community Health Clinic found that group medical visits for patients with diabetes both increased the frequency of obtaining recommended diabetes tests and preventive medicine measures (Fig. 9.13) and resulted in very high patient satisfaction (Figs. 9.14 and 9.15). These results provide a compelling argument for integrating group medical visits into both chronic illness treatment programs and outpatient clinical practice settings—i.e., regardless of whether or not access is a problem.

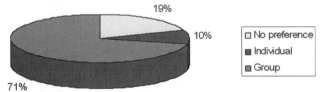

Fig. 9.14 Patients at Dartmouth–Hitchcock Community Health Center were asked, if they were offered the choice of a group or individual appointment for the same reason they were seen today, which type of appointment would they prefer?

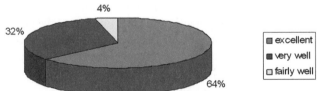

Fig. 9.15 Patients at Dartmouth–Hitchcock Community Health Center were asked to rate how well they liked the experience of sharing with and learning from others in the group. (1 = not at all to 5 = excellent)

Study 12: PSMAs for Women Seeking Consultation for Breast Reduction Surgery—The BRITE Visit

The following contribution was submitted by Carolyn L. Kerrigan, MD, Professor of Surgery, Dartmouth College. Dr. Kerrigan has been championing SMAs at Dartmouth–Hitchcock since 2003. She discusses her use of the PSMA model for surgical intake visits for women seeking consultation for breast reduction surgery, which she terms the "BRITE" visit. By so dramatically increasing the efficiency and quality of the intake process, she was able to retool her master schedule to dedicate more time to surgery during her workweek. Because of the remarkable success that she was able to achieve for breast reduction surgery intakes through application of the PSMA model, Dr. Kerrigan has expanded this work to carpal tunnel surgical intake visits as well. In fact, she has been so satisfied with her SMA that she once told me: "This has been so successful that I cannot compete with myself in the quality of care that I am able to offer my patients. Therefore, I am going to shift to doing group visit intakes almost entirely for these patient populations."

How I Got Started

I participated in a teleconference series on patient access to care put on by the Institute for Healthcare Improvement in January 2002. Although many strategies were discussed to help address issues of access, the one that most strongly caught my interest was that of Shared Medical Appointments (SMAs). I followed up by reviewing the literature on SMAs and, in particular, read several articles by Dr. Ed Noffsinger published in *Group Practice Journal*. Despite traditional thinking that SMAs are not intended for initial consultations, I felt that there was significant potential for this model of care in a subset of my own patients. My next step was to assemble a team that would help explore and design this care model for women seeking consultation regarding surgical correction of symptomatic breast hypertrophy.

The Team

Our team included two surgeons, our practice manager, two nurses, and an administrative supervisor. Over time we have added a scheduling secretary to our group. Our first task was to map out in detail the components of a typical patient visit and to perform a cycle time analysis.

This allowed us to visualize each professional's role and time allocation to the care of the patient. We did some brainstorming about the flow of the visit, each professional's role, and dreamed about how we could improve the quality of care for this group of women. We also analyzed past demand for consultations so as to plan for an appropriate frequency of SMAs and an optimal census for each visit.

Assessment of Quality of the Old Model

In reflecting on the quality of care delivered in a traditional one-on-one visit, I often felt somewhat rushed and, by the end of the visit, I was not always convinced that the patient had a full understanding of the merits and perils of surgery. In a typical clinic I had 4–6 new consultations of this sort and, by the end of the day, would be losing my enthusiasm and feeling like somewhat of a broken record. I'm sure that on occasion I left out useful information and, even if I did not, I'm sure that many patients retained only a fraction of what I was trying to convey to them—i.e., despite my best efforts and use of visual aids. A final reflection that I made was that I frequently felt that I was providing certain components of care that other professionals in the team could do just as well, or even better.

Redesign of the New Model

All these reflections were included in our redesign—which has evolved over the 4 years since we have been holding BRITE (*Breast Reduction Informative Team Encounter*) sessions. Essentially this redesign followed that of the Physicals Shared Medical Appointment model as designed by Dr. Noffsinger, but for a very homogenous group of patients. The visit begins with registration, welcome, and orientation. Four patients are then shown to exam rooms while others remain in the group area until it is their turn for the exam. During this time, those in the group room are watching an educational video on breast reduction surgery, plus receiving information about perioperative details from our nurse facilitator. I made this 12-minute video, and in it I explain the three major procedures for breast reduction surgery (the liposuction, the "lollipop," and the "anchor" surgeries) plus show actual pre- and post-op photos of women who have had these surgeries. The video also includes a frank discussion of potential surgical complications, including graphic photographs of wound healing problems and nipple areolar complex loss.

In the meantime, I am going from exam room to exam room providing private individual breast examinations upon all group attendees in turn; however, when doing so, I try to minimize the amount of discussion that occurs in this inefficient individual exam room setting—deferring such discussions instead to the interactive group segment of the visit which follows. After all the exams are completed, I join the patients in the group room for discussion of questions and support for decision-making with regards to the optimal surgical technique for each patient.

The "Mock" and "Actual" Initial Session

Our first BRITE session, which was held in March 2003, was actually a *mock* session with practice managers and nurses from elsewhere in the hospital serving as patients. This helped us to smooth out several bugs in the process—plus it better prepared us for our first live BRITE session in April 2003. We have continued to have monthly sessions and have increased this to one session every 2–3 weeks, depending on demand.

Multiple Iterations

Two to three days before a BRITE session, the team has a briefing session. Then, immediately after the session, we debrief to review what went well and what still needs improvement.

We Have Continuously Improved the BRITE Program:

Each visit has been slightly better than the previous one, and we continue to do mini-improvement cycles. In the early sessions, the majority of the group session with the surgeon was spent on education using a PowerPoint presentation. However, at the end of such sessions, even though patients were well informed, they had not yet had a chance to do individual decision-making with the surgeon. In addition, the nurses were spending most of their time gathering and organizing health surveys—and entering patient responses into an electronic medical record template. Our administrative support person found herself responding to more and more medical questions—questions which she was not adequately trained to respond to. We therefore revisited roles and made several changes, including conversion of a live PowerPoint presentation to a 12-minute video recording of the same information.

The Current Flow of a BRITE Visit:

In our current iteration, during the first hour (while I am providing the private breast examinations on patients individually in the various exam rooms), the unroomed patients' activities include watching the video and

spending time with our nurses to learn about postoperative care and planning (as well as with a secretary who is responsible for getting insurance pre-authorization). During the second half of the visit, women spend up to a full hour in the group room together with me as their surgeon. During this hour, while I work individually with each woman in turn, questions are addressed, patients learn from both my comments and each other, and each woman makes a decision with regards to her preferred choice of technique. This provides an excellent forum for a thorough discussion and disclosure of the risks and benefits of breast reduction surgery.

An Unexpected, but Much Appreciated, Benefit:

One unexpected side-benefit of our BRITE PSMA format came for those women whose primary reason for seeking surgery was cosmetic as opposed to relief of physical symptoms of shoulder and neck pain. Previously, I was spending considerable time each week repetitively explaining that their insurance would not pay for the procedure they desired—something which few, if any, wanted to hear. In the group setting, these women are surrounded by others truly needing breast reduction surgery for medical reasons, and those seeking a cosmetic solution can now immediately see the differences from their own situation. As a result, they will often self-select out of having the surgery or understand the need for out of pocket expenses—which greatly reduces the need for my involvement in telling them "no" because their insurance will not pay for the procedure they want, a task that I personally disliked.

After 45 BRITE Sessions, I Am Convinced that the Quality of Care Is Superior

In reflecting on this model of care now that I have lead more than 45 SMAs for this patient population, I am absolutely convinced that I can provide superior quality care in this model compared to traditional one-on-one visits. In fact, I no longer offer the traditional one-on-one visit. For women who decline participation in the SMA, they are offered a one-on-one visit with one of our other providers.

Patient Satisfaction

Over the last 4 years, we have collected anecdotal stories as well as prospective survey data from our patients. An early e-mail from a patient stated very eloquently the benefits of this model of care: "Hello. Thank you very much for making my recent visit with you and the staff so welcoming, informative, and worthwhile. I felt very comfortable in the group setting and think it is an excellent format for providing information and attention to women who have individual needs but shared concerns. Thank you again."

How One Initially Reluctant Patient Ultimately Benefited:

Another woman came to me for a second opinion and at first declined to participate in my BRITE PSMA. After seeing me one-on-one, she requested an additional appointment as she remained uncertain about proceeding with surgery. At this next visit, it was clear that she had a high level of anxiety and that the information I was giving her was still not adequate. As it happened, I was holding a BRITE visit on that very day, so I persuaded her to participate in the PSMA as I thought it might be helpful to her. She was hesitant but did agree to join us—and by the end of the visit, she was a convert. She expressed the wish that she had attended the SMA initially, as it addressed her concerns. Just knowing that other women were going through the same issues made it much more comfortable for her.

Patient Satisfaction Data:

But for the scientist, what is the evidence that this care is as good as or better than traditional care? A patient satisfaction survey (which was mailed to patients' homes after their surgical intake visit) was custom designed for

this PSMA. This survey could be used by patients to evaluate their breast reduction surgery intake visit—regardless of whether that visit was in my SMA or in an individual visit. The patient satisfaction data shown in Fig. 9.16 was collected on an early cohort of consecutive patients during the first 3 months of our BRITE visits.

Discussion of Results

The results depicted in Fig. 9.16 are based on responses from 27 patients involved in the BRITE SMA and 30 patients involved in one-on-one visits. Those patients attending the SMA reported equivalent or higher satisfaction than those attending individual visits on almost all dimensions. The question that was rated with slightly lower satisfaction in SMAs compared to individual visits was in response to satisfaction with *time* spent with your doctor. This finding was surprising to Dr. Noffsinger, as his experience with most prior SMAs has been increased satisfaction with time spent with provider; therefore, we will continue to monitor this trend. Other than this, the most striking findings seen in patient satisfaction were timeliness of getting an appointment, having all questions discussed, comfort with their decision as to whether or not to have the surgery, and receiving the amount of information that they wanted. As can be seen in Fig. 9.16, SMA attendees consistently responded with higher satisfaction than one-on-one attendees on these four important dimensions.

My greatest surprise with regard to this data was that patients felt that they got all of their questions answered and discussed in the SMA—which outscored individual intakes on this dimension by a considerable margin. This

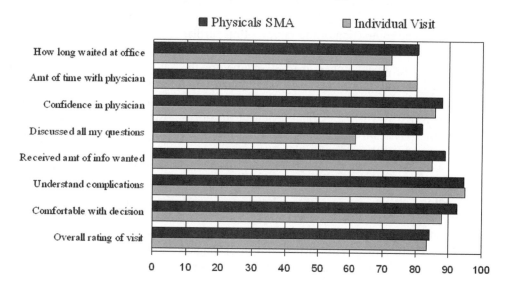

Fig. 9.16 Average level of patient satisfaction for breast reduction surgery intake visit (SMA vs. individual intake) at Dartmouth–Hitchcock

was a surprise to me because I was spending 45–60 minutes with patients seen individually, during which there was a great deal of question and answer time. Granted, I was sometimes bored answering the same questions repetitively for one patient after another all week long, but I was still spending 45–60 minutes with each patient—i.e., as opposed to seeing 8–12 (average 9) patients in 2 hours, as was the case for my BRITE SMA. The *questions answered* piece above really speaks to the strength of the SMA as I think women realized that they were fortunate to receive answers to important medical questions of interest to them which they did not know to ask themselves (and therefore did not know the answer to)—but received these answers because other patients did ask these questions.

Documentation Support

One of the biggest challenges to the physician in this model of care is the efficient and timely documentation of the encounter. Different groups have developed alternate creative solutions for this challenge. In our situation, we are fortunate to have a relatively robust electronic medical record. In addition, for several years, we have been using standardized templates to document consultations for breast hypertrophy. We have also had patients complete a paper-based health survey to collect standardized information as part of a research study. We found that this systematic collection of data was useful for medical decision-making, and have now fully incorporated this into a standard visit. The physicians typically transcribed the information from the paper forms to the electronic record, but we have now gradually shifted most of this responsibility to the support staff attached to the SMA.

As the volume of SMAs has grown in our section, we have hired and trained a medical assistant to perform this role. We have designed, and are currently testing, a prototype for online completion of the survey—thus further streamlining the intake and documentation process. Much of the documentation is carried out before the visit, and additional data points—such as physical exam measures and final medical decision-making—are added during the SMA by a *scribe*. A final review of the document by the physician at the completion of the SMA ensures accuracy of the content.

Maintaining Census

Our target census for a BRITE visit is nine patients. Therefore, 11–14 patients are invited and prescheduled as we typically have several no-shows. This leverages my time by 340% or more over individual breast reduction surgical intakes, which I used to schedule for 45 minutes each (which also led to a great deal of physician downtime when there was a no-show). On the occasions when our census has been low (five—six patients), we have noted that the group dynamics never work as well as when we have a full census. The whole team works hard to ensure a process that will support a full census at each and every visit so as to optimize the experience for the participants—as well as to optimize efficiency for the providers and support staff.

Other Applications of SMAs in Our Practice

As we gained experience with our first SMA model, we began to experiment with other patient populations—and to engage other providers in trying this new model of care delivery. I run a twice-monthly SHAKE clinic (Shared Hand Assessment Klinic Encounter) which is designed to address common hand problems. Most attendees at this SMA have carpal tunnel, with others having diagnoses such as cubital tunnel, trigger finger, or osteoarthritis. It is not uncommon that several diagnoses are present in one patient. A colleague has introduced NOGGIN into his practice, a SMA attended by babies with plagiocephaly (misshapen heads) and their families. We have two providers offering SMAs for patients who are post massive weight loss and seeking consultation for body contouring (PRIDE), and one provider offering SMAs for women seeking consultation for breast reconstruction. Our two newest models, which are still in the planning stages, are designed around individuals seeking consultation for facial rejuvenation and those with "lumps and bumps".

The Business Model for SMAs in Our Practice

During the time that I introduced SMAs into my practice, I reduced my FTE equivalent from 1.0 to 0.8, yet was able to not only maintain my clinical volume but increase it. By using the BRITE and SHAKE SMAs, and by implementing parallel efficiencies in the operating room, I have been able to improve patient access and increase my productivity. BRITE has averaged a 204% increase in consultation revenue (averaging $2580 per SMA compared to $843 for one-on-one visits in an equivalent time period) and SHAKE a 175% increase ($3091 compared to $1124). With more consultations completed in a timely fashion, more patients are requesting surgery. The increase in surgical volume is 34% and the impact on overall gross billings is an increase of 75%.

Obstacles That We Still Face

The most important challenges that we face at the Dartmouth–Hitchcock Medical Center as we attempt to move our shared medical appointment program forward are appropriate space and facilities; institutional support for a program (program manager, etc.); and documentation support (scribe).

Most Frequently Asked Questions by Medical Staff

The most frequently asked questions by medical staff considering SMAs have to do with HIPPA and confidentiality as well as with billing—issues that are addressed more fully elsewhere in this book (see Chapters 2 and 10).

Conclusion

SMAs have redefined for me what quality means in a consultation. I can provide much more information, have richer dialog with patients, truly believe that they are much more informed about their decisions, and I love how this has re-energized my support staff and me. I honestly wish that more providers were aware of this model of care and offering it to their patients. I have a son with a seizure disorder and would love to find a neurologist who offered SMAs as a way to more fully engage and inform patients about the different options for medical management and surgical intervention as I almost always leave appointments with residual questions unanswered. I continue to champion the SMA concept throughout the hospital and know that in many other areas patients will greatly benefit from SMAs. They are not for all patients, all providers, or all health conditions, but their penetration will definitely increase.

Using DIGMAs to Solve an Entire Department's Access Problems

This is an important section for both larger integrated healthcare delivery systems and midsized medical groups because it clearly demonstrates how DIGMAs (and, by extension, PSMAs) can be used to solve an entire department's (or medical group's) access problems. Furthermore, this access benefit can be achieved by DIGMAs and PSMAs alone (i.e., without any other departmental changes), although using them in conjunction with other access solutions such as Advanced Clinic Access to optimize scheduling would undoubtedly accelerate the entire backlog reduction process.

Another interesting point that can be inferred from this study is that the dramatically increased physician production that the DIGMA and PSMA models provide can be directly translated into additional physician full-time equivalents (FTEs), but without the additional cost of actually having to hire additional physician staff—or the extra support staff required to support them. In addition, because these additional physician FTEs are in effect created by the DIGMA/PSMA program out of current physician staffing by leveraging existing resources (i.e., without the need of actually hiring additional providers), the additional equipment, office space, exam rooms, and recruitment costs that extra providers would entail would not be necessary. As can be seen, a well-run DIGMA and PSMA program can improve access, increase productivity, contain costs, and save money in many ways—plus, most importantly, enhance quality and patient satisfaction.

Study 13: DIGMAs Can Be Used to Solve an Entire Department's Access Problems

This study (which was published in AMGA's Group Practice Journal in November–December, 2001) was the first of its kind to demonstrate that when all providers within a medical department simultaneously start a DIGMA program for their practice, access problems for the entire department can sometimes be completely solved—and that this can be accomplished through use of existing resources and the DIGMA model alone (i.e., without hiring any additional physician staffing and without use of other access improvement tools such as Advance Clinic Access) (17). Of course, this can only be accomplished when the added capacity and reduced demand provided by the DIGMA program is sufficient to balance supply and demand—and to therefore overcome the department's access problems over time.

Setting

This study examined, in actual practice, the impact of the DIGMA model upon access, physician productivity, service, the patient–physician relationship, and patient as well as physician satisfaction in a severely backlogged Neurology Department of a large health maintenance organization (HMO) in Northern California. The three neurologists in this department were responsible for the neurological care of approximately 200,000 patient members; however, the system lacked the resources to hire the additional neurology staff that was needed. Because this department had a severe and worsening access problem (yet lacked the resources required to solve this problem through traditional individual office visits alone), the DIGMA model was employed in the hopes that it would be able to sufficiently increase productivity and leverage the neurologists' time in order to solve these departmental access problems through use of DIGMAs and existing resources alone.

It is important to note that this study could equally well have been performed with virtually any primary or specialty care department—i.e., in fee-for-service, capitated, community health, VA, or DoD settings. However this HMO's Neurology Department was chosen because of its severe and growing return appointment access problem, its manageable size, and the willingness of all three neurologists in the department to simultaneously launch a weekly 90-minute DIGMA in their respective practices.

Problem

Because the DIGMA model was specifically developed to enhance the patient's healing experience, improve access, increase physician efficiency and productivity, and to provide high levels of both patient and physician professional satisfaction, this study was designed to examine the impact that DIGMAs could have in actual practice when applied to an entire department that was severely backlogged and impacted as a result of access problems. Since this healthcare organization lacked the funds to hire the additional physician and support staff that would be necessary to solve these problems through traditional means alone, the decision was made to try and create the equivalent of extra physician full-time equivalents (FTEs) from existing staffing by dramatically leveraging the neurologists' time through a carefully designed and properly run DIGMA program.

The backlogs, wait lists, and serious access problems experienced by this Neurology Department had resulted not only in insufficient availability of return appointments to meet the demand, but also in growing patient dissatisfaction as reflected in increased patient complaints about poor access, a heavy patient phone call burden, and the need to *force-book* (i.e., to *work-in* or *double book*) as many as five additional appointments per day into these neurologists already full schedules. These conditions were not only resulting in inadequate service to patients, but adversely affecting the quality of the neurologists' professional lives as well. There seemed to be no obvious solution to this problem which, if left unchecked, was likely to develop into even more severe access problems and patient (as well as staff) dissatisfaction in the future.

Methodology

A cost–benefit analysis was done at 1 month, 2 months, and 1 year for simultaneously initiated DIGMAs conducted by all three neurologists in the Neurology Department at a large staff model HMO that services approximately 200,000 patient members. Each neurologist conducted one 90-minute DIGMA per week, with the three Neurology DIGMAs being held back-to-back on Fridays—with a 30-minute break separating groups. The same group room and adjoining exam room were used in each case, with the author being the DIGMA champion and acting as the behaviorist for all 3 of these Neurology DIGMAs.

Patients and Measures

The patients in this study were the neurologists' own return patients needing a follow-up appointment—i.e., patients who voluntarily attended a DIGMA session in lieu of an individual return visit. Measurements documenting the effectiveness of the DIGMA program upon access included: (1) the number of return patients on the Neurology Department's waiting list; (2) the number of waitlisted patients *past due* for their return appointment; (3) the number of return appointments available to the Neurology Department; (4) the number of available return appointments added via these three Neurology DIGMAs; (5) the leveraging of neurologists' time; (6) the subtype of the DIGMA model used initially and after 1 year; (7) the number of DIGMA visits patients attended on average per year; and (8) the results of patient and physician satisfaction surveys.

The Three DIGMAs Were Customized to Each Neurologist's Specific Needs

Each of the Neurology DIGMAs was customized to the specific needs, goals, practice style, and patient panel constituency of the three individual neurologists. Therefore, all three Neurology DIGMAs were expected to gradually evolve over time as the neurologists learned how to best use them for their practices and as these programs were continuously adapted to better meet the neurologists' changing needs. The Chief of the Neurology Department initially chose a heterogeneous DIGMA design—in which every session would be open to all of his neurology patients, regardless of condition or diagnosis—in order to keep sessions full and to make them open to all of his patients. This was because he had a large practice but relatively few return appointments available due to his multiple responsibilities regarding departmental administration, running the electrophysiology laboratory, and the many regional administrative activities that he was involved with.

The other two neurologists initially chose the same mixed DIGMA design—i.e., one in which all of their neurology patients could attend any group session they wanted, but for which each weekly session of the month focused upon a different cluster of neurological diagnoses and conditions. For these two Neurology DIGMAs, the first Friday of the month focused on headache; the second upon multiple sclerosis, seizure disorders, and younger neurology patients; the fourth focused upon Parkinson's disease, dementia, stroke, and older neurology patients; and the third and fifth sessions of each month (i.e., for those couple of months each year having five Fridays) were general in scope and open to all of these two neurologist's patients, regardless of diagnosis. The caveat here was that all of these two neurologist's patients were invited to schedule any other of the DIGMA sessions held each month should the one that best fit their needs not be convenient or possible for them to attend. For these two mixed Neurology DIGMAs, the scheduler attempted to match patients (both from the waiting list and those calling in for a return appointment) with the appropriate group session.

This mixed DIGMA design was structured so as to simultaneously accomplish several goals: (1) to make groupings sufficiently broad to cover the neurologist's entire patient panel during the four weekly sessions held each month; (2) to ensure that all group sessions had enough patients qualifying to attend to consistently meet minimum group census requirements; (3) to have just four different types of sessions each month (one for each week of the month), so that patients could easily remember which group session(s) of the month best focused upon their condition; and (4) to ensure that no neurology patient needed to wait longer than a couple of weeks for an appropriate DIGMA session. As so often happens with the mixed DIGMA design in actual practice, these two mixed Neurology DIGMAs were observed to gradually evolve into a heterogeneous DIGMA design over a year's time. In other words, it was observed that these distinctions between group sessions in the mixed Neurology DIGMA design tended to become less important over time—the net result being that patients with a wide variety of neurological conditions soon attended virtually every Neurology DIGMA session for all three neurologists (so that the heterogeneous subtype ultimately prevailed).

Scheduling

To maximally leverage neurologists' time and reduce the department's return appointment backlog, emphasis was placed upon directly booking patients into DIGMA sessions instead of individual return office visits whenever possible and appropriate. Nonetheless, because DIGMAs are meant to be voluntary to patients and are designed to work together with individual appointments (rather than to completely replace them), any patient preferring an individual appointment was given one—and this option was always made available to them. Patients could enter these Neurology DIGMAs in six different ways: (1) by being booked directly from the neurologists' waiting lists through telephone calls by the neurology scheduler; (2) by invitation from the neurologist and/or support staff during regular office visits (i.e., to have their next visit be in a DIGMA session); (3) by direct referral via DIGMA promotional materials; (4) by existing patients who call in to schedule a return appointment being encouraged by scheduling staff to attend the DIGMA; (5) by simply *dropping-in* whenever they have a medical need and want to be seen; and (6) by being referred from the DIGMA setting (i.e., once they actually attend a DIGMA session) to have their next follow-up visit scheduled back into a future DIGMA session if they would like.

However, patients who did drop-in were encouraged to telephone the office at least a business day in advance in order to inform staff that they were coming so that: group size could be monitored; paper medical charts could be ordered; and patients could verify that the DIGMA was in fact going to be meeting that week. Also, in the event that the DIGMA needed to be cancelled at the last minute (perhaps because the neurologist was ill), the patients could then be telephoned by staff and advised not to come in since the DIGMA was not going to be held—thus avoiding the frustration of an unnecessary trip into the medical center. Patients were also invited to bring a partner or support person to the DIGMA appointment. Although group sizes were anticipated to be smaller at first (until patients became familiar with, and accepting of, the DIGMA concept), all three neurologists targeted an ideal group census of 10 patients.

The regular scheduler for the Neurology Department telephoned patients from the wait list that had been pre-approved by the neurologist, starting with patients past due for their return appointment in order to give first priority to this already delayed group of patients. The scheduler would explain the DIGMA program to patients and offer them the choice of either a 90-minute group appointment with their neurologist that week or the next available 15-minute individual return appointment—which was often a month or more into the future. This differential in availability between these two appointment types was especially pronounced during the early part of this study—i.e., before the DIGMA program also made individual office visits much more available to patients. The neurology scheduler then directly booked all patients choosing to attend a DIGMA session into the next appropriate group session. This telephone invitation by the neurology scheduler was then followed up (i.e., both for patients accepting this offer and for patients who could not be reached and for whom a message was left) by a personalized, computer-generated invitation letter incorporating the neurologist's signature and containing all necessary information about the program.

In addition, the scheduler was to telephone all these patients the day before their scheduled DIGMA session to remind them that they were scheduled to attend that Friday. Regrettably, due to conflicting departmental duties, the neurology scheduler often lacked the necessary time each week to telephone and invite sufficient appropriate patients from the waiting list to ensure full groups—i.e., let alone to call all scheduled patients the day before DIGMA sessions and remind them to attend. The unfortunate consequence of this was that group sessions all too often went unfilled, that less than optimal census was achieved during most DIGMA sessions, and that the group census of sessions was substantially less than it could have been if only adequate scheduling support had been provided. This underscores the need for having a specially trained dedicated scheduler attached to every DIGMA session if it is to be optimally successful—i.e., one with adequate time allocated to the program each week to achieve full census).

Scheduling staff for the Neurology Department would often invite patients to attend the DIGMA in lieu of an individual office visit when they called the office to schedule an appointment—although making this offer was unfortunately all-too-often forgotten, which again reduced group census from what it otherwise could have been. In addition, some patients self-referred themselves based upon the promotional materials used for the program—especially the professional appearing framed wall posters on the neurologists' lobby and exam room walls, and by taking a program description flier from the adjacent plastic flier dispenser.

Neurologists—as well as the various members of their support staffs—also invited appropriate patients seen during routine office visits to have their next follow-up visit be in an appropriate future Neurology DIGMA session. After briefly explaining the DIGMA program and some of its benefits to their patients, the neurologists would give them a flier describing their Neurology DIGMA in more detail and then personally invite them to attend the group for their next visit—a process that

seldom took more than a minute or so to complete. Patients accepting this offer were directly booked into the appropriate future DIGMA session in lieu of an individual return appointment. Similarly, neurologists invited appropriate patients seen during routine office visits who did not require a follow-up appointment to attend a DIGMA session "the next time they have a medical need"—thereby off-loading individual office visits onto DIGMAs whenever appropriate and possible. Unfortunately, neurologists sometimes forgot to perform this important function of personally inviting all appropriate patients seen during regular office visits, with the net result again being a reduction in group census from what it otherwise might have been.

Professional Appearing Marketing Materials

High-quality, professional appearing marketing materials were developed to inform patients about the DIGMA program and its many advantages. These promotional materials included large framed wall posters prominently mounted on the neurologists' lobby and examination room walls, which were accompanied by an adjacent plastic flier holder containing approximately 100 program description fliers having a matching graphical design (to make an eye appealing wall display) for patients to take home with them. The warm and inviting image of these posters and accompanying fliers (see examples of each in the forms section of the DVD attached to this book) were designed to: (1) catch the patient's eye and cause them to go over and read the poster; (2) explain the program and encourage patients accustomed to individual office visits (i.e., not group visits) to attend a DIGMA session; (3) increase patient familiarity and comfort with the DIGMA concept; (4) accurately represent the high-quality medical care that was being delivered in these sessions; and (5) encourage patients to remove a flier from the adjoining dispenser and take it home to read. Experience has consistently demonstrated that once patients attend a DIGMA and experience its many patient benefits, they are almost always willing to return to the DIGMA setting for future follow-up care.

Assessing the Scope of the Neurology Department's Access Problems

Before the three neurologists launched their DIGMA programs, the maximum number of regularly scheduled individual return appointments offered per week was first determined for the entire Neurology Department. This was accomplished by first counting the total number of individual return appointments of all types available on average per week on all three of the neurologists' schedules combined. Because they rotated on-call duties on a weekly basis, the three neurologists' initial weekly regular and on-call schedules were used in this calculation—i.e., before 1 ½ hours was blocked off each week for their Neurology DIGMA. In effect, this number represented the maximum number of regularly scheduled individual return appointments available on average each week to the entire Neurology Department—i.e., without double-booking any extra return appointments.

This conservative calculation assumes that the neurologists would never be sick, on vacation or education leave, leading DIGMAs, or otherwise absent from currently scheduled clinic duties for any reason—which of course was not true, but this difference would be somewhat difficult to estimate. This is a conservative calculation in that it tends to overestimate the actual number of regularly scheduled return appointments originally available each week to the entire Neurology Department, and therefore to correspondingly underestimate the percentage increase in return appointments made available to the department via the Neurology DIGMA program. It was the author's intent throughout this study to always error on the conservative side with regard to the productivity and access improvement numbers generated from this Neurology DIGMA program.

The Neurology Department's backlog of individual return appointments was determined by tabulating each neurologist's *booking list*—i.e., the computerized monthly posting of patients due or past due for an individual return appointment. These booking lists consisted mostly of 3- to 12-month follow-up appointments. Because it was deemed especially critical to promptly address the *past due* booking list (i.e., the worst part of the wait list as these patients were already past due for a return appointment, often by months), these patients were given first priority in this study—and were therefore the first patients on each neurologist's waiting list to be called by the scheduler and invited to attend a DIGMA session. At the beginning of this study, when all three neurologists' schedules were severely impacted and completely full for the next 3 months (the computer could only schedule appointments a maximum of 3 months ahead) and no return appointments remained available on any of their schedules to put patients into, the due and past due booking list simply represented each neurologist's accumulated individual return appointment backlog. Therefore, the backlog for the entire Neurology Department was simply the sum of the three neurologist's individual due and past due booking lists.

Finally, in order to demonstrate the rate of improvement in access over time through the Neurology DIGMA program, the Neurology Department's return appointment backlog was determined: (1) at the start of this study; (2) after 1 month of operations; (3) after 2 months; and (4) again after 1 year of running the DIGMA program.

Patient Satisfaction

In order to determine how satisfied patients were with the DIGMA program, anonymous questionnaires were issued to 102 consecutive patients attending these three Neurology DIGMAs during the last month of this study. Because there were times when the neurologists were absent due to meetings, vacations, illness, etc., their DIGMAs did not meet each week—which included the last month of this study, when the patient satisfaction questionnaires were issued. On this patient satisfaction questionnaire, patients were asked (among other things): "Overall, how satisfied were you with today's visit?" Possible responses ranged along a 5-point Likert scale from "very dissatisfied" (=1) through "very satisfied" (=5). Each patient was limited to a single patient satisfaction questionnaire. If patients attended more than one session during the last month of this 1-year study (although the study stopped after 1 year, the Neurology DIGMA program still continued for many years afterward),), then no additional questionnaires were given to these patients during subsequent sessions. Group attendees were asked to anonymously deposit their completed patient satisfaction questionnaires (i.e., without their names or any other identifying information on them) into a slotted, covered box outside the door as they left the group room after the DIGMA session. The Neurology Department's reception staff exhibited their creativity by neatly and attractively decorating this box.

During the same 1-month time period at the end of this study, the same anonymous patient satisfaction questionnaire was given to 70 consecutive return patients seen for individual office visits by each of the three neurologists (for identification purposes, these forms were a different color for each of the three neurologists)—which amounted to 210 completed forms in total. These patients similarly deposited their completed questionnaires anonymously into the same slotted, covered, and neatly decorated box (this time, it was kept in the department's lobby) as they left the examination room in which their individual return visit was held.

To evaluate the effect of the program on the patient–physician relationship, the anonymous questionnaire also asked the same 102 consecutive patients seen in Neurology DIGMAs toward the end of the study to rate the following on a 5-point Likert scale: "As a result of today's visit, I feel that my relationship to my doctor has deteriorated a lot (=1); deteriorated somewhat (=2); remained unchanged (=3); improved somewhat (=4); or improved a lot (=5)." At the end of the study, similar data were also collected from the same 210 patients after their individual office visit with their neurologist.

Results

Let us now turn our attention to the results of this pioneering DIGMA study—the first ever to be conducted for an entire department (i.e., a department with severe access problems and no obvious solution that could get them out of this dilemma).

Return Appointments Available to the Department Each Week

This study examined return appointments only—i.e., not initial evaluations, one-time consults, administrative meetings, on-call commitments, time spent either in headache programs or in the electrophysiology lab, etc. The mean initial maximum weekly total of available return appointments of all types for the entire Neurology Department (excluding double bookings) prior to any DIGMAs being held was 74.0—or a mean of 24.7 available return appointments per neurologist per week. Of these available appointments, 78% were 15-minute and 22% were 30-minute return appointments.

Because two neurologists were full-time and one worked 9/11ths time, subsequent analyses prorated the number of available return appointments to a mean maximum (i.e., following the above-stated *conservative* strategy of not deducting for unscheduled meetings, vacations, illnesses, etc.) of 26.3 return appointments per week per full-time neurologist. Given the time used for all sources of absences combined (sick time, education leave, vacations, etc.), the realistic number of available return appointments per week for the entire department was probably closer to 60 than 74.0. Had this smaller (but undoubtedly more accurate) number been used in subsequent analyses, the increased gain in productivity provided by the Neurology DIGMA program would have been determined to be even larger than that actually calculated by the conservative analyses that follows.

Increased Throughput, Backlog Reductions, Access Gains, and Physician FTEs Generated

On October 30, 1997, just prior to launching the Neurology DIGMA program, it was determined that the department as a whole had a backlog of 131 patients on the combined booking list of return appointments due or past due (of which 45 were past due)—with no individual return appointments being available on any of the neurologists' schedules during the next 3 months, which was as far out as the computer scheduled. At the start of this study, patients were upset because they were telephoning the office all-too-frequently in vain attempts to schedule return appointments. The truth was, the department was impacted and return patients could not schedule an appointment to get in to see their neurologist (except by being *worked in*, or *double booked*) until the beginning of the next month, at which time the computer opened up yet another month's schedule—i.e., which was 3 months further into the future.

This future month's schedule would then be completely booked within a couple of days, and then it would not be until the beginning of the following month that patients could once again attempt to schedule a follow-up visit—which would once again still be another 3 months away. As a result, patients frequently complained about this lack of access through formal channels to their neurologist's schedules. Worse yet, many of the more savvy neurology patients started to *defensively schedule* return appointments 3 months into the future whether or not they needed one—just in case they might need an appointment, because patients knew that they could not otherwise see their neurologist in a relatively timely manner should they subsequently develop a medical need.

Mean weekly DIGMA attendance data during the first year of operations were examined for each of the three participating neurologists. During the year of this study, total mean weekly DIGMA attendance for the entire Neurology Department (i.e., for all three DIGMAs combined) was 22.25 patients, or an average 7.42 patients per 90-minute weekly DIGMA session—plus an additional weekly mean of 8.65 support persons, yielding an average total of 30.90 attendees per week.

The Results Would Be Even Better with Dedicated Scheduling Support

Although these numbers are respectable, they could have been much higher. As previously mentioned, had a dedicated scheduler with adequate time available to the DIGMA program each week (perhaps an average of 2 hours per DIGMA each week) been available to telephone and invite the necessary number of patients, to fill all sessions, and to call the day before to remind patients of their upcoming DIGMA appointment, then these totals could clearly have been a great deal larger. If this resource had been available, then the targeted census levels of 10 patients per DIGMA session could undoubtedly have been consistently achieved—i.e., rather than the 7.42 patients who did in fact attend.

This is a case of one of the least expensive resources in the clinic being able to leverage the time of the most expensive resources. Unfortunately, this much needed resource was not available to the Neurology DIGMA program, and census suffered as a result—and therefore, the productivity and access gains of the DIGMA program were correspondingly reduced. While the results of this study were remarkable, they could nonetheless have been even better if only this important resource were available. The same is true regarding personal invitations from the neurologists and support staff, who often forgot to personally invite all appropriate patients seen during regular office visits to have their next neurology follow-up visit be in a DIGMA.

A 26% Increase in Departmental Return Appointments Per Week

Despite deducting the 3.0 individual return appointments originally lost on average per week to the Neurology Department as a whole as a result of the DIGMA program (i.e., by blocking off 4.5 hours total time per week from the neurologists' schedules for these 3 weekly 90-minute Neurology DIGMAs), the department was still provided with a net gain of 19.25 extra return appointments per week as a result of the DIGMA program. In terms of return appointments available to the Neurology Department as a whole, this gain through the DIGMA program constituted an overall average weekly increase of 26% more return appointments to the Neurology Department.

In Terms of Return Appointments, This Was Equivalent to Hiring an Additional 0.7 FTE Neurologist

Assume that any additional neurologist to be hired would be just as productive in terms of individual return appointments as the current three neurologists initially were—i.e., prior to starting the DIGMA program. In that case, an extra full-time neurologist's schedule would also include the same number of individual return appointments as the three current neurologists initially averaged, prorated to working full time—i.e., 26.3 individual return appointments per week. Then the net gain of 19.25 extra

neurology return visits per week provided by the DIGMA program slightly exceeds the return appointment workload that an additional 7/10th-time neurologist would theoretically provide—assuming that this neurologist just offered individual appointments, and not DIGMAs. In other words, at least in terms of return appointments, the Neurology DIGMA program in effect created the equivalent of an extra 0.7 FTE neurologist out of existing resources.

Because this benefit was created out of existing resources by the Neurology DIGMA program, it did not entail the extra cost of hiring an additional 0.7 FTE neurologist—for which the necessary funds were not available within the system. In actuality, the savings generated by the DIGMA program would be approximately 50% greater than just this additional 0.7 FTE neurologist's salary, as this additional manpower is being created from existing resources—so that the additional office, extra exam rooms, extra nursing and support staff, as well as extra durable medical equipment and recruitment costs would not be necessary to house and support this 0.7 FTE neurologist. As a result, assuming that a 0.7 FTE neurologist was to cost $120,000, the overall savings provided by this Neurology DIGMA program would have been approximately 150% larger (or $180,000) during the first year of operations alone—at least in terms of return appointments.

Had a 0.7 FTE Neurologist Actually Been Hired, then the Benefits of the DIGMA Would Have Been Lost

It is important to note that the same net benefit in terms of improved return appointment access to the Neurology Department could have theoretically been achieved by hiring an additional 0.7 FTE neurologist—assuming that the extra funds were available within the system (which was not the case) to hire a 0.7 FTE neurologist and the required support staff, plus provide the fully equipped office and exam room space that would be necessary. This potential solution would have simply thrown more physicians at this access problem in an attempt to solve it through traditional means alone. It is important to note that such an inefficient approach would have failed, however, to provide the many additional benefits that the DIGMA program delivered: max-packed visits; freedom of choice; patient support; help from the behaviorist; attention to mind as well as body needs; the opportunity for neurologists to do something interesting and different, etc. It would also have precluded the development of the DIGMA program, which was much liked by patients and neurologists alike.

On Average, the Neurologists' Return Appointment Productivity Was Increased 650%

In terms of return appointments, these three Neurology DIGMAs were determined to leverage the neurologists' time and increase productivity in delivering return appointments by more than 650% in actual practice during the first year of operations. Note that this 650% figure was generated by looking only at the number of follow-up visits that the physician was actually providing individually on average during 90 minutes of clinic time as the workweek was constructed, and then comparing it to the number of group follow-ups offered on average during a 90-minute DIGMA. It is important to note that this differs from the types of calculations that I now do when determining the percentage increase in physician productivity.

What I currently do is to look at the number of individual follow-up visits that the neurologist would typically provide in 90 minutes of clinic time in the event that the physician provided only individual follow-up visits during that amount of time (i.e., using the same types of follow-up appointments and relative ratios in which they are currently being offered on the physician's schedule in the clinic). I then compare the number of follow-up visits provided on average in each 90-minute weekly DIGMA session to the number of individual return visits that would typically be seen on average during 90 minutes of clinic time devoted to follow-up visits, and multiply that ratio by 100%.

When the latter type of calculation is performed, it is somewhat unusual for the DIGMA model to increase physician productivity by more than 200–400% (i.e., in the delivery of group vs. individual return appointments on average during 90 minutes time), which is what the DIGMA model was originally designed to typically achieve. However, the large increase in productivity found in this study was possible because of this study's method of calculation—and because of its singular focus upon return visits, especially when coupled with the low initial throughput of individual neurology return visits prior to starting the Neurology DIGMA program. This low initial throughput of follow-up visits in the Neurology Department was in turn due to a large variety of factors: one neurologist being on-call at all times; multiple administrative, electrophysiology laboratory, and headache program commitments; many intake and one-time consultation appointments; etc. Therefore, it is recommended that future DIGMA programs at other integrated healthcare delivery systems use the latter method for calculating increased provider productivity, and that they target to increase physician productivity by the more realistically achievable goal of 200–400% (usually 300%) in DIGMA vs. individual return appointments in most primary care and medical sub-specialty applications.

Access Problems Were Completely Solved in Less than 1 Year

The improvement in productivity (and thus capacity) that the Neurology DIGMA program offered was nonetheless sufficient to solve the Neurology Department's access problems to return appointments within one year through use of existing resources alone. One year after the Neurology DIGMA program began, it was determined that no patients were *past due* for their return appointments—in fact, no patients had been past due for their return appointments since the end of the second month of this study. Moreover, after just 1 year of DIGMA operations, all three neurologists had completely solved their access problems. In fact, at the end of 1 year, all patients coming due for a return appointment during the next 2 months on any of the three neurologists' booking lists had already been scheduled for either an individual return visit or a DIGMA visit—yet 46 individual return appointments remained unfilled on the three neurologists' schedules during the next 2 months, and were still available for the Neurology Department to schedule additional patients into. In other words, so much extra capacity had been generated by the DIGMA program that the Neurology Department had eliminated all return appointment wait lists, and completely caught up on its access problems within a year of DIGMA operations. In fact they were now *ahead of the game* as all patients coming due for a return appointment during the next 2 months already had one scheduled, yet 46 return appointment slots still remained open to put additional patients into.

This study demonstrated the remarkable power of the DIGMA model—both in solving departmental access problems and as a practice management tool. In short, by using only the DIGMA model and existing resources, the Neurology Department's large and growing wait list for return appointments was completely caught up within just a year—in fact, the department was even 2 months ahead by year's end. Furthermore, after the conclusion of this 1-year study, it was expected that the Neurology Department's access problems would remain solved into the foreseeable future through continuation of this DIGMA program—except for such unforeseen difficulties as loss of staff, additional workload commitments, failure to continue to adequately promote the program to patients over time, or unexpected increases in either panel sizes or patient demands for service and care.

Additional Departmental Benefits Included Decreased Phone Calls, Patient Complaints, and "Work-Ins"

By the end of the first year of this study, the Neurology Department's support staff was also reporting a host of additional benefits from their DIGMA program (i.e., beyond improved access and increased neurologist productivity): (1) a substantial reduction in patient phone call volume (Why call when you can come in and be seen?); (2) the virtual elimination of previously frequent patient complaints regarding poor accessibility; (3) a greatly reduced need to force-book extra return appointments into the neurologists' already full schedules; (4) high levels of patient as well as physician professional satisfaction; (5) enhanced patient–physician relationships; and (6) a tool enabling the neurologists to better manage their large patient panels and busy practices. As early as the first monthly Neurology Department meeting after starting the Neurology DIGMA program, the departmental scheduler stated that even after only two weeks of operations, the Neurology DIGMAs were "already significantly reducing our booking lists (i.e., waiting lists)."

Then, in a personal conversation just 1 month after the start of the program, the neurology scheduler added: "It feels good to be able to offer the group to patients, especially if they're on a booking list past due or if they're scheduled for a return appointment that needs to be cancelled and no return is available for a month or more. Also, we're no longer having to force-book by chipping away 15 minutes from consultation times to make more return appointments available." Clearly, the DIGMA program dramatically and immediately benefited the Neurology Department in multiple ways—including alleviating its substantial and growing backlog of return patients—and these benefits continued to accumulate throughout the first year of operations and beyond. Certainly, this reduction in patient phone call volume, complaints about poor access, and double-bookings was most appreciated by all—patients and staff alike. It is worth noting that, because of both the enhanced physician professional satisfaction and the numerous benefits that the Neurology DIGMA program provided, all three neurologists chose to continue their DIGMAs—both initially after this study had concluded and a year and a half later, after the author took an early retirement package and another behaviorist was assigned to these groups.

Patient Satisfaction Was Very High

The response rate regarding patient satisfaction questionnaires for the Neurology DIGMAs was 91.2%, and the mean response score was 4.77 out of 5—with 80.6% of respondents rating themselves as "very satisfied," 16.1% as "somewhat satisfied," and 3.2% as "neutral." Not a single patient reported being either "somewhat dissatisfied" or "very dissatisfied" with a DIGMA session. These results clearly show that overall patient satisfaction with the Neurology DIGMA program was very high.

For individual return visits at the conclusion of this study, the response rate was 81.9% and the mean response score was 4.625—also indicating high levels of patient satisfaction. Although not statistically significant, the mean overall patient satisfaction score was in the direction of showing greater satisfaction with Neurology DIGMA visits (4.77/5) than with traditional individual office visits (4.625/5). Unfortunately, I only measured patient satisfaction with individual office visits at the end of this 1-year study—i.e., after the Neurology Department's access problem had been completely solved by the DIGMA program and patients were able to obtain timely individual as well as DIGMA visits. Had I measured the level of patient satisfaction with routine follow-up visits before this study actually started—i.e., when access to individual return office visits was poor and patient complaints were common—the level of patient satisfaction with individual office visits would have undoubtedly been demonstrated to be significantly lower than for DIGMAs.

Patients Reported an Improved Patient–Physician Relationship

The questionnaire assessing the patient–physician relationship yielded an 82.4% response rate for Neurology DIGMA visits and a 69.5% response rate for individual return visits. No patients reported a deteriorating relationship with their neurologist as a result of their Neurology DIGMA visit, although the same could not be said for individual office visits. With respect to patients' responses regarding their Neurology DIGMA experiences, 64.3% reported that the relationship to their neurologist had improved "a lot," 17.9% reported that it had improved "somewhat," and 17.9% reported that it "remained unchanged"—although approximately half of these latter respondents voluntarily wrote on the questionnaire that their relationship with their neurologist remained unchanged because it had always been excellent.

The mean score was 4.46 out of 5 for the Neurology DIGMAs and 4.18 out of 5 for individual office visits. This result indicated that patients felt that their DIGMA as well as individual return visits improved their relationship with their neurologist (at least once the Neurology Department's serous access problems had been eliminated by the DIGMA program)—again in the direction of greater improvement for patients attending Neurology DIGMAs than for traditional office visits. Had this measure been assessed at the beginning of this study (i.e., long before the DIGMA program solved the Neurology Department's serious access problems and patient complaints were common), scores for individual office visits would almost certainly have been much lower than for highly accessible DIGMA visits—and a statistically significant difference would almost certainly have been achieved.

During focus group debriefings after sessions, patients reported appreciating the many benefits that they felt the Neurology DIGMA program offered to them: increased accessibility to their neurologist; the greater amount of time they were able to spend; the increased attention to *mind* as well as *body* needs; the closer follow-up care that could be provided; the help and support provided by the behaviorist, other patients, and support persons in attendance; and the additional healthcare choice that they now had available to them.

Physician Professional Satisfaction Was Also High

Similar to the case for patients (who reported both a high level of satisfaction with the Neurology DIGMA program and an improved relationship with their neurologist), the neurologists themselves reported that the Neurology DIGMA program enhanced their own level of professional satisfaction. All three neurologists reported that the Neurology DIGMA program actually increased their professional satisfaction.

They cited the following reasons for their improved professional satisfaction: (1) substantially improved access to their practice and reduced patient complaints about poor access; (2) the increased level of mind–body and follow-up care that they were able to provide; (3) the greater amount of patient education and disease self-management skills that they were able to impart to their patients; (4) the reduced patient phone call volume and force bookings that they had to deal with; (5) the decreased need to repeat the same information over and over to different patients individually; (6) the opportunity to do something different, interesting, and fun while getting to know their patients better; (7) the help provided by the behaviorist; (8) the ability they now had to appropriately schedule patients best seen in group to highly efficient DIGMA sessions while reserving more costly individual office visits to those patients truly requiring them; and 9) the increased ability that they now had to better manage their large and busy practices.

In addition, the neurologists pointed out that their Neurology DIGMAs proved to be an ideal venue for better managing some of their most information seeking, psychosocially needy, problematic, and time-consuming patients—especially those with extensive informational, emotional, and psychosocial needs. Finally, neurologists as well as patients appreciated the opportunity for patients requiring routine follow-up care to simply *drop-in* to a DIGMA session any week that they happened to have a medical need and wanted to be seen—i.e., without any barriers to care whatsoever.

For Ideal DIGMA Group Sizes to Be Achieved, There Needed to Be More Dedicated Scheduling Support and Physician Invitations

It is important to note that the dramatic results achieved in this study reflect only a fraction of what the Neurology DIGMA program could have accomplished had the necessary dedicated scheduling support (as well as invitations by physician and staff) just been consistently provided. I say this because all three DIGMAs could have accommodated substantially more patients than actually attended, which would have resulted in even greater efficiency and productivity gains (plus a more rapid reduction in access problems).

Ideal Group Size

The first year's experience led the author and the three neurologists to conclude that the ideal Neurology DIGMA group size would be between 10 and 16 patients, plus 3–5 support persons. It was found that Neurology DIGMA sessions could be conducted successfully with as many as 27 attendees (patients and support persons combined) with relatively high levels of patient satisfaction. In fact, after one particularly large and busy group, the patients actually stood up and spontaneously applauded the physician.

Certainly, if you were to ask these patients whether they would have preferred 90 minutes alone with their physician, some undoubtedly would have responded in the affirmative; however, this would not have been a realistic or economically viable option. The main point here is that patients were able to be successfully seen in large DIGMA groups, and that this could be done with high levels of patient satisfaction. However, because it was found that 90-minute Neurology DIGMA sessions that included more than 16 patients (i.e., a total of about 20 attendees, when support persons were also counted) imposed an excessively large workload demand upon the neurologist, such large groups are generally not recommended. I say this because physician professional satisfaction has always been one of the major goals of any well-run DIGMA program, and because physicians appear to be tired when more that 16 patients are seen in a single session. Thus, it appears that the limiting factor with regards to maximum DIGMA group size is excessive physician workload, not patient satisfaction.

Need for a Dedicated Scheduler and More Personal Invitations from Physician and Staff:

Another factor contributing to low census was the fact that it is always important for all physicians conducting DIGMAs to remember to invite all appropriate patients seen during regular office visits to attend their DIGMA the next time they have a medical need. Unfortunately, this invitation was all-too-often forgotten by the neurologists (as well as their support staffs) during this study. In addition to this frequent failure of neurologists and their staffs to invite all appropriate patients into a future DIGMA session whenever they next had a medical need, the other great difficulty faced throughout the entire year of this study was consistently obtaining the necessary 6 hours of dedicated scheduling time per week (i.e., an average of 2 hours per week for each of the three Neurology DIGMAs to *top-off* and fill all sessions to targeted levels of 10–16 patients). This was needed in order for the neurology scheduler to telephone and invite a sufficient number of appropriate patients approved by the neurologists to consistently fill all DIGMA groups, and then to call all scheduled attendees a business day or so prior to the session in order to remind them to attend.

This amount of time dedicated to the program would also have enabled the dedicated scheduler to pre-book patients accepting this offer into a future DIGMA session in lieu of an individual return appointment whenever possible and appropriate, and to make the necessary number of *reminder calls* to patients the day before the sessions were to be held each week so that full groups could consistently be achieved. Certainly, the combination of 2 hours of dedicated scheduling support per week for each DIGMA—plus greater attention to personal invitations of all appropriate patients seen during traditional office visits by the neurologists and support staff—would have been most helpful in consistently achieving desired group sizes. In turn, this would have increased even further virtually all of the already remarkable results reported in this study.

Conclusions

This was the first study to clearly demonstrate that the many benefits that the DIGMA model was originally designed to achieve for the individual physician could also be achieved at the departmental level. After just 1 month, the Neurology DIGMA program had already substantially alleviated the Neurology Department's wait list and shortage of available return appointments. It had especially reduced that part of the wait list which was of greatest concern (i.e., of patients *past due* for a return appointment) because that was the initial focus of this

study. In fact, the wait list of patients past due was reduced by 67% after the first month, and completely eliminated by the end of the second month of this study—and this problem has not, to my knowledge, re-emerged since.

By the end of this 1-year study: (1) the Neurology Department's access problems were completely solved by the DIGMA program; (2) all patients coming due for a return appointment during the next 2 months already had their appointment scheduled; and (3) 46 unfilled individual return appointment slots (plus numerous DIGMA appointments) were still available to put patients into on the three neurologist's schedules during the next 2 months. Also of interest, patients did not abuse this privilege of improved access by frequently coming in unnecessarily simply because they could—i.e., as it was observed that patients who attended these Neurology DIGMA sessions only came in for an average of two visits during the entire year of this study. In other words, after just a year, the DIGMA program enabled the neurology department to not only get caught up but actually be 2 months ahead in their scheduling of follow-up appointments. This contrasted sharply with the situation that existed for the entire Neurology Department just prior to the start of this study, at which time a substantial wait list existed and no return appointments remained available to schedule patients into as far out as the computer was able to book (i.e., for 3 months in advance). Plus, all of this was accomplished while patient phone call volume was greatly decreased, patient complaints about poor access were completely eliminated, the need for double booking patients was substantially reduced, and high levels of patient as well as physician professional satisfaction were achieved.

Clinical Outcome Studies Involving DIGMAs and PSMAs

We now turn to some clinical outcome studies and reports involving DIGMAs and PSMAs, studies that are just now beginning to emerge due to the relative newness of these models.

Study 14: Using DIGMAs in a Chronic Illness Treatment Paradigm for Diabetes—The Kansas City VA Medical Center Experience

This case study, which discusses the Kansas City VA Medical Center's experience with DIGMAs in a chronic illness treatment paradigm for diabetes, was submitted by

Janet M. Carroll, RD, LD, CDE, DIGMA Coordinator and Wayne L. Fowler, Jr., M.D., Ph.D., FACP, Endocrinologist. This discussion is important because, to my knowledge, the Kansas City VA Medical Center was the first healthcare system in the country to use the chronic disease population management paradigm that I developed which makes full use of group visits—a chronic disease management model that is discussed in detail in Chapter 7 of this book.

In addition, because the KCVA is estimated to serve approximately 20,000 veterans with diabetes, their Diabetes DIGMA program can potentially become very large—and can therefore be of considerable importance. Of particular interest is their preliminary clinical outcomes data in which they note that "Even at this early point of operations, this data made it clear to us that patients seen in our diabetes DIGMA program were able to achieve better control over their diabetic symptoms." For example, for the 196 patients with diabetes who attended their Diabetes DIGMAs during the first 3 months of implementation, overall HbA1c levels were found to decrease from 8.59% in January 2003 to 7.36% by September 2003—which represented an average decrease in hemoglobin A1c of 1.23 percentage points. The lessons that they have learned, as well as the anticipated future growth of their Diabetes DIGMA program, will also likely be of interest to the reader.

Background

The Veterans Health Administration (VHA) consistently strives to improve patient access, without sacrificing the highest quality medical care. Over the past decade, group medical visits have emerged as a means to provide better access, excellent patient satisfaction, and more complete care at lower costs, particularly in the area of diabetes (18). The specific "shared medical appointment" (i.e., DIGMA and PSMA) models described by Dr. Noffsinger (19) have several patients meeting with the same physician at the same time. This allows interactive targeted education and medical care delivery. There is a high level of patient-to-patient empowerment as well as direction from clinician to patient. The concepts of the Drop-In Group Medical Appointment (or DIGMA) and Physicals Shared Medical Appointment (or PSMA) group visit models were presented by Dr. Noffsinger to the Kansas City VA (KCVA) staff in the fall of 2002 as a means of providing improved access, increased patient education, and high-quality clinical care with the potential for improving clinical outcomes through use of these efficacy enhancing models.

SMAs Offer Many Potential Benefits, Including Recognizing and Treating PTSD

The VA serves those who have experienced military service, especially combat Veterans who have unique characteristics. Those who have served have an understanding of "trusting a buddy with their lives." This deep level of trust is linked to survival. The DIGMA affords medical care in the presence of Veteran buddies who reinforce trust, because they have "walked the walk." Trust is a huge part of the relationship between provider and patient. Health issues now have a "face," because the Veteran is not alone. Can you imagine a clinic without walls with providers, pharmacists, nurses, dietitians, psychologists, etc. and the camaraderie of military veterans? These patients have consistently remarked that they feel more comfortable in shared medical appointments, because other Vets understand their situations and are helpful.

One situation that is unique to the VA system is that a large percentage of the Veterans we treat are dealing with Post Traumatic Stress Disorder (PTSD) issues. According to the VA National Center for Posttraumatic Stress Disorder, PTST is experienced by approximately 30% of male and female veterans who have been in war zones, with an additional 20 to 25% experiencing partial PTSD in their lifetimes. "Clinically serious stress reaction symptoms" have been experienced by approximately 50% of male and almost 50% of female Vietnam veterans. Among Gulf War veterans, PTSD has been estimated at 8% (20).

One of the hallmark symptoms of PTSD is lack of trust. The DIGMA and PSMA shared medical appointment (SMA) models provide a comfortable venue for comrade Veterans to share, support, and help one another. The information that was previously shared in the waiting room is now shared with qualified staff that are present to "clinically coach," if you will. Patients can formulate and begin to take steps toward targeted goals for their care. With DIGMAs and PSMAs, the entire group acts as a witness and supports one another in their individual disease management.

Project Implementation

In December 2002 and January 2003, Dr. Ed Noffsinger, offered two workshops to interested staff. Staffs from Eastern Kansas (Topeka and Leavenworth) and KCVA were mentored in the SMA process and developed an action plan to start SMAs in medical subspecialty care. KCVA had an existing diabetes team, which included an endocrinologist, 2 RN Certified Diabetes Educators (CDEs), two Doctors of Pharmacy, and a Dietitian CDE.

In March 2003, the KCVA launched its pilot diabetes DIGMA program—which included a program specialist (also a CDE) who was detailed half-time to this SMA program. The medical center director and chief of staff enthusiastically supported the project. An unoccupied patient activity room was converted to house DIGMA sessions. Detailed action plans, promotional brochures, closed circuit television (CCTV) announcements, posters, and a VA-Intranet Website were developed for this new SMA diabetes population management program. Confidentiality release forms were developed in concert with the privacy officer and legal counsel in compliance with HIPAA regulations. Patients were gleaned by each clinician, invited, and scheduled into the new Diabetes DIGMA program.

Patient Education

Patient self-management booklets for goal setting were developed for each SMA—as well as individualized lab reports (health summaries), which explained lab and vital sign status as well as desired targets to patients. For all group attendees, this information is regularly updated to comply with clinical guidelines and state of the art research. As the physician moves about the room, each patient's situation and personal goals offer a point of education for the fellow attendees. Each patient leaves the session with specific written goals for the next visit. The patient education committee reviews/updates educational pamphlets and packets for each SMA.

Computer Technology

The VA's Computerized Patient Record System (CPRS) lends itself well to SMAs. Progress note templates were developed to incorporate pertinent history as well as treatment goals for each patient. This electronic progress note is actually a "mini-chart" prepared for each patient prior to the SMA. A hard copy is printed for each clinician to use. These progress note templates have greatly expedited the documentation process, which is important as timely documentation is imperative to quality care. Clinical reminders are noted prior to each DIGMA session, and all materials are prepared for each patient having reminders due. A wireless laptop on a cart was obtained to provide the clinician in the DIGMA with the added flexibility of moving freely from patient to patient—a process that is greatly expedited by having patients seated in a circle. Coders, computer applications coordinators, and staff networked to ensure appropriate workload and billing information for this unique style of medical care delivery.

Staff

A nephrologist and endocrinologist successfully conducted pilot DIGMAs in May 2003 with the assistance of the RNs and Clinical Pharmacists. A psychologist was initially used as a facilitator. However, once the process was perfected, each SMA could operate with 2 staff members, regardless of discipline. The physician or other lead clinician generally develops good group management dynamics in 10 sessions or less. While it would be helpful to have a behaviorist and a documenter in each DIGMA on an ongoing basis, that resource is not available at present. As it turned out, both the endocrinologist and the nephrologist proved to have wonderful skills in this area.

Because the initial pilot sessions proved to be an unqualified success, the SMA program was expanded on an ongoing basis to three Diabetes DIGMAs and one Nephrology DIGMA—which were launched on a weekly basis in June 2003. A full-time SMA coordinator was hired for the endocrinology DIGMA program shortly thereafter, i.e., in December 2003.

Rollout Timeline for the DIGMA Program

Since that time, additional DIGMAs have been launched at KCVA in the following areas: nephrology, obstructive sleep apnea, diabetes podiatry, posttraumatic stress disorder, infectious disease, depression, Parkinson's disease, heart disease, pulmonary disease, gastroenterology, and a variety of Diabetes SMAs (including insulin pump).

Outcomes

KCVA was the first VA in the nation to launch DIGMAs for diabetes, hypertension, and sleep apnea. The KCVA has also been the first healthcare system to utilize Dr. Noffsinger's chronic illness population management paradigm which makes full use of group visits in a systematic approach to chronic disease management. SMAs have been offered to Veteran patients on a regular basis at the KCVA since June 2003. By the end of FY 2006, 26 different DIGMAs were operational within our medical center.

Patient Satisfaction

Patient satisfaction surveys were collected over the first 12 months of the SMA program from every new patient who attended. Outcomes data are regularly analyzed according to a variety of parameters based on clinical guidelines. The VA is mandated by Congress to obtain patient satisfaction surveys on a regular basis in all VA Healthcare Facilities for both in-patients and out-patients. Additionally, a DIGMA-specific survey was used. Overall, patient satisfaction ratings were found to be "good" or better 100% of the time, with 92% of patients rating SMAs as "very good" or "excellent" (Fig. 9.17). Because the results of the Patient Satisfaction Surveys were so consistently "very good" or "excellent," the DIGMA-specific survey has been eliminated and used only if a veteran requests one. However, Medical Center surveys are still conducted on a regular basis and reflect the same positive outcomes for our DIGMAs.

Satisfaction Overall

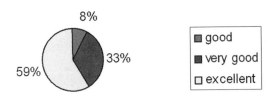

Fig. 9.17 DIGMA-specific survey used for the Kansas City VA Medical Center showed overall patient satisfaction ratings were "good" or better 100% of the time, with 92% of patients rating SMAs as "very good" or "excellent."

Decrease in Wait Times—Open Access

In January 2003, the average wait time to be seen in our Diabetes Clinic was 60.3 days. Diabetes education classes allowed for entrance into the program; however, follow-up was a problem. Eighteen months later (1 year after DIGMAs were initiated in our Diabetes Program), the wait time had dropped to 17.5 days. In other words, appointment wait times to enter our Diabetes Program had decreased by slightly more than 42 ½ days through use of DIGMAs. In addition, a Diabetes Hot Line was established for patients to call. Urgent problems can be managed by patients simply dropping into any one of our three Diabetes DIGMAs each week, which can typically be done within a day or two.

The Podiatry SMA provides another means of accessing care for foot problems, including the ongoing foot care needs of diabetic patients. Patients with problematic changes in foot integrity are able to simply drop-in and obtain immediate care for foot problems—i.e., in concert with care received in other surgical and medical clinics. The importance here is that patients "are seen" and care is appropriately provided at the earliest possible time as a result of our diabetes DIGMA program.

Productivity (Workload Production)

As a result of our growing DIGMA program, there has been a considerable increase in the number of patients seen—which is reflected in Table 9.7. The percent increase in patients seen can be extrapolated to productivity as follows. If a DIGMA has an increase of 100%, the provider is seeing twice as many patients as would be seen in traditional clinics. For every 100% increase, the provider is as productive as another physician working side by side. All numbers are compared to the provider's baseline workload in existing traditional style clinics.

As seen in Table 9.7, over half of the SMAs increased provider productivity by at least 200%—in other words, they substantially increased productivity. "DM Survival" was held at a Community-Based Out-Patient Clinic (CBOC). Staff was able to see 14 patients in each of these three single session DIGMAs, which were held on Fridays. SMAs, which are held on a periodic basis, continue to be a valuable clinical tool for the CBOCs. As a result of the SMA program, the endocrinologist's enrollment has dropped and is being supplemented with patients from the Diabetes Nurse Educators, who have been overly scheduled.

Table 9.7 Increase in workload since SMA began June 2004 as of 4th quarter FY06 at the Kansas city VA

SMA	Percent increase pts seen 2004*	Percent increase pts seen 2005*	Percent increase pts seen 2006*
Diabetes MD/ PharmD	103	106	160
Diabetes RN/ PharmD	178	176	167
Renal MD/RN	240	291	197
Sleep apnea RT	30	175	152
Renal 2 MD/RN	250	170	158
Posttraumatic stress disorder MD/SW	397	744	685
Podiatry DPM	152	103	150
Infectious Disease Nurse	33	Closed	Closed
Depression MD/ ARNP	7	308	277
Diabetes pump RN		33	656
Diabetes insulin start RN		59	67
Diabetes insulin F/U RN		90	108
Diabetes CGMS RN		44	91
Diabetes survival (1 × sessions at community-based outpatient clinics or CBOC's) RN / RD		1300	Replaced with a diabetes education class
Nutrition carb counting RD/RD		98	141

* Where a "100% increase" means that productivity was doubled.

For the DIGMA model, it is recommended that the goal be to increase provider productivity by 300% (i.e., 3x the number of patients normally seen individually in the clinic during the same period of time). Our PTSD, PTSD Significant Other, Depression, and DM Survival SMAs (which are single session DIGMAs), have exceeded this goal—and most of our DIGMAs have improved the rate at which patients are seen. The Infectious Disease DIGMA, which focused on patients who were HIV +, was closed because the patients desired one-to-one appointments to preserve their anonymity. The Diabetes DIGMAs which fall below 300% are extremely high-tech sessions—e.g., the insulin pumps group. Because this technology was very new to KCVA, these DIGMAs were found to have a slow growth.

Preliminary Clinical Data

One hundred ninety-six patients with diabetes attended our Diabetes DIGMAs during the first 3 months of implementation. Overall, their HbA1c levels were found to decrease from 8.59% in January 2003 to 7.36% by September 2003—which represented an average decrease of 1.23 percentage points (Fig. 9.18). Even at this early point of operations, this data made it clear to us that patients seen in our diabetes DIGMA program were able to achieve better control over their diabetic symptoms. The data for January 03 reflects the FY quarter before the DIGMA program was implemented and traditional one-to-one visits were utilized. September 2003 data were reflective of the first quarter that the DIGMA program was implemented.

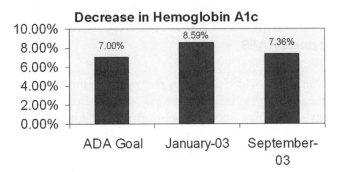

Fig. 9.18 Decrease in hemoglobin A1c in the Kansas City VA Diabetes DIGMAs

Lessons Learned

We have learned several lessons from the KCVA Diabetes DIGMA program, including the following:

- Administrative support, which needs to include a Program Coordinator and/or Champion, is a key to success. There must be one person to take responsibility for the implementation and administration of any comprehensive SMA program. This person must not only take on overall responsibility for the entire SMA program, but also be willing to do all the clerical tasks such as scheduling. until appropriate staff can be hired.

- A scribe is essential for all DIGMAs and PSMAs, especially in systems using electronic medical records.

- Back up plans for vacations and cancellations must be communicated and established. An e-mail group for all clinicians and support staff doing SMAs is helpful. Set a 30-day limit for notices of planned vacations.

- Heterogeneous groups are likely the way of the future. The most successful and flexible SMAs are those that encompass a wide variety of patients. Example: The Renal DIGMAs invite patients with hypertension, renal diseases, renal failure, and post transplantation. Commonality of chronic disease is the underlying factor that makes groups work. Do not limit your patients by selecting singular diagnosis (think broader, such as the whole spectrum of disease).

- Patients hesitate to attend SMAs that force them into "rush hour" traffic.

- Serve decaffeinated coffee all day! It provides a welcoming atmosphere and does not elevated blood pressures and nervous tension.

- Have handouts specifically outlining steps that patients can take to achieve goals set by clinicians. Write out individual instructions for patients. Always be succinct and do not waste time with long verbal explanations. The written words will stay with patients when they go home and work on their individualized disease management program.

- The more humor you can inject, the better. One of my favorite SMAs included the following anecdote: One day, one of the nephrologists was a few minutes late to the DIGMA. Feeling that he had to apologize for his lateness, he stepped into the middle of a room of 19 patients and said, "Welcome to Oprah for Kidneys!"

- The more "reality" that can be reached during SMA sessions, the better the results.

- In the Sleep Apnea DIGMA, a young man was handing in his machine. Of course, this meant he would be giving up. Another patient who was in a motorized wheelchair spoke about how he had worked hard to commit to the cumbersome treatment. He had set a goal to see his grandson graduate from college. In the process of committing to his treatment, he reduced his insulin requirements for his diabetes and delayed the possibility of needing dialysis. The young man shook his hand and promised him that he would try again to use his CPAP machine. This encouragement was palpable, and tears were visible throughout the room.

- Caring is sharing—A SMA for patients with depression was brightened by a veteran who brought flowers that he had grown for each group member.

In a world where society is run by anxiety, is it not wonderful that we can provide targeted, cost-effective, positive medical care in a live talk-show format for patients?

Conclusion

Having started DIGMAs in June 2003, the KCVA now regularly runs approximately 25 different DIGMA sessions per week with focuses that include diabetes, hypertension, nephrology, obstructive sleep apnea, diabetes podiatry, PTSD, cardiology, congestive heart failure, heart disease, infectious disease, depression, Parkinson's disease, pulmonary disease, gastroenterology, and a variety of diabetes-related SMAs (such as insulin pump). In our chronic disease management paradigm for patients with uncontrolled diabetes, patients typically enter the program through our diabetes education class and then attend a variety of diabetes DIGMAs as needed (usually every 3 months) until their HbA1c levels reach 7—at which time they are able to graduate from our program and return to their primary care providers for follow-up care. Because DIGMAs enable individualized medical care and education to be delivered by the same provider to many patients at once during a 90-minute group session, we have found this innovative new model of care delivery to not only be cost effective and highly productive, but also result in improved outcomes and highly satisfied patients.

We have found our DIGMA program to be effective in meeting all of the goals that we initially had for the program: improved access to care; decreased wait times; improved clinical outcomes; increased patient satisfaction; and more educated and empowered patients who are now better able to set their therapeutic goals and manage their disease. We have documented improvement in all of these areas. Overall, we have found the DIGMA model to be very successful at the KCVA: wait times for diabetic patients decreased by 42.5 days during the first 18 months; diabetic patients showed a significant decrease in HbA1c from 8.59% in January 2003 to 7.36% by September 2003; 92% of participating patients have rated their DIGMA experience as "very good" or "excellent"; and we have been able to handle a large increase in workload without the need of hiring additional staff.

The Future

Proposed new SMAs include: Erectile Dysfunction; Spinal Cord Injury; New Patient Orientation; Low Vision; PACT (Prevention of Amputations); etc. Other VA staffs from Wichita, Columbia, and Topeka have come over to observe the KCVA SMA program—which was also featured on Fox 4 WDAF News. The KCVA SMA program coordinator also participates in the VA National SMA Workgroup. "Re-inventing the wheel" is not necessary in this process as Dr. Noffsinger has defined all the necessary steps to success.

Recent news has heightened our awareness of our Veterans' medical, emotional, and psychological needs for care. We in the VA system are charged with supporting our hero Veterans in their quest to re-enter society and the American workforce as they return from war. The numbers of returning Veterans, who will seek care immediately upon discharge from the military, will stretch the resources of the VA system. Group medical appointments will serve as a high-touch and high-tech, cost-effective venue for their medical care.

The future of group medical appointments depends on thorough research evaluating their usefulness and outcomes. Further in-depth study is needed to determine the efficacy of SMAs vs. traditional one-to-one medical appointments. A study team has been formed and a retrospective study for patients with diabetes is underway at KCVA. It is our great honor to serve our Veterans in this exciting new venue for healthcare.

Study 15: Pharmacist Managed Group Medical Appointments at the 1st Medical Group, Langley AFB

This study, which addresses pharmacist managed group medical appointments at the 1st Medical Group, Langley AFB, was received from Brian E. Logue, Maj, USAF, BSC, Chief Clinical Pharmacy 1st Medical Group, 1st Fighter Wing, Air Combat Command, Langley Air Force Base, who is a Clinical Assistant Professor at the Medical College of Virginia. I believe that the reader will find this contribution regarding the successful SAR, URI, and Lipid DIGMAs run at Langley AFB to be of interest because of its implications for applying DIGMAs to urgent care, cold and flu, allergy, and primary care settings—especially when there is a need to treat and triage facility-overwhelming acute infections in order to relieve workload from overcrowded and inundated ER, urgent care, and primary care clinics.

In addition, the reader will find it interesting that, as good and helpful as their SAR and URI DIGMAs were for acute care in treating and triaging potentially facility-overwhelming acute infections (and in relieving workload from the overcrowded ER, urgent care, and family practice clinics), they found DIGMAs to be even more helpful for chronic conditions such as hyperlipidemia. The successful Lipid DIGMAs run at this facility underscore the benefits of DIGMAs in the treatment of chronic health conditions such as hyperlipidemia with regard to educating and empowering patients—and to improving clinical outcomes. Also, their findings show that—in addition to improving access to care and patient as well as provider satisfaction with care—a DIGMA can improve a patient's medication use, treatment outcomes, and the efficiency of healthcare.

Background

The 1st Medical Group at Langley AFB implemented pharmacist managed walk-in group medical appointments to treat seasonal allergic rhinitis (SAR) in April of 2004. Our group medical appointments (GMAs) were adapted from Dr. Noffsinger's DIGMA model to fit our unique practice environment. SAR, along with upper respiratory

tract infections (URI), was among the most common reasons for patient visits to our hospital during certain periods each year (see Fig. 9.19A and B). Through the use of GMAs, we were able to remove uncomplicated SAR cases from our busy family practice clinics—which allowed those clinics to see patients with more urgent needs, while simultaneously decreasing patient wait times for SAR treatment.

Patient Recruitment for Our New SAR DIGMA Program

Concerned with patient recruitment, at the start of our new SAR DIGMA program we actively advertised in the base newspaper and sent a mailer to the home of every patient treated for SAR at Langley in 2003. We initially attracted a small number of patients to the service. Patient outcomes and satisfactions were high, and we were able to convert 80% of patients to the preferred formulary antihistamine in a patient friendly manner. A credentialed pharmacist provider led the GMA and was assisted by Red Cross volunteers, pharmacy students, pharmacy technicians, and other pharmacists. The DIGMA created an ideal venue for communication at multiple levels. We found that word of mouth on base about easy access and quality of care turned out to be our best patient recruitment tool.

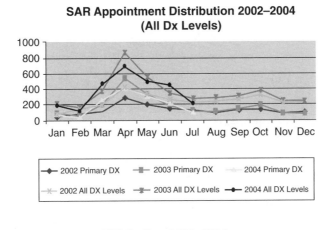

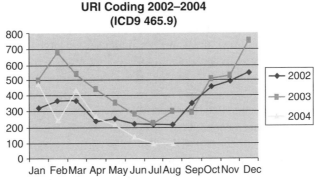

Fig. 9.19 (A and B) SAR and upper respiratory tract infections were among the most common reasons for patient visits to 1st Medical Group at Langley Air Force Base hospital during certain periods each year

Rationale for Starting Our URI DIGMA

Faced with a shortage of flu vaccine in the fall of 2004, we implemented a pharmacist managed walk-in GMA to treat upper respiratory tract infections (URI). This was not a class or an over the counter (OTC) medication-only program. Our DIGMAs operated seasonally based on tracked influenza activity, pollen count, and patient appointment trends. This URI service was designed to treat and triage facility-overwhelming acute infections in order to relieve workload from the overcrowded ER and family practice clinics. In the winter of 2005, our DIGMA increased our military MTF (medical treatment facility) surge capability to treat URI, including influenza, in a controlled manner.

DIGMAs Can Be Used to Address the Global Health Issues of Influenza, SAR, and URI

Due to many variables, the threat of influenza remains an issue of great global health and economic concern. This DIGMA model was able to deal with an increased number of influenza cases among our beneficiaries, and was a great addition to our excellent existing services for improving both infection control and access to care. We were able to reduce "presenteeism" at work—i.e., people at their job but not working at full speed because they were distracted by the symptoms of allergic rhinitis or the loss of energy and symptoms of an upper respiratory tract infection. By improving access to care, we improved readiness and productivity.

Patient Satisfaction with the SAR and URI DIGMA Programs

Both the SAR and URI DIGMAs were evaluated based on a simple patient assessment form (Fig. 9.20A and B) completed during the DIGMA. I have attached the URI form in the event that the reader might find it helpful. The URI DIGMA used the same form as our family practice clinic. This improved the transition of complicated patients out of our DIGMA and on to more care when needed. We successfully treated and triaged 1421 patients for SAR and URI using pharmacist managed DIGMAs between December 2004 and May 2006. The majority of the patients were seen during the flu season of 2004–2005. The clinics were only open seasonally when needed. Pharmacists frequently treat multiple patients concurrently, and are accepted in that role by patients for the treatment of SAR and URI. Results of 447 patient satisfaction surveys assessing pharmacist interaction (labeled RPh) and other parameters are summarized in Table 9.8 and

Fig. 9.21. By protocol, credentialed pharmacists prescribed prescription and non-prescription medications, performed rapid strep tests, and made test recommendations such as chest X-ray for patients that were triaged in the GMA and transitioned into more care. This improved appropriate antibiotic use to treat viral colds and provided an opportunity for patient education about antibiotic resistance. The Center for Disease Control (CDC) "Get Smart" series was used.

Providers Were Also Very Satisfied with This New Service

Following protocol, the pharmacist URI DIGMA triaged and treated influenza, viral colds, strep throat, pharyngitis, otitis media, bronchitis, pneumonia, and SAR. The family practice clinic sent us patients they initially assessed as uncomplicated and all the walk-in patients that they were unable to fit into their schedule. Our service was needed and appreciated, as verbalized on a hectic day by one busy family practice provider who stated jokingly, "Brian, get 'em off me, man." A more common statement heard was "Whatever you can do to help as a provider would be greatly appreciated." Only 10.7% of patients treated in our URI program had another MTF (medical treatment facility or hospital) appointment 2 weeks post-DIGMA. No patients that required a return appointment had a positive rapid strep test or throat culture. We found that 77% of the patients we treated had attempted over the counter medication self-care before coming to our URI DIGMA. Non-pharmacist provider (MDs and PAs) survey results are shown in Table 9.9 and Fig. 9.22.

Although Existing Resources Were Used, Creativity Was Sometimes Required

Our DIGMAs operated in the main lobby of the 1st Medical Group hospital. We used a small room in the lobby for privacy when needed. Our clinic was one of the first pharmacy clinics in the USAF to go live on a worldwide electronic medical record system. We had immediate access to complete information on each walk-in patient, including past medical history, allergies, medication profile, and previous encounter electronic SOAP notes. When we completed an electronic SOAP note in each patient's electronic profile, it was immediately available to their primary care manager following the DIGMA session. When the electronic SOAP note was signed, the appointment was coded. There was no front-end scheduling or back-end coding to our walk-in GMA. These were keys to our efficiency.

Our Biggest Concern: Medication Errors

A primary concern of pharmacists is medication errors and identifying, resolving, and preventing them. When our DIGMA sessions were busy, we sent patients to the pharmacy for their medications. When we were slow, we handed the medications to the patient in the DIGMA area. Some types of dispensing medication errors, such as handing a medication to the wrong patient, polypharmacy, and drug interactions are reduced if the patient is treated in a pharmacist DIGMA. Having a pharmacist engaged in the open treating multiple patients improves patient interaction with the pharmacy—and can enhance interactions during the future treatment of other conditions, follow-up care, or the care of family members. The contribution of Doctor of Pharmacy students from the Medical College of Virginia and Hampton University—along with the professionalism of Air Force pharmacy technicians—helped make our new pharmacist DIGMA program successful.

DIGMAs Permit Important Psychosocial Aspects of Care to Be Better Addressed

I originally thought that the psychosocial aspect of the DIGMA model was secondary in importance to the

3059567982

Cold/Flu/Sore Throat Assessment
Symptoms, Diagnosis and Treatment
Patient Questionnaire

1st Medical Group
Langley AFB Pharmacy Clinic

Today'sDate ☐☐ / ☐☐ / 200☐

Sex ☐ Male ☐ Female   Age ☐☐ years

AreyouEnrolledatLangleyAFB? ☐ No ☐ Yes

DeploymentRelated? ☐ No ☐ Yes

Recenttraveloutofthelocalarea? ☐ No ☐ Yes

Didyoureceiveaflushotthisyear? ☐ No ☐ Yes

Forhowlonghaveyouhadyoursymptoms? ☐☐ days

Main Symptom/Concern:

☐ Cold Symptoms
☐ Cough
☐ Sore Throat
☐ Other (specify) ____________

TobaccoUse?
☐ No ☐ Yes → DesiretoQuitSmokinginnext6months? ☐ No ☐ Yes

Allergies?
☐ No ☐ Yes → ____________

AreyouCurrentlyonanAntibiotic?
☐ No ☐ Yes → ____________

Other Current Medicines: ____________

Pain? ☐ No ☐ Yes → LocationofPain ☐☐☐☐☐☐☐☐☐☐
PainIntensity(1-10) ☐☐

Fever? ☐ No ☐ Yes → HowHighwasyourTemp? ☐☐☐.☐ degrees
HowwasTempTaken?
☐ By Mouth ☐ In Ear
☐ By Rectum ☐ Under Arm
☐ On Forehead ☐ Other

Other Symptoms (Mark all that apply.)

☐ Rash ☐ Diarrhea
☐ Cough ☐ Hoarseness
☐ Nasal Congestion ☐ Pressure in ears
☐ Nasal Drainage ☐ Ear pain
☐ Nausea ☐ Shortness of Breath
☐ Vomiting ☐ Wheezing

Patient's Name ____________

Relationship to Sponsor ____________ Status ______ Rank/Grade ______

Sponsor's Name ____________ Sponsor's SSN ___/___-___-___

Dept/Service ____________ Patient's DOB ____________

Please turn the page over and answer the questions on the back page.

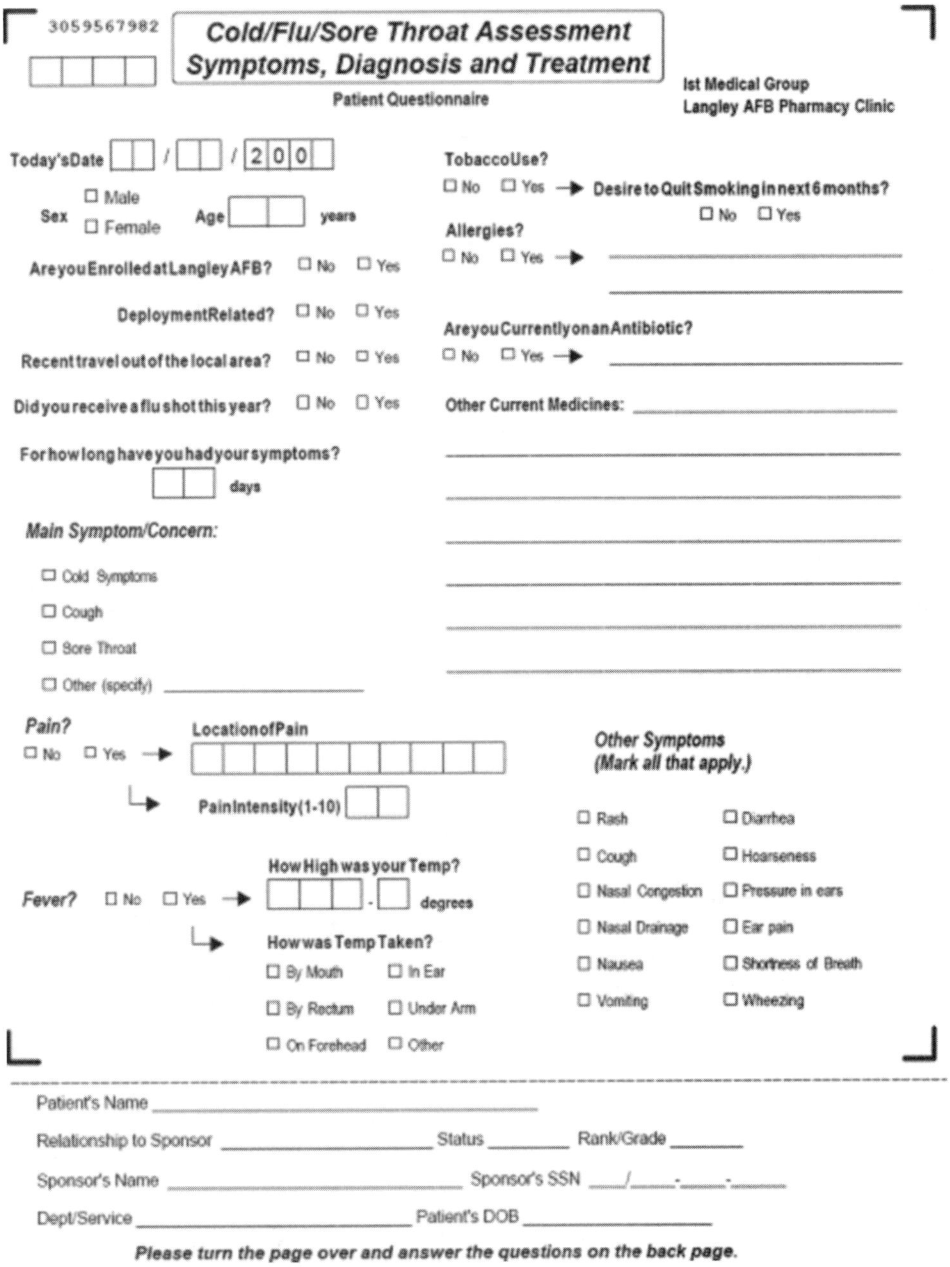

Fig. 9.20 (A and B) Simple patient assessment forms for SAR and URI DIGMAs at 1st Medical Group at Langley Air Force Base

Fig 9.20 (continued)   9674567981

Which of the following medical conditions do you currently have?

☐ Emphysema/COPD   ☐ On Cancer Treatment

☐ Asthma   ☐ On Immunosuppressive Drugs

☐ Diabetes   ☐ History of Rheumatic Fever

☐ HIV/AIDS   ☐ High Blood Pressure

Females: Are you pregnant?   ☐ No   ☐ Yes

Have you had any recent exposure to an illness?   ☐ No   ☐ Yes   →   Describe: _____

_____

Please Place an "X" Near the Appropriate Response: _____

Signs and Symptoms:	For each sign and symptom check one choice from either column that best applies to you.	
Onset	☐ Sudden	☐ Gradual
Fever	☐ High, lasting 3-4 days (over 101°F)	☐ Rare
Cough	☐ Dry, severe	☐ Hacking
Headache	☐ Prominent	☐ Rare
Myalgia (muscle aches & pains)	☐ Usual, often severe	☐ Slight
Tiredness and weakness	☐ Can last up to 2-3 weeks	☐ Very mild
Extreme exhaustion	☐ Early and prominent	☐ Never
Chest discomfort	☐ Common	☐ Mild to moderate
Stuffy nose	☐ Sometimes	☐ Common
Sneezing	☐ Sometimes	☐ Usual
Sore Throat	☐ Sometimes	☐ Common

I UNDERSTAND THAT THIS IS A PHARMACIST RUN GROUP MEDICAL APPOINTMENT IN WHICH OTHERS MAY BECOME FAMILIAR WITH MY MEDICAL CONDITION AND HISTORY. I WILL FOLLOW UP WITH MY PCM IF MY SYMPTOMS CONTINUE OR WORSEN.

Signature of Individual Completing Questionnaire: _____

Table 9.8 Patient satisfaction with pharmacist led SAR and URI (cold/influenza) DIGMAs

Patient Satisfaction Surveys $N = \sim447$ (1 = low, 5 = high)	SAR	URI
1. Access to the pharmacy clinic	4.58	4.44
2. The quality of the interactions with pharmacist in the clinic	4.60	4.67
3. My overall opinion of this pharmacy clinic	4.70	4.67
4. My overall opinion of the quality of care I received	4.75	4.33
5. My experience in a walk-in clinic group appointment	4.80	4.35
6. The amount of time it took me to have a prescription ordered and pick it up	3.85	3.82
7. I would use this clinical pharmacy service again	4.85	4.33

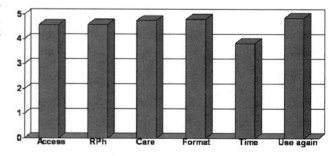

Fig. 9.21 Graph of results from 447 patient satisfaction questionnaires for the SAR and URI DIGMAs. Scale 1 (low) to 5 (high). RPh, pharmacist interaction

Table 9.9 Results of non-pharmacist provider surveys evaluating satisfaction on a 5-point Likert scale with new walk-in pharmacy cold/flu clinic, winter, 2005

This clinic served a need at this medical treatment facility	Average = 4.89
By mildly ill patients being seen in this clinic, additional appointment slots were made available with medical providers for sicker patients	Average = 4.63
The level of care provided by this clinic compared to the standard of care at this MTF	Average = 4.86
I was satisfied with the service provided by this clinic	Average = 4.29
Patients seen in this clinic were appropriately triaged	Average = 4.29
I would like to see this clinic continued	Average = 4.88

Scale: 1 (low) to 5 (high). Number of non-pharmacist providers, $N = 12$.

model's ability to improve access to care. Regularly observing the buddy support of active duty warriors committed to their mission—e.g., talking on chairs in the main hospital lobby while filling out a form or interacting with the team—emphasized another aspect of the model. Commiserating about their frustration of being diminished by a virus or illness for a few days and kept away from duty, they edify each other and encourage each other to heal. This model improved patient care by adding an additional built-in support component to their visit to the MTF that does not always occur in a traditional appointment—and it never occurs at all if they do not seek or receive a timely appointment. It costs nothing and improves quality of care.

Infection Control

By spreading patients out in the main lobby in a controlled manner and making those deemed infectious wear masks,

we improved infection control in the facility. By providing increased access to care, we were able to decrease the spread of infection by placing the infected on quarters and sending them home to rest and recover rather than back to their duty section where the infection could spread and reduce mission readiness. At the same time, the "*working sick*" were in and out quickly and back to the mission.

This Model Can Help All Healthcare Systems Meet Increased Needs for Appointments During the Annual Influenza Season

Development of pharmacist URI DIGMAs can help meet the increased needs that all healthcare systems have for numerous additional medical appointments during the annual influenza epidemic. In addition, it can help train patients to increase optimal use of the existing infrastructure and the distribution capacity of pharmacy networks in the event of a pandemic. Development of URI and SAR DIGMAs can improve access to care while simultaneously addressing some of today's healthcare limitations—and, by doing so, they can help to meet future access challenges facing the U.S. healthcare system.

Our New Lipid DIGMA

In August 2006, we began referring all active duty personnel with hyperlipidemia to a GMA. All patients were mailed a letter (plus received an automated phone call) directing them to their new appointment venue. In doing so, we noted that we needed to invite more than 30 patients in order to have 20 or more show up. We see the Lipid DIGMA as an excellent way to augment

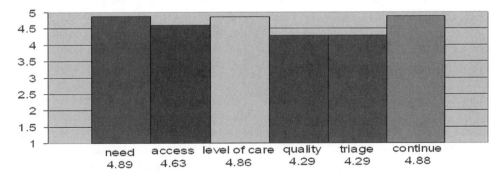

Fig. 9.22 Graph of results of non-pharmacist provider surveys evaluating satisfaction with new Walk-in Pharmacy Cold/Flu Clinic (Winter 2005) at 1st Medical Group at Langley AFB

traditional care; however, participation is voluntary and we do not plan to deny a patient's preference to have a one-on-one appointment with their primary care manager. In our experience, many patients do not regularly have routine follow-up with the same physician thru months or years of treatment anyway, so the Lipid DIGMA works very well for them.

DIGMAs Are an Ideal Venue for Treating Chronic Conditions such As Hyperlipidemia

Hyperlipidemia treatment fits the shared medical appointment venue extremely well. We found that our new Lipid DIGMAs were even better suited for treating high cholesterol than our SAR and URI DIGMAs were for treating acute conditions like seasonal allergic rhinitis, upper respiratory tract infections, and the annual influenza epidemic. Through these group visits, it became possible to avoid repetitively counseling patients individually on lifestyle management—repetition that seems to be a hallmark of the traditional office visit model of care for patients with issues such as high cholesterol. Reviewing the importance of diet and exercise, describing the difference between LDL (*bad cholesterol*) and HDL (*good cholesterol*), and discussing the importance of quitting smoking can all be completed by the pharmacist at one time in the DIGMA setting—i.e., for a dozen or more patients at once. During Lipid DIGMA sessions, patients are given an individual assessment of their cholesterol goal, their medical and medication histories are taken, and their blood pressure is screened.

Our Lipid DIGMA Program Has Grown, and Patient and Provider Satisfaction Are High

Our patient (N = 289) and provider (N = 6) surveys (Figs. 9.23 and 9.24) showed that this is rapidly becoming both a provider and patient preferred way of treating high cholesterol. Our group clinic expanded as referrals increased. We began using a conference room in the 1st Fighter Wing clinic in the NASA Langley Research Center. To improve access to care in the NASA clinic, we began treating retirees and family members of active duty personnel via shared medical appointments. Results of patient satisfaction surveys showed that both active duty and retiree patients accepted this new appointment format (Fig. 9.23).

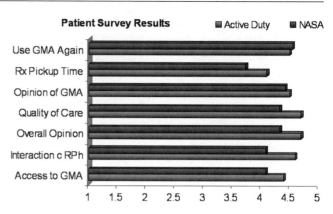

Fig. 9.23 Results of patient satisfaction survey conducted on Lipid DIGMA program at 1st Medical Group at Langley AFB

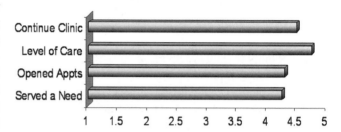

Fig. 9.24 Results of provider survey evaluating satisfaction with our Lipid DIGMA program at 1st Medical Group at Langley AFB

Methodology

We performed a detailed medication use analysis of all active duty patients identified with an assigned ICD code for dyslipidemia (272.0–272.9) between January 1, 2005 and December 31, 2005 to assess the level of medication non-adherence. 716 patients were identified and 348 of these patients were on a cholesterol lowering medication. Patients on a cholesterol medication were taking an average of 3.5 prescription medications, including non-cholesterol lowering medications. 81.8% of the patients taking a cholesterol lowering medication were taking a HMG-CoA reductase inhibitor, often called a "statin". 94.8% of the patients were male.

Medication adherence was defined and assessed four ways: Medication Possession Ratio (MPR); Length of Therapy (LOT); Persistency Rate; and Median Gap Analysis. MPR shows the percentage of days a patient has the medication they should be taking every day. LOT is the sum of medication days supplied for a patient being treated for a new episode of care. Persistency rate shows the number of patients remaining on a medication at specific time points after therapy was started—i.e., 3 months, 6 months, 12 months, etc. Median Gap Analysis is the median number of days that the patient should have run out of a medication and the actual fill date of the subsequent refill.

Results

We turn now to the results of the data analysis of our Lipid DIGMA program. In patients that we had complete data to evaluate, the average MPR for patients on statin therapy was 80% (with the range being 9–100). 41% of patients had a MPR of <80%. The median gap analysis of patients taking a statin was 15.5 days. The average LOT for a patient on a statin was 291 days. The persistency rate for a patient on a statin was 98% at 3 months, 94% at 6 month, 83% at 9 months, and 69% at 1 year. The persistency rate for fibrates at 1 year was 49% and niacin at 1 year was 38%. It was clear from these results that, with traditional medical appointments, in terms of money spent on prescription medications and pharmacy efforts, drug therapy was not optimized in our hyperlipidemia population.

A primary target in the treatment of high cholesterol is low-density lipoprotein (LDL) goal attainment. Prior to the use of a Lipid DIGMA, our LDL goal attainment was 76% for a patient with a goal of <160 mg/dl, 45% for <130 mg/dl, 30% for <100 mg/dl and 13% for <70 mg/dl. The literature has shown that percent decreases in LDL may equate linearly with a percent decreases in morbidity and mortality.

Six months after we began our Lipid DIGMA we reassessed the MPR, median gap analysis, and LDL goal attainment in the patients we treated in our lipid DIGMA. The average MPR, available on our patient assessment form to aid in developing treatment plans (Form 2), improved to 99% in our Lipid DIGMA patients. The median gap analysis improved to 2.3 days. LDL goal attainment improved to 84% for a <160 mg/dl goal, 75 % for <130 mg/dl, 50 %< 100 mg/dl, and stayed at 13 % for <70 mg/dl (Fig. 9.25). In addition, the mean LDL cholesterol for patients treated in our lipid DIGMA was reduced from 138.3 mg/dl in August of 2006 to 124.0 mg/dl in January of 2006. Our findings have shown that, along with improving access to care (and patient and provider satisfaction with care), a DIGMA can improve a patient's medication use, treatment outcomes, and efficiency of healthcare. *(Note: Carl Tullio PharmD and John Ostrosky PharmD assisted with data analysis and graphs.)*

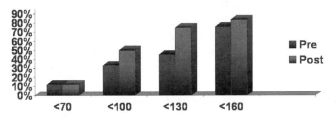

Fig. 9.25 LDL cholesterol goal attainment pre- and post-DIGMA at 1st Medical Group at Langley AFB

The Business Case for Group Visits

Our lipid DIGMA varies in attendance (range, 5–34). When fully staffed and with good attendance, we were able to see an average of 22 patients during 90 minutes of a day. By doing this 4 days a week, we were able to free up 440 individual appointments per month (and 5280 appointments per year) through our Lipid DIGMA program—thereby improving access to care for all other conditions. This represents a dramatic increase in capacity, and is achieved solely through our lipid DIGMA program and use of existing staffing and facilities resources. We have had over 700 patient referrals to date. The lipid DIGMA is open year round, which helps in familiarizing patients, students, and staff with the format.

DIGMAs Can Help Busy Pharmacies Provide Medication Therapy Management to Improve Outcomes from Drug Therapy

Group medical appointments can provide an effective way for more busy pharmacies to provide Medication Therapy Management (MTM), a distinct service or group of services that optimizes therapeutic outcomes for individual patients. MTM services are independent of, but can occur in conjunction with, the provision of a medication product. MTM services include: assessment of a patient's health status; formulating a medication treatment plan; monitoring a patients response to drug therapy; performing a comprehensive medication review (to identify, resolve, and prevent medication-related problems); and providing education and information.

Since January 2006, the American Medical Association's Current Procedural Terminology (CPT) Editorial Panel has approved three CPT billing codes for pharmacists to use for billing third-party payors when providing MTM services. The codes can be used to bill any health plan that provides MTM services, including those covered under Medicare Part D prescription drug benefit. Third party payors will individually determine the reimbursement rates and criteria for MTM services. The DIGMA group medical appointment format may allow busy dispensing pharmacies to provide MTM services to improve patient outcomes from drug therapy. Furthermore, the increasing availability of electronic medical records in pharmacies will likely increase the opportunities for collaborative practice with pharmacists.

Conclusion

We have been very pleased with the increased service to patients and improved clinical outcomes that we are achieving through our SAR, URI, and Lipid DIGMA group programs—especially because it occurs in a format that is satisfying to patients and providers alike. Anticipated future demands upon our healthcare system—driven by an aging American population in need of more medical appointments coupled with fewer healthcare providers to take care of them—increases my advocacy of group medical appointments. Today's practitioners must develop and implement new techniques now—and immediately begin training students and new practitioners in these methods—in order to prepare healthcare workers for the practice environment they will be working in, and responsible for, during the coming decades.

Study 16: Use of Physicals Shared Medical Appointments for Heart Failure Patients

This study will be of interest to the reader because it demonstrates how the PSMA model can be used in a heart failure clinic to reduce hospitalizations among this costly high-risk patient population, while simultaneously achieving high levels of patient satisfaction and enhancing other outcomes as well—such as improved medication utilization, increased use of cardiac rehabilitation services, improved compliance with lifestyle recommendations, decreased depression, and enhanced quality of life. This study was submitted by Andrew H. Lin, M.D., Jeffrey J. Cavendish, M.D., and Daniel F. Seidensticker, M.D. from the Department of Internal Medicine and Division of Cardiology at the Naval Medical Center San Diego in San Diego, California.[*]

Background

The American Heart Association estimates that it costs the United States over $28 billion a year for the treatment of heart failure (21). This disease is complex and multi-factorial, requiring the services of multiple medical

[*]Disclaimer: The views expressed in this article are those of the authors and do not reflect the official policy or position of the Department of the Navy, Department of Defense, or the United States Government.

disciplines: pharmacy; psychiatry; nursing; physical therapy; nutrition; social work; and physicians. It is well established that a multi-disciplinary approach improves results and outcomes in these patients (22,23), so the Cardiology Department at the Naval Medical Center San Diego (NMCSD) set about to establish such a clinic.

Need and Rationale

The physical layout, clinic manpower, and logistics made a traditional individual-appointment model impractical and inefficient. First, the clinic consisted of seven staff cardiologists, with each staff physician having only one exam room. Because of the lack of physical exam room space, it would have been physically impossible for each patient to be seen individually by the multi-disciplinary team in an efficient amount of time. Second, the clinic usually has two corpsmen checking in patients, obtaining vital signs, and performing ECGs in a central "vital signs room." On a typical day, the clinic only has three registered nurses who also act as the clinic director, conscious sedation nurses, and patient relation representatives. Although one nurse could be dedicated to a traditional heart failure clinic, the standard check-in process and lack of exam-room space greatly limit the potential efficiency of such a clinic.

Therefore, in order to use a traditional model for a heart failure clinic, the physician clinic schedules would have needed to be rescheduled—and 30-minute appointments would have needed to be created in order for the other disciplines to teach each patient individually. This would have created an inefficient and labor-intensive clinic that would not have survived. There were many challenges in establishing this clinic with this particular format. The primary challenge was overcoming the inertia of the traditional model. At NMCSD, both physicians and patients had no experience with group medical visits for such chronic conditions. Fortunately, our leadership gave us great latitude to pilot this project. For the Physicals Shared Medical Appointment (PSMA) heart failure clinic to work, at least four patients are needed for it to be efficient and useful. The clinic originally started with an initial recruitment of 20 patients to be able to support a minimum of three clinics.

We Used the Physicals SMA Model

In 2004, the Cardiology Department at the NMCSD started a heart failure clinic using Dr. Noffsinger's Physicals Shared Medical Appointment (PSMA) model. The

NMCSD PSMA heart failure clinic was based upon this model as utilized by Drs. Bronson and Maxwell at Cleveland Clinic (24).

The heart failure patient is a very complicated patient with polypharmacy needs and multiple co-morbidities. In the PSMA format, multiple complicated decisions have to be made by the physician in front of a group of patients; therefore, easy to follow, space efficient flow sheets and documentation were created for the patient chart.

Another important aspect to this clinic was working with the coders to make sure appropriate documentation and maximum credit was recorded for the clinic. It was initially difficult and complicated for nutrition and mental health to maximally code for each appointment.

Finally, with the current Navy operational requirements, all areas of the hospital have had people deployed overseas. Not only have there been multiple physicians participating in this clinic, but there have been many different pharmacists, nurses, and nutritionists attending this clinic. This format takes time to develop a comfort level that allows for rapid succinct dissemination of information to our patients.

Goals

Numerous studies have shown that multi-disciplinary heart failure clinics work, but none have used the PSMA format. The cardiology department set up a PSMA heart failure clinic with the goal to reduce re-hospitalization rates, increase ACE inhibitor and beta-blocker use, and improve diet and medication compliance.

Methodology and Flow

The program was designed to incorporate two 90-minute PSMAs each week. In each session, six to eight patients are scheduled. The appointments begin with each patient checking in at the front desk, where vital signs are taken. The patients then congregate in a conference room, where their medication lists and focused histories are recorded by a RN and a corpsman on standard forms designed specifically for the heart failure clinic. Afterward, the physician takes each patient back to a private exam room for a focused physical exam. Upon returning to the conference room, a pharmacist, psychologist, and nutritionist are present to provide further individual instruction before beginning the group session.

Once all of the exams are completed, all of the patients and the multidisciplinary team start the group discussion. The physician discusses each individual's assessment and plan, while incorporating input from the other medical providers. During these discussions, important general concepts concerning heart failure—such as monitoring daily weights, recognition of symptoms, depression, and side effects of medications—are always reviewed. These discussions are always open-ended, and the patients are invited to participate in the discussion and to give advice, support, and encouragement. The questions often lead to more in-depth discussions concerning such topics as end-of-life issues, sexual dysfunction, and stress management.

During the discussion, the patients' labs and medication changes and renewals are ordered in the computer, follow-up appointments are scheduled, and sheets with written instructions are given to the patients. This whole process should take 2 hours. We do two sessions every Friday morning, and see 12–14 patients each morning.

Patients

Patients are eligible for the heart failure clinic if they met one of the following criteria: NYHA class III or IV symptoms at initial presentation; history of multiple heart failure admissions; specific high-maintenance needs; or aggressive initiation or titration of target medications with cardiomyopathy (Table 9.10). Patients with either diastolic or systolic heart failure could participate. However, prior to enrolling, each patient would have to agree to the open group discussion format of the PSMA, which includes filling out a confidentiality waiver and appropriate Health Insurance Portability and Accountability Act (HIPAA) paperwork.

Table 9.10 Eligibility for PSMA heart failure clinic

Any one of the below criteria*:

1) NYHA class III or IV heart failure symptoms at initial presentation
2) History of multiple heart failure admissions
3) Specific high-maintenance needs
4) Aggressive initiation or titration of target medications with cardiomyopathy

* To qualify for the PSMA heart failure clinic, patients must meet at least one of these criteria.

Measures

Prior to each patient's initial visit, prospective surveys and indexes on depression, left ventricular dysfunction, self-care management, and health partnership were measured. At completion of 6 months, these same surveys were re-mailed to the patients. The first survey completed was a NMCSD cardiology clinic produced survey which was called the Heart Failure Clinic Satisfaction Survey. The rest of the surveys used were validated indexes: The Left Ventricular Dysfunction-36 Questionnaire; The Self-Care Management Index; The Beck Depression Inventory; and the Health Partnership Scale. Other performance measures, such as hospitalization rates, ACE inhibitor use, and beta-blocker use were also measured.

Demographics

The demographics of the patient population were an average age of 73 years and over 73% males. Over 40% of the patients were between the ages of 76 and 85 years old, with the oldest patient being 90 years old. Approximately 70% of the patients were Caucasian, 9% African American, 9% Asian/Pacific Islander, and 6% Hispanic. Over 60% were married, 17% widowed, and 11% divorced. The average ejection fraction (EF) was 33%, with only five patients with diastolic dysfunction (EF >40%). Over 58% of the patients had New York Heart Association Class III or IV symptoms (Table 9.11).

Table 9.11 Demographics of patients attending the PSMA heart failure clinic

Mean age (yrs)	73
Males	78%
Average ejection fraction	33%
Systolic dysfunction (EF <40%)	28/33

Results

Many important results were demonstrated. In addition to high levels of patient satisfaction, several positive clinical outcomes were demonstrated in this Heart Failure Clinic PSMA study: reduced hospitalizations; improved medication utilization; increased use of cardiac rehabilitation services; improved compliance with lifestyle recommendations; reduced depression; and enhanced quality of life.

Patient Satisfaction Was High

By February 2005, over 56 patients had been enrolled into the program with 33 patients having completed

6 months. The 6-month data for the heart failure clinic were recently submitted for publication in the Mayo Clinic Proceedings. Of the patients to have completed at least 6 months, it was noted that 96% felt the "the group visit format was more educational than a regular cardiology visit" and "the time frame for the group visit was satisfactory." All patients felt that "the discussions about each patient's health and treatment plan was helpful in understanding my own condition and plan," "it was beneficial to have members of a multidisciplinary team present," "time spent with me individually was adequate," and "the time spent in the Heart Failure Clinic was worthwhile" (Table 9.12).

Table 9.12 Percentage of patients responding "agree" or "strongly agree" to each item on the patient satisfaction questionnaire

	Percentage (%)
The group visit format was more educational than a regular cardiology visit.	96
The time frame for the group visit was satisfactory.	96
The discussion about each patient's health and treatment plan was helpful in understanding my own condition and plan.	100
It was beneficial to have members of a multidisciplinary team present during heart failure clinic.	100
The time spent with me individually was adequate.	100
The educational material is valuable in learning about heart failure.	100
The time spent in the heart failure clinic was worthwhile.	100
I was overall satisfied with the heart failure clinic.	100

Improved Clinical Outcomes—Reduced Hospitalizations

One of the most powerful results from the Heart Failure PSMA has been a decreased number of hospitalizations. By comparing inpatient records for the 6-month period prior to the 6-month period after enrollment, the Heart Failure PSMA was able to decrease admissions for all causes from eleven to eight. In addition, admissions for heart failure alone decreased from four to two. Although 12-month data are not available at the time of publication, our data continue to show significant decreases in readmission rates.

Improved Clinical Outcomes—Improved Medication Utilization, Program Attendance, Compliance, and Quality of Life

The use of ACE inhibitors increased from 77 to 96%, while the use of beta-blockers increased from 73 to 93%. The number of patients participating in a cardiac rehabilitation program increased from 7 to 42%. The survey and index questionnaires showed significant improvements in patient symptoms to include less fatigue, exhaustion, and limitations to activities of daily living. Patients reported improved compliance with daily weights (55 to 80%), diet (70 to 90%), and exercising three times weekly (47 to 70%). Patients also expressed increased "hope for the future," interest in sex, and decreased feelings of sadness. Clinical depression decreased from 77 to 48%, and all patients felt the format to be more "educational and an appropriate use of their time" (Table 9.13).

Table 9.13 Improved outcomes data from the heart failure physical shared medical appointment vs. traditional care

↓ ACE inhibitor use	77 – 96%
↓ Beta-blocker use	73 – 93%
↓ Cardiac rehabilitation participation	7 – 42%
↓ Compliance with daily weights	55 – 88%
↓ Compliance with diet	70 – 90%
↓ Exercising three times weekly	47 – 70%
↓ Clinical depression	77 – 48%

Discussion

Perhaps the greatest testament to impact of the clinic has been the establishment of other group medical visits in the hospital. Rheumatology and endocrinology have both started group clinics modeled after the heart failure clinic, while a new tobacco cessation clinic has been established using a different group visit model. The physicians involved in these clinics have expressed great personal satisfaction at the level of comprehensive care they have been able to provide to some of their sickest patients.

Personal Observations—Dr. Seidensticker

Participating in the heart failure clinic is the highlight of my week. It is gratifying seeing patients walk in to clinic when they initially were wheeled into the clinic. It is invigorating to hear people talk about trips to Las Vegas that before were only dreams, and endearing to hear how a patient adjusted his lasix after eating out at a restaurant. Likewise, helping patients move into a hospice program and having a peaceful death with their family present is no less satisfying.

The group medical visit has shown me how clearly inadequate the individual appointment model is for treating such complex patients. Ten- to twenty-minute appointments with an individual provider simply cannot meet the needs of these sick, symptomatic patients.

By participating in this format, I have learned so much from the nutritionists, pharmacists, and mental health providers. After listening to the patients and the group discussions, I have also gained a whole new level of appreciation for the complexity of heart failure and its impact on every aspect of life for these patients.

Conclusion

The Physicals Shared Medical Appointment is a proven model that has been used effectively in other chronic disease processes; however, it has not previously been employed and studied in a heart failure clinic setting. This small pilot project at NMCSD highlights the benefits a PSMA can have to improve medication compliance, enhance utilization of services, make positive lifestyle changes, and—most importantly—reduce hospitalizations.

Study 17: Going from Good to Great: Using Group Medical Care to Change Healthcare Outcomes

The following contribution was received from James B. Sutton, RPA-C, Director of Clinton Family Health Center in Rochester, New York (a large outpatient Medicare and Medicaid provider in the Rochester area). He serves as Adjunct Clinical Faculty for the Rochester Institute of Technology (RIT) Physician Assistant Program and precepts PA students in Family Medicine. He has been the Director of Clinton Family Health Center since 2006.

This write-up will be of interest to readers because it demonstrates the remarkable benefit that even severely backlogged and overloaded healthcare systems can realize when they simultaneously launch Open Access (or Advance Clinic Access, ACA) and well-designed shared medical appointments (SMAs) in their system—i.e., even if there is considerable initial skepticism and push-back from staff to these progressive ideas. Although consistent with the findings of other systems, the outcomes data here are remarkable because they reflect what properly designed and run SMA models can do in the public health sector for serving the poor and underserved.

For me, it was singularly gratifying to see my DIGMA and PSMA models being used in such a special manner—i.e., not only in reaching out to the underserved and in overcoming the treatment challenges posed by this unique patient population, but also in delivering a modality of care that effectively and efficiently met their medical needs—and with both high levels of patient satisfaction and reduced no-show rates. Mr. Sutton points out that, as a result of the SMA and ACA programs they instituted in their community health center, the number of diabetics in their practice that are at ADA goals on their hemoglobin A1c and LDL-cholesterol has actually doubled. In addition, patient no-show rates have dropped from approximately 50% to less than 5%. A further result of the SMA and ACA programs they instituted has been a substantial drop in the average HbA1c levels of the center's diabetic patients—which dropped from 8.5 to 7.4 between 2003 and 2006. Much of this improvement is attributed to group medical visits and use of the Institute of Healthcare Improvement's chronic care model.

A Growing Problem

Clinton Family Health Center (CFHC) is a Community Health Center located in a predominantly Hispanic area of Rochester, New York. In this area, some 50,000 people face enormous obstacles, including poor health. With a median household income below $22,000, 35% of residents in this Northeast section of Rochester live in poverty. The acuity of medical conditions and frequency of hospital admissions for patients in this part of an otherwise progressive Upstate city was alarming.

Two major studies of the area (1998 and 2001) showed growing health disparities. Residents were 20 to 50% more likely to be hospitalized for diabetes, asthma, and hypertension than those living in the city as a whole, and four to five times more likely to end up in a hospital bed for these conditions than nearby suburbanites. Prior to redesigning its delivery system, CFHC (owned and operated by Rochester General Hospital) was plagued by low show rates for appointments, poor health outcomes, and the lack of continuity of care since patients were seen utilizing a traditional "clinic" model. The center, though, had the potential to make an impact. Patients who sought healthcare at the center were mostly Hispanic (86%); walked to their appointment (53%); and (of greatest importance) were most likely to get all their healthcare needs at that facility only (70%). Therefore, the effect of the any redesign of the delivery system at CFHC would be felt directly by the community that the center served.

In November 2003, CFHC undertook an ambitious and aggressive approach, and totally redesigned the way care was delivered in an effort to reduce these health disparities. The innovations that were imbedded within the redesign, such as open access scheduling and group medical care, were in some ways counterintuitive to traditional healthcare delivery—and were initially met with skepticism and frank disbelief by the center's providers and staff.

A Possible Solution

It was hypothesized that, if patients living in this impoverished area had full open access to their primary care provider, emergency room visits would decrease. Then, through the redesign of the health center's delivery system, better chronic disease management would ensue and lead to better patient self-management. The group medical visit was the critical component of this new delivery system at the health center. The combination of better access, better continuity of care, and better chronic disease management was believed to be a solution to these growing health disparities. These innovations, in total, had the potential of affecting thousands of lives in the community.

The redesign involved four major areas of change over a 2-year period of time: multidisciplinary teams; open access; IHI's chronic care model, and group visits.

Team Formation

Teams were formed that consisted of a provider, nurse, and secretary. A panel of patients was assigned to that team, and all patient care and patient matters were handled by the team members. This both personalized care and increased continuity of care.

Open Access

With open access, all patients requesting care received a same-day appointment, no matter the person's ailment or request. Each morning, all the providers in the building started their day with an empty schedule—and then built their schedule with the phone calls that came in that day. Patients were seen the same day of their phone call regardless of whether they had an acute problem, required routine follow-up, or needed a physical. Thus, nurse triage was eliminated because acute problems did not have to be overbooked on top of routine care. This provided patients unfettered, full open access to their primary care provider regardless of their request for care.

Chronic Care Model

All elements of the Institute for Healthcare Improvement's (IHI.org) chronic care model were instilled into daily practice. Staff met weekly to discuss patient care and plan better care for their patients. Chronic disease prevention was embedded into daily practice. Preventive care was provided to every patient during every visit, regardless of the reason for the visit.

Group Medical Visits

Providers began seeing patients with chronic illnesses in groups instead of individually for their routine follow-up appointments. Instead of seeing one patient after another with the same condition in separate rooms (and answering the same question over and over again), 10–15 patients with the same condition were brought in at the same time for their follow-up care—and were seen in a group room for a DIGMA for one and a half hours. Patients did not undress or divulge private matters and, if they wanted personal time with the provider, they could have that time toward the end of the group visit. The theme of the group visit consisted of the various aspects of the chronic medical condition the patients came for that day. If the condition was diabetes, then the whole time was spent discussing diabetes and delivering individualized care to each of the attendees.

Patients who joined the groups for their care loved them, and most wanted to continue their chronic disease management in a group setting. Medical providers at CFHC began to discover the joy of extended interaction with a group of their patients—and the opportunity to teach their patients more about their disease. The group visit model led to better disease self-management by patients at the facility.

Data Tracking

First by paper and pencil, and later by computer, patients' hemoglobin A1c, blood pressure, LDL cholesterol, attendance, and overall sense of well-being were tracked. Tracking was vital to show others in the community if the changes we had implemented were having any impact on health disparities—plus, to also assist in the spread of successful ideas through the collection of evidence-based data.

Putting It All Together

Clinton Family Health Center has utilized open access scheduling since January 2004. Shortly thereafter,

CFHC began a homogeneous version of the DIGMA for patients with diabetes. What makes it a DIGMA is the sequential individualized medical care being delivered to each patient individually throughout the group session. The patients attending these groups did so with the same group of patients over a 2 year period of time. [Note from Dr. Noffsinger: Although a DIGMA is typically open to many or most patients in a physician's practice or in a chronic disease management program—and usually has different patients attending each session—the same group of patients can be followed over time in a DIGMA although, in this case, sessions would typically not meet daily or weekly and would usually meet say monthly or quarterly instead (i.e., according to best practices and when patients have an actual medical need for being seen). The main point is that DIGMAs are run like a series of individual office visits with observers from start to finish, and are therefore a series of one doctor–one patient interactions attending to each patient's unique medical needs individually.]

Every time I get enough patients (say 10–16) to start another group, I usually start another Diabetes DIGMA. We typically meet monthly for 9 months, then quarterly for 6–9 months, and then twice a year thereafter as this is a chronic disease that will require lifelong care. Since then, group care for other chronic diseases has been instituted as well. In 2006, the more traditional heterogeneous DIGMA model, that is not disease specific, was also started at the center. In 2007, CFHC added OB/GYN care at the facility and began delivering prenatal care in groups.

Patients receiving care at CFHC were tracked for 2 years prior to the implementation of these changes and have been continually tracked since that time. Patient satisfaction, practice growth, arrival rates, access, and medical outcomes have been the key markers followed. The most studied chronic illness at the facility has been diabetes since it is the most common and most complex chronic illness at the center.

Results—Better Access

Prior to open access scheduling, only 50% of scheduled patients arrived for their appointments. With the open access model, the show rate at the center has remained above 95% since January 2004 (Fig. 9.26). All established patients that seek care at CFHC are given appointments on the day that they call, regardless of the reason for the appointment. An industry standard used to measure the maximum time a patient has to wait for an appointment is the third next available long appointment. CFHC has established and maintained a waiting time of zero days

Fig. 9.26 The show rate at the Clinton Family Health Center, Rochester, NY

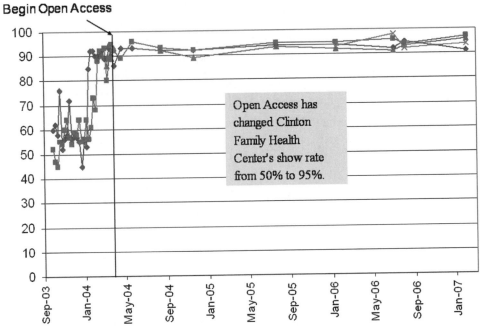

for the third next long appointment since instituting the new open access scheduling system (Fig. 9.27). In 2004, as a result of open access, there was a 24% decline in all emergency room visits, and a 30% decrease in the number of patients going to the emergency room for non-urgent care. For a variety of reasons, CFHC has not been able to sustain or replicate this dramatic decrease in emergency room visits in the years since, but continues to study ER visits for patients registered at the facility and continues to explore the effect of open access scheduling on such visits.

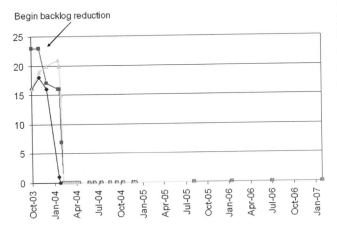

Fig. 9.27 Number of days until third available long office visit at the Clinton Family Health Center

Results—Better Clinical Outcomes

The number of diabetics in the practice that are at ADA goals on their hemoglobin A1c and LDL-cholesterol has doubled (Fig. 9.28) as a result of our ACA and DIGMA

programs. The average hemoglobin A1c of the center's diabetics has dropped from 8.5 to 7.4 between 2003 and 2006 (Fig. 9.29). Many of these improvements can be attributed to group medical visits and use of the chronic care model.

The social component and peer support that the DIGMA has over a traditional individual visit is often the key to success. Patients receiving care in a DIGMA have an opportunity to see (in a nonjudgmental way) how their medical care and self-management compares to that of another patient with the same disease. Medical providers are often afraid (or shy away from) such intense patient-to-patient interaction, but, in our experience, patients prefer to openly discuss their condition and treatment in a group setting and do not seem to share the fears that providers sometimes have about group care. At some point in a DIGMA there is always a *moment of truth* when one patient leans over and sees the hemoglobin A1c of another patient and says "Wow!" The effect of that *wow* on both the patient with a normal A1c and the patient with an abnormal A1c cannot be overstated.

Results—Better Patient Satisfaction

Many say that practice growth is a sign of patient satisfaction. In fact it is commonly said that patients vote with their feet. Within 6 months of CFHC changing the way care was delivered, the facility had to shut down to new patients until more personnel could be hired to

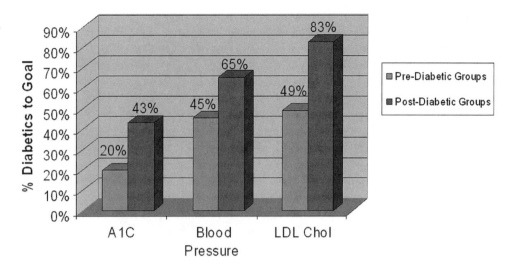

Fig. 9.28 Clinton Family Health Center diabetic groups' percentage of diabetics to goal (as of January 2007)

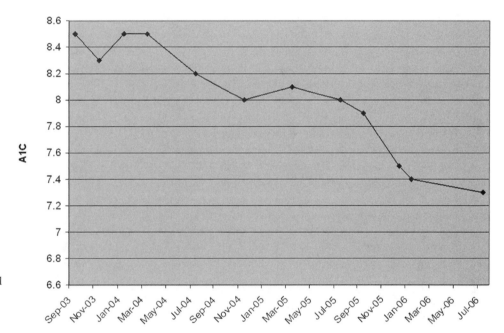

Fig. 9.29 Average HbA1c of all diabetic patients at Clinton Family Health Center from 2003 to 2006

accommodate the rapid growth. Since opening to new patients in June 2005, the center has had an increasing number of new patient requests. In fact, just having as many patients wanting to join a practice now as the month before would be great. However, in the case of CFHC, each month brings even more requests to transfer care to the center than the month before (Fig. 9.30). This growth shows that patients are drawn to the new delivery system design. Even within the medical practices that Rochester General Hospital owns and operates in the Northeast section of Rochester, CFHC is outpacing others for growth (Fig. 9.31).

In late 2006, a leading insurance carrier in the region, Monroe Plan for Medical Care, looked at patient satisfaction at the largest outpatient Medicaid providers in the

Rochester area. Their results showed that CFHC led in overall satisfaction (Fig. 9.32). Rochester General Hospital has recognized these changes. The unprecedented patient growth rate at our facility has led the hospital to double our operating space in 2006. Data from CFHC has inspired other health centers regionally and nationally to adopt similar changes.

Conclusion

Clinton Family Health Center has demonstrated that the triad of team formation, open access scheduling, and group medical care can significantly change medical outcomes and decrease health disparities.

Fig. 9.30 Clinton Family
Health Center new patients
entering the practice per quarter

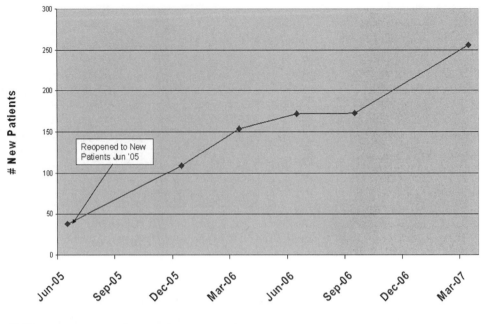

Fig. 9.31 Percentage of new
patients entering Rochester
General Hospital practices in
2006. CFHC, Clinton Family
Health Center

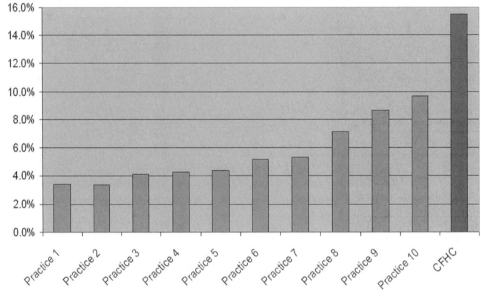

Fig. 9.32 Monroe Plan
member perception of overall
quality (fall 2006). CFHC,
Clinton Family Health Center

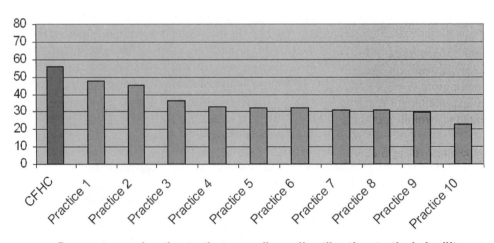

From Good to Great

In 2006, U.S. Department of Health and Human Services Secretary Michael Leavitt said "this ambitious project has yielded impressive results since its inception in 2003." The facility has been recognized locally and nationally for the changes it has undertaken, and the resulting positive outcomes. Clinton Family Health Center was one of only nine programs nationally that received the 2006 Department of Health and Human Services "Innovation in Prevention Award," and was the sole winner in the Healthcare Delivery category. The center also received the 2007 HANYS (Health Association of New York State) "Community Health Improvement Award," and again was the sole winner among all programs in New York State.

This is an example of how an average Community Health Center can transform itself *from good to great* through the use of progressive ideas such as group medical care. We did it, and so can you—plus have some fun in the process.

Study 18: Two Previously Unpublished Outcomes Studies at ProMed Healthcare

The following two outcomes studies, which have not been published elsewhere, were provided by Dr. Ed Millermaier, MD, MBA (Chief Medical Officer, Ambulatory Care, Borgess Health and Medical Director of ProMed Healthcare in Kalamazoo, Michigan) for publication in this book. These are interesting and important studies because they underscore how DIGMAs and PSMAs can be successfully employed to: (1) significantly enhance the likelihood of consistently updating screening tests, performance measures, and routine health maintenance for chronically ill patients in attendance (in this case, diabetic patients); and (2) improve clinical outcomes for diabetic patients attending DIGMAs and PSMAs (as shown in the second study).

With regards to the second study, I found it particularly interesting that—for all clinical outcomes that were measured—the trend in every case was for SMA patients to outperform those receiving usual one-on-one office care, even when the results were not statistically significant. The reader will also find another interesting component to Dr. Millermaier's contribution to this book—i.e., an innovative approach taken at ProMed that permits 10 women's health physicals to be delivered during a single 90-minute Physicals SMA session (and with high levels of patient satisfaction), but which only requires 60 minutes of the patients' time. I then close this section of the chapter by briefly referencing other reports that cite improved clinical outcomes for chronically ill patients (typically patients with diabetes) who attend group visits as opposed to traditional office visit care.

Shared Appointments at ProMed Healthcare

Shared medical appointments at Borgess Health's ProMed Healthcare, a medium sized (predominantly primary care) multispecialty group with 59 physicians and 34 non-physician providers in Kalamazoo Michigan, began in February 2003. Dr. Noffsinger's Drop-In Group Medical Appointment (DIGMA) and Physicals Shared Medical Appointment (Physicals SMA, PSMA, or Shared Physicals) group visit models were the two group visit models selected for use. DIGMAs and PSMAs were chosen for two primary reasons: (1) because they have been shown to dramatically improve both physician productivity and access to busy, backlogged physicians' practices; and (2) because they have been successfully employed in many other fee-for-service systems like our own.

Many of Our Physicians Run DIGMAs and/or PSMAs

During the week that we initially launched our shared medical appointment (SMA) program, eight primary care physicians (family practitioners and internists), including approximately one-third of the largest family practice group, began with weekly 90-minute DIGMAs and/or PSMAs for their practices—some running just a DIGMA, others a PSMA, and still others choosing to run both. As clinic demands and providers have changed over time, additional providers have been added and subtracted as the SMA program has evolved. Now that we are 4 years into our SMA program, we currently have nine different primary care providers running shared medical appointments for their practices. As our SMA program has evolved, it has expanded to include disease specific, homogeneous DIGMAs as well as the traditional heterogeneous and mixed DIGMAs—plus Physicals SMAs that we have been running from the start.

Our Goals Have Always Been to Improve Quality, Access, and the Bottom Line

The initial motivation for instituting SMAs was to improve access, augment the system of care, and improve quality. In addition, when good census is maintained in the groups, SMAs also make good business sense by improving the bottom line.

In Less than a Year, Access Improved Dramatically

With regards to access for traditional individual office visits in our SMA physicians' practices, prior to beginning our SMA program, the third available appointments for physicals were 12 weeks out and return appointments were 5 weeks out. Within 10 months of instituting the SMA program, the availability of third available appointments in the SMA physicians' practices at ProMed was reduced to just 10 days or less for both physicals and return appointments. Furthermore, as is always the case for weekly heterogeneous DIGMAs, return appointments are promptly available in the group any week that patients have a medical need and want to be seen.

Therefore, even when individual return appointments within the clinic might not be available for 2 weeks or more, return appointments are virtually always available in the heterogeneous DIGMA group setting every week (i.e., within 1–5 days). In addition, there is almost always an available physical examination appointment that can be arranged in the PSMA within 2–3 weeks or less—even though an individual physical examination appointment might not be available in the clinic for several weeks or months.

Improved Screening Test and Outcomes Are a Major Focus

In every case, close attention is paid to measurable disease management outcomes—both for the percentage of patients getting their screening tests, injections, and health maintenance, and for actual clinical outcomes. Here at ProMed, outcomes are tracked in asthma, hypertension, heart failure, obesity, and diabetes. A check list of screening tests, injections, health maintenance, and outcome measures is used to assess gaps in care prior to the SMA visit. Where appropriate, the gaps are closed by the appropriate member of the care team during each and every SMA visit. Most often, this is done by the nurse specialist attached to the DIGMA or PSMA. Because they represent a multidisciplinary team-based approach to care, a major advantage of DIGMAs and PSMAs over traditional office visits is that they provide real, meaningful help to the physician. For example, it is not unusual for a provider to enter into a SMA at Borgess ProMed Healthcare to find that all of the patients have had an immunization provided, a diabetic management screen accomplished, and/or an appropriate preventive health screen ordered.

Although some benefits come from the group setting itself (e.g., reduced repetition and overbooking sessions to compensate for no-shows and late-cancels), it is primarily this off-loading of physician responsibilities onto less costly members of the care delivery team—i.e., whenever possible and appropriate—that so dramatically increases our physicians' productivity in the SMA setting. It is simply built into the nursing protocol for the SMA to have all appropriate injections, routine health maintenance, and disease management protocols updated during each and every SMA visit. In this way, the nurse attached to the DIGMA or PSMA can ensure that these nursing functions are consistently conducted on all patients in attendance.

To Optimize Productivity, Physicians Must Delegate Fully to the SMA Team

As just discussed, it is by maximizing the nurse's role (and then consistently off-loading onto the nurse such things as updating injections, health maintenance, and performance measures) that physicians are then able to focus on those elements of care that are unique to them and which they alone can do. It is by fully delegating to the multidisciplinary team that physician productivity within the DIGMA or PSMA is optimized. With the understanding that the success of a DIGMA or PSMA depends upon off-loading from physicians all the work that can be done by other, less costly members of the healthcare team, a distinct position (the Shared Medical Appointment Specialist) was created and staffed at ProMed.

The SMA Specialist

At ProMed, it is the SMA Specialist that occupies the nursing role for many of the DIGMAs and PSMAs that are run. However, the primary role of the SMA Specialist is to review the medical records of all patients to be seen in upcoming SMA sessions. The successful applicant for this position was an LPN with several years experience in ambulatory care nursing. The focus of the review is to make sure—in every case—that all dimensions of disease management in HTN, CHF, Asthma, obesity, and diabetes are successfully accomplished during the upcoming DIGMA or PSMA visit.

Because the Shared Medical Appointment Specialist is a nurse, care can be provided at a very high level when patients arrive for the DIGMA or PSMA session—which typically occurs before the physician sees the patient. The physician is thus able to spend all of his/her time in activities that are unique to that provider—and which the physician alone can provide. Everything else is off-loaded either to the SMA specialist or another member of the care team—such as the behaviorist, documenter, or dedicated scheduler. This new SMA nursing specialist role was necessary to ensure consistency in the application of disease management protocols, to enhance physician productivity, and to assure the long-term sustainability of the SMA program.

The Dedicated Scheduler

For larger and midsized medical groups in which multiple providers participate, there is additional staffing required for a successful shared medical appointment program—such as a scheduler dedicated to the SMA program. The Borgess ProMed SMA scheduler has a marketing background and possesses excellent interpersonal and telemarketing skills. Consistent with the theme of enhanced outcomes through an altered model of care, the scheduler is empowered to identify appointment gaps in patients in need of care, such as diabetics in need of their periodic evaluations; women in need of appropriate screening (such as pap, pelvic, and breast exams, as well as bone densitometry studies or mammograms); or patients with chronic illnesses in need of appropriate follow-up care.

The scheduler must have an outgoing, *up-beat* personality and be willing to make *cold* calls on behalf of the providers. When done properly, the SMA scheduler (referred to as the ProMed SMA Marketing/Scheduler) can be very helpful in maintaining the census of shared medical appointments. Of course, the most effective way to maintain census in the shared medical appointment is by personal invitations to all suitable patients from the provider.

The Behaviorist

A mix of individuals is used in the behaviorist (or SMA facilitator) role at Borgess ProMed. Initially, all the facilitators were behavioral health professionals—i.e., either licensed psychologists or MSWs from the ProMed behavioral health division. Over time, there have been nurses and even a diabetes educator that have become involved in the facilitation of SMAs. The diabetes educator is specifically utilized to facilitate disease-specific shared medical appointments for diabetics. In these visits, the patient record is marked regarding the topics covered, so that a different topic can be discussed, time permitting, at a subsequent visit. Patients and providers find this very satisfying. It should be pointed out, however, that the use of a diabetes educator as a facilitator for a SMA is not a substitute for formal diabetes education. Rather, the educator as facilitator helps to reinforce this education as the primary purpose of a DIGMA or PSMA is the efficient delivery of quality medical care.

The behaviorist/facilitator has many primary responsibilities during DIGMA and PSMA sessions: arrive early to warm the group up and write down patient concerns; assure that confidentiality/HIPAA forms are signed; start the group on time with an introduction; handle group dynamic and psychosocial issues; keep the group running smoothly and on time; temporarily take over the group, focusing upon behavioral health issues, when the physician documents a chart note or steps out of the group room for brief private discussions or exams; and stay after the group for a few minutes to address last minute questions, clear the room, and straighten up the group room.

The Program Coordinator (and the Physician Champion)

One of the most important members of the SMA team at Borgess ProMed is the SMA program coordinator. At all times, the program coordinator assists—and works closely with—the physician champion to ensure the success of the SMA program. Responsible for maintaining the staffing of the program, the coordinator also aids the transition of new providers into doing shared medical appointments. The coordinator makes sure there is a facilitator and, from time to time, also facilitates a DIGMA or PSMA when there is a need for this (such as when the regular behaviorist is out ill or on vacation).

There have been two coordinators at Borgess ProMed Healthcare, both LPNs. While management experience is helpful, it is not an absolute requirement. The attributes for success in the program coordinator position are willingness to be creative, good *people* skills, ability to learn, knowledge of the DIGMA and PSMA models (and what it takes for them to be successful), and a flexible attitude—plus, an undying commitment to maintaining group census and high standards in patient care. Borgess ProMed has been fortunate in that both SMA coordinators have had these essential attributes. Because the SMA program is still relatively small with only 9 providers running DIGMAs and/or PSMAs for their practices, the current coordinator also occupies the role of the SMA nursing specialist and has managed both positions well.

The Business Case for the SMA Program

The business aspect of DIGMAs and PSMAs is intuitive. DIGMAs and PSMAs offer a multidisciplinary team-based approach to care that off-loads work that is not unique to providers onto the SMA team—thereby increasing provider efficiency and enjoyment of the process (as physicians are thereby freed up to focus upon what they alone can do and which they typically most enjoy). Our SMA program provides patients with the benefit of a one-stop shopping experience in which immunizations and routine health screenings are updated, more time with the provider and greater patient education are delivered, and easy access to this informative setting are all provided—along with a relaxed environment that can be a lot of fun! We have found that patient satisfaction with the SMA program is very high. Once patients actually attend a DIGMA or PSMA session, almost all say they would come back—and 95.6% of surveyed patients reporting that they would refer family and friends to a SMA.

Because DIGMAs and PSMAs leverage the time of the provider, improve throughput, and increase production without the expense of adding additional providers, they make business sense. In other words, because throughput is increased per unit of time, there is additional productivity. One must be aware, however, that the additional staffing required to run a successful SMA program (program coordinator, dedicated scheduler, nursing specialist, documenter, and behaviorist) all add to cost, and therefore directly contribute to overhead. Therefore, it is important to assure good fill of all DIGMA and PSMA sessions—as full SMAs are successful SMAs (because this additional overhead is thereby more than compensated for, and a profit margin for the SMA program is thereby achieved). Put another way, SMA care is more expensive care; however, because of its efficiency and quality benefits, it can actually save money—provided that groups are kept full.

Another aspect of our DIGMA and PSMA program that makes business sense is the power of these models in efficient and effective chronic disease management. To date, we have used DIGMAs and PSMAs to effectively manage several chronic conditions and diseases: diabetes; CHF; hypertension; asthma; headache; COPD; depression; hyperlipidemia; obesity; and women's wellness issues (such as menopause, osteoporosis, and pap, pelvic, and breast exams). Furthermore, because of the additional time available (plus the support of the behaviorist and other patients), greater patient education around disease self-management can be provided in the SMA setting. In addition, this education can be reinforced by other patients and the team, which helps to reduce noncompliance. Fig. 9.33 depicts how the ProMed SMA program is designed to better meet patients' needs.

Our strategy at Borgess ProMed has been to: (1) combine the specialist and program coordinator positions; (2) cross-train the scheduler to schedule for both SMA and non-SMA appointments, when appropriate; and (3) to avoid setting up or scheduling SMAs in such a way that it would be difficult to keep sessions full—e.g., not using providers with less than full practices, not starting SMAs that are too homogeneous to fill, and not running SMAs during seasonal times when appointment demand is low. While this has proven to be a viable approach at a mid-sized medical group such as ours, we recognize that this might not be the appropriate strategy in larger systems—especially when the number of DIGMAs and PSMAs being run each week exceeds 25, 50, 100, or more.

In terms of billing, we treat DIGMAs and PSMAs just like a standard office visit (except that we do not bill for counseling time or the behaviorist's time). We bill according to services rendered and documented, and review coding just like any other visit. Patients are informed of our billing policy in both mail communication and in all promotional materials.

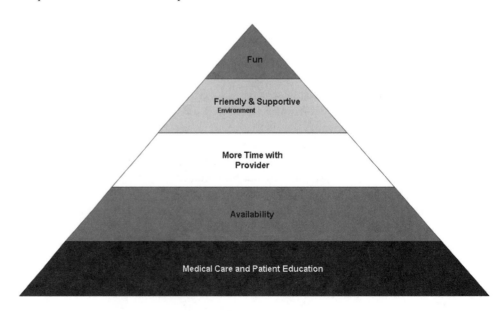

Fig. 9.33 The ProMed SMA program is designed to better meet patients' needs

Each DIGMA and PSMA Is Customized to the Individual Provider

Each DIGMA and PSMA is customized to the specific needs and practice of the individual provider. At Borgess ProMed, all of the SMA providers elected to do PSMAs. In addition, several do either heterogeneous DIGMAs or disease-specific DIGMAs—i.e., according to their interests and the needs of the patients. One family physician does bone health DIGMAs to allow time for discussion of bone densitometry results. Here, the shared setting: facilitates individual results presentation (coupled with a detailed, individualized plan of care); promotes discussion of the interpretation of bone densitometry; and enhances education regarding the care and maintenance of healthy bones. Both patients and the provider achieve high satisfaction with the experience.

Innovative Gynecology PSMA Design

In the Women's Health division, one of the GYN providers decided the 90 minute duration of the shared physicals was too long for her patients. She recognized, however, that she would need the entire 90 minutes to accomplish the usual elements of care required for a routine pap, pelvic, and breast exam for the number of patients she wanted to have in attendance. She therefore created a PSMA model of care where the patients spend 60 minutes in the office, yet the traditional 90 minutes of total time is still used for the shared physical model. In the design that she uses, five patients initially arrive at once—at which time they are received, roomed, and examined. Thirty minutes later, when all five exams are efficiently done with minimal talk, these first five patients are joined by five additional patients for the shared portion of the appointment.

It is during this interactive group segment that the provider sequentially addresses the individual medical concerns and questions that each patient has, but does so while fostering some group interaction. In addition, each patient's physical findings are discussed, data from lab tests and procedures are reviewed, and expectant care is provided. Thirty minutes later, the second five patients are roomed and examined; however, the first group is then free to leave after spending only 60 minutes in the clinic. Because they enter the PSMA 30 minutes into the session and then leave when it is over, the second group of patients also needs to only spend 1 hour in the clinic (i.e., total time for both the interactive group and private exam segments).

This model provides a shorter length of stay while optimizing the time of the provider. As a result of her customized PSMA, this gynecologist was able to work through and eventually eliminate an extensive backlog of more than 250 women waiting for their health exams by using this model. *[Note from Dr. Noffsinger: As discussed earlier in this book in the Physicals SMA chapter, be certain that you are capable of being an efficient time manager before you use this design format. Otherwise you might have difficulty finishing on time, as the last group of five patients that you give private physical examinations to could still have "just a few more questions" for you to answer after the interactive group segment is over—i.e., when they later see you alone in the individual exam room setting. This can lead to time-consuming and inefficient one-on-one discussions in the exam rooms that make it difficult to finish on time. Also, I would recommend spending 45 minutes in the interactive group segment—rather than 30 minutes—whenever possible because of the educational benefits and efficiency gaints that occur there. This would mean that the two physical examination groups of five women each would need to be reduced from the 30 minutes employed here to just 22½ minutes each for a 90-minute PSMA session (unless you wanted a 2-h PSMA, in which case the 30 minutes spent on the physical exmination of each group of five women could remain at 30 minutes, although the group census would then need to be correspondingly increased to maination the desired productivity gain).]*

Diabetes Outcome Study 1

We at Borgess Health's ProMed Healthcare have been exceedingly pleased with the significant improvements we have documented in screening measures for our diabetic patients as a result of our SMA program. The disease management review process that the Shared Medical Appointment Specialist undertakes on all patients coming in for a DIGMA or PSMA appointment has had a very positive impact upon our chronically ill patients. As an illustrative example, consider our diabetic patients—as we have demonstrated significantly improved diabetic screening outcomes for our diabetic patients (i.e., for diabetic patients treated in DIGMAs and PSMAs vs. those receiving usual care alone).

Diabetic Screening Outcomes Are Significantly Better for SMA Patients

As seen in Table 9.14, there is a statistically significant difference between SMA and non-SMA care for diabetic patients in terms of consistently achieving disease management performance measures—e.g., the consistency with which we were able to achieve screening measures

Table 9.14 Comparison of outcomes for diabetic patients attending SMAs vs. a control group of diabetic patients receiving usual care only (i.e., traditional individual office visits) with the same physicians from ProMed Family Practice, Borgess Health, Kalamazoo, MI

Outcome measures	$N = 60$ SMA(%)	$N = 60$ Non-SMA(%)	Probability level
Urinary microalbumin*	95	69	$<.001$*
Influenza vaccination*	71	37	$<.001$*
Pneumococcal vaccination*	93	50	$<.001$*
Foot exam*	88	53	$<.001$*
Eye exam*	84	64	0.0125*
BP<130/80	33	24	0.274
HgA1C< 7%	57	60	0.739
Total cholesterol at target	67	60	0.426
LDL < 100	52	44	0.38
HDL >45 M, >55F	52	39	0.153
Triglycerides < 150	51	40	0.226

* = Statistically significant at the $P < 0.05$ level.

such as nephropathy assessment and eye exams. Significant improvements in microalbumin, pneumonia and influenza vaccination, foot exam, and eye exam were achieved. The blood pressure and lipid data showed improvement. The only area that did not improve is in diabetes control, as reflected in the HgA1c. We believe that such benefits as these build upon and extend other patient benefits from the SMA program—extra time, improved access, greater patient education, help from other patients and a multi-disciplinary team, improved doctor–patient relationships, improved patient satisfaction, etc.

I did like to give you my initial impressions of the data. First, the data validate the system we put in place. We use a nurse specialist, who is an LPN, in our office to review charts prior to visits for diabetic patients seen in shared medical appointments in either the shared physical or DIGMA model. The nurse completes these tests or services without the need for physician approval. The physician reviews the foot exam after she completes it.

Second, the blood pressure and lipid data suggest the group process encourages better compliance with treatment plans. Several times I have witnessed the engagement of patients by members of the group to encourage others to take their medicines, focus on what the targets are, and be comfortable with managing their chronic diseases. It is not unusual for a DIGMA to have patients with well-controlled lipids on statin medications set an example for others to follow. In addition, the greater amount of time in a SMA allows me to fully articulate the need to place target goals higher in priority than avoidance of medication or delay in lifestyle modification. We also hand out many more educational materials in SMAs than we do in standard office visits.

Third, I would like to point out that, in this case, SMAs did not necessarily improve the medical decision-making of physicians in diabetes care. The HbA1c did not improve. No matter the format of clinical care delivery, we need to be encouraged to improve diabetes control in our patients.

Fourth, I would like to indicate that we intend to take what we have learned from SMAs—i.e., with respect to the quality improvement we have seen in diabetes control—and export it to the rest of the practices. ProMed has over 6000 diabetics. We will need to use computerized registries to manage these patients. We can use the prospective chart review and the tools created to do that review as our template for the other clinics in ProMed. I am thankful to Dr. Noffsinger for guiding us in our efforts to improve care by the use of shared medical appointments, and most especially in the proper application of his DIGMA and PSMA models. We are excited about what we have done, and look forward to advancing what we have learned.

Why Screening Outcomes Are Significantly Improved in Study 1, but Clinical Outcomes Are Not

In the data presented in Table 9.14, the results for 60 diabetic patients seen by eight providers in their SMAs were compared with 60 diabetic patients seen by the same providers with the same frequency, but who had never been to a SMA. While there was no significant difference in the clinical outcomes of Study 1, there was a significant improvement in the consistency with which all appropriate diabetic screening measures were achieved in the SMA program.

This improved screening data suggests that the DIGMA and PSMA models of care would ultimately also result in measurably improved outcomes for diabetic patients—notice how all but one of the clinical outcome measures are already in the direction of favoring SMA group care. However, since the same physicians were involved in both groups (i.e., with the same number of patients in both the SMA and the usual care control groups), significant differences in outcomes that are dependent upon physician medical decision-making would not be expected between the SMA and usual care groups. In addition, many of the SMA patients also received usual care from the same providers, which is another factor that could tend to reduce any differences between these groups. Therefore, the only statistically significant differences achieved in study 1 were in the outcomes connected with the work of the shared medical appointment specialist. However, in and of itself, this is certainly an important accomplishment of the SMA program.

What Surprised Me the Most About Our Data

I would like to mention that my greatest surprise from our SMA program was not that doctors and patients liked it. That had been so demonstrated with the DIGMA and PSMA models that we expected it. We were likewise not surprised at their remarkable productivity gain, as we anticipated that as well. What surprised me the most was that, even though we have a clinic standard of every patient having their pneumonia and tetanus vaccinations updated as appropriate during every office visit, a retrospective chart review of 60 patients spread among eight providers conducting SMAs in either a DIGMA or a PSMA format revealed that only 50% of patients attending a non-SMA visit had pneumonia vaccinations completed while 93% were up to date after the SMA (Fig. 9.34). The data for tetanus updates were similarly

distributed. These data are likely due to the improved system of care manifested in the work of the nurse specialist.

However, the important point here is that the SMA provides an opportunity to put protocols and systems in place that members of the SMA team will then systematically and uniformly conduct on all patients in attendance. SMAs mandate efficiency and consistency in patient care. Putting a process in place to identify the need for the service (in this case, immunizations of diabetic patients)—and then empowering the appropriate clinical team member to get the vaccinations consistently done on all appropriate patients in attendance per protocol—improves outcomes for this population of patients. Shared Medical Appointments made this not only possible but also necessary for the optimal success of the program.

Diabetes Outcome Study 2: SMA Outcomes Compared to NCQA/ADA Standards

Outcomes data for the alternative clinical care delivery model of DIGMAs and PSMAs were evaluated against national standards for diabetic care—i.e., using the National Committee for Quality Assurance (NCQA)/ American Diabetes Association (ADA) criteria for the Diabetes Physician Recognition Program. A separate study at ProMed (i.e., which we are calling study 2) involved two hundred patients with type two diabetes who had never been to a shared medical appointment, and compared them with 50 patients who had been to at least one shared medical appointment.

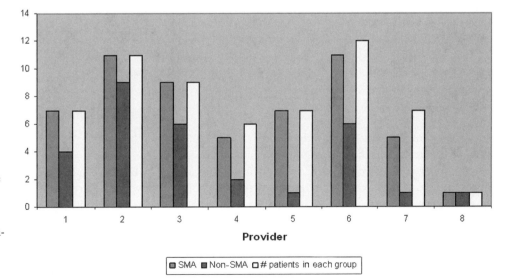

Fig. 9.34 Comparison of ProMed SMA vs. traditional care outcomes for pneumonia vaccination updates in diabetic patients seen by eight different providers. The number of patients seen by each provider was the same in SMA as in non-SMA (the total number of patients was 60 each for SMA and non-SMA)

Figure 9.35 presents the data from study 2. It should be noted that every outcome in this study trends positively in the direction of SMAs over usual care, and with many of these differences achieving statistical significance—including an improved clinical outcome for blood pressure control (BP < 130/80), as well as increased annual lipid, eye exam, and nephrology screenings. When the data are measured against the 2005 NCQA/ADA criteria, the non-SMA data only generated 17 out of 80 points, which was inadequate for recognition. When the data from the SMA patients were measured against the NCQA/ADA criteria, all 80 points were achieved. This made the SMA section of Borgess ProMed Healthcare recognizable for the Diabetes Physician Recognition Program.

What does it take to make a successful SMA program happen? We found that it takes vision, will, and the appropriate resources. I would like to conclude by pointing out that, as depicted in Fig. 9.37, properly run SMAs can positively impact all dimensions of patient care, plus the bottom line. With proper attention to the team supporting SMAs, and a combination of vision and will, shared medical appointments can be a reality in any setting. In terms of ideas we are considering for future SMA programs, we are looking at starting chronic pain, medication refill and update, cardiac risk, snow bird, and comprehensive respiratory SMAs for smokers, asthmatics, and COPD.

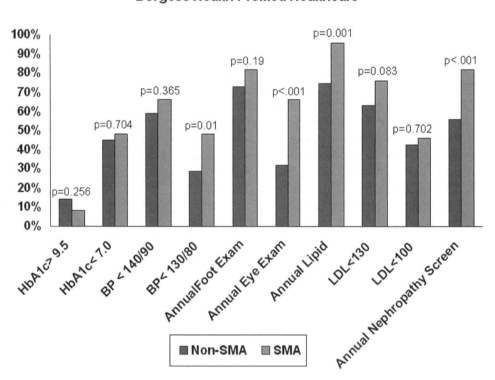

Fig. 9.35 Outcomes data for ProMed SMA vs. non-SMA (usual) care, which favors SMA care in every case

Conclusion

In conclusion, we have found that our DIGMA and PSMA program has benefited our patients in many ways, not the least of which are improvements in many areas of care delivery, as depicted in Fig. 9.36. It should be clear that shared medical appointments can be a very important tool for improving access, enhancing quality, improving clinical outcomes, redesigning the model of care, increasing productivity, and improving the bottom line.

Other Relevant SMA Studies Show Improved Clinical Outcomes for Diabetics

A 2002 article in the *Minnesota Medicine* journal gives the following report regarding the high-quality care that group visits can provide to diabetic patients: "DIGMAs and other group visits have not yet caught on in Minnesota, but David Agerter, M.D., has experimented for 2 years with diabetes group visits at Mayo's Family Practice Clinic in Kasson. 'We decided to give group visits a

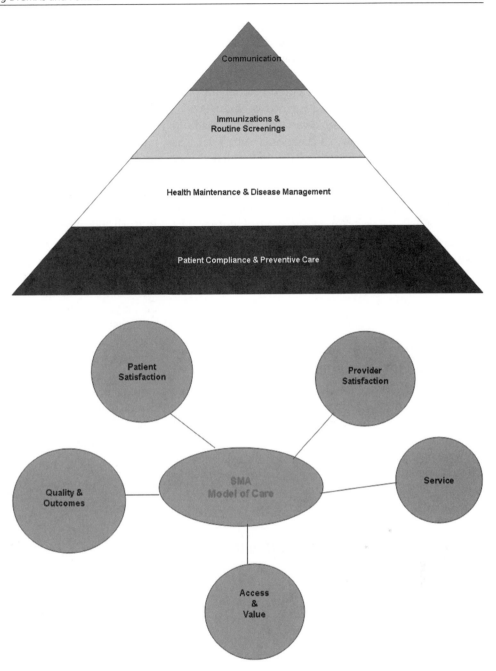

Fig. 9.36 The DIGMA and PSMA program at ProMed has provided many benefits to our patients which have resulted in improvements in many different areas

Fig. 9.37 Properly run SMA programs can favorably impact all aspects of patient care, plus the bottom line

try because we were frustrated,' says Agerter. 'Many of our patients were not adequately managing their condition.' After attending four 60- to 90-minute group visits over a period of 6–8 weeks, all 30 patients who participated had lower blood glucose levels, better blood pressure control, and better compliance monitoring their own glucose levels. They were more likely to manage their diet and schedule recommended eye exams. 'Patient satisfaction is quite high for group visits,' says Agerter, who says the clinic may someday offer group visits for other diagnoses" (25).

One study from a diabetes management group in an HMO that used cluster visits, another type of group appointment, reported improved A1c levels and reduced inhospital and outpatient visits.(26) Another study that compared patients attending a diabetes group visit with those receiving standard care reported that the average A1c level decreased to 6.3% in the group visit from 7.3 or 7.7% in 2 two groups receiving standard care.[Sawyer D, Benson D. The group visit: innovation in multidisciplinary, resident driven patient care. Unpublished manuscript.]

Masley et al. who ran a diabetes group visit, reported that after a year, total cholesterol/HDL ratios were reduced by 32%; HbA1c levels were reduced by 30%; and costs were reduced by 7%. (27)

Trento et al. who reported on a randomized controlled 4-year study of 112 patients with type two diabetes who were not treated by insulin, compared shared visits to usual care.(28) "The mean hemoglobin A1c level was 7.4% at baseline: it decreased to 7.0% in the shared-visit cohort and increased to 8.6% with usual care, a statistically significant difference. Weight decreased in the shared-visit patients by an average of 2.6 kg compared to only a 0.9 kg decrease in the control group. The patients who had shared visits were able to decrease their dosages of hypoglycemic medications and had more slowly progressing retinopathy than the usual-care patients" (28).

DIGMAs and PSMAs Are Beginning to Be Used Internationally

Although international applications are just beginning and are still in their earliest stages, DIGMAs and PSMAs are starting to find their way onto the international scene. In this section, we will look at two early international implementation studies—one from Canada and another from the Netherlands.

Study 19: DIGMAs at Northern Health in British Columbia, Canada

The following article was submitted by Alice Domes, RN, BScN, Regional CDPM Coordinator for Northern Health in Canada, and Judy Huska, Executive Director, Health Services Integration, Northern Health in Canada. Northern Health is one of six Health Service Delivery Areas in British Columbia, Canada. Their catchment area encompasses almost two-thirds of the upper portion of the province and delivers healthcare to a population of over 300,000, many of whom live in northern and rural settings.

Background and History of Group Visits at Northern Health

In an effort to improve the care delivered to patients in the region, representatives from Northern Health attended an Institute for Healthcare Improvement (IHI) conference and were intrigued by a presentation on group visits. In it, Dr. Noffsinger had described two group medical appointment models (the DIGMA and Physicals SMA models) that would address access problems, improve the quality of patient care, and increase patient and professional satisfaction. Northern Health already had a network of primary healthcare teams, and group medical appointments offered the potential of further improving the quality of patient care in the region.

In February 2006, Dr. Noffsinger was invited to Northern Health to introduce the concept of Group Medical Appointments to interested healthcare professionals. In April 2006, he returned to provide intensive training on the DIGMA model and launched the first three DIGMAs in two communities in Northern Health. Following Dr. Noffsinger's visit, several physicians around Northern Health began offering Group Medical Appointments on a regular basis. The DIGMAs have been either homogeneous or heterogeneous, depending on the group's purpose. DIGMAs and Physicals Shared Medical Appointments in Northern Health have addressed a variety of health issues, including asthma, hypertension, cardiovascular disease, diabetes, drug and alcohol dependence, women's wellness, and general health problems. DIGMAs are also being offered to patients who require follow up for a chronic health conditions.

DIGMAs Address Access and Physician Shortage Problems

DIGMAs have allowed one physician in a rural community to address access problems due to a severe physician shortage in the more rural and remote areas of our region. In one small community, it is not uncommon for patients to wait 3–4 weeks to book a regular office visit. This physician stated, "With the shortage of family doctors, group visits are a great way to provide more care to more people."

DIGMAs Have Been Liked by Patients and Providers Alike

Patient satisfaction with our DIGMA and PSMA group medical appointment programs is high. The patient satisfaction surveys completed at the end of each session are overwhelming positive. Some patients call the physician's office asking when the next DIGMA will be held. Patients who prefer an individual office visit over a group visit are in the minority. In one office, a group visit addressing women's health issues was particularly successful. The female patients found the relaxed group atmosphere, coupled with the group sharing and the professionals' expertise, effectively addressed many of their questions and issues.

Healthcare providers are also generally very happy with the DIGMAs. As one team stated, "With DIGMAs there is satisfaction 'plus' for all involved." Physicians offering DIGMAs find they are one way to deliver comprehensive medical care and education to patients in a relaxed group environment. "Group visits provide for increased efficiency, increased availability, and proactive care," commented a physician who regularly offers DIGMAs to his patients.

Positive Clinical Outcomes Are Beginning to Appear

Group visits are also showing some positive clinical results. One physician schedules group medical appointments for "blood work" discussions with his patients. These individuals have a range of health issues—including diabetes, arthritis, and high cholesterol levels. After conducting group visits for more than 6 months, the physician started to see some positive clinical results. Out of a total of 105 patients who attended the groups, 54% decreased their total cholesterol, 48.5% increased their HDL, 50% decreased their triglyceride levels, and 45% showed improved cholesterol/HDL ratios.

Challenges That Needed to Be Addressed

Some creative solutions have been needed to address challenges encountered in offering group visits. Often physicians in remote areas only have a small office and one medical office assistant, which makes obtaining the necessary personnel and facilities resources for doing group visits somewhat of a challenge. In some communities, the role of behaviorist has been filled by healthcare providers from a variety of backgrounds and areas of expertise. Nurses, medical office assistants, mental health workers, and dieticians have functioned as behaviorists, but this has not detracted from the outcomes of the group.

A second challenge lies in finding an appropriate space in which to hold group medical appointments. Some physicians use their waiting room areas, whereas others are using space outside of their offices. Northern Health is helping to address this issue by leasing rooms in the large clinics of some of the more major communities in the region. Physicians with offices in these clinics will use this space to provide group medical appointments. To sustain the delivery of DIGMAs and PSMAs, Northern Health is providing ongoing training and support. A manual complete with all the resources needed to hold shared medical appointments is

available to any healthcare provider in the region (see the attached DVD). Monthly teleconferences provide support to the DIGMA teams. Champions in the region help train and support teams new to offering group medical appointments, plus Dr. Noffsinger is also available for support when needed.

While Improved Access and Patient Satisfaction Are Important, Quality Care Is Paramount

Northern Health is committed to improving the quality of care delivered to patients across northern British Columbia. Those engaged in implementing DIGMAs and PSMAs are excited about the potential that these models hold for helping us to achieve this goal. As the number of physicians offering group medical appointments to their patients continues to grow, the anticipated outcomes are increased satisfaction levels, reduced access problems, and (most importantly) improved patient care and clinical outcomes.

Study 20: Introduction of Shared Medical Appointments in the Netherlands and First Results

This contribution was submitted by Stan Janssen RN, MS, Senior Advisor Radboud University, Nijmegen, the Netherlands, and Femke Seesing, MSC, Advisor, Dutch Institute for Healthcare Improvement (CBO).

Background

Until recently, group visits were completely unknown in Dutch healthcare. There has, however, been experience with group therapy—especially in mental health—where group education together with the support of companions is provided during group sessions. As a result, in June 2005, the Dutch Institute for Healthcare Improvement (CBO) invited Dr. Ed Noffsinger to the Netherlands to give several lectures on the subject of group visits—one was for general interest, whereas other talks were part of collaborative working sessions on Advanced Access, Flow, and Diabetes. These presentations raised interest amongst specialists, outpatient clinic co-workers, and general practitioners. As a result, six medical specialists from five different Dutch hospitals asked the CBO to help them introduce group visits into their outpatient clinics. After this successful introduction of shared medical appointments in the Netherlands, the CBO has trained another 10 medical specialists in two different training sessions to set up shared medical appointments in their outpatient clinics. Also, at the University Hospital in Nijmegen and the Gelderse Vallei Hospital, specialists are trained by in-company training.

DIGMA Training Was Provided

For the first six teams willing to introduce group visits into their practices, the CBO then organized a follow-up training program led by Dr. Noffsinger the following fall. The aim of this training for the CBO was to find out if shared medical appointments could be successfully translated to the Dutch healthcare system. This training program further introduced group visits to staff, provided the teams with necessary skills, assisted teams in planning their own group visit programs, and helped teams to begin making group visits a part of the care program in their organizations. They accomplished this by custom designing their DIGMAs, forming group visit teams, involving management, addressing operational issues, selecting the facilities, informing and inviting their patients, etc. Then, these teams had a 2 day follow-up training program with Dr. Ed Noffsinger.

After they had introduced group visits into their own practices, the CBO organized a learning session in which experiences, along with tips and lessons learned, could be shared. After these initial training sessions, the group visit teams (as well as their patients) seemed to be very pleased with this new form of medical care delivery. In addition, subsequent training sessions were offered to other interested teams which focused upon the methodology of correctly implementing group visits—plus, they were offered additional follow-up training as needed after they had actually launched their group visit programs.

From a Patient's Perspective, DIGMAs Offer Many Potential Benefits

What advantages do we see for group visits, from the patient's perspective? During the first training, the teams brought the results from the satisfaction survey that they had given to their patients after their initial SMA sessions. The patients from all six teams were asked their opinion about consulting their doctor through a group visit. The results showed that more than 80% of the patients who attended a group visit: were better (or just as well) informed as during a one-on-one visit with their doctor; said that they had learned a lot from the other patients; said they would choose a shared medical appointment

again the next time they made an appointment with their doctor; and said they would recommend the SMA to others (relatives, fellow patients, friends).

Group visits offer many other patient benefits as well. From a patient's perspective, the following are but some of the other SMA benefits reported by patients:

- Patients receive considerable information beyond that obtained during a traditional one-on-one visit (i.e., besides the medical information, there is more attention paid to the psychosocial part of their disease, plus they got expert information from fellow patients experiencing similar things).
- Group visits help them to see things in perspective because they recognize that they are not alone and that others are often worse off than they are.
- The extra time and greater education enables group visits to help patients better self-manage their health problems.
- Patients can make an appointment at the outpatient clinic for a group visit themselves (this fits nicely into our strategy of patient initiated care, which has won tremendous popularity in outpatient care during the past couple of years).
- They can spend more time with their physician.
- The average consultation time during a traditional individual office visit is only approximately 10 minutes, which limits the number of questions that can be answered. Although the actual time spent on a single patient in a group visit is less, the patient experiences "his" or "her" doctor much longer in the 90-minute group setting.
- Although some patients are very busy and cannot stay for the entire session, this is fine as they can be treated first and then be left free to leave whenever they want.
- Patients enjoy the encouragement and help of other patients in the group visit setting, and psychological needs can be better addressed.
- Patients listen to other patient's questions and the answers, and thus learn from each other in the educational setting that the group visit provides.
- The USA experience shows a high rating with regards to patient education and empowerment, especially in homogeneous groups.

DIGMAs also offer many benefits from a provider's perspective

From the provider's point of view in the Netherlands, the group visit teams report the following benefits:

- They provide an efficient and innovative new method of delivering care, i.e., compared to the traditional healthcare model of one to one consultation.

- Group visits reduce the need to repeat the same information to different patients individually, and accomplish this while also providing a milieu that enhances education and empowers patients in their own disease self-management.
- They increase the quality of care that we are able to deliver.
- A medical specialist in a university hospital says that he sees more patients with a rare disease in 2 hours than other providers see in years (as a result, he can identify new disease-related problems and discuss them with the patients—plus also discover new research questions).
- Shared medical appointments provide greater flexibility in our ability to provide appropriate and timely medical care to our patients.
- Group visits can improve both patient and provider satisfaction.
- They provide a multidisciplinary team-based approach to care.
- Group visits can be used as part of the education provided to medical students and fellows.

Confidentiality and Billing Have Not Been Problems in the Netherlands, but Staffing Resources and Group Room Space Are

The privacy and confidentiality aspects of group visits did not prove to be a problem in the Dutch system. Some group visit teams choose to have patients give their written consent prior to the shared medical appointment session. But this is not officially accepted by law. So some group visit teams also gave information about privacy and confidentiality during the behaviorist's introduction at the beginning of the session. If patients were not OK with this, they could always leave the room; however, to date, this has never happened. In addition, financing group visits was not expected to be a problem. This is because, during a group visit, the unique medical needs of each patient are met individually so that the visit can be billed like a one-on-one visit (or as a day care tariff, if the DIGMA/PSMA takes longer than 2 hours).

On the other hand, getting the required staffing resources—especially for filling the role of behaviorist—has been more problematic as behaviorists are not common in Dutch healthcare. Therefore, the group visit teams all choose a behaviorist that is best suited to them, which means that we have nurses, psychologists, specialized nurses, dieticians, and nurse practitioners who have acted in the role of behaviorist. Additional challenges have included securing the necessary facilities and inviting sufficient patients to fill groups to desired capacity. Because of the additional staffing and facilities requirements that

DIGMAs entail, the involvement of the higher management was crucial to introducing group visits in Holland, a process that CBO facilitated.

DIGMAs Are Beginning to be Accepted as Part of Our Healthcare Environment

Since the early beginnings of our group visit program, it seems like DIGMAs are gradually becoming a natural part of our healthcare environment for patients in the Netherlands. After the initial meetings that we originally had with the first six interested doctors, members of the six original group visit teams concluded that it seemed like DIGMAs could really work for patients in the Netherlands. The remarkable thing was that soon thereafter, even during the earliest group visit sessions (i.e., when the doctors and group visit teams were still working out what the best ways were for them to do group visits, and were not yet feeling totally comfortable in doing their DIGMAs), they all still wanted to continue. They wanted to continue running their DIGMAs because they noticed that their patients were very excited and satisfied with the care they were receiving in the groups. After doing just two or three DIGMA sessions, the teams asked us to plan another meeting a few months later on so that we could evaluate how the groups were progressing after half a year.

From the Start, Patient Satisfaction with DIGMAs Was very High

As it turned out, by the time we held that follow-up meeting 6 months later, all the teams had made group visits a part of the regular care they were giving. By that time, most of the doctors were feeling more secure in doing their DIGMAs. We found it interesting that, by then, every team had made their own customized designs for their DIGMAs. All the teams gave their patients a satisfaction questionnaire after the DIGMA. When the results of all the teams were taken together, the results—which are depicted in Table 9.15—were really exciting to all.

Although Still New, DIGMAs Are Already Receiving Much Positive Publicity in the Netherlands

Furthermore, even though our group visit program is still quite new, there has already been a lot of positive publicity about DIGMAs over here—even during the early stages of our program. One of our internal medicine doctors was interviewed for national television about his DIGMA.

Table 9.15 Patient satisfaction results for group visits in The Netherlands

	Yes (%)	No (%)	Do not know (%)	N
For my next appointment with my doctor, I would choose a DIGMA again.	82.5	5.8	11.7	103
I am better informed about my disease and my health after a DIGMA than after a one-on-one visit.	42.8	16.2	41.0	105
All questions I had were answered during the DIGMA	87.9	12.1	0	99
I would recommend family, friends, or others to go to a DIGMA, if they asked me to.	96.0	4.0	0	100
I learned from my fellow patients and the questions they asked during the DIGMA.	91.9	8.1	0	99
The information that I received during the DIGMA was clear to me.	92.9	7.1	0	42

From Dutch Institute for Healthcare Improvement CBO, with permission.

Another physician, a neurology professor, was interviewed about his DIGMA on the radio and in nationwide newspapers. In addition, we wrote an overview article on the first six pilot teams and their results—which was published on the 30th of June, 2006, in a magazine that is published in the Netherlands that is read by most doctors as well as by other people in healthcare (29). In addition, there has been a lot of smaller articles in magazines, including one by a daily newspaper, that have also been written about them (all of which are in Dutch) (30–41).

Plans for Formal Outcomes Research in the Netherlands

The future for DIGMAs in the Netherlands looks very positive and involves plans for future outcomes research. Together with the doctors running DIGMAs, we are now looking for a way to do more scientific research in the Netherlands as to the effects of DIGMAs upon our healthcare delivery system. Our DIGMA program is continuing to grow, although doctors here still find it difficult to imagine themselves doing a DIGMA (and this despite the fact that reports and stories from their colleagues who are already running them are very good).

Some Concluding Thoughts on Group Visits in the Netherlands

Although it seems that group visits in the Netherlands are indeed successful, it is *not* primarily because of their efficiency gains—at least this is what the participating doctors tell us every time. Therefore, it would not do SMAs justice to say that this is true. It is their quality, access, and camaraderie benefits that are most appreciated—especially their quality benefits and the fact that they provide a means of giving patients and caregivers more tools for disease self-management. Our SMA providers like to offer group visits to their patients because they think they can enhance the quality of the care they provide, and because it is an interesting and nice way of delivering care for the caregivers themselves.

It is a pleasure to provide such a nice way of giving medical care, and for working together as a team. The doctors who participate in shared medical appointments feel that the way they used to give care (i.e., one-on-one visits alone) could not adequately help all of their patients in managing and coping with their own diseases. They feel that shared medical appointments provide them with an efficient means of giving patients the medical care and disease self-management skills that they need in order to better manage their own health problems.

However, it is important to keep in mind that group visits could be a more expensive form of care to deliver—i.e., if an adequate group size is not maintained so as to offset the additional personnel and facilities costs they involve. A study comparing the cost of group vs. individual visits has yet to be done in the Netherlands; however, the outcome of such a study will clearly be dependent upon maintaining desired census levels. Clearly, the success of introducing group visits in the Netherlands will ultimately depend upon whether they: contribute to enhancing the capacity of outpatient clinics; reduce access time; are seen by healthcare professionals as a helpful innovation in delivering care; and, last but not least, are appreciated and embraced by patients. According to the results obtained in the USA, these goals are anticipated to be quite achievable. Assuming that our group visit program continues to be successful, the CBO will continue to provide ongoing training to interested physicians and their teams on a regular basis—training that will likely include clinicians already doing them.

References

1. Noffsinger EB. Enhance satisfaction with drop-in group visits. Hippocrates. February–March 2001;15(2):30–36.
2. Noffsinger EB. Physicals shared medical appointments: a revolutionary access solution. Group Practice Journal. Jan 2002; 51(1):16–26.

3. Noffsinger EB. Operational challenges to implementing a successful physicals shared medical appointment program. Part 1: Choosing the right type of shared medical appointment. Group Practice Journal. Feb 2002;51(2):24–34.

4. Noffsinger EB. Operational challenges to implementing a successful physicals shared medical appointment program. Part 2: maximizing efficiency. Group Practice Journal. Mar 2002; 51(3):32–40.

5. Noffsinger EB. Operational considerations for a successful physicals shared medical appointment program. Part 3: Hints and guidelines. Group Practice Journal. Apr 2002;51(4):22–26.

6. Atkins TN, Noffsinger EB. Implementing a group medical appointment program: a case study at Sutter Medical Foundation. Group Practice Journal. March 2001; 50(3):32, 34–39.

7. Noffsinger EB, Atkins TN. Assessing a group medical appointment program: a case study at Sutter Medical Foundation. Group Practice Journal. April 2001;50(4):42–50.

8. Noffsinger EB, Atkins TN. A business plan for implementing a group medical appointment program: a case study at Sutter Medical Foundation. Group Practice Journal. May 2001;50 (5):31–32, 34–38.

9. Mary P. Patients visit doc together. The Commercial Appeal. May 2004;A1 and A2.

10. Daniel C. Combat vets reach out to each other in VA appointments. The Commercial Appeal. April 2007; C1, C2.

11. Congressman Ford's Office. Ford introduces Veteran's Health Legislation. July 2004.

12. Meehan K, Hill JM, Root L, et al. Group medical appointments: organization and implementation in the bone marrow transplantation clinic. Supportive Cancer Therapy. 2006;3:84–90.

13. Noffsinger EB. Increasing quality of care and access while reducing costs through drop-in group medical appointments (DIGMAs). Group Practice Journal. Jan 1999;48(1):12–17.

14. Bronson DL, Maxwell RA. Shared medical appointments: increasing patient access without increasing physician hours. Cleveland Clinic Journal of Medicine. May 2004;71(5):369–70, 372, 374.

15. Trento M, Passera, P, Bajardi M, et al. Lifestyle intervention by group care prevents deterioration of type ii diabetes: a 4-year randomized controlled clinical trial. Diabetologia. 2002;45:1231–9, with kind permission of Springer Science + Business Media.

16. Wagner EH, Grothaus LC, Sandhu N, et al. Chronic care clinics for diabetes in primary care: a system-wide randomized trial." Diabetes Care. 2001;24:695–700.

17. Noffsinger EB. Solving departmental access problems with DIGMAs. Group Practice Journal November/December 2001;50(10):26–28, 30–32, 34–36.

18. Funnell M, et al. Implementing an empowerment-based diabetes self-management education program. The Diabetes Educator. 2005;31(1):53–61.

19. Noffsinger E. Shared medical appointments. American Academy of Family Physicians. June 14 2005 (Web article).

20. VA National Center for Post-Traumatic Stress Disorder, http://www.ncptsd.va.gov/facts/general/fs_what_is_ptsd.html.

21. American Heart Association. Heart disease and stroke statistics: 2005 update. Dallas, TX: American Heart Association; 2005.

22. Rich MW, Beckham V, Wittenberg C, Leven CL, Freedland KE, Carney RM. A multidisciplinary intervention to prevent the readmission of elderly patients with congestive heart failure. The New England Journal of Medicine. 1995;333:1190–1195.

23. Rich MW. Heart failure disease management: a critical review. Journal of Cardiac Failure. 1999; Mar(1):64–75.

24. Bronson D, Maxwell R. Shared medical appointments: increasing patient access without increasing physician hours. Cleveland Clinic Journal of Medicine. 2004;71:369–77.

25. Howard B. Group appointments—just what the doctor ordered. Minnesota Medicine (published monthly by the Minnesota Medical Association). June 2002;85(6):59.

26. Sadur CN, Moline N, Costa M, et al. Diabetes management in a health maintenance organization: efficiency of care management using cluster visits. Diabetes Care. 1999;22:2011–2017. 27. 2002.

27. Masley S, Sokoloff J, Hawes C. Planning group visits for high-risk patients. Family Practice Management. Jun 2000;7(6):33–7.

28. Trento M, Passera P, Bajardi M, et al. Lifestyle intervention by group care prevents deterioration of type 2 diabetes: a 4-year randomized controlled clinical trial. Diabetologia. 2002;45: 1231–9. Epub 2002 Jul 11.

29. Seesing FM, Janssen SFMM, Westra E, Moel JPC de. Samen naar de dokter: groepsgewijs consult lijkt goed alternatief voor individueel spreekuur. Medisch Contact. 2006;61:1080–2.

30. Harmsen A. Individueel consult of Gezamenlijk Medisch Consult? Afstudeeronderzoek voor de studie bedrijfscommunicatie aan de Radboud Universiteit Nijmegen. 2006.

31. Kraan GM. Evaluation of shared medical appointments; the first experiences of group consult teams in the Netherlands. Research for the Master of Public Health, Department of Health Care Studies, Universiteit Maastricht. 2006.

32. Loon J van. Met z'n tienen op consult. Algemeen Dagblad, 30 juni 2006.

33. Cate A ten; Patiënten in groep naar het spreekuur, Telegraaf 12 august 2006.

34. Exters S.; Uit de Schaduw. Plexus, oktober 2006.

35. Cort de W; Samen sterk op spreekuur van de medisch specialist. Gelderlander 10 augustus 2006.

36. Meeussen J; Arts gaat als simultaanschaker langs de patiënten. Radbode 9, 2005.

37. Groepsconsult: Een nieuwe vorm van poliklinische zorg. Gelderse Valei 2006 maart. ZGV informatie.

38. Een nieuw fenomeen in de zorg: Gezamenlijke op consult: Kwaliteitsjournaal; april 2006, jaargang 8.

39. Tien patiënten tegelijk op consult bij neuroloog; artsen experimenteren met 'gezamenlijke medische afspraken'. Mednet Magazine, nr. 10, 18 mei 2006.

40. Kragten P. De meerwaarde van een Gezamenlijke Medische Afspraak. In Beweging.

41. Nieuw: op consult met lotgenoten. Gezondgids maart 2006. 69.

Part II
Implementing Group Visits

Chapter 10
Twenty Essential Steps to Implementing a Successful Group Visit Program

Let us now pull together all that we have learned so far in this book to: (1) establish 20 essential steps to implementing a successful group visit program (in this chapter); and (2) develop the "pipeline" for launching all new DIGMAs and PSMAs in the organization, which we cover in the following chapter.

Representing a new biopsychosocial model of care that provides high levels of patient and physician professional satisfaction, shared medical appointments can significantly impact the economics, efficiency, accessibility, quality, and outcomes of healthcare services rendered. To be fully successful, they carry their own special support requirements for proper implementation—in terms of budget, design, training, promotion, personnel, facilities, and program evaluation. The 20 key steps discussed in this chapter are critical to the successful implementation of any DIGMA or PSMA program (many of these key steps apply to CHCCs as well), which are the two group visit models that are best envisioned as a series of individual office visits with observers—and which are currently in widespread use in both fee-for-service and capitated healthcare systems. Although this chapter will primarily focus upon DIGMAs and PSMAs, CHCCs require most of these same steps to be taken; however, they do not require certain resources (such as a behaviorist and documenter).

This chapter is dedicated to laying the basic foundation for your SMA program. It systematically addresses each of 20 essential steps required for developing both a successful shared medical appointment program in actual practice and an overall strategy for moving your program forward (in a step-by-step manner) toward organization-wide implementation (Table 10.1). You must first establish the groundwork for your program by addressing these 20 keys to success: first, by obtaining the required degree of administrative support; next, by securing the necessary personnel, facilities, promotional, and budgetary supports for the program; then, by conducting a pilot study; and finally, by expanding your SMA program to organization-wide implementation.

Once you have laid the groundwork to a successful group visit program by successfully addressing the 20 macroscopic keys discussed in the first section of this chapter, you can then review the 24 practical tips for physicians to use in creating and running a successful DIGMA or PSMA program—as well as 10 common beginner's mistakes to avoid—which are discussed later on in this chapter. Finally, Chapter 11 discusses the detailed *pipeline* by which all SMAs are launched—which represents a microscopic look at the entire sequence of steps that must be taken prior to, during, and after the launch of each and every new SMA implemented within the system—i.e., in primary care as well as the various medical subspecialties.

Step 1: Secure High-Level Administrative Support

Do not even consider implementing a group visit program within your integrated healthcare delivery system without first securing the necessary administrative support from the highest levels of executive leadership, unless, of course, you are either a solo practitioner or in a small group practice. Obtaining the required degree of high-level support within the organization is the first and—with the singular exception of selecting of the best possible champion for the entire program—most important step to implementing a successful DIGMA and PSMA program.

Give Presentations to Executive Leadership and Submit a Business Plan

In order to secure high-level administrative support, thoughtful but succinct presentations on DIGMAs, CHCCs, and Physicals SMAs must first be given to upper

E.B. Noffsinger, *Running Group Visits in Your Practice*, DOI 10.1007/b106441_10,
© Springer Science+Business Media, LLC 2009

Table 10.1 Twenty steps to a successful DIGMA or PSMA program

1. Secure the necessary high-level administrative support and budget for the SMA program first (through presentations and a business plan given to upper management), before attempting to launch any group visits.
2. Achieve organizational consensus to proceed at the executive leadership level, despite any initial dissension or diverse opinions.
3. Select the best possible champion (and program coordinator) for your group visit program—i.e., in larger systems.
4. Establish a comprehensive billing policy first—i.e., before starting a group visit program.
5. Have your corporate attorney or risk management department draft an appropriate confidentiality release for all attendees to sign.
6. Develop computer codes and scheduling procedures for your group visit program.
7. Pre-establish and consistently meet *minimum*, *target*, and *maximum* census goals for each SMA that is established.
8. Promote the program effectively to patients: (a) through personal invitations from providers and staff; and (b) through use of high-quality marketing materials that accurately reflect the quality care patients can expect to receive in the SMA.[a]
9. Use comfortable, well-equipped group, and exam rooms.
10. Max-pack all DIGMAs and PSMAs to maximize the amount of quality medical care delivered during each session—plus provide brief individual exams and private one-on-one discussions with the physician as needed.
11. Optimize the mix of individual and group appointments in the provider's practice.
12. Select your initial SMA providers with care.
13. Carefully select and train the behaviorist for each SMA.
14. Select the best possible treatment team for each SMA—a dedicated scheduler, a documenter (whenever possible), and one or two nursing personnel (RNs, LVNs, MAs, Nursing Techs, etc.) in addition to the behaviorist.
15. Custom design each SMA to the specific needs, goals, practice style, and patient panel constituency of the individual provider.
16. The physician must learn to delegate as much as possible and appropriate to the skilled and trained SMA team.
17. Develop policies that will ensure success, promptly solve any problems that arise, and avoid making common mistakes.
18. Most systems will want to start with a carefully designed pilot study and then evaluate its success.
19. Expand the SMA program from successful pilot study to system-wide implementation.
20. Determine how rapidly you want to move the program forward throughout the system—i.e., how many new SMAs do you want to launch each year?

[a] Note: Downloadable templates/examples of all necessary forms and documents for your SMA program are included in the DVD attached to this book (although they are not to be used "as ia")—confidentiality releases, patient satisfaction surveys, announcement letters, invitations, wall posters, program description fliers, chart note templates, etc. (which should prove most helpful in enabling you to develop your own forms).

management in order to: update them on these models; make them aware of the multiple benefits these SMA models can offer; discuss the respective strengths and weaknesses of these group visit models; and cover key personnel, facilities, promotional, and budgetary supports that are required for success.

Submit a proposed business plan that includes DIGMAs and PSMAs as efficient, cost-effective tools for better achieving critical organizational objectives: increased productivity; improved accessibility; the leveraging of existing resources; improved job doability; enhanced quality of care; improved outcomes; increased patient and physician professional satisfaction; a strengthened bottom line; and enhanced value in medical services rendered.

Administrative Support Means Real and Meaningful Support for the SMA Program

Administrative support must include not only your organization's blessing and best wishes, but also the required budget, personnel, support staff, promotional materials, and facilities that are mandatory for launching a successful DIGMA and/or Physicals SMA program. For example, in larger systems, the required support personnel for a

successful DIGMA or PSMA would include a carefully selected champion (and a program coordinator), a skilled and specially trained behaviorist well matched to both the physician and the physician's practice, one or two nursing personnel capable of efficiently dispatching the expanded duties of this role, and a documenter (especially for systems that have shifted to electronic medical records).

In addition to properly training the physician's own scheduling staff, well-trained dedicated scheduling personnel typically also need to be assigned to the group visit program (perhaps one dedicated scheduler for every 15–25 SMAs that are established)—and given sufficient time dedicated to each DIGMA or PSMA every week to make certain that targeted census levels will consistently be attained for every session that is held. Proceeding without these critical supports first being in place—supports that only high-level administrative authorization can ensure—could undermine the success of the entire program.

Inadequate Support Undercuts Attendance and Productivity

Healthcare organizations frequently try to skimp in various ways on the supports necessary for a well-run group visit program, which all too often results in patient and staff resistance to the program, poor group attendance, and reduced productivity. Some organizations design their group visit programs around utilizing the cheapest, rather than the best available, SMA personnel. Some systems want physicians to run their DIGMAs and PSMAs without behaviorists, while others refuse to provide schedulers, adequate nursing support, documenters, dedicated schedulers, or a champion. Other integrated healthcare delivery systems avoid making necessary *up-front* investments—e.g., in appropriately training the physician's support staff, in the high quality and professional appearing marketing materials needed for promoting the program to patients, or in a program coordinator to assist the champion by handling most of the SMA program's administrative and operational details. Still other medical groups provide only an inadequate *shoestring* budget for the program, fail to provide the needed facilities, or refuse to put the necessary priority on the SMA program to ensure that the support needs required for success are adequately met on a consistent basis.

There are appropriate ways to save money in your SMA program, but the foregoing are not among them. All such deviations from what is being recommended for the successful implementation of a group visit program will likely have the same ultimate net effect—reduced census during sessions, decreased efficiency, and frustration for patients, physicians, and support staffs alike. And with decreased group census comes reduced productivity and economic gains for the program—and all too often, reduced group interaction and patient bonding as well.

Budget

An adequate budget for the program (as well as the necessary personnel, group and exam room space, and professional appearing and informative promotional materials) is required for success. The necessary budget for the program should be outlined in the business plan submitted to executive leadership, which should carefully and realistically estimate all costs for the program—at least in its early stages (e.g., for the pilot study), with projections of budgetary needs as well as potential cost savings thereafter. Although the costs of personnel, facilities, promotional materials, and forms will in the long run be more than offset by the cost savings from the increased productivity of a well-run DIGMA and Physicals SMA program (see financial analysis at end of Chapter 2), these costs are nonetheless real and need to be secured during the early, start-up stages of the program.

With DIGMAs and PSMAs, much of the hard work comes at the very beginning of the program, which is one of the main reasons that everybody isn't doing them. In the beginning of the program, promotional materials as well as chart note templates and all necessary forms need to be developed (examples of which are included in the DVD attached to this book). In addition, the champion's job in larger healthcare systems (as well as that of the program coordinator) in terms of recruiting providers, custom-designing SMAs, training staff, and establishing the pilot study will likely be the most time consuming in the beginning—as patients, physicians, and staff will likely be largely uninformed about group visits and the multiple benefits they offer (and therefore be most resistant to them). Furthermore, it is at the beginning of the SMA program that the *pipeline* and systems necessary for efficiently conducting DIGMAs and PSMAs will not yet have been developed and put into place.

Personnel

The personnel requirements for a successful DIGMA or PSMA include the following: (1) an appropriate and specially trained behaviorist; (2) one or two nursing personnel (RNs, medical assistants, LVNs, nursing techs, etc.), which typically includes the physician's own nurse or MA; (3) a documenter (optional, but highly recommended); (4) a dedicated scheduler attached to the program to ensure that all sessions are filled to targeted census levels (perhaps one full-time dedicated scheduler for every 15–25 DIGMAs and PSMAs that are established); and, in larger systems, (5) a champion with primary responsibility and the commensurate authority for overseeing the entire SMA program (as well as a carefully selected program coordinator to assist the champion by handling most administrative and operational details). Most of these personnel resources will likely be available internally in larger integrated healthcare delivery systems, especially during the early stages of the program when personnel demands are smallest; however, in the long run (as 10, 20, 50, 100, or 1000 or more DIGMAs and Physicals SMAs are implemented within larger systems), additional personnel resources will likely need to be hired on an as-needed basis.

Although optional, it is important to note that having a documenter (who is trained to meet the physician's specific charting requirements, using the physician's own chart note template) to assist with the extensive documentation requirements of a DIGMA or PSMA can be most helpful—especially for PSMAs and systems using electronic medical records (EMR). A documenter is helpful not only in increasing physician efficiency, but also in obtaining physician *buy-in* to the group visit concept—especially in the case of systems using electronic medical records. This is because one of the greatest physician resistances to group visits is the amount of documentation that they fear will be incurred after the session is over (even though the goal of every DIGMA and PSMA session is to complete all work during the session). In addition, having a documenter permits a superior chart note to be generated—one that is both comprehensive and contemporaneous in nature, and uses the physician's own chart note template—on each patient during the available group time.

Facilities

In terms of facilities, DIGMAs typically require a large furnished group room capable of comfortably seating 15–25 persons plus a nearby exam room. PSMAs typically require a group room that is only half as large; however, they might also need 2–5 (most commonly 4) exam rooms—although they need not be near to the group room (as is the case for the exam room used in a DIGMA) and can even be in the physician's own office area. These usually include the physician's own exam rooms, plus a couple of additional exam rooms from a colleague who is not in the clinic at the time the Physicals SMA is scheduled.

Step 2: Reach Organizational Consensus Despite Dissension

Various administrators and members of the organization's executive leadership team are likely to initially hold widely differing opinions with regard to whether or not to launch a SMA program. Therefore, it is important that organizational consensus first be achieved at the management or executive committee level—despite anticipated dissension and diverse initial opinions.

Expect Dissension Because SMAs Represent a Major Paradigm Shift

In many integrated healthcare delivery systems, resistance will likely occur in part because some will feel that the physicians and staff have already undergone *too much change* recently—perhaps changes in external/internal review processes or standards, performance measures, panel sizes, reimbursement policies, electronic medical records, advanced clinic access goals, etc. In addition, executive leadership might experience *push-back* regarding group visits from some of their most conservative members—perhaps the chief financial officer, billing and compliance experts, or certain *old school* physicians. Furthermore, some leaders and administrators might hold the view that they would not want to personally attend a group visit session, and therefore assume that many others would feel likewise, despite the well-established fact that patient satisfaction with group visits properly designed, supported, and run has consistently been very high.

Despite Dissension, Agreement Must Be Achieved Before Proceeding

Whatever the source of disagreement, the important point is that the organization's leadership needs to successfully resolve this internal dissension before moving forward with group visits. The last thing that anyone would want is for leaders and administrators who do not want to proceed with the SMA program to feel unheard, dismissed, or overruled—and then to *lay in wait*, perhaps for years, so that they can pounce with righteous indignation when something eventually does go wrong with the program.

Certainly, things can go wrong with almost any new program, especially with one that differs as dramatically from traditional individual office visits as group visits do—and one that can be expected to stress the system as much as DIGMAs and PSMAs will (i.e., because of the large amount of change they introduce and their dramatically increased productivity).

Overcome Dissension by Giving Presentations, Information, and a Business Plan to Leadership

In larger healthcare organizations, a good starting point for any SMA program is to first provide thoughtful, succinct presentations on DIGMAs, CHCCs, and Physicals SMAs to upper management (preferably even a business plan) to secure high-level administrative support, to answer any questions, and to address any resistance to the program. If dissension and disagreement with the program persists, then perhaps a balanced follow-up presentation to the leadership team addressing the points of disagreement as well as the multifarious potential benefits that group visits can offer to patients, physicians, and the organization—along with their support requirements—might be helpful.

These presentations should allow adequate time for questions and answers—plus in depth discussions pertaining to any concerns or resistances regarding the proposed SMA program. A business plan covering the SMA program would help to clarify the potential benefits and costs of the program, as well as the resource and support requirements necessary for success. In addition, a couple of relevant articles published about group visits (and, most especially, this book) will undoubtedly prove beneficial in overcoming this impasse posed by dissension. In any case, it is imperative to recognize that, before any group visit program is initiated, it is critical to the ultimate success of the SMA program that a working degree of organizational consensus to be achieved despite initial dissension.

Step 3: Select the Best Possible Champion and Provide the Required Amount of Time

Once the necessary administrative support has been secured and consensus to proceed has been achieved, the next step in larger healthcare organizations is to carefully select the best possible SMA champion—one who has the necessary skills plus adequate time available to dedicate to the program. The thoughtful selection of a SMA champion is only important to the development of a successful SMA program in larger and mid-sized integrated healthcare delivery systems—perhaps those having approximately 20 or more physicians. The champion must become intimately familiar with the DIGMA and PSMA models through this book, recently published articles, and by attending existing successful group visit programs in other organizations. Select the champion carefully as this is the person who will assume overall responsibility for the entire SMA program, and must therefore be capable of multitasking and handling the substantial responsibilities of this position.

Not having any champion at all in a larger system would be a serious error because SMA programs will seldom migrate from one provider in the organization to the next (or from site to another) without the ongoing efforts of the champion. Because everybody is already so busy dealing with existing tasks, if SMAs do migrate at all (i.e., from provider to provider, from department to department, and from facility to facility), it will likely be at a much slower rate than if the active efforts of an effective champion are involved.

Because of the importance of the role of SMA champion, it is critical that remuneration be commensurate with the extensive responsibilities of this position. This will ensure that, once the multiple duties of this job are well learned and being efficiently dispatched, the champion will be motivated to stay in this position (and with the organization) for a long time.

The Champion Has Many Responsibilities and Must Have Appropriate Qualifications

The champion needs to be respected by—and able to work closely with—administrative leadership, physicians, and medical staffs alike. The champion (with the program coordinator's assistance) needs to serve as *point person* for: the entire SMA program. This includes assuming primary responsibility for: (1) recruiting new providers to run group visits for their practices; (2) custom designing each provider's SMA around their own particular needs, goals, practice style, and patient panel; (3) developing the entire SMA program and rapidly expanding it throughout the system; (4) overseeing the myriad of operational, training, and measurement details necessary to ensure the program's success; and (5) ensuring that everything goes as smoothly as possible and proceeds in a timely manner.

In addition, the champion plays a critical role in designing, conducting, and evaluating an effective pilot study to establish feasibility of concept within the organization—and, assuming that the pilot is successful, in expeditiously moving the SMA program forward from pilot study to facility–and organization-wide implementation. Clearly, the champion must have a strong working knowledge of the various group visit models, be a strong and tireless advocate of SMAs, have an understanding of the culture of the organization and be able to work within it, and be cable of moving the SMA program forward throughout the system—i.e., despite various operational challenges, physician and staff resistances, and possible opposition from a number of sources (all of which can be expected with any new innovation that introduces as much change to the modus operandi as group visits do).

In addition, we are currently setting up the "Noffsinger Institute of Group Visits" at Harvard Vanguard Medical Associates/Atrius Health to train executive leaders, physicians, allied health providers, SMA champions, SMA program coordinators, behaviorists, nursing personnel, documenters, and dedicated schedulers from interested medical groups around the nation (indeed, the world) on how to optimally dispatch their duties in a successful group visit program within their own organization. Whenever possible, it is also advisable that the champion should try to visit one or two other healthcare organizations that are already successfully conducting a substantial group visit program in order to witness what they are doing and learn firsthand from their experiences—i.e., from what they are doing *wrong* as well as what they are doing *right*.

Most Systems Select a Psychologist or Social Worker as SMA Champion

Most integrated delivery systems prefer to have a highly skilled, experienced, and motivated mental health professional (such as a skilled health psychologist or experienced medical social worker) as SMA champion. Clearly, this person must be highly respected by physician colleagues and administration alike. The champion will need a detailed working knowledge of the various group visit models, considerable experience in running and managing large groups, a solid understanding of the psychosocial issues faced by medical patients and their families, and an ability to work closely with physicians, staff, and administrators.

A Mental Health Champion Can Act as the Behaviorist at the Start of Each New DIGMA and PSMA

A psychologist or social worker champion would have the advantage of being able to train the behaviorist for each new DIGMA or PSMA that is established. Although this is optional, the mental health champion could even temporarily act as the behaviorist for the first couple of sessions at the start of each new DIGMA or PSMA as it is being launched—i.e., while simultaneously training the replacement behaviorist who will ultimately take over the program once it is established. While the champion is temporarily acting in the behaviorist role, the replacement behaviorist (who also attends the early sessions and watches the champion in action) is then able to gain important training as to the intricacies of this new role—all of which can ultimately prove invaluable when later taking over as the behaviorist.

The champion needs to have exceptional communication and behavioral health skills, and be able to quickly and tactfully address group dynamic and psychosocial issues during group sessions. The champion also needs to be empathic toward medical patients and their families, while being a knowledgeable and patient teacher. Once the SMA is running smoothly and all system problems are resolved, and once the behaviorist is sufficiently trained and the physician is comfortable with the new program, the champion can then gracefully exit this newly established DIGMA or PSMA to start additional group visits with other providers (i.e., with the next cohort of interested primary and specialty care providers in the system).

Seasoned Nurses, Administrators, and Educators Are Sometimes Selected as Champions

If you do not have an appropriate mental health professional available to champion your SMA program, then consider anybody else who might be qualified and available to you—someone who could adequately fulfill the multiple responsibilities of the champion's role. For example, some organizations have an abundance of experienced nurses, seasoned administrators, solid diabetes nurse educators, or capable health educators who know the physicians and patients well, understand how to get things done in the organization, and would be highly motivated to become the SMA champion.

However, champions who are not mental health providers would probably not be able to temporarily act as behaviorist when new DIGMAs and PSMAs are launched. In addition, champions without a mental health background would likely need additional training in such areas as: managing large groups and fostering group interaction; understanding the emotional and psychosocial issues of medical patients; developing, managing, and overseeing a rapidly expanding SMA program; and gaining the behavioral health skills needed to train behaviorists for their active roles within DIGMAs and Physicals SMAs.

Another Possibility Is to Have Both a Physician and a Mental Health Champion

Some larger healthcare organizations find that they would like to have a physician champion to head their SMA program, but recognize that their physician staff is already too busy to take on the multiple added duties that this position entails. A couple larger integrated healthcare delivery systems have solved this conundrum by having two champions: (1) a mental health champion, such as an experienced psychologist or social worker, tasked with the time-consuming, front-line responsibilities of managing the day-to-day operations of the entire SMA program; and (2) a higher level physician champion (one who is highly respected by administration and physician colleagues alike) in the less time-consuming role of having broad oversight responsibilities for the SMA program and reporting directly to administration and executive leadership. Such a physician champion would have oversight responsibilities for the SMA program, but in the more limited and less time-consuming role of reporting on the program's progress directly to organizational leadership. All of the other time-consuming, day-to-day operational, and administrative responsibilities for initiating, developing, managing, evaluating, and expanding the program would then go to the mental health champion. Clearly, the physician and mental health champions would need to get along very well and be able to work closely together.

If No Qualified Internal Candidate Exists, Then Go Outside for Your SMA Champion

As has been discussed, there are many reasons for having a SMA champion in larger healthcare systems, and the selection of champion is critical to the overall success of the program. If your organization cannot identify and recruit a qualified person internally to act as SMA champion, then larger systems should consider going outside to hire the right person for this absolutely critical role.

The Champion Starts by Recruiting Willing, Motivated Physicians on an Ongoing Basis

To develop the SMA program effectively and foster physician acceptance and buy-in, the champion needs to network and frequently attend appropriate primary care and medical and surgical subspecialty departmental meetings. At these meetings, the champion gives presentations to: familiarize physicians with today's major group visit models; answer physicians' various questions; address common physician concerns; discuss the multiple benefits that well-run SMA programs can offer (to physicians, patients, and the organization); and call for physicians to volunteer to start a SMA for their practice—preferable busy physicians with substantial patient backlogs and access problems, as it will be easier to keep their group sessions filled. Once providers (physicians, nurse practitioners, osteopaths, pharmacists, physician's assistants, podiatrists, etc.) have indicated that they have an interest in possibly starting a DIGMA, CHCC, and/or Physicals SMA for their practices, the champion then typically follows up promptly by meeting with them individually.

The Champion Then Meets with Interested Providers Individually

After attending departmental meetings in an effort to recruit interested providers, the champion then arranges one-on-one follow-up meetings with those providers who indicate interest in establishing SMAs for their practices. During these initial one-on-one meetings, the champion encourages providers to try SMAs for their practices while: familiarizing them with the various SMA models and their respective strengths and weaknesses; answering any questions or concerns; addressing any operational and implementation issues; and clarifying the many benefits that well-run SMAs can offer to these providers and their practices. The champion also makes clear that, while much will be done by the champion and program coordinator to minimize the front-end time commitment that the physician will need to make in order to get the SMA launched, there is one ongoing responsibility that every provider must assume in order to have a successful SMA program—i.e., they must take primary responsibility for keeping all sessions filled to desired capacity, which requires inviting all appropriate patients seen during regular office visits (i.e., via a 30–60 second personal, positively worded invitation) to have their next visit be in the SMA. In addition to extensive verbal discussion, it is helpful if videotapes on SMAs are shown, copies of relevant published articles are provided, and a copy of this book is given to interested providers. Subsequent to these initial meetings, at least in integrated healthcare delivery systems, the champion

would likely set up a meeting with each physician's department chief and site administrators to discuss the proposed program—and to secure administrative input and approval.

Physicians Must Trust that the Champion Will Be Sensitive to Their Needs

The champion must be able to develop strong relationships of trust with physician colleagues. The champion must spend a great deal of time recruiting physicians, which means: getting to know them; understanding the challenges they are faced with on a daily basis; recommending the appropriate SMA model to them; addressing any concerns physicians might have about SMAs; and making clear the multiple benefits that DIGMAs, CHCCs, and PSMAs can offer to physicians, patients, and the bottom line. For the SMA champion to be successful, it is important that the physician and champion genuinely grow to like and trust one another—which takes time and a certain degree of contact.

Next, the Champion Customizes the SMA to the Particular Needs of the Physician

Once physicians elect to run one or more SMAs for their practices, the champion then meets with them individually to custom design each DIGMA, CHCC, or PSMA according to the physician's own particular needs, goals, practice style, and patient panel constituency. The champion and program coordinator also schedule some additional follow-up meetings with the provider, and then with the provider's staff. These meetings should be scheduled, whenever possible, during lunch or non-clinic hours so as to minimize the physician's down time. During these meetings, the appropriate SMA model and subtype are selected; the DIGMA team members are chosen; the group and exam rooms are identified; all forms and promotional materials are developed; and any handouts to be used during the program are selected.

In addition, appropriate training is provided to the physician—as well as the physician's support staff—during these meetings on how to run the SMA and successfully recruit patients on an ongoing basis so as to consistently fill all sessions. It is also in these meetings that the champion explains what responsibilities the provider must fulfill for success (e.g., the importance of staying succinct and focused at all times, as well as of personally inviting each and every appropriate patient seen during traditional office visits to attend the SMA for their next medical visit) and what supports will be made available by the SMA Department.

Once the heterogeneous, homogeneous, or mixed subtype is selected and the patient populations for each session are identified, a variety of additional parameters for each DIGMA and PSMA needs to be selected: frequency; weekday; time of day; session length; and start date. The group and exam rooms are chosen, members of the SMA treatment team are selected (behaviorist, nursing personnel, documenter, and dedicated scheduler), and a realistic start date is picked. Finally, the provider's input is necessary for: specifying which patients will and will not be included in each SMA session; selecting and developing any patient education handouts that are to be used during the SMA; determining whether a Patent Packet will be used and, if so, precisely what its contents will be; and creating various forms and promotional materials for the provider's SMA from established templates already developed for the SMA program. Such forms include the chart note template that the provider will ultimately use in the SMA as well as the various promotional materials and handouts that will be employed.

Once Customized, Numerous Other SMA Details Need to Be Attended to

After these initial meetings with the provider, the SMA team, and the provider's support staff, the champion (in larger systems, with the assistance of a program coordinator) then needs to attend to the numerous details itemized in the *pipeline* described in Chapter 11 in order to minimize the physician's outlay of time in the design and planning stages of the group visit. This includes developing the handouts, Patient Packet, and promotional materials that will be used in the program—as well as training the physician, schedulers, and the support staff regarding how to successfully refer patients into the DIGMA or Physicals SMA.

Directing appropriate patients seen in the SMA into future DIGMA and PSMA sessions whenever possible (i.e., for their next follow-up visit or private physical examination, respectively) maximally leverages the physician's time and increases the productivity of the SMA—plus plays an important role in maintaining group census targets during future sessions. It also increases the physician's ability to manage a large patient panel—both by scheduling patients that can appropriately be treated in a SMA into that highly efficient and cost-effective venue (rather than into more costly and less efficient individual office visits) and by making valuable individual appointments more available to those patients who truly need them. Nonetheless, it is important that patient attendance be voluntary, as SMAs are meant to always be voluntary to patients and providers alike.

In larger systems, the champion is actively involved in the launch of every new SMA. Once the provider has been recruited and the SMA program has been custom designed to the provider's specific needs, then the champion (together with the program coordinator) must do everything possible to move the SMA smoothly through its design, development, training, implementation, and evaluation phases. This enables the group visit to be successfully launched as rapidly as possible and with a minimum amount of the provider's own time being committed to the process. When the physician's involvement in the planning process is necessary, all such meetings need to be set up with sensitivity to the physician's busy schedule—and must therefore be thoroughly prepared for by the champion and program coordinator, as well as efficiently conducted.

The Champion Often then Participates in the Actual Launch of the SMA

In larger systems, the champion typically needs to actually participate in the launch of each new DIGMA and Physicals SMA, handling any systems or operational problems that might arise, training the physician and behaviorist as needed, addressing any issues that the nursing and documentation personnel might have, making certain that census requirements are achieved, and ensuring that each new program runs smoothly and on time. However, this is done with the knowledge that initial SMA sessions often finish late at first (and sometimes quite late), despite everyone's best efforts—i.e., until everyone becomes more comfortable with their new SMA roles and responsibilities, everyone's anxieties gradually disappear, and the treatment team becomes more succinct and coordinated. To accomplish this, it is recommended that the champion actually sit and observe the first couple of sessions—or actually participate by acting as the behaviorist during these initial sessions, while the group visit is getting started. In addition, whenever possible, it is important that the champion debriefs for approximately 10–20 minutes after each of these initial sessions with the physician, behaviorist, documenter, and nursing personnel to discuss how to make future sessions even better and more efficient.

In Larger Systems, a Program Coordinator Is Also Needed to Leverage the Champion's Time

Many larger systems will also need to provide a program coordinator (who is often a seasoned administrator, manager, clinical supervisor, etc.) to assist the champion in every way possible. It is important to carefully select the program coordinator, as this is the person who will work closely with the champion and will leverage the champion's time by handling most planning, operational, management, and administrative details. The program coordinator's responsibilities will include: helping to launch all new SMA programs; assisting in the development of templates for all forms and promotional materials used in the program; supervising the SMA nurses and dedicated schedulers (and possibly even behaviorists); dispatching most of the SMA program's administrative, management, and operational details; generating the weekly, or twice weekly, pre-booking census reports on all SMAs that have been implemented; and developing weekly, monthly, quarterly, and annual reports that are necessary to properly evaluate the SMA program on an ongoing basis.

The Champion and Program Coordinator Develop a Pipeline for All New SMAs

In larger systems, the champion and program coordinator will also need to develop a *pipeline* for all new SMAs (see Chapter 11), which consists of the entire sequence of discrete steps that must be completed to successfully launch each and every new DIGMA or PSMA within the system. Once this pipeline has been developed within the healthcare organization, the same series of steps and processes detailed therein can then be utilized for designing, launching, running, and evaluating all subsequent SMAs that are implemented—although some minor alterations might be required from time to time. In this manner, efficiency is gained, as one does not need to waste time and energy continuously *recreating the wheel* for every new group visit that is implemented within the system.

During the initial planning and start-up phases of the DIGMA or Physicals SMA, the physician can delegate many of the associated time-consuming tasks to the champion—who can, in turn, delegate a lot of these duties to the program coordinator. Likewise, during the actual group visit sessions, the physician delegates heavily to the various members of the SMA team. In order to minimize the outlay of the physician's time outside of the actual group visit sessions, the champion and program coordinator—not the physician—should oversee most of the operational details and time-consuming tasks associated with the planning, training, implementation, and evaluation phases of each new SMA that is established.

Step 4: Address Billing Issues First, Before Starting SMAs

Before starting any group visit program, healthcare organizations must first come to a clear decision as to how they will address the issue of billing, a matter that is still evolving and is not completely resolved for group visits, and which undoubtedly differs for the various types of group visit models. Therefore, you will want to first contact local representatives of your contracted insurers as well as the appropriate governmental agencies to let them know what your are doing, why your have decided to offer SMAs, and what benefits they offer to patients and insurers alike—and to understand what the reimbursement ramifications are as well as any possible billing issues or concerns.

Because no CPT codes currently exist that are specific to SMAs, the entire issue of billing for group visits is still evolving. Nonetheless, DIGMAs and PSMAs have been successfully used for many years in both fee-for-service and fully capitated systems, as well as in systems that are partially fee-for-service and partially capitated. Other types of group visit models may have different types of billing issues in the fee-for-service world because, unlike DIGMAs and PSMAs, they are not run as a series of one doctor–one patient encounters with observers throughout the entire session. In addition to the fee-for-service and capitated healthcare organizations within the private sector, these two group visit models have also been used nationwide as well as internationally in a variety of applications in other settings as well—such as VA, DoD (Air Force, Army, Navy), and public healthcare settings. Although group visits are still in their early stages, they have been around for many years and are already widely deployed by early adopters nationally (and more recently, internationally). They are rapidly expanding, both in the number of group visit programs offered and in the variety of applications in primary care and the medical and surgical subspecialties.

In part, the success of DIGMAs and PSMAs in the fee-for-service world is the result of the fact that, from start to finish, these two group visit models are run throughout like a series of one doctor–one patient encounters with observers attending to each patient's unique medical needs individually. In other words, these two SMA models are run throughout just like a sequence of individual office visits with observers. Additionally, the same medical services (and often more) are provided in properly run DIGMAs and PSMAs as in traditional individual office visits. Well-run DIGMAs and PSMAs are best envisioned as a series of individual doctor visits with other patients as observers that are conducted in a supportive group setting—where all present can simultaneously listen, learn, and interact.

Billing Can Be Straightforward in Capitated Systems

Clearly, all three of today's major group visit models discussed in this book (DIGMAs, CHCCs, and PSMAs) appear to work well and present no significant billing issues in capitated healthcare delivery systems—i.e., beyond whether or not the system chooses to offer group visits and, if so, how much to charge for the co-payment.

DIGMAs and CHCCs Were Developed in a Capitated System

In fact, the DIGMA and CHCC models (but not the PSMA model) were originally developed at Kaiser Permanente, a large, fully capitated, staff model HMO. The author was a psychologist at the Kaiser Permanente Santa Clara and San Jose Medical Centers from 1973 to 1999, where he served as Director of Oncology Counseling and Chronic Illness Services as well as the Team Manager of the Affective Disorders Team—and participated at the regional level in Kaiser's adult primary care redesign. Dr. John C. Scott developed the CHCC model at Kaiser Permanente in Colorado in 1991, whereas I independently developed the DIGMA model at Kaiser Permanente in San Jose in 1996. On the other hand, the author developed the PSMA model in 2001 at the Palo Alto Medical Foundation, which at that time was a largely fee-for-service (but partially capitated) healthcare organization in which he served as Director of Clinical Access Improvement and as champion of their SMA program from 2000 to 2003.

Capitated Systems Often Have the Internal Resources Needed for Group Visits

Although capitated systems present their own unique challenges, they have the advantage of being largely self-contained—because all of the necessary ingredients for a successful DIGMA, CHCC, or Physicals SMA program are often available in-house. They often have the staff necessary to support the program (providers, behaviorists, nurses, schedulers, documenters, champion, program coordinator, etc.) as well as the required group and exam room facilities. In fact, many capitated systems already have considerable experience in both providing a multidisciplinary team-based approach to care and running large group treatment programs (for example, in their psychiatry, behavioral medicine, substance abuse, and health education departments as well as in chronic illness population management programs).

Capitated Systems Nonetheless Face Potential Challenges

However, capitated systems can sometimes face their own particular challenges as well—such as understaffing issues, heavy patient demand, large patient panel sizes, over-extended physicians and support staffs, access problems, relatively short appointment times, backlogs and delays, heavily booked group and exam room space, an organizational structure that can be compartmentalized into many discrete *silos*, and multiple competing demands upon budget, facilities, and personnel.

Competing resource demands can make it difficult to acquire the resources—and the necessary degree of priority on these resources—that properly run group visits require. Some capitated systems might try to run a group visit program with minimal support, with little if any investment in training time and promotional materials, and by utilizing the least expensive (rather than the best possible) personnel—all of which could severely undercut the quality and efficiency of their DIGMA and PSMA programs. Furthermore, this can also lead to potential abuses of group visits—such as groups being too large, physician panel sizes being further increased, or group visits not being voluntary to patients and staff alike (which has always been a fundamental maxim of today's major group visit models).

Capitated Systems Often Have Considerable Experience in Running Group Programs

On the positive side, capitated systems often have large population management programs and care pathways in place for the various types of chronic diseases and conditions—although these programs often do not make full use of group visits. These are largely group programs that offer a multidisciplinary team-based approach to care (often involving mid-level providers) for such chronic conditions as diabetes, congestive heart failures, depression, hypertension, asthma, etc. In addition, capitated systems often have solid group programs in their psychiatry, behavioral medicine, health education, and nutrition departments—such as group programs for the cognitive behavioral treatment of depression and anxiety, smoking cessation classes, nutrition classes, weight loss programs, exercise classes, etc.

Because fully capitated systems assume risk and are pre-paid for services to be rendered, the payment model in such organizations eliminates many of the billing issues surrounding group visits that could prove problematic in other types of healthcare delivery systems. It also incentivizes the use of midlevel providers, of a multidisciplinary team-based approach to care, and of gaining efficiency by off-loading as many physician duties as possible and appropriate onto less costly members of the care delivery team. In addition, their philosophy regarding health maintenance, disease self-management, prevention, self-efficacy, and patient education and empowerment fits nicely with the philosophical underpinnings of group visits.

Billing for Group Visits in Fee-For-Service Systems

In fee-for-service (FFS) organizations, the issue of billing for group visits is still evolving—and some uncertainty still exists. At present, I am not aware of any billing procedures or specific CPT codes that exist either for group visits in general or for the different types of existing group visit models. Therefore, FFS systems must address this uncertainty as best they can through use of existing billing and compliance codes and procedures. As a result, FFS healthcare organizations may vary in their decision as to whether they choose to proceed with a group visit program at this time—and, if so, what guidelines, safeguards, billing procedures, and documentation requirements they will put into place for their SMA program. It has been the author's experience that many billing and compliance experts in fee-for-service systems around the country have pointed out that properly run DIGMAs and PSMAs are conducted from beginning to end to be like a series of individual office visits with observers occurring in a supportive group setting—with basically the same types of care being delivered in both settings.

They also point out that current billing codes neither address the issue of how many observers you are allowed to have in a medical visit nor limit the setting in which care is delivered—i.e., in an exam room, a group room, or a doc-in-the-box at the local Costco, K-Mart, or pharmacy. Patients already sometimes bring spouses, family members, friends, and caregivers to their individual office visits, so a precedent already exists for observers in traditional medical visits. Furthermore, mothers already sometimes take multiple siblings to a traditional pediatric office visit during which they all simultaneously receive care—so that there are even precedents with individual office visits for having other patients as observers. DIGMAs and Physicals SMAs simply extend this concept of observers to include all other patients and support persons in attendance at the group. SMAs also formally broaden the concept of appropriate medical setting to include the group room as well as the exam room. Neither the number of observers present nor the setting in which care is delivered appears to be addressed in current billing regulations and procedures.

FFS Systems Often Bill DIGMAs and PSMAs by Level of Care Delivered and Documented, but Not for Counseling Time

At present, it is the author's understanding that many fee-for-service systems currently running DIGMA and PSMA programs are billing for these visits according to the level of care delivered and documented—but only for care actually delivered to each patient individually within the group or exam room setting. There appears to be just a couple of differences relative to billing for SMAs versus individual office visits. First of all, these systems bill according to history, exam, and medical decision making only—i.e., not according to counseling time, which certainly provides a benefit to insurers. This is because many patients could simultaneously be benefiting from the same counseling in the group visit setting, and it would be egregious (and probably outright fraudulent) to simultaneously bill multiple patients for the same block of counseling time. However, if the counseling were specific to the single patient that the physician was working with at any given time, then it would seem that a case might be made for billing that particular patient for the specific counseling being delivered—but other patients acting as observers who happened to fortuitously benefit from this particular counseling could not be simultaneously billed.

The Behaviorist's Time Is Typically Not Billed

Second, these FFS systems apparently do not bill for the behaviorist's time—which represents a substantial benefit to both patients and insurers. This is because, if one were to bill for the behaviorist's time, then patients could conceivably receive two bills with co-payments for a single medical visit—which is potentially problematic and certainly could make patients angry. Therefore, fee-for-service systems typically do not bill for the behaviorist's time and instead treat it as an overhead expense to the SMA program—relying instead on the remarkable physician productivity gains that properly run DIGMAs and PSMAs offer to more than compensate for the additional personnel, facilities, and promotional costs that the program entails.

Billing for Group Visits Remains a Work in Progress

Billing for DIGMA and Physical SMA visits through use of existing CPT codes according to the level of medical care delivered and documented, regardless of the number of observers present, might seem like a reasonable approach to take. However, one must keep in mind that billing issues for group visits in fee-for-service systems are still evolving and have not yet been fully resolved—i.e., they remain *a work in progress*. In addition, they could potentially be complicated by the lack of specific E&M billing codes for DIGMA and PSMA visits.

On the other hand, there are billing and compliance experts nationwide who question the need for additional billing codes specific to DIGMAs and PSMAs. Instead, they view these two group visit models (but only these two group visit models) as being very much like a series of individual office visits with observers—i.e., because they involve delivery of the same types of medical care throughout. They differentiate these two SMA models from other group visit models that are designed to be more educational or supportive in nature (or are designed for mid-level providers), as DIGMAs and PSMAs are specifically designed to be highly efficient replacements for the traditional individual office visit itself. As a result, these billing and compliance experts conclude that the current billing codes for individual office visits are sufficient for these two group visit models alone.

Billing Issues Will Likely Vary for the Different Types of Group Visit Models

Let us now examine how the issue of billing differs for the various types of shared medical appointment models.

How Some Organizations Actually Bill for DIGMAs and PSMAs

Because they so closely resemble individual office visits throughout the whole session, it is my understanding that most systems currently bill for DIGMAs and PSMAs according to the level of care delivered and documented, using existing billing codes—except that they do not typically bill for either counseling time or the behaviorist's time. Thus, different patients attending these two types of group visits will likely be billed at different levels (i.e., based upon the level of care actually delivered and documented for each patient). Table 10.2 presents an approach to billing that some organizations are actually using for their DIGMA and PSMA program, an approach that I personally like (although I am not a billing and compliance expert) because it is open and transparent, and because the rationale seems to be reasonable.

In the June 2002 issue of *Minnesota Medicine*, which is published monthly by the Minnesota Medical Association, the issue of getting paid for DIGMAs is discussed in the following quote: "Many private insurers pay for DIGMAs and other group visit models. So does Medicaid....Medicare pays for them too, but has no specific CPT code for group visits. Existing CPT codes say nothing about how many observers can be present or in what settings care can be delivered, so many clinics bill for the level of care provided during the group visit. 'We can't find anything in the rules that prohibits observers,' says David Hooper, M.D., vice president of Palo Alto's

Table 10.2 Rationale and approach used by some organizations for billing DIGMAs and PSMAs[a]

- First, notify all insurers (including Medicare) about the new DIGMA or PSMA program, and the reasons for it.
- DIGMAs and PSMAs represent complete follow-up visits and physical exams, respectively.
- Like the individual office visits they so closely resemble, the focus from start to finish is upon delivery of medical care.
- Throughout, DIGMAs and PSMAs provide a series of one doctor–one physician encounters with observers (e.g., there is no preplanned educational presentation).
- DIGMAs and PSMAs sequentially address the unique medical needs of each patient individually.
- They offer the added benefits of greater patient education and the help and support of the behaviorist and other patients.
- There are currently no existing billing codes for group visits in general, or for the various specific SMA models.
- Capitated systems typically do not involve any significant group visit billing issues, other than whether or not to assess a co-payment—and, if so, how much the co-payment should be.
- Because of their similarity to individual office visits, many fee-for-service systems bill DIGMAs and PSMAs like traditional office visits—i.e., according to the level of care provided and documented.
- But they bill for history, exam, and medical decision making only—using existing billing codes.
- They do not bill for counseling time, which is difficult to allocate between patients.
- They also do not bill for the behaviorist's time, which is treated as an overhead expense to the SMA program.
- Not billing for counseling time or the behaviorist's time provides a clear benefit to insurers.
- Use a documenter to increase efficiency and generate comprehensive, contemporaneous chart notes. In every case, the documentation must support the bill, and the bill must cover only those services actually provided to each person individually.
- For every new SMA, review all billings for accuracy and compliance during the first 2 months.
- Spot check SMA billings thereafter to ensure that documentation and care delivered comply with all existing current billing standards.
- Provide specific remedial training for any physicians who fail to bill SMAs properly.
- Adjust to any future changes that might occur in the rules and regulations regarding billing for group visits.

[a] Note: To my knowledge, this approach is currently only being used for DIGMAs and PSMAs due to the uniqueness of these two group visit models, because—from start to finish—they alone are run like a series of individual office visits with observers.

clinical operations. 'Family members are often present during a one-on-one visit, so that sets a precedent'"(1).

Unlike CHCCs, with DIGMAs and PSMAs there is: (1) no formal warm-up segment; (2) no structured educational presentation; (3) no formal working break; (4) no question and answer period; and (5) no planning for the next session segment. Instead, properly run DIGMAs and Physicals SMAs are straight-out delivery of individualized medical care from start to finish. Unlike CHCCs, all of the patient education that occurs in the DIGMA and Physicals SMA models comes in the context of the doctor working with each patient individually—while other patients are privileged to listen, learn, and interact—rather than in any type of formal educational presentation to the group as a whole. In addition, unlike CHCCs, virtually all of the medical care that is delivered in a DIGMA or PSMA is provided in the group setting—where all presentcan listen, interact, and benefit.

The CHCC Model

In the CHCC model, the same 15–20 high utilizing, multimorbid geriatric patients are followed on a monthly basis over time. The visit itself is divided into two parts. First, there is the 90-minute group that is largely educational, although it does have a care delivery component during the working break (where vital signs are taken, some medical care can be delivered to patients individually, and it is determined which patients need to be seen during the approximate hour of individual care that follows the group). Although flexible, the group segment itself is structured and divided into warm-up, educational presentation, working break/care delivery, question and answer, and planning for the next visit components. Second, the group session is followed by approximately an hour of individual care for the roughly one-third of patients (typically 4–7 patients) that might need to be seen individually.

Although billing problems might be unlikely for the patients seen individually after group (however, little, if any, efficiency gain over individual office visits occurs here), there are questions as to how to appropriately bill for the approximately two-thirds of patients who attended just the group segment of the CHCC due to its largely educational and class-like nature. This would be particular problematic for any patients who might not happen to have an actual medical need at the time of the CHCC visit. Should some providers be calling these patients out of the group segment of the CHCC—one at a time—just to deliver one-on-one medical care to each patient individually in order to fulfill their understanding of FFS billing requirements, that would seem to be a case

of the *tail wagging the dog*. I say this because, when taken out of the group room, patients would then be missing out on what is then transpiring in the group room. Worse yet, all the other pateints in attendance would not be able to listen and learn from what the physician is discussing with each patient individually outside of the group room. It is important to note that, in the CHCC, the actual delivery of medical care in both the *working break* and the *individual care* segments typically occurs outside of earshot of other patients, so that the many efficiency and educational benefits of delivering medical care in the group setting are lost with the CHCC model.

Insurers Can Also Benefit

Clearly, not billing for either the counseling time or the behaviorist's time in DIGMAs and PSMAs constitutes a clear benefit to insurers, which seems appropriate. Personally, I view the fact that insurers can also benefit through properly run DIGMAs and PSMAs in fee-for-service systems as a positive. I have always felt that there is enough gain in carefully designed, properly run, adequately supported, and appropriately reimbursed DIGMA and Physicals SMA programs to benefit patients, physicians, healthcare organizations, third-party insurers, and corporate purchasers alike. Personally, I feel that it would be beneficial if all were to share to some degree in the multiple benefits that well-run group visit programs can offer.

Appropriate Reimbursement Is Required in FFS Systems for Group Visits to Survive

Nonetheless, should specific billing codes eventually be developed (either for group visits in general or for certain types of group visit models), one can only hope that the final reimbursement structure put forth will be fair, equitable, and appropriate—so that the economic viability of properly designed and run group visit programs, which can offer so much to our patients, is assured into the foreseeable future. Simply put, because they provide so many patient benefits, one can only hope that properly designed and conducted group visits will not be undermined in the future by potentially adverse reimbursement policies or issues—such as over- or under-incentivizing them, as discussed in Chapter 8. Furthermore, despite the fact that they can be so productive and efficient, one must recognize that group visits were originally designed to provide our patients with better and more accessible care—and that they do require additional personnel, facilities, and budgetary resources. Therefore, they need to be appropriately reimbursed in order for their future economic survival to be assured—i.e., to not be either under-reimbursed (which would kill group visit programs in FFS systems) or over-reimbursed (which could force physicians to run them in order to compete economically, even though they might not want to).

Recognize that Substantial Program Costs Are Associated with SMAs

It is important to recognize that, whereas there are many benefits to a successful group visit program (including economic benefits), there are also substantial risks, changes, and expenses involved with the program. Furthermore, it is only because DIGMAs and PSMAs can so dramatically ratchet up physician productivity and efficiency that a substantial net gain in economic benefit can be achieved—but only if predetermined targeted census levels are consistently attained. Nonetheless, the additional personnel, facilities, and promotional costs of the SMA program reduce these potential economic benefits considerably—so that adequate reimbursement is required for SMAs to succeed in the long run.

Miscellaneous Up-Front Costs

Organizations must first evaluate whether or not they want a DIGMA and PSMA program and, if so, whether or not they are willing to make the necessary initial front-end investments required for success. Although some corners can be cut on the pilot program in order to establish feasibility of concept (as pilot studies often need to make use of existing resources), once the decision has been made to proceed with organization-wide implementation, the appropriate investments in facilities, personnel, and promotion must necessarily be made in the program—investments that are detailed below.

However, even in the pilot study, certain investments must be made in the program from the outset—e.g., in quality promotional materials, the best possible champion, and appropriate personnel for the SMA teams. On the other hand, other investments can temporarily be curtailed—e.g., group rooms with nearby exam rooms (i.e., by using existing facilities, such as the lobby, during off hours for the group room as well as existing exam rooms). In addition, healthcare organizations must always keep in mind that DIGMAs and Physicals SMAs are census driven programs. In order to attain the desired economic benefit, minimum and targeted census levels must be pre-

established (based upon both medical economics and group dynamics) for each and every SMA that is implemented—and must then be consistently maintained by promoting the program effectively to patients.

Promotional Costs

Because DIGMAs and PSMAs represent a major departure from the traditional individual office visits that patients have grown to expect, maintaining census requires that the program be effectively promoted to patients—and this involves additional costs. Costs can be minimized by creating standardized templates for all marketing materials, so that only minor alterations are required for use with any particular SMA program. Nonetheless, there are substantial promotional expenses involved—especially for the framed posters that are to be displayed on the walls of the physician's lobby and examination rooms (a one-time expense), and the program description fliers and invitation letters (which represent an ongoing expense as these materials must constantly be replenished). In addition, it is advisable that—at the start of each new DIGMA or Physicals SMA—letters announcing the program be mailed to all appropriate patients in the physician's practice, which involves copying and mailing costs.

While the associated costs are small compared to the substantial economic benefits that well-run DIGMA and PSMA programs can provide, they are nonetheless real and must therefore be budgeted for—as all marketing materials need to be of high quality so as to accurately represent the high-quality care that patients can expect to receive through the SMA program. To encourage patients to attend, all promotional materials must convey a professional image that accurately reflects the warm, caring, and high-quality medical care that properly run and adequately supported DIGMAs and PSMAs do in fact provide.

Personnel Costs

In addition to promotional expenses, there are substantial personnel expenses attached to DIGMA and Physicals SMA programs. These personnel costs include a highly skilled champion and program coordinator (in larger systems), behaviorists (typically a halftime behaviorist for approximately every 9 or 10 DIGMAs and PSMAs established), 1–2 nursing personnel per SMA (MAs, RNs, LVNs, nursing techs, etc.), documenters (for which providers are expected to see an additional patient or two in the

DIGMA or PSMA in order to cover this additional expense), and dedicated schedulers (typically a fulltime dedicated scheduler for every 15–25 DIGMAs and PSMAs launched, charged with the responsibilities of *topping-off* sessions and assisting the program coordinator in every possible way). It is important to note that the use of nursing personnel in the SMA usually does not involve an extra expense as: (1) the physician's own nurse is normally attached to the DIGMA or PSMA; and (2) there may actually be a net cost savings to the system as the nursing personnel's time is also leveraged by seeing 2–3 or more times as many patients in the same amount of time (although, on the other hand, the nursing role is typically much expanded in a DIGMA or PSMA).

Because as many as 15–25% or more of DIGMA or PSMA sessions might not be held during the year due to the physician being absent (vacation, meetings, illness, sabbatical, etc.), one might consider hiring SMA personnel contractually so that they only need to be paid for sessions that are actually held—at least when the required flexibility for this exists on their schedules. The fact that a substantial number of SMA sessions are not held each year, coupled with the desire to only pay for sessions that are actually held, presents a strong argument for hiring SMA behaviorists, documenters, and nursing personnel on a contractual basis. On the other hand, one might have less control over contracted personnel—at least, as compared to employed staff. An alternative would be to use staff behaviorists, documenters, and nursing personnel for these SMA responsibilities, but have them go back to normal clinic duties whenever SMA sessions are not being held so that the SMA program is not assessed with this oppressive overhead expense.

Additional Costs (Including Facilities Costs)

There are also additional costs to the DIGMA and Physicals SMA program, such as the costs associated with planning the entire program, launching each new SMA, training all personnel associated with the DIGMAs and PSMAs, developing all the templates and forms that are needed, making copies of all forms utilized on an on-going basis, and reproducing handouts as they are used. In addition, there are mailing and telephone costs, as well as the costs of all the facilities that will be used in the program. In the case of a DIGMA, the necessary facilities include a large group room capable of handling 25 people plus a nearby exam room. In the case of a Physicals SMA, a smaller exam room is required (perhaps only half as large); however, 2–5 (most commonly 4) exam rooms are typically needed—although they can usually be in the physician's own office area rather than necessarily being adjacent to the group room.

Step 5: Draft a Confidentiality Release

Physicians and administrators invariably inquire as to how confidentiality is to be handled during SMAs. Before launching your SMA program, have your corporate attorney or medical risk department develop an appropriate, comprehensive (but relatively brief, understandable, and patient friendly) confidentiality agreement and release form for the SMA program—for all patients and support persons in attendance to sign before the start of every visit. It is imperative that this confidentiality waiver/release of information form be comprehensive and appropriate to the SMA program—and that it be updated as often as needed. In addition, ensure that this confidentiality release meets all applicable privacy regulations and that it is HIPAA (Health Insurance Portability and Accountability Act) compliant by first getting it approved by your organization's HIPAA compliance officer.

Some sample confidentiality release forms are included on the DVD attached to this book; however, these are strictly to be used for illustrative purposes only, and are not meant to be used *carte blanche* (also see Table 10.3 for many of the types of points that need to be covered in the release). Try to keep your confidentiality release form as short, simple, and patient friendly as possible; however, be certain to include all of the major points discussed herein—and ensure that the form your organization ultimately develops meets all applicable standards, policies, and regulations. Consider having administration tone down any harsh rhetoric or complex legalese in this waiver and try to keep it in fifth grade language that is clearly understandable to all.

By incorporating a separate line at the bottom of the form (i.e., either above or underneath the patient's signature line) for the date and the support person's signature, a single confidentiality release form can be used for both patient and support person (i.e., the spouse, adult family member, friend, or caregiver that might accompany the patient to the SMA session). Try to keep the confidentiality form brief (i.e., no longer than one page in length, and preferably only 2–3 paragraphs). The signed document can then be kept and stored as a hard copy (either in the patients' paper charts or in a separate file), or else scanned into patients' electronic medical records. In

Table 10.3 Some important points for your corporate attorney or medical risk department to consider incorporating into your confidentiality release form[a]

- Much of the medical care that the patient will receive will be delivered in the group setting.
- Patients' medical conditions and issues will be discussed in front of others, which is OK with the patient.
- Patients are welcome to bring a support person with them (i.e., if the physician agrees to this).
- All attendees must agree to keep the setting safe by not identifying others in attendance, either directly or indirectly, and by not discussing other patients' medical issues once the session is over.
- Everyone (patients as well as any support persons accompanying them) must sign the release prior to actually entering the SMA group setting.
- The confidentiality release can also spell out that, during SMA sessions, patients are always welcome to request private one-on-one time with the physician for brief private exams or to discuss any truly private matters—although this time will typically be made available toward the end of the group session so as to not interrupt the flow of the group.
- In addition, the release can point out that
  - The choice as to whether or not to attend a DIGMA or Physicals SMA is a completely voluntary, as is whatever they choose to discuss in the group
  - Patients are free to leave the session any time they wish, without any repercussions whatsoever for doing so
  - Subsequent to attending a DIGMA or PSMA session, individual office visits will continue to be made available to patients in the future—just like before
  - The DIGMA or PSMA is meant to provide patients with an additional healthcare choice.

[a] These points are provided to be helpful to you; however, there can be no warrantees as to their accuracy or comprehensiveness. Therefore, each medical group must have its own corporate attorney or medical risk department develop its own Confidentiality Agreement and Release Form in order to ensure that it is: (1) comprehensive and properly updated; (2) in full compliance with all of your local, state, regional, and national regulatory requirements; (3) inclusive of all your corporate standards; and (4) complete and fully appropriate to your organization's purposes and circumstances.

the case of paper charts, the confidentiality waiver can even be printed on the backside of the SMA chart note. For more information on how confidentiality is handled, see Chapter 2.

Step 6: Develop Computer Codes and Scheduling Procedures for the SMA Program

Prior to launching your SMA program, be certain to develop appropriate computer codes and scheduling procedures for DIGMAs, CHCCs, and PSMAs so that patients can be scheduled into them and so that time can be reserved for the program on the master schedules of the physician and all SMA team members. Computer codes need to be developed for a variety of reasons, including the following, so that: (1) patients can be scheduled into future SMA sessions; (2) the group time can be held weekly on the master schedules of the physician, behaviorist, documenter, and nurse/MA(s); (3) the group and exam rooms can be reserved for the SMA on an ongoing basis; (4) SMAs appear appropriately on the schedulers' computer screens; and (5) the SMA is appropriately labeled and referred to as the organization wants it to be (i.e., according to its own particular name for the SMA program).

Involve IT as to How the SMA Is to Appear on Schedulers' Computer Screens

The precise manner in which next available group visit appointments and individual appointments are to appear on schedulers' computer screens needs to be determined. Clearly, the IT Department will likely need to be involved in this process. Furthermore, all support staff will need adequate training in order to appropriately schedule SMA appointments, and to do so with minimal errors.

These computer codes for the group visit program could be as simple as "DIGMA", "CHCC", and "PSMA" for DIGMAs, CHCCs, and Physicals SMAs, respectively—or "SMA" and "PSMA" for DIGMAs and Physicals SMAs. However, these computer designations would also need to somehow incorporate the subtype of the SMA model being utilized (at least in the case of homogeneous and mixed DIGMAs and PSMAs), so that only appropriate patients will be booked into each session. Or they could be designed so as to reflect the name that the organization has chosen for these models in order to brand these group visits within their system—for example, different systems have referred to DIGMAs in various ways (such as SIGMAs for Scheduled In Group Medical Appointments and RAMAs for Rapid Access Medical Appointments).

Install Computer Code on the Master Schedules of the Physician and SMA Team Members

At the beginning of each new SMA, the program coordinator must ensure that the physician's master schedule is changed so as to reserve the appropriate time each week for the program (i.e., by suitably placing the computer code for the DIGMA, CHCC, or PSMA onto the physician's schedule on a regular basis). For homogeneous and mixed DIGMA designs, each different type of session might also need to be individually coded (perhaps by adding an additional alphanumeric character), so that patients can easily be scheduled into appropriate future sessions according to their diagnosis or health condition. Similarly, this computer code must also be installed on the weekly master schedules of the entire SMA team—behaviorist, documenter, nursing personnel, and possibly even the dedicated scheduler (who needs flexibility as to how much time is necessary to dedicate to the SMA each week).

Once the Computer Code Is Installed, Patients Can Be Scheduled into the SMA

Inserting the computer code for the DIGMA or PSMA onto the physician's schedule each week will permit suitable patients to immediately start being booked into appropriate SMA sessions—often weeks or months ahead. From this point forward, all appropriate patients seen by the physician during regular office visits (i.e., who need a subsequent appointment for a follow-up visit or physical examination) should immediately be invited to attend a future DIGMA or PSMA session, respectively, for their next visit. Patients accepting this offer should then be promptly booked into the appropriate future session of the DIGMA or Physicals SMA.

Determine How the SMA Will Appear on Schedulers' Computer Screens Before the SMA Begins

This issue of how group visit appointments will be coded and displayed on the schedulers' screens must be resolved prior to actually launching the SMA program. Computer codes are developed for SMAs for three reasons: first, so that the group visit time can be held each week on the master schedules of the physician, behaviorist, nurse/MA, and documenter; second, so that the group and exam rooms can be reserved for the SMA; and third, so that patients can be appropriately scheduled into future group sessions. One might choose to have the *next available* appointment pop up on the scheduler's computer screen, irregardless of whether it is a DIGMA/PSMA or a short/long individual appointment. Although this approach has the advantage of making it easier to fill SMA sessions, it also has disadvantages when the next available individual office visit is weeks or months away. For example, in the event that an individual follow-up appointment needs to be scheduled—but the first available individual appointment is weeks or months away—it requires the scheduler to first scroll through several DIGMA sessions (i.e., this week's SMA, next week's SMA, etc.) before the next available individual appointment appears.

On the other hand, should the next available appointment be displayed for both appointment types—i.e., with the next available DIGMA and individual appointment both being simultaneously displayed side by side on the scheduler's computer screen? If this option is selected, then make certain that schedulers receive the necessary training to properly inform patients that their DIGMA or PSMA visit is a shared medical appointment that includes other patients and will be held in a group setting. Believing that they have the unbelievable good fortune of scheduling a 90-minute individual office visit that week with their own doctor—but later finding out on arriving that they instead have a 90-minute group appointment with a dozen other patients—is one thing that will really upset patients and make them angry. However, this problem can easily be avoided by using skilled schedulers who have been properly trained.

A third possibility is to have only the next available individual appointments displayed on schedulers' computer screen—i.e., for follow-up visits and physical examinations. This requires that schedulers remember which physicians have SMAs on their schedules and that they need to recommend the SMA to appropriate patients (plus search availability of upcoming SMA appointments as well). This is generally an undesirable option, because too few DIGMA and PSMA appointments will likely be scheduled by the organization's scheduling staff, thereby making the program susceptible to failure. Schedulers will all too likely soon forget about the physician's SMA program and therefore fail to schedule patients into it.

Insufficient census to achieve economic viability of the program will then be the probable result. This is because the organization's scheduling staff would not be likely to schedule SMA appointments in this case, unless the scheduler were to: (1) remember which providers are offering SMAs; (2) enter the appropriate computer code for their DIGMA or PSMA; (3) take the time to search for the next available appropriate SMA session; and finally (4) take the time to sell the SMA to patients. All this is highly unlikely, especially when an off-site Call Center exists in which schedulers know little about the SMA program, have no accountability to it, and are being evaluated on how quickly they can schedule patients and how short their telephone queue line is.

Train Support Staff Well with Regard to Scheduling Patients into the SMA

All support staff needs to be adequately trained regarding how to correctly schedule SMA appointments—and to do so with minimal communication errors both between staff members and with the patients themselves (a problem that can be considerably reduced by providing schedulers with sample scripts and talking points regarding the program, which are included on the attached DVD). It is important to ensure that all scheduling staff receives the necessary training to properly inform patients that their DIGMA or PSMA visit is a shared medical appointment that includes other patients and will be held in a group setting.

Step 7: Pre-establish and Consistently Meet Census Targets

The next step, before any DIGMAs or Physicals SMAs are launched, is to predetermine the census requirements for each and every group visit that is to be launched—i.e., the number of patients that one desires to have attend all group visit sessions. It is only by so doing that the cost-effectiveness—as well as the desired productivity and efficiency gains for the program—can be consistently achieved. DIGMAs and PSMAs are census driven programs, with consistently maintaining adequate census being the key to success and economic viability of these programs. As long as pre-established census targets are consistently met, the DIGMA and PSMA models have repeatedly been demonstrated to increase productivity and efficiency, improve access, and leverage existing resources. Furthermore, it also ensures a sufficiently large group size so that the group moves along at a pace that maintains everyone's interest and fosters important group interaction.

It is for this reason that I am fond of saying that the most important part of a DIGMA or PSMA program occurs outside of the group room and in-between sessions—i.e., before the physician ever enters the group room for the SMA—because that is when patients are scheduled into the SMA and census for the session is determined. Almost any physician, upon entering a full DIGMA session of 10–16 patients (or, in the case of PSMAs, of 6–8 women or 7–9 men in primary care, or 10–13 patients in the medical and surgical specialties), will have a very lively, interactive, enjoyable, and successful group that meets the medical needs of all patients in attendance. On the other hand, if the best physician in the world enters a DIGMA session with only three to five patients in attendance, it will likely be a failure—an *economic failure* because the physician could have seen more patients individually during 90 minutes of clinic time (i.e., and without the overhead costs of the DIGMA program), and a *program failure* because such a small group is likely to be less interesting, less interactive, less informative, and possibly even boring (especially if the few patients in attendance are reticent to speak and have little in common).

Equally unfortunate is the fact that physicians who have run such small groups report that, because the workload just expands to fill the amount of time available, they frequently end up doing more work than they do in a fast paced, highly interactive larger group due to the fact that patients are actively involved and carry some of the workload. Therefore, this issue of consistently maintaining pre-established census levels is an ongoing challenge that must be addressed during each and every SMA session—even years after the DIGMA or PSMA has been launched. This is much less of an issue for CHCCs as the same 15–20 patients attend all sessions over time, and some of these groups have already been running for 10 years and longer—although even with CHCCs, group size can easily be too small for both economic viability of the program and effective group dynamics. In other words, sufficient patients must be initially recruited into each new CHCC that is launched, and then replacements must be added as enrolled patients drop-out, move, become too feeble to attend, or pass away.

The Keys to Successfully Filling Group Sessions

Consistently meeting pre-established census targets requires focusing attention upon all of the important steps involved with successfully scheduling patients into the DIGMA or PSMA. Table 10.4 depicts the key steps involved with consistently filling SMA group sessions.

Table 10.4 Keys to successfully filling all DIGMA and PSMA sessions

- Use the best possible marketing materials to promote the program, including professional appearing framed posters and accompanying fliers prominently displayed on the physician's lobby and exam room walls.
- Send an announcement letter to all appropriate patients just prior to the launch of the SMA program—perhaps in batches of 50 announcements being mailed out per week so as to spread self-referring patients out over the first few DIGMA or PSMA sessions.
- Have the physician and staff constantly invite all appropriate patients seen during regular office visits to attend a future DIGMA session for their next follow-up visit (or a PSMA for their next physical examination)—the most important part of which is a positively worded, personal invitation from the patient's own doctor.
- Have receptionists give all appropriate patients registering for a regular office visit an invitation for the physicians DIGMA or PSMA program to read while they are waiting in the lobby—plus say some positive and encouraging words about the program.
- Have the physician's nurse or MA *talk up* the DIGMA or PSMA when rooming patients for a regular office visit, plus give them a program description flier to read in the exam room while waiting for the doctor to arrive.
- Train the physician's front and back office staff (as well as any schedulers in the Call Center) to recommend, refer, and schedule all appropriate patients into future DIGMA or PSMA sessions.

Table 10.4 (continued)

- If the provider runs a PSMA, have scheduling staff also check to see whether patients calling in to schedule a follow-up visit might be due for a physical examination and, if so, invite them to attend the next appropriate PSMA session (i.e., along with giving them the follow-up appointment they desire).
- Have a specifically trained, dedicated scheduler call the patients that the physician wants invited into future DIGMA sessions in order to *top-off* all sessions and ensure that they are consistently filled.
- Have the physician, nursing personnel, dedicated scheduler, champion, and program coordinator all monitor the census of upcoming group sessions on an ongoing basis (with the program coordinator typically generating twice weekly pre-booking census reports) and work together to promptly backfill any future sessions that are not yet adequately filled.
- Develop the procedures necessary to ensure that census targets are constantly met during each and every DIGMA session.

When SMAs Fail, It Is Almost Always Due to Poor Attendance

If there is a weak point in the DIGMA and Physicals SMA models, inadequate census is certainly it. Because different patients typically attend each DIGMA and PSMA session, ongoing attention to promoting the program and consistently filling all sessions is critical to success. In fact, full census is the single most critical ingredient to achieving the remarkable economic, productivity, efficiency, and access benefits that well-run DIGMA and PSMA programs can provide. When inadequate census for upcoming sessions begins to occur, alarms must immediately go off—and all involved (especially the physician and support staff, but also the dedicated scheduler) must promptly redouble their efforts for inviting patients and filling these sessions. It is important to remember that group visits are dramatically different from the individual office visits that patients are familiar with, and must therefore be carefully promoted to patients if they are to be successful. On the other hand, once patients do in fact attend a SMA session, they are very likely to be willing to return to the group setting for their next appointment—i.e., provided that they are invited to do so.

I would estimate that approximately 15–25% of all DIGMAs and Physicals SMAs ultimately fail, almost always due to inadequate census during sessions. Poor SMA census is symptomatic of insufficient planning, a poor design, scant training, or inadequate promotion of the program by the physician and staff—especially by the physician and scheduling staff. A major source of this difficulty is that physicians, especially busy and heavily backlogged physicians, are not used to personally inviting patients. All that they need to do with regular individual office visits is to show up in the morning–at which time they always find that their schedule is full. This is not true for DIGMAs and PSMAs, as the physician's personal invitation is the single most important ingredient to getting patients to attend–and thus to having full groups and a successful SMA program. However, with practice (and the help of support staff and quality promotional materials), this personal invitation should not take the physician any longer than 30–60 seconds. It is important to note that failures of DIGMAs and PSMAs are almost always due to inadequate census and are not the result of either patient or physician dissatisfaction.

If You Have a Problem with Your SMA, Examine the Design and Supports

On occasion, I have heard from physicians in different parts of the country regarding some problem they were having with their SMA—often asking for my help and, on rare occasions, even suggesting that the model might be flawed. Typically, they point out that they are not meeting their census targets—although they much less frequently report that they are finishing late or having some type of personal, patient, or staff dissatisfaction issue with their program. Whenever this has happened—at least when we were able to ferret out the underlying causes and carefully examine them—it has inevitably turned out that the program was prematurely launched, poorly designed, inadequately supported, or incorrectly run. Such complaints by physicians, infrequent as they are, often result from a flaw in the design of the program, inadequate planning, insufficient training, or an off-site Call Center without accountability for scheduling patients into the SMA—almost all of which ultimately produce the same net result, insufficient census.

There might be a lack of appropriate promotional materials, a failure on the part of the provider or staff to enthusiastically promote the program, or inadequate attention paid to census. Or there might be a lack of critical administrative support, some unsolved operational problem, a lack of appropriate facilities, or a staffing issue such as a poor choice for a behaviorist (or perhaps the lack of a documenter, adequate nursing support, or a dedicated scheduler). For example, there might be a problem due to selecting the behaviorist based solely upon available staffing rather than based upon choosing the best possible person for the job.

If an announcement letter is not initially mailed to all appropriate patients, if eye-catching posters and fliers are not prominently displayed in the physician's lobby and exam rooms, if receptionists do not hand out invitations when patients register for regular office visits, if nurses/MAs do not recommend the SMA and distribute fliers to all appropriate patients when rooming them during regular office visits, if scheduling staff does not consistently promote the SMA and invite patients, if a dedicated scheduler is not used, or (most importantly) if the physician does not personally invite all suitable patients seen during normal office visits to have their next appointment be in the SMA, then the DIGMA or PSMA will ultimately be at risk for failure due to inadequate census. Furthermore, all of these promotional efforts become even more important for physicians who work part-time, have small practices, or do not have access problems. Also, if the physician does not truly believe in the SMA program, if the support staff is not enthusiastic about it, or if someone is not held accountable for monitoring census on an ongoing basis, then the inevitable result will likely be failure to consistently achieve predetermined census targets—which, in turn, can frustrate the physician and support staff, plus put the SMA at high risk for failure.

Once the underlying source of such a problem can be diagnosed and corrected, the SMA program can once again be put onto a secure foundation and made successful. However, whenever the root causes of these problems are not addressed, then the inevitable result will ultimately be some type of failure of the program—perhaps in meeting its financial goals, or else in fully achieving the multiple objectives for which the DIGMA and PSMA models were originally designed. Most likely, all such problems will inevitably have the same net result—insufficient census—and consequently a SMA program that is at risk for failure.

The Single Most Effective Means of Filling SMAs: Positively Worded, Personal Invitations from Physicians

Experience has demonstrated that there is nothing more important in persuading patients to attend a DIGMA or Physicals SMA for the first time (i.e. the next time they need a follow-up visit or physical examination, respectively) than a positively worded, personal invitation from their own doctor during regular office visits—an invitation that should only take 30–60 seconds to make. Although patient satisfaction with DIGMAs and PSMAs tends to be very high for those patients who actually do attend (as once there, patients almost always

like this new venue of care delivery and the many benefits it provides), the challenge lies in getting patients to attend the SMA for the first time. This is because group visits are something that patients simply are not used to and that, for the most part, they know nothing about.

It has also been observed that when the physician fails to assume this basic responsibility of personally inviting (on an ongoing basis) all appropriate patients to attend the SMA the next time they have a medical need, even remarkable efforts on the part of the schedulers, nurses, and receptionists to promote the program and invite patients to attend are insufficient to compensate for the physician's failure to do so. This ultimately puts the SMA at risk for failure due to inadequate census. More common, however, is the finding that if the physician is unmotivated to personally invite patients, then the physician's support staff will likely also be just as unmotivated in this regard.

Patients Enter into DIGMAs and PSMAs in Six Different Ways

Before patients can be directly booked into a DIGMA or PSMA session, the physician must first determine which patients are appropriate candidates for their DIGMA. These appropriate patients can then be invited to enter into future DIGMA or PSMA sessions in any of the following six ways: self-referral; dropping in whenever they have a medical need; being scheduled by staff; being invited by the physician or staff; by the efforts of the dedicated scheduler; or by being scheduled in a SMA for a follow-up visit in another SMA.

Establish and Consistently Meet Three Different Census Levels

Efficient use of the physician's time is critical to the success of any DIGMA or Physicals SMA. Therefore, *minimum*, *target*, and *maximum* census levels—based upon medical economics, effective group dynamics, and the number of patients that the physician can comfortably see in the group setting once experience is gained—must be pre-established before each SMA is ever launched. Furthermore, it is imperative that these three pre-established census targets then be consistently maintained once the program is implemented.

Minimum Census Level

The *minimum* census is simply the minimum number of patients that can be seen while maintaining the economic viability of the program—i.e., below which sessions would simply not be held. I usually set the DIGMA's minimum census to be either 10 patients or a 200% increase in the physician's average productivity for the same types of patients seen individually during 90 minutes of clinic time during the previous 6–12 months (i.e., for the types of appointments that will be seen in the DIGMA)—whichever is larger.

Target Census Level

The *target* census is simply the number of patients that the physician ideally wants to see during each and every DIGMA or PSMA session. It is pre-established prior to launching the DIGMA or PSMA and is generally set so as to ensure a productivity gain of between 200 and 400% over the physician's normal productivity for similar types of patients seen during normal clinic hours—with 300% being typical. Do not forget to add an extra one or two patients (just as the airlines do) so as to overbook sessions according to the expected number of no-shows and late cancels—less the anticipated number of drop-ins in the case of DIGMAs. For a Physicals SMA in primary care, the target census is typically between 7 and 9 male or 6 and 8 female patients; however, the target census is most commonly between 10 and 13 patients in the medical and surgical subspecialties, where the physical exam is often more limited in nature and thus quicker to perform.

Maximum Census Level

The *maximum* census is simply the maximum number of patients that the physician is willing to see during any given DIGMA or PSMA session. The maximum census must take into account the expected number of no-shows and late cancellations for the DIGMA or PSMA—a number which must be empirically determined in practice and then added to the maximum census. On the other hand, the maximum census must also take into account the number of last-minute drop-ins anticipated for each DIGMA session. This is taken into account by deducting the expected number of drop-ins from the maximum census, and then adding to this number the expected number of no-shows and late cancels.

For example, if you want a maximum census of 16 patients in attendance but typically have two more *no-shows* and *late-cancels* than *drop-ins* per DIGMA session, then you will need to set your maximum census to be 18 patients actually scheduled. On the other hand, if the opposite is true and you should happen to have say four drop-ins and only two no-shows and late-cancels on average, then you would only want to schedule 14 patients

into the DIGMA session—i.e., if your maximum census is 16 patients. Doing this makes the SMA program basically immune to no-shows and late cancels. This is definitely an advantage over individual office visits as it virtually eliminates this vexing and costly source of physician downtime due to no-shows and late cancellations. Although it can initially make physicians nervous to overbook their group visit sessions by a patient or two (and occasionally more), they quickly find out that the numbers do not lie and that everything works out in the long run—and, if not, that they can easily compensate for this by simply making the necessary readjustments later (based upon accumulated experience) to the numbers being used as the expected number of no-shows, late-cancels, and drop-ins.

How to Calculate These Census Targets for Your DIGMA or PSMA

Let us now examine how to calculate the minimum, target, and maximum census levels for your DIGMA or PSMA program.

First Determine the Provider's Current Average Productivity During Regular Clinic Hours

The first step in the process of calculating the census targets for your DIGMA or PSMA is to accurately determine the physician's actual current average productivity for individual office visits during the same amount of clinic time—and for the types of patients and appointments that will be seen in the DIGMA or PSMA. In the case of DIGMAs, this calculation needs to include both short and long return appointments in the clinic, and in the ratio in which they are currently being provided.

In addition, this calculation must take into account the deleterious impact of no-shows and late cancellations (as well as any unfilled appointment slots and downtime on the physician's schedule), which in combination can reduce the average number of patients actually seen during 90 minutes of clinic time substantially below the number of patients that have actually been scheduled. Consider physicians primarily having 15 minute office visits for the follow-ups of established patients—which is often the case in primary care (although some longer return appointments might also be available, perhaps 20 or 30 minutes in length). For 15-minute appointments, the result of this average productivity calculation in most cases is that between 3.9 and 4.7 patients are actually seen on average during 90 minutes of clinic time—i.e., not the six patients that many physicians might believe they see because they can potentially schedule that many 15-minute return appointments into 90 minutes of clinic time. This number could even be further reduced if there are also some longer return appointments on the physician's clinic schedule, such as some 20 or 30 minute returns—or if the physician has some unfilled follow-up appointment slots.

For physicians primarily on 20-minute office visits, this average productivity range typically drops to approximately 3.0–4.0 patients actually seen on average during 90 minutes of clinic time—which is substantially below the 4.5 patients that could potentially be scheduled into that amount of clinic time. Again, this is due to the combined effect of no-shows, late-cancels, unfilled appointment slots, and some downtime during the physician's workweek. This number could be even further reduced if there are also some longer return appointments on the physician's clinic schedule—such as 30 or 40 minute returns. Similarly, for physicians on 30-minute office visits, this average productivity range often drops to an average of between 1.9 and 2.6 patients actually seen per 90 minutes of clinic time—i.e., versus the three 30-minute appointments that could potentially be scheduled into that amount of clinic time.

Next, Multiply the Provider's Average Clinic Productivity by the Percentage Increase You Want the DIGMA or PSMA to Achieve

More specifically, the target census level is established for the DIGMA or PSMA by multiplying the physician's average current clinic productivity for the types of patient appointments that will be seen in the SMA by the percentage increase in productivity that is ideally desired for the SMA—which is typically between 200 and 400%, and most commonly 300%. Therefore, if the goal is to increase physician productivity in a DIGMA by 300%, we will typically need to set the target census between 11.7 and 14.1 patients for physicians who are primarily on 15-minute office visits—and between 9.0 and 12.0 patients for physicians primarily on 20-minute office visits.

In the case of physicians having 30-minute return office visits, this range would correspondingly be only between 5.7 and 7.8 patients (as physicians with 30-minute office visits would typically only see between 1.9 and 2.6 patients during 90 minutes of clinic time), which generally speaking is too small for a vibrant DIGMA program. Therefore, I would recommend raising the DIGMA's target census level in this case to 10 patients—i.e., in order to have a lively, informative, and interesting group visit program (which would correspond to approximately

a 400–500% increase in physician productivity). This is because we also want this calculated DIGMA and PSMA census level to fall within the ideal range for these models—i.e., between 10 and 16 patients for DIGMAs and 7–9 male patients or 6–9 female patients for primary care PSMAs (or 10–13 PSMA patients in the medical and surgical subspecialties).

Two Final Steps for Refining the Minimum, Target, and Maximum Census Levels

Two final steps still need to be taken in order to refine and fine-tune the *minimum, target, and maximum* census levels for your DIGMA or Physicals SMA—i.e., to determine these numbers with the greatest possible accuracy.

First, overbook sessions by adding (i.e., to the number of patients calculated in the *minimum, target*, and *maximum* census level calculations above) the anticipated number of patients expected to *fail-to-keep* or *late-cancel* each session. The expected number of no-shows and late-cancels can be established empirically with reasonable accuracy after only a couple of month's experience has been gained in running the DIGMA or PSMA. This number typically varies widely between physicians and organizations and ranges from approximately 0.5 patients per session (on the low side for some providers) to as many as 4.0 or even more patients in the case of physicians having large DIGMAs with a high no-show and late-cancel rate.

Second, in the case of DIGMAs only, deduct the number of patients that are expected to *drop-in* to each session from the *minimum, target* and surgical census levels just calculated. The number of drop-ins will undoubtedly be negligible when the DIGMA is first started and patients do not yet know about the program or the fact that they can just drop in, but will likely gradually increase over time until it ultimately plateaus off—perhaps eventually accounting for as many as 10–25% of all attendees for DIGMAs that have been running for some time.

The Most Common DIGMA and PSMA Goal Is to Increase Productivity by 300%

As discussed, the minimum, target, and maximum census levels need to be predetermined and then consistently met during every session. While the minimum census level of the session is often set so as to double (or somewhat less than triple) the provider's productivity over individual office visits, the target census level for most DIGMAs and PSMAs is usually set so as to at least triple the provider's actual productivity, on average, for individual office visits and the same type of appointments during normal clinic hours. For full-time physicians running one 90-minute DIGMA or PSMA per week, increasing productivity by 300% typically translates into an 8–9% increase in productivity for the entire week (or a 16–18% increase for half-time providers). In a similar manner, running daily DIGMAs or Physicals SMAs could conceivably increase the full-time provider's productivity for the entire week by as much as 40–45%—and accomplish this while simultaneously increasing provider and patient satisfaction, and without the need of having the provider spend extra hours in the clinic.

In consulting with medical groups around the country, I have often been confronted by physicians—particularly primary care physicians—who say that they see return patients in 15-minute appointments, and therefore see six patients in 1½ hours of clinic time. They argue that, in order for a DIGMA to leverage their time by 300%, they would need to see 18 patients during every DIGMA session—which falls outside the recommended range of 10–16 patients that I state is ideal for most DIGMAs. These physicians point out that this is an unrealistically large number of patients and that a DIGMA will therefore not work for them. One might therefore ask: "If this is so, then why is a 300% increase in physician productivity a realistic goal for most DIGMA programs?"

As explained previously, a different picture emerges when one examines the actual historic throughput of primary care physicians who primarily schedule 15-minute return appointments. The key here is to first accurately measure the true number of established patients of the type seen in the DIGMA (or Physicals SMA) that the provider actually sees during 90 minutes of clinic time dedicated to follow-up or physical examination appointments, respectively, averaged over the past 2 months–2 years. As pointed out above, such an analysis typically reveals that the average number of follow-up patients actually seen during 90 minutes of clinic time by most internists, family practitioners, and nurse practitioners on 15-minute office visits usually ranges between 3.9 and 4.7 patients—which is far from the 6.0 patients that many physicians on 15-minute office visits believe they are seeing. Also, for those physicians who are on 20-, 30-, 40-, or 60-minute office visits, the target census level for the DIGMA is correspondingly reduced even further (although it is generally recommended that the target census not be allowed to go below 10 patients in order to keep the DIGMA group session interesting and interactive for all in attendance).

Let us briefly review the many reasons that the average number of patients actually seen during 90 minutes of clinic time is often much less than what physicians believe. Some patients fail to keep their office visit appointments, while others cancel too late for their appointment slots to be refilled. Furthermore, some appointment slots might go unfilled. In addition, physicians often have some longer return appointment slots in their schedules, which must also be weighted into this average (i.e., in the same proportion as they occur on the physician's office visit schedule), which also reduces the physician's actual productivity. Finally, physicians sometimes have various sources of *downtime* during their normal clinic hours wherein they are not actually seeing patients, which further reduces their actual productivity.

It is because actual physician productivity for 15-minute visits so often lies in this 3.9–4.7 patient range (i.e., rather than being the 6.0 patients which could theoretically be scheduled) that we are so frequently able to triple physician productivity during a DIGMA. Notice that in order to triple the productivity of primary care physicians on 15 minute office visits, we would typically need to achieve an average DIGMA census of between 11.7 (= 3 × 3.9) and 14.1 (= 3 × 4.7) patients. Serendipitously, this is within the ideal range of 10–16 patients for a DIGMA, and a perfect target census level to strive for. Tripling productivity also becomes easier as the length of the traditional office visit becomes longer—say 20, 30, or 40 minutes as opposed to 15 minutes—where productivity gains through the DIGMA or PSMA can often be as great as 400% or more. In the case of one physician with 60-minute intake appointments (who actually saw 1.2 patient intakes on average in 90 minutes of clinic time during the previous 2 months), we were actually able to increase productivity by 800% during the first PSMA session—and to do so while simultaneously enhancing patient satisfaction. To my knowledge, this is the greatest leveraging of physician time that has ever been achieved to date through a well-run DIGMA or PSMA program. During the past couple of years, this surgical specialist has since titrated her group census back to 8 patients actually seen per 90-minute PSMA session, which still increases her productivity over individual office visits by 667%.

In Certain Situations, Physician Productivity Can Only Be Increased 200%

It is important to keep in mind that there are a few providers who are already so productive in their pace of delivering individual office visits that the most that DIGMAs and PSMAs can leverage their time is 200%, rather than the 300% that is more typically set as the desired productivity increase for DIGMAs and PSMAs.

Extremely Productive Primary Care Physicians Having Only 10-Minute Office Visits

While many providers on 15-minute office visits might believe that they see six patients in 1½ hours of clinic time, to date I have only encountered one primary care physician whose actual average productivity was measured to be six or more patients per 90 minutes of clinic time. In fact, his average productivity in the clinic was actually determined to be 7.05 patients per 90 minutes. However, he was the most productive primary care provider that I have ever launched a DIGMA with. This result only occurred because this family practitioner saw all of his established patients in short 10-minute follow-up appointment slots—and had no 15 or 20 minute appointments whatsoever on his weekly schedule in which to see established patients.

That said, it is still important to note that even in this extreme case, the physician's actual clinic productivity was 7.05 patients per 90 minutes, and not the 9.0 patients that one might postulate—i.e., due to his being able to schedule nine 10-minute appointment slots available during 90 minutes of clinic time. Even for such a highly productive physician as this, the DIGMA model was still able to work well. However, to be realistic we need to set the targeted percentage increase in productivity for such highly efficient physicians at only 200%, rather than the 300% increase that could typically be achieved for most physicians.

Certain Highly Productive Specialists Can Similarly Only Increase Productivity by 200%

Similarly, there are a couple of highly productive medical specialties for whom a 200% increase in productivity is the most that can realistically be achieved through a DIGMA or PSMA program, e.g., for specialized and general dermatology DIGMAs, for prenatal exams in obstetrics, and for well baby checks (as well as school, camp, and sports physicals) in pediatrics. The reason that a 200% increase in productivity is the most that can typically be achieved in these instances is that the baseline productivity for these physicians during normal clinic hours is already very high. This limits the percentage increase in efficiency that a DIGMA or PSMA can realistically achieve while still staying within recommended census range of between 10 and 16 patients for a DIGMA (or 6–9 patients and 10–13 patients in primary and specialty care PSMAs, respectively).

In certain cases, other factors can impose a less than optimal 300% increase in productivity, such as: the lack of adequately sized group rooms in many facilities; a limited number of exam rooms being available for PSMAs (say one or two instead of the normal ideal of four exam rooms, which will likely slow the physician down); the chaos and large group size of Pediatrics PSMAs in which parents bring siblings into the visit; etc.

Think Twice Before Launching DIGMAs or PSMAs that Only Increase Productivity by 200%

It is important to be cautions about launching DIGMAs and PSMAs that can only increase provider productivity by 200% because the profit margins can be much less in such cases, which could result in the SMA just breaking even or possibly posting a loss. True, it is very helpful to double the productivity of extremely productive physicians such as dermatologists, pediatricians (for well baby checks; school, camp, and sports physicals; etc.), obstetricians (e.g., for pre-natal exams), and highly productive primary care physicians having only 10-minute follow-up appointments. However, one must be certain to take into account the actual revenues generated as well as the additional overhead expenses that such a DIGMA or PSMA entails (including the added personnel, facilities, promotional, training, and monitoring costs.)—i.e., so as to ensure that the program will still be economically viable in actual practice. By so doing, it might turn out that the typical RVU reimbursement for a typical dermatology appointment is so much larger than for a typical primary care appointment that a 200% increase in productivity turns out to be economically viable for the former, but not for the latter.

For Some Providers, Productivity Can Be Increased by 400% or More

On the other hand, DIGMAs and PSMAs can increase the productivity of many medical and surgical specialists (e.g., neurologists, nephrologists, oncologists, rheumatologists, physiatrists, general surgeons, plastic surgeons, cardiologists, etc.) by 400% or more, particularly when they have longer clinic appointments. This is also the case for the intake appointments of many plastic, orthopedic, and general surgeons. The reason for this is that such medical and surgical specialists often tend to have longer intake and/or return appointments, i.e., individual intake appointments of between 40 and 60 minutes, or follow-up appointments of 30 minutes or longer. This is also often the case for private physical examinations, which can usually be effectively and efficiently handled in a PSMA. The same is true for primary care physicians having appointment slots that are 30 minutes or longer—which is often the case for physical examinations, and sometimes the case for follow-up visits (at least in certain healthcare systems where complex, multi-morbid patients are frequently seen).

Therefore, the baseline productivity for these providers (i.e., the average number of patients actually seen individually during 90-minutes of clinic time) tends to be correspondingly less than for their faster-paced physician colleagues on 10- or 15-minute office visits—so that it is correspondingly easier to leverage their time through a DIGMA or PSMA. For these medical and surgical specialists (and primary care providers having longer clinic appointments), it is often possible to increase physician productivity through a DIGMA or PSMA by as much as 400% or more. This is because the census required in order to leverage the productivity of such physicians by 400% or more still lies well within the ideal range of 10–16 patients for a DIGMA program, 7–9 patients for a male Primary Care PSMA, 6–8 patients for a female Primary Care PSMA, or 10–13 patients for a medical or surgical subspecialty PSMA.

Whenever Possible, Try to Increase Physician Productivity by 300% or More

Whenever possible, I always like to at least triple the provider's productivity during the 90-minute DIGMA or PSMA session because: (1) the first 100% of the SMA patients would have been seen anyway if they were being seen individually in the clinic during the same 90 minutes' time; (2) the second 100% of patients seen should more or less cover the complete overhead costs of the DIGMA or PSMA program (personnel, facilities, promotion, snacks, handouts, patient packets, etc.); and (3) the third 100% would be the economic profit margin for the program. Clearly, without that profitable third 100%, the potential profit margin for the program will be much smaller, if not non-existent. Therefore, I would recommend starting with those DIGMA and PSMA programs that can clearly increase physician productivity by at least 300% or more. In fact, try to start first with some DIGMA and PSMA programs that can increase physician productivity by 400%—beginning with busy and backlogged providers, who will have an easier time consistently filling their group sessions to targeted census levels.

Only later, after experience has been gained and you have become comfortable with running profitable DIGMAs and PSMAs that increase productivity by 300% or more, should you consider trying SMA programs that only increase productivity by 200%—and then only if you feel absolutely confident that you can do so with some degree of economic gain. Always be cautious about starting a

DIGMA that can only leverage provider time by 200%, especially when it also requires additional resources—such as a pediatrics well-baby check Physicals SMA needing a sitter to baby sit siblings that parents bring to the visit because they cannot find a sitter at home. It is possible that having such a sitter could eat up any thin profit margin that the program might provide.

A 300% Increase in Productivity Creates Three Extra Hours of Physician Time Per Week

Consider the physician who is, on average, able to increase productivity by 300% during a 1½ hour weekly DIGMA or Physicals SMA. This translates into the physician actually seeing as many patients during the 90-minute SMA as could normally be seen during 4½ hours of clinic time through individual office visits alone. This represents a net gain of 3 hours of physician time per week for each weekly DIGMA or PSMA that is run (as 4.5–1.5 = 3.0), which is equivalent to the physician having the help of a colleague for 3 hours every week, but not just any colleague. Rather, it would be equivalent to 3 hours of help per week from a colleague who is just as skilled, productive, and hard working as the physician is, because it is, in effect, the physician's own time that is being leveraged.

Similarly, physicians running a weekly DIGMA or PSMA that increased their productivity by 200% would leverage their time by 1½ hours per week, whereas a 400% increase in productivity would result in a net gain of 4½ hours per week (again, less the net overhead cost of the program). Also, running multiple DIGMAs or PSMAs per week could correspondingly multiply these gains by two, three, four, or five times.

There Are Many Ways that Physicians Can Use this Benefit

The physician can use this 3-hour weekly benefit provided by the 300% increased productivity of the DIGMA or PSMA in any number of ways. To date, physicians have used this benefit in a multitude of ways:

- To increase productivity and income
- To improve access to their practice by using this increased capacity to eliminate patient backlogs and wait-lists
- To open up more appointments of the type that the physician most enjoys
- To go home an hour or two earlier by reducing the number of clinic hours worked
- To convert short 15-minute individual appointments on their clinic schedule into 20-minute appointments

- To open up more time on their schedule for surgeries or procedures
- To convert an hour or two per week from clinic time to desktop medicine time for reading journals, teaching, administration, research, phone calls, e-mails, etc.
- To grow a practice and increase panel size
- To open practices that have heretofore been closed

In addition, the physician can use the DIGMA or PSMA as a practice management tool—for example, by off-loading many patient phone calls onto the group and by offering prompt access to DIGMA visits even when the first individual office visit might be weeks away. This percentage increase in the physician's weekly productivity would be correspondingly larger for healthcare organizations requiring less than 36 clinic hours per week (such as 34 or 32 hours).

300% Increased Productivity Translates into an 8–9% Overall Increase in Weekly Productivity

For systems where 36 hours of clinic time is the standard for a full-time physician, a single weekly 90-minute DIGMA or Physicals SMA that increases provider productivity by 300% results in the full-time physician's productivity for the entire week being increased by approximately 8–9%—i.e., assuming that the physician does not reduce productivity elsewhere on his or her schedule. Presumably, the physician whose salary is 100% productivity based in a fee-for-service system could theoretically increase revenues by approximately this 8–9% amount—i.e., less the cost of the program. This, of course, assumes that the physician's current levels of productivity are maintained during the remaining clinic hours, that DIGMAs and PSMAs are able to be billed out and reimbursed at the same rates as traditional office visits, and that the overall number of hours spent seeing patients in the clinic is not reduced.

Caution, Do Not Correspondingly Reduce Productivity Elsewhere on Your Schedule

If the intent is to use the increased productivity of the DIGMA or PSMA to improve access to the physician's practice, one must caution against reducing either productivity elsewhere on the physician's schedule or the number of hours actually worked in the clinic (plus recommend keeping the overhead costs of the SMA program as reasonable as possible). Correspondingly cutting back on clinic time by 2–3 hours during the workweek might translate into the physician enjoying an improved quality of professional and family life, but it would not likely translate into increased overall productivity for the week—nor, as a result, would it improve access to the physician's practice (or increase

revenues) because the net overall impact of the SMA program would then be productivity neutral. Nevertheless, some physicians might to choose to use this gain in productivity provided by the DIGMA or PSMA to improve the quality of their professional life—i.e., by reducing hours spent in the clinic, going home early, lengthening short individual appointments, spending more time on teaching or desktop medicine, or having some additional research or administrative time (that is, rather than by using this increased productivity to improve revenues, overall weekly productivity, or access).

This actually happened in one FFS system, where the first eight physicians to launch DIGMAs and PSMAs in their practices all chose to increase the quality of their professional life while remaining revenue and productivity neutral by cutting back their workweek by a couple of hours for each SMA they started. Thereafter, administration in this organization made it a practice not to allow physicians to cut back their workweek according to the number of DIGMAs and PSMAs they started—i.e., so that the dramatic productivity and access benefits of well-run SMAs could instead be captured. Perhaps an intermediate ground could be struck in such managed-care organizations by permitting SMA physicians to cut back clinic hours by 30–60 minutes (and use this time instead for desktop medicine) for each weekly 90-minute DIGMA or PSMA run that increases productivity by 300% or more.

While Financial Benefits Might Be Less, Providers in Capitated Systems Enjoy Many of the Same Benefits from Their SMAs

Physicians in capitated systems will generally not capture the same direct financial benefits from a highly productive DIGMA or Physicals SMA that providers in fee-for-service systems can enjoy (at least in the case of those whose FFS salaries are close to 100% productivity based). However, physicians in capitated systems might nonetheless enjoy some monetary gain through the increased productivity that the SMA provides because their performance evaluations, bonuses, salary, etc. might be positively affected to some degree.

In Other Ways, Providers in Capitated Systems Enjoy Many of the Same Benefits from Their SMAs

However, physicians in capitated systems do enjoy many of the other potential benefits from their DIGMAs and PSMAs as providers in fee-for-service systems, such as:

- The opportunity to do something new, different, and interesting
- Real, meaningful help (as well as collegiality) from a multidisciplinary team
- A documenter to assist in charting
- Better patient education and closer attention to patients' psychosocial issues
- Fewer patient complaints regarding access
- Reduced patient telephone call volume
- Decreased need to double book and work-in patients
- Closer follow-up care, when appropriate
- Improved doctor–patient relationships
- High levels of patient and physician professional satisfaction

A Word of Caution to Administrators in Capitated Systems

However, there is one point that is critical to the overall success of a DIGMA or PSMA program in capitated systems. As discussed in Chapter 8, it is imperative that administrators in capitated systems do not correspondingly increase the physician's patient panel size by 8–9%—thereby effectively eliminating any net productivity benefit whatsoever to the physician for running a DIGMA or PSMA each week. In my work as a consultant to healthcare systems around the nation, I have found that one of the great fears regarding group visits among physicians in capitated systems is that any net gain in productivity that their SMA might provide to them would be completely offset by a subsequent management decision to correspondingly increase the patient panel sizes that physicians would be expected to manage. Such a decision would, of course, completely negate any net gain that the SMA might otherwise have provided to the physician—thereby completely stripping away (to the benefit of the organization) all of the benefit that the physician might otherwise have achieved by choosing to alter her/his care delivery style and taking the risk of running a DIGMA or PSMA in her/his practice.

Perhaps some compromise here might be possible—one that involves an equitable sharing of this net benefit by the physician and the system. In any case, if a SMA program is to succeed in a capitated system, then it is imperative that the physician always be left with some substantial net benefit for taking the risk of undergoing the change in practice style that implementing a successful DIGMA or PSMA entails—and for investing the requisite time and energy into the SMA program in order to ensure its success.

Do Not Settle for Less than Full Benefit from Your DIGMA Program

Physicians and high-level administrators at various medical groups have occasionally told me that even if their DIGMA or PSMA programs were cost-neutral (i.e., even if predetermined census targets were not met, or only minimally met), they would still want to develop the program anyway. They say this because of both the increased quality and patient satisfaction that SMAs can provide and the uplifting effect they can have upon the morale of physicians actually running them (as well as their staffs). This being the case, organizational leaders have sometimes stated that they felt that this was reason enough to continue the SMA program—and that these benefits were sufficient, in and of themselves, even if no increase in productivity was achieved.

Be Cautious About Rationalizing Small Groups

Personally, I recommend against implementing DIGMAs and PSMAs solely for these reasons—i.e., when you are having difficulties filling sessions and group sizes are smaller than recommended. Yes, improved patient and physician professional satisfaction can still be achieved through your SMA program—as can enhanced quality of care, attention to psychosocial issues, and the amount of patient education provided—even if the group size is smaller than the target census level. However, my recommendation is to always meet your predetermined census targets so that you can also simultaneously achieve the economic, productivity, and access benefits that the DIGMA and PSMA models were originally designed to provide—and so that the result is in a lively, interesting, and interactive SMA experience for all (which is something that full groups can best provide). If you are going to go through all the effort of starting a DIGMA or PSMA in your practice, then why not put in the small amount of extra work required to ensure that all sessions are filed to desired capacity?

Be Cautious About Lowering Pre-established Census Requirements

I similarly caution against reducing desired census levels below pre-established targets. Should you ultimately decide to reduce census requirements for your SMA, be certain to only do so very slowly. It is important to the success of the DIGMA and PSMA program that pre-established minimum, target, and maximum census levels be held whenever possible—at least they should be held until all other viable options have been thoroughly tried, and no other reasonable option exists except to lower the SMA's census requirements. When initial DIGMA or PSMA sessions fail to finish on time (which is often the case for the first couple of months of implementation, while the physician and SMA team are still learning to be coordinated and efficient in their efforts), physicians and staffs alike can quickly become frustrated. As a consequence they all too often immediately reduce the program's pre-established census requirements to a substantially lower level—which should actually be their last choice, not the first.

Unfortunately, lowering census requirements is often the first (rather than the last) solution considered by physicians and behaviorists when any type of problem arises—such as finishing late, not completing all charting by the end of the session, feeling rushed, having unfilled sessions, etc. When this is done, the next thing that starts to happen is that the physician and staff begin to like this smaller group size—thus becoming comfortable with a census that is insufficient to provide the multiple benefits that DIGMAs and PSMAs were originally designed to achieve. It is for this reason that I recommend providers start with their DIGMAs and PSMAs filled to capacity, and thus learn from the outset to adapt to this high workload volume—and that they not make the common beginners' mistake of starting with small groups with the intent of later working up to full groups, which is an approach that seldom works. This seldom works because physicians and SMA teams become comfortable at some point with a less than optimal group size, and therefore never increase census beyond that point—so that that the increased productivity benefits that could otherwise occur are never achieved.

It Usually Takes a Couple of Months to Become Comfortable with Large, Full Groups

Because the learning curves are quite steep, it usually only takes physicians a couple of months (i.e., by debriefing after sessions with their SMA team) in order to adjust to running DIGMAs and PSMAs that are filled to capacity. However, once this is achieved, they quickly grow to enjoy these full groups and the multiple benefits they offer. This result contrasts sharply with the approach of starting with small groups and then gradually working up to larger groups, an approach that has seldom been observed to succeed in actual practice because pre-established census targets are then infrequently, if ever, achieved.

Debrief with Your SMA Team for the First Couple of Months

For the following three reasons, I strongly recommend that you do not reduce pre-established census targets during the first 2 months after launching your DIGMA or PSMA: (1) It takes a couple of months for the physician and SMA team to become comfortable with this new and dramatically different modality of delivering care; (2) because of their remarkably increased productivity, DIGMAs and PSMAs tend to exacerbate any pre-existing system problems, so that it often takes a couple of months for the *bugs* to get worked out of the new SMA program; and (3) it usually takes a couple of months for the physician, behaviorist, nurse(s), and documenter to learn their respective roles and responsibilities and to coalesce into a coordinated, efficient, and well-functioning team—and to begin to finish on time with all charting completed. Therefore, just accept the fact that you will likely finish late at first, and possibly even quite late. Instead of reducing pre-established census requirements, debrief with your team for 15–20 minutes after sessions for the first couple of months after launching your new DIGMA or PSMA program—having frank, honest, and creative discussions while focusing upon how to make future sessions even better and more efficient. These team debriefing sessions can typically be discontinued a couple of months after launching the DIGMA or PSMA; however, it might be advisable to still hold them from time to time afterwards—i.e., on an as-needed basis.

If You Continue to Finish Late, Try to Determine Why as There Are Many Possible Causes

Always strive to make the next session even better than the last—especially in the beginning, during your initial sessions. Make every effort to refine and improve your DIGMA or PSMA each week by incorporating the recommendations that you and your team come up with during these debriefing sessions. In addition, continue trying to do everything possible to finish each session on time while continuing to meet your pre-established census targets. Always focus upon optimizing quality and census.

Above all, if you are finishing late, try to find out why. Are you or your team arriving late? Is your behaviorist failing to arrive early to warm the group up and write down patients' reasons for today's visit? Is the behaviorist taking too much time for the introduction or occupying too much time during sessions on behavioral health interventions and psychosocial issues? Is the exam room located near to your DIGMA group room? Are you using two nurses, or just one? Are you wasting time looking for forms or equipment? Are you using a documenter to increase your efficiency and productivity? Are you unnecessarily taking patients out of the group room for "private" discussions and exams that could equally well be conducted in the group room and, when it is necessary, are you keeping such discussions and examinations as brief as possible? Are you as coordinated as possible with your SMA team, and are you fully delegating to them?

Have you carefully designed an efficient chart note template for your SMA? If you are spending too much time reviewing the EMR chart note after working with each patient in the SMA setting, can you streamline your review and modification process—perhaps by having only those segments of the chart note that are individualized or typed in by the documenter (as opposed to complete templates for normal physical exams or stock text on diabetes, hypertension, hyperlipidemia, etc. that are dropped into the chart note by keystroke shortcuts) highlighted in color or bolded so that you can quickly go to that which is most important in the chart note, and do not waste time reviewing a lot of standardized text? Are you spending too much time on social chit-chat or in fostering too much group interaction? Are you staying focused and succinct throughout the session, or are you sometimes rambling and entering into lengthy academic or tangential discussions? Do you need additional help from your behaviorist in pacing the group? Are you letting a couple of dominating patients control the group? Are you spending too much time on the first couple of patients (or on patients with your favorite conditions)?

Have you removed as much clutter as possible from the group room, especially tables or other potential obstacles that might slow you down? Do you have all the equipment, forms, handouts, etc. that you need and are they organized and accessible? Are you delegating as many responsibilities as possible to the nurse/MA(s), behaviorist, and documenter? Are you consistently debriefing with your SMA team after all sessions during the first 2 months of implementation, focusing upon increasing efficiency and quality during future sessions? All of these sources of inefficiency can end up costing you precious time during DIGMA and PSMA sessions, and ultimately contribute to your finishing sessions late—perhaps even quite late.

If You Must Cut Back on Census, Do so Slowly—But Only After All Other Options Are Exhausted

Only after you have done everything else possible should you consider cutting back on your pre-established census levels—but, even then, wait for a couple of months and only do so very slowly. In other words, reduce census targets only after all other options have been fully tried, yet you nonetheless find that you are still consistently running late in your DIGMA or PSMA. Then, should you ultimately make the decision to cut back on census, be sure to do so by just one or two patients at a time. If you later find that you are still finishing late after a couple more months of running your SMA with this slightly reduced census level, then you could try cutting your census back once again by another patient or two—and see how that works for you during the next month or 2.

Stay Within Recommended Group Sizes, Even Though Considerably Larger SMAs Can Be Run

Even though much larger DIGMAs are possible and have been run successfully, I would recommend that you try to keep your group size within the ideal range of 10–16 patients—especially at first, until you and your team have gained considerable experience with this new paradigm of care. One example of large group sessions occurred when the regional multimedia department came out to videotape all three of the DIGMAs that I happened to be a behaviorist in during a single day just prior to my retirement at Kaiser Permanente in June 1999. At that time, I was the behaviorist in 12 DIGMAs per week at the Kaiser Permanente Medical Center in San Jose, California. On that particular day, it turned out that three physician-led DIGMAs were run and videotaped. All three of these physicians were quite experienced in running their DIGMAs as they had been conducting one or two sessions per week for over 2 years.

As it turned out, during the 4½ hours of physician time that these three DIGMAs took that day, the three physicians in combination saw 60 patients and 14 family members—and these groups did not finish late or feel particularly rushed. Nonetheless, even though substantially more than the recommended 10–16 patients were seen by these physicians (keep in mind that they were all very experienced in running their SMAs), I would recommend keeping DIGMAs between 10 and 16 patients—i.e., to keep sessions from tiring physicians out due to excessive workload and documentation demands and to ensure that SMAs are an enjoyable experience for all (including the physician).

Continue Filling All SMA Sessions, Especially After Initial Success

Approximately 10–25% of all DIGMAs and Physicals SMAs fail, almost always due to a lack of sufficient attendance. Although some physicians and support staffs never succeed at filling their initial SMA sessions to desired capacity, others enthusiastically fill the first couple of DIGMA and PSMA sessions when they first start their program; however, they sometimes soon become complacent and stop consistently inviting and scheduling all appropriate patients. When this happens, the inevitable result is that subsequent sessions are eventually no longer filled to targeted census levels—putting them at risk for failure. Consistently meeting targeted census levels takes constant vigilance and ongoing effort on the part of the physician, support staff, and all personnel associated with scheduling the patients into SMA. Each person must learn to do their part in promoting the SMA program—and in informing, inviting, and scheduling all appropriate patients.

Step 8: Promote the Program Effectively to Patients

Prior to actually launching a DIGMA or PSMA program, integrated delivery systems (for profit, not for profit, group practices, HMOs, PPOs, IPAs, VA and DoD systems, public health systems, etc.) need to make the necessary investment in quality promotional materials (posters, fliers, announcements, invitations, patient packets, "Ask me about SMA" buttons, etc.) to ensure that census targets can consistently be met (examples of all these materials are contained in the DVD attached to this book). These quality promotional materials are meant to familiarize patients with the SMA program, *sell* them on the concept, and encourage patients to attend for the first time. They also enable the physician to personally invite, in just 30–60 seconds, patients seen during regular office visits to have their next visit be a DIGMA or PSMA visit—i.e., because the promotional materials have already helped to inform patients of the SMA program and its many patient benefits. Such marketing materials are needed for DIGMAs and PSMAs because these SMA models represent a major paradigm shift to a form of treatment that patients are not familiar with and could initially resists—and because, unlike CHCCs and Specialty CHCCs, different patients typically attend each session (which makes patient recruitment an ongoing issue over time).

Once patients do in fact attend a SMA, experience has repeatedly demonstrated that they will almost invariably like it and be willing to return. The use of high-quality promotional materials is critical to getting patients to attend a DIGMA or PSMA for the first time and therefore to achieving desired group census targets during all sessions. In addition, all staff (physicians, schedulers, receptionists, nurses, etc.) associated with the group visit must fulfill their role in promoting the program to patients and in keeping all sessions filled.

Develop High-Quality Marketing Materials that Look Expensive but Are Not

Be sure to enlist the help of your public relations or marketing department in developing these promotional materials as they often have much experience in this area. Although these materials will likely look expensive, their cost can in fact be kept quite modest by using reasonably priced materials and printing processes, by procuring all promotional materials in bulk, and by initially developing all such promotional materials in template form. It is also important that all promotional materials have a warm, inviting, and eye-catching appearance and that they be graphically coordinated so as to make a wall display that is appealing to the eye (Fig. 10.1). Because these marketing materials will create the trademark image for the SMA program as it is launched throughout the organization, they must be informative and promotional in nature—plus hold eye appeal for patients. In addition, they must: (1) convey the impression of quality care that SMAs do in fact provide; (2) possess the desired look for the organization; and (3) fit into the budget for the program.

The promotional materials should focus on the enhanced quality, service, medical care, and educational benefits that patients can expect to receive from a well-run group visit program. Be certain to have the theme of your promotional materials focus upon patient benefits, the doctor–patient relationship, the warmth of the group visit experience, and the quality medical care that SMAs offer—for example, by incorporating positive photographs of doctors talking to, and caring for, their patients into the wall posters (Figures 3.5 and 10.1). In other words, the graphic design and wording of the framed wall posters, program description fliers, invitations, announcements, and follow-up letters must all convey a professional image that is commensurate with the warm, supportive, informative, and high-quality healthcare experience that patients can expect to receive from the SMA. The same graphic design should permeate all of the system's promotional materials for the SMA program, so that it eventually becomes the trademark look for the program.

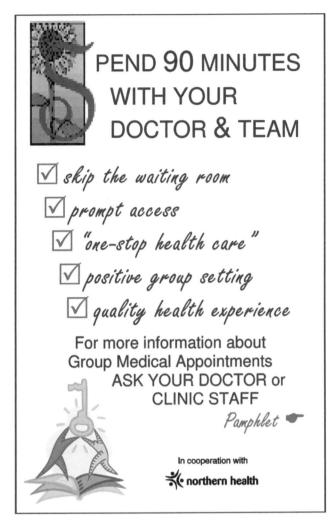

Fig. 10.1 Promotional materials should have an inviting appearance and inform the reader of what they can expect in a group visit (Courtesy of Northern Health, Prince George, British Columbia, Canada)

The Budget Must Include Adequate Funding for Quality Promotional Materials

It is therefore imperative to the success of the DIGMA and PSMA programs that the budget include adequate funding for these high-quality, professional-appearing promotional materials—ones that exude warmth and caring, and are appealing to patients. On the other hand, costs can be kept down somewhat by developing templates for all marketing materials (framed wall posters, fliers, invitation letters, etc.) and then simply making copies of these materials for all future DIGMAs and Physicals SMAs—i.e., after modifying them slightly according to the particular needs and SMA design of each provider. Nonetheless, there will be significant expense incurred in developing these initial templates, and thereafter for making quality copies from these templates for each DIGMA and PSMA

that is implemented—costs that include paper, printing, mounting and framing, mailing, etc.

Quality Marketing Materials Make It Easier for Physicians to Refer Patients

In addition to effectively recruiting patients in their own right, these promotional materials are meant to minimize the amount of physician time that will be required to successfully invite established patients to attend a DIGMA or PSMA. Some physician time and effort will always be required to consistently meet SMA census targets, as nothing is more important in persuading a patient to attend a DIGMA session for the first time than a personal and positively worded invitation from their own doctor. Nonetheless, the amount of physician time required to do so can be minimized through effective use of posters, fliers, announcements, invitation letters, and other promotional materials—and through the help of all support staff associated with the SMA program in inviting patients to attend.

This is because, by the time the physician invites the patient to attend a SMA (i.e., in the exam room during a regular office visit), the patient should already have: (1) received the original announcement letter prior to the start of the DIGMA or PSMA; (2) seen the wall posters in the physician's lobby and exam rooms; (3) been invited to attend a future SMA session by the receptionist (by being handed the "You Are Invited..." letter and through a few positive words about the program); and (4) been strongly encouraged to attend by the nurse/MA rooming the patient (who gives all appropriate patients both the program description flier and a strong personal recommendation). In addition, the physician and entire support staff could wear a clearly visible "Ask Me About SMAs" button as a lapel pin so that many patients will have already asked staff about what a SMA is—and would, as a result, have been told about the program.

Examples of all these promotional materials are included in the DVD attached to this book. It is strongly recommended that you not use these templates in their present form *carte blanche*, but rather that you update and customize them to your own particular needs, specifications, regulations, requirements, and corporate culture.

Develop All Promotional Materials in Template Form

One example of how to save money for your SMA program is to design and develop all forms and promotional materials that are to be used in the program in template form. With the help of the pilot physicians, the program coordinator, and the marketing department, the champion will need to design and develop templates for all of the promotional materials, forms, and reports to be used in the program. These include wall posters, program description fliers, announcement letters, patient invitations, chart note templates for each medical discipline, patient packets, follow-up letters, attendance logs, signs directing patients where to go, patient satisfaction forms, the confidentiality waiver, the format of periodic reports to evaluate the program, etc. (Please note that examples of all of these forms and promotional materials are included in the DVD attached to this book.) All of these SMA materials can then easily and inexpensively be adapted to each provider that subsequently runs a DIGMA or PSMA for his or her practice—i.e., from the original templates first developed for the program. This saves time and money, as the *same old wheel* does not need to be recreated over and over.

Templates of Promotional Materials Save Time and Money

Once developed, quality templates will help the champion and program coordinator to rapidly and systematically launch all new DIGMA and Physicals SMA programs in the future—and to thereby move the SMA program forward throughout the organization. They also save time, frustration, and money by avoiding the need to recreate them over and over as the group visit program is expanded—and as evermore SMAs are launched throughout the system. The guiding principal here is to invest the time and energy required to do the template right the first time (i.e., during its first application)—and then to later have all other physicians who subsequently choose to also run a group visit for their practice simply *fine-tune* the appropriate templates and adapt them to their particular needs and writing style.

Also Develop Chart Note Templates in Primary and Specialty Care

By carefully designing the chart note template for the first primary care DIGMA or PSMA that is run in your system, the same documentation template can then subsequently be used over and over for all future primary care SMAs implemented throughout the organization (internal medicine, family practice, nurse practitioners, physician assistants, etc.)—that is, with only minor modifications according to each provider's specific needs. The same is true for the initial chart note template that is developed for the first

SMA implemented in each medical subspecialty (e.g., rheumatology, cardiology, oncology, endocrinology, nephrology, etc.), because all other providers in these departments could subsequently use the same chart note template (or some variant of it) as it was originally developed for that specific medical specialty.

Tips on Designing Your DIGMA Wall Poster

Before any new DIGMA is launched, a large framed wall poster should be prominently displayed on the walls of the physician's lobby and exam rooms—one that announces the program and informs patients about it. The wall poster displayed in the lobby should be perhaps 30 by 36 inches (or 36 by 40 inches); whereas the smaller version of the same poster used in the exam rooms could be only 20 by 24 inches (or approximately 24 by 30 inches). Although the poster could be in a template form that allows for the physician's name and photograph, as well as the name of the group (and the time that it meets), to be inserted and then printed out for any particular physician's DIGMA or PSMA, most healthcare systems choose a different approach. They instead use the same poster for all DIGMAs and PSMAs, which means that there is no information pertaining to a particular physician or SMA contained in the poster (physician's name, name of SMA, day and time it meets, etc.)—instead such personalized information only appears on the adjacent program description flier. I prefer using the same poster for all SMA providers because it is easier and cheaper—i.e., because the same poster can always be used, even if various changes are subsequently made to the design of the SMA, or to the time and place that it is held (see Figures 3.5 and 10.1).

The wall posters also create a distinctive trademark image for the SMA program, a look that can then be carried forward to all other marketing materials subsequently developed for the program. As more and more of these SMA posters and fliers begin to be prominently displayed in different physicians' lobbies throughout the organization, patients will gradually become more familiar with—and accepting of—the DIGMA and PSMA programs. Eventually patients will begin to view these group visit programs as an important part of the way in which care is being delivered throughout the system and should therefore gradually become evermore willing to attend.

The poster for the SMA program should be tastefully laid out and have a professional appearance; however, it will also need to have a notable *hook* imbedded in it (in large font) that represents the single most important selling point of the SMA program to patients in that system.

Different systems have used various hooks, with the following being fairly representative: *"Imagine Spending 90 Minutes With Your Doctor Any Week You Want!"*; *"Spend More Time With Your Doctor!"*; *"No Appointment Necessary!"*; *"See Your Doctor Any Week You Want To— and for 90 Minutes!"*; *"Medical Care With A Warm, Personal Touch!"*; *"Would You Like to Just Drop-In the Next Time You Want an Appointment?"*; *"Why Wait For An Appointment?"*; *"You Can Feel Better!"*; *"Tired of Hurrying Up and Waiting?"*; etc. In addition, the major selling points of the SMA program should also be listed on the poster as bullet points.

The poster's background should reflect the high-quality medical care that patients can expect to receive, perhaps by including two or three classy photographs of doctors examining and interacting with their patients—with everyone smiling and appearing happy. You might want to have 3 different sets of photos for the wall poster: (1) one showing a mixed assortment of adult patients and male as well as female providers for general use; (2) another showing pediatricians and children (as well as adolescents) for use in pediatrics; and (3) a third set of female patients and predominantly female providers for use in Ob-Gyn and Women's Health. Also, the fact that it is a group should be made clear, even if this is downplayed somewhat—for example, by having three photographs in the poster, with two showing doctors interacting with and examining individual patients—and one smaller photo showing the doctor interacting with a group of patients. Please note that a couple of excellent examples of DIGMA and PSMA wall posters appear in the DVD attached to this book.

Tips on Drafting Your Program Description Fliers

A program description flier should also be developed for your SMA program with a graphic design that matches and coordinates with the wall poster—so that, when taken together, the poster and flier make an eye-appealing wall display. Although wall displays are generally preferable, there are occasions when table or floor displays are the only workable option in the provider's lobby/or and exam rooms. In this case, make the posters in stand-up form (either self-standing or mounted on an easel or tripod)—ensuring that the poster and attached flier dispenser are displayed as prominently as possible. For each new DIGMA or PSMA that is launched within the system, it is typically the program coordinator that develops the initial draft of the program description flier for that physician from the existing SMA template for the program description flier previously developed for the program. However, the physician then needs to examine this flier prototype very carefully and to make the necessary edits and modifications so that the final draft meets with the physician's approval.

The fliers are usually printed on a single sheet of paper and can be printed on heavier than normal paper stock. Although customized bi- or tri-folded fliers printed in brochure form in three or four colors (i.e., on both sides of high quality, glossy paper) are very nice and elegant, they are unfortunately also quite expensive. Therefore, it is wise to select a reasonably heavy paper for fliers that looks expensive, but are in actuality quite reasonably priced—and then buy in volume.

An Inexpensive but Highly Functional Type of Program Description Flier

One of the cheapest, yet nicest, types of flier that I have ever seen used consists simply of an unfolded single page of 8 ½ × 11 inch paper that has been preprinted in volume on one side—i.e., with a soft design in one color (typically in a vertical band along the left edge or horizontally at the top of the sheet) that matches the graphic design and color of the wall poster. These preprinted sheets of paper (which are blank other than the preprinted graphic design either along one edge or in the background) can be produced in bulk by the thousands at minimal cost—provided that they are printed in a single color on nice appearing, inexpensive, and heavier than normal weight paper.

Later, all of the detailed information regarding the physician's DIGMA or PSMA (including the physician's photograph) can be printed or photocopied onto one side of this preprinted sheet of paper, which makes for an inexpensive and immediately available SMA flier. Another advantage of this approach is that the same preprinted paper can be used for the fliers of all providers who subsequently choose to launch a DIGMA or PSMA for their practice—plus the same preprinted paper can also be used as letterhead stationary for the SMA program. Furthermore, neither time nor money needs to be spent on bi- or tri-folding these fliers. The end result here is an inexpensive but nice looking flier that can make a graphically coordinated and eye-appealing wall display with the framed poster.

Start with an Initial Run of 300 Fliers

Once the physician approves the program description flier that is to be used, start with a small run of approximately 300 copies—i.e., of the flier that has been modified according to the exact specifications of the provider from the original SMA department flier template, and then approved by the physician. After approximately 300 copies of the final, approved flier have been photocopied or printed, the physician and staff can immediately start distributing the flier and inviting patients—typically starting this process weeks before the DIGMA or PSMA is actually launched. Do not print more than 300 copies at this early point in time, as providers frequently make substantive changes during the first few weeks of running a SMA—changes that will need to be carried over into the flier. Please note that some excellent examples of program description fliers are contained in the DVD attached to this book.

Mount Flier Holders Adjacent to the Wall Poster in the Lobby and Exam Rooms

One then needs to purchase the necessary flier holders that are to be mounted adjacent to the poster in the lobby and exam rooms—i.e., which will contain perhaps 100 copies of the program description flier. Personally, I like to use thick, clear plastic flier holders with high edges (to keep fliers upright so that they do not droop over) that are custom made for the SMA program (i.e., eye-appealing wall dispensers that will hold approximately 100 fliers at a time)—holders which look elegant and expensive, but are handmade by a local vendor for only $50 each.

Designate One Person to be Responsible for Refilling Flier Holders as Needed

Finally, be sure to assign one person the responsibility of keeping all of the physician's flier holders filled at all times. In order to ensure that the flier holders in the lobby and exam rooms are consistently kept full with approximately 100 fliers each, arrange for a member of the physician's support staff to be given primary responsibility for keeping the dispensers stocked with fliers at all times and making certain that they are never empty. Typically, this task is assigned to a motivated receptionist, nurse, medical assistant, or office manager who is willing to take on this responsibility; however, it could also be the dedicated scheduler attached to the SMA program. The program coordinator must then check periodically to ensure that the all flier holders are in fact being kept full and should take prompt corrective action if the flier dispensers are ever found to be empty.

Tips Regarding the Announcement Letter

To *kick start* the DIGMA or PSMA, it is very helpful to send an announcement letter to all appropriate patients before the SMA starts. In other words, the first step in promoting each new group visit program should be to send a letter announcing the physician's new DIGMA or PSMA to all appropriate patients in the physician's practice—or possibly to all suitable patients with a particular chronic illness in the event that the SMA is part of a chronic illness population management program. Somebody on the physician's support staff needs to be given primary responsibility for this task of sending out the announcement letter either by traditional mail or by secured e-mail—often a motivated clerical or administrative person, but occasionally a nurse or medical assistant.

What is the recommended content of the announcement letter? The announcement should be relatively short (typically just a single page, and preferably less, so that patients will read it), uncluttered, laid out neatly, and signed by the physician—and could even include a small black and white photo of the physician smiling pleasantly. In can be printed or photocopied on the SMA Department's letterhead—i.e., the same preprinted paper as the fliers are being photocopied onto. The announcement should include a brief description of the program in understandable, patient-friendly, and positive terms—which should be written in such a manner that it motivates patients to attend. Like the wall poster and adjacent program flier, the announcement letter should saliently outline a few of the DIGMA or PSMA's most important benefits to patients in bulleted format (e.g., prompt access, more time with the doctor, a more relaxed pace of care, drop-in convenience, extensive patient education, answers to important questions that you did not know to ask, help and support from the behaviorist and other patients, etc.).

The announcement should clearly explain that this is a group visit and that other patients will be in attendance. It should also make clear all of the important information that patients need to know about the program in order to attend (starting date, when and where it is to be held, the cost, how to sign up, where to register, etc.) and should close with an invitation to attend the next time that the patient has a medical need in the future—plus conclude with the physician's signature. As previously mentioned, an appealing black and white photo of the physician and a personalized tone to the announcement is also recommended. An example of an announcement letter can be found on the DVD attached to this book (see Invitation Letters folder).

While the announcement letter, which can be sent out either all at once or weekly in batches of 50 or so, will not cause many patients to attend the DIGMA or PSMA in and of itself, it does let the patient know about the existence of the physician's new SMA program. It also makes it more likely that patients will later accept the physician's invitation to attend a future DIGMA or PSMA session when they next come into the office and are invited by the physician and staff to attend. In addition, it tends to reduce the amount of time that it will typically take for the physician to successfully invite the patient to attend. Patients will often accept the physician's invitation by saying something like: "Oh, yeah. I read about that program when you sent me a letter on it. I remember it now. Thanks for thinking about me."

Tips Regarding the Invitation

It is important to have receptionists give invitations to all appropriate patients seen during regular office visits (see sample invitations on the attached DVD). As soon as the starting date for the group visit has been established, the physician's receptionist(s) needs to start giving out invitations to all appropriate patients as they register for regular clinic visits with the physician—pointing out, in a friendly manner, that the doctor personally requested that it be given to the patient and that the doctor would like for them to read it while they are waiting in the lobby. Actually, the invitation letter is typically very similar to the announcement letter that has previously been sent to patients. Receptionists should also personally recommend the SMA to patients when giving out the invitation—including a few carefully chosen words about the program as well as any positive comments that other patients might have made to the receptionists regarding the SMA (along with receptionist's own positive observations when sitting in on a session or two regarding what a warm and informative experience the DIGMA or PSMA provides).

The receptionist(s) should also be trained to answer, in positive terms, a few of the most common questions that patients frequently ask about SMAs (see related material on frequently asked questions included in the DVD attached to this book). From that point onward, the receptionist(s) should begin saying a few positive words about the program to all suitable patients as they register, and then giving them an invitation letter to read in the lobby while waiting to be roomed for today's office visit. This is especially helpful because receptionists often chat briefly with patients when they register anyway, and patients will often be open to listening to their recommendations.

Promote SMAs Through Newsletters and the Local Mass Media (Radio, TV, Newspapers, etc.)

The organization can further accelerate the rate at which patients become familiar with the SMA program by publishing articles on DIGMAs and Physicals SMAs in their patient newsletter, by utilizing any other promotional opportunities that might exist within the system, and by alerting the mass media to their new SMA program and its many patient benefits. The organization's public affairs or marketing department can be most helpful in *getting the word out* to the local mass media outlets (radio, television, and newspaper)—all of whom have historically tended to be quite positively disposed toward DIGMAs and PSMAs, so long as the focus remains upon patient benefits and enhanced quality of care. In addition, the physician could create a brief (say 10–30 minutes in length) video on the DIGMA or PSMA program that could be shown in the physician's lobby as a continuous loop videotape (or DVD) in order to promote the new program to patients and inform them about it.

The Nurse/MA Gives Fliers to Patients During Regular Office Visits and Invites Them to Attend

Upon calling patients from the lobby and rooming them in the exam room for a traditional office visit, the nurse/MA/nursing tech. needs to tell all appropriate patients about the physician's DIGMA or Physicals SMA in positive terms—explaining that the nurse is part of the program and that patients seem to really like it. The nurse can then recommend the program and invite the patient to attend the next time they have a medical need and want to be seen. The nurse/MA can state that, in the event that the physician invites them to attend, the patient might seriously consider attending—and that, should the physician forget to invite the patient to attend the DIGMA or PSMA for their next medical visit, the patient might then ask if it is something that the doctor would recommend for them). Pointing out the poster in either the lobby or the exam room, the nurse/MA then goes over and—taking a program description flier from the wall dispenser next to the poster—hands it to the patient, asking that the patient read it while waiting in the exam room for the physician to arrive. In addition, the nurse/MA should also check and make certain that the receptionist gave the patient an invitation. If for some reason the patient did not receive one, the nurse could then also give the patient an invitation letter at that time—plus let the receptionist know that this lapse had occurred.

What Patients Need to Know Before Attending a Group Visit

Before attending a group visit, it is important that patients know several things about the program—i.e., in order to fully benefit and be able to make an informed choice about whether or not to attend. The SMA program's promotional materials should therefore address these points:

- This is a group medical appointment—several other patients of the physician will also be in attendance
- This is an extended 90-minute medical appointment, not a class or support group
- Most of the same medical care will be provided as in regular office visits, but with others present
- One-on-one time with the doctor is available as needed for brief private talks and exams
- You will get help and support from other patients, plus have some fun
- To gain the full patient education benefit from the program, patients should stay for the entire visit
- If this is not possible, come anyway and simply let the provider know that you must leave early
- Patients can pre-schedule their DIGMA appointments, or they can simply drop in
- Before dropping in, call the office at least a day ahead

  - to let staff know you're coming
  - to check and make certain that the DIGMA will be meeting

- You can bring a support person with you (spouse, friend, adult child, caregiver)
- All who attend are encouraged to ask questions, interact, and actively participate

One Physician's Strategy for Successfully Promoting—And Filling—All DIGMA Sessions

One physician I worked with was exceptionally successful at promoting his DIGMA, and at referring patients into it, from the very start of his program. In fact, he had 19 patients scheduled into his second DIGMA session. I believe that we all can learn an important lesson from this physician's approach to successfully inviting patients to his SMA.

His Staff Was Fully Engaged in Referring Patients

When I asked for his secret to success, he said that he instructed his staff to refer all appropriate patients into his DIGMA—and to not invite patients only when there was a compelling reason to do so. "If in doubt, go ahead and invite them" is what he told his staff. Wanting to do today's work today, he would instruct his staff to also offer his upcoming DIGMA session to all patients calling for an appointment that he was not able to see individually that day (or certainly for any patients that he was not able to schedule during that

week). In addition, all patients calling for a routine follow-up appointment were offered their choice of either the first available 15-minute office visit (which was typically weeks away) or a 90-minute DIGMA group appointment that week, which was briefly described by staff in positive terms. However, even though patients need to be informed about the DIGMA/PSMA program and encouraged to attend, patient attendance must at all times be voluntary.

Patient Phone Calls Were Referred Directly into the DIGMA Whenever Appropriate and Possible

If a patient telephoned his office and asked to speak to him regarding a non-emergent issue, he would—whenever appropriate and possible—have his staff offer the patient his 90-minute DIGMA that week in lieu of a return phone call. His staff would point out that this would allow the physician to personally speak with the patient, take vital signs, update injections and routine health maintenance, and even examine the patient, if necessary. They further explained that patients would get answers to not only all of their medical questions, but also questions they might not have known to ask—because others often will ask. This approach had the added advantage of converting uncompensated telephone calls into compensated DIGMA visits. Because these telephone calls often needed to be made at the end of the day (i.e., at the expense of personal or family time), it was especially helpful to the physician when these patients could be referred into the provider's SMA. This was also important because these calls were often made at the end of the day, when insufficient information about the patient might be available and when the physician was tired—and therefore at greater risk for making a mistake.

This Physician Would Personally Invite Every Appropriate Patient Seen During Office Visits

This physician was so successful because he believed himself that the DIGMA was the best approach for many patients, and he would give every appropriate patient seen during regular office visits a personal, very positively worded invitation to attend his DIGMA the next time they had a medical need and wanted to be seen. His invitation was certainly not tepid or weak—i.e., it was nothing like "You can have either an individual or group visit for your follow-up, just schedule it when you leave."

Instead, his referrals were positively worded and very persuasive. He would say something like "John, you have diabetes and I think that you should come back in 3 months for follow-up to see how you are doing. I would like to invite you to my new DIGMA program, as it is open only to my own patients and was specifically designed for people like yourself. It will give us 90 minutes together, so that I can go into more detail than I normally could during a rushed office visit—and I can even talk more about the latest treatments for diabetes. Not only will we have more time together in a setting that fells less rushed, but it will also give you a chance to meet some of my other patients dealing with similar issues. It will probably include some of my patients who have been successfully dealing with diabetes a lot longer than you have, so they might have some helpful tips for you. There is a strong focus upon patient education and empowerment so that my patients can learn how to take the best possible care of themselves. You will probably get answers to medically important questions that you might not have thought to ask. If you would like, you can bring your wife or a support person along with you, as they will likely also find it to be interesting. It's lively, informative, and fun—heck, we even serve up some Starbucks coffee and healthy snacks. Would you like to attend my DIGMA for your 3 month follow-up and give it a try?" If the patient accepted this offer, then the physician promptly scheduled the patient into the appropriate future DIGMA session.

Finally, this physician had developed a very successful innovation—an extra step he would take with those few patients who initially balked at his invitation to schedule their next follow-up appointment in the DIGMA. If the patient was still reluctant to attend the DIGMA after this positively worded, personal invitation from the physician explaining the many patient benefits that the DIGMA offered, then this physician would ask the following question: "Would you be willing to try it once for me, as I really believe it will help you?" He never had a patient refuse to try it once "for the doctor." Almost invariably, the patient would say something like "Sure, if you feel that strongly about it, I'll try it once and see."

Once Patients Did in Fact Attend a Session, They Almost Invariably Liked the DIGMA

Of course, once patients actually attended a DIGMA session, they almost always liked it. Patient satisfaction scores with DIGMAs and Physicals SMAs have quite consistently been found to be very high—typically between 4.4 and 4.7 on a 5-point Likert scale. Therefore, the key to success lies in getting patients to try the SMA for the first time. Because perhaps only 1 in 20 will say after attending the DIGMA that it was not for them and that they preferred individual office visits (whereas it is not uncommon for 4–6 patients out of 20 to state afterwards that they prefer the DIGMA to traditional office visits, while the remainder say they are willing to attend

either, depending upon which is more available), patients will almost always be willing to return to the DIGMA setting the next time they have a medical need—provided that they are invited to return to the SMA for their next follow-up visit.

Step 9: Use Comfortable, Well-Equipped Group and Exam Rooms

Because group visits are relatively lengthy and provide medical care in a non-traditional manner (i.e., to many patients at once in a supportive group setting), they require appropriate and comfortable facilities in order to be conducted properly. DIGMAs require a group room that is sufficiently large and contains enough comfortable chairs to accommodate 15–25 people (staff and attendees)—typically 10–16 patients, 2–6 support persons, and three staff members (physician, behaviorist, and documenter). It is important to ensure that the group room will be consistently set up and properly prepared in advance of each session—which includes setting up enough comfortable chairs for the expected number of attendees, typically in a circular or elliptical configuration for DIGMAs and PSMAs (or a horseshoe arrangement for CHCCs). In addition, there needs to be a properly equipped exam room nearby the group room used for the DIGMA. On the other hand, PSMAs will require a group room approximately half as large with 12–15 comfortable chairs, and typically 4 exam rooms—although they can be in the physician's own office area.

Make Certain that the Group Room's Ventilation Is Adequate and that the Temperature Is Comfortable

Be cautious to set the temperature of the group room at a comfortable level and check to ensure that the ventilation in the room is adequate for the expected number of attendees. It is important to keep in mind that it is sometimes poor ventilation, rather than inadequate room size, that is the limiting factor regarding the number of patients that the group room can comfortably accommodate. If this is the case for your group room, consider adjusting the thermostat so that the room is on the cool side when the group starts, so that it will only be mildly warm and stuffy when the group ends—i.e., rather than feeling like an uncomfortable *steam bath* by the time the group is over.

What to Do When No Group Room Is Available to You

If you do not have a group room large enough to accommodate the expected number of attendees, then consider using any suitable space that is available—such as a conference room, staff lounge, portion of the cafeteria, storage room, or even the lobby during off-clinic hours. If you have a group room that is not large enough, then consider another solution—i.e., running a 60-minute DIGMA, with its correspondingly lower census requirements, rather than one that is 90 minutes in duration. Or consider running two 60-minute DIGMAs per week rather than one 90-minute DIGMA, or perhaps three weekly 60-minute DIGMAs rather than two 90-minute DIGMAs.

Or else consider running a PSMA, which typically requires a group room only half as large as that required for a DIGMA. However, keep in mind that a PSMA often requires 2–5 exam rooms (and most often 4, especially for complete physical examinations on women in primary care), although they do not need to be adjacent to the group room—even though that would be preferable. While utilizing whatever space happens to be available might prove to be a workable short-term solution when you first launch your DIGMA or PSMA, the best long-term solution is to have the appropriate group and exam room space made available by retooling the physical plant so as to provide that space.

Decorate the Group Room so as to Create a Comfortable Ambiance

Try to avoid a cold, sterile, or clinical appearance to the group room. Hang some pictures on the walls, bring in an artificial tree or two, and clear out the clutter. A group room can be pleasantly decorated at little cost to provide a warm and comfortable ambiance. Try not to have tables or other obstructions in the midst of the elliptical or circular arrangement in which the DIGMA patients, support persons, physician, and behaviorist are seated. Such clutter makes it difficult for the provider to walk over to individual patients during group time and can create psychological barriers for patients to hide behind—barriers that can actually interfere with patients' candor and the group process. It is sometimes advisable to have a light box in the group room (for the physician to examine X-rays), some basic medical equipment (such as a stethoscope and a filament for diabetic foot exams), a couple of anatomical models, a few medical wall charts, and a selection of patient education handouts—along with anything else that might prove helpful.

Many providers will want an assortment of handouts regarding available internal and external resources—such as nutritional classes, smoking cessation classes, depression programs, community support groups, chronic illness groups, health education classes, behavioral medicine programs, etc. It is also helpful to have relevant educational handouts on issues as such as PSA, hormone replacement therapy, breast self-exams, good nutrition, exercise, and diabetes. Be certain to select handouts that are not only relevant to the patients in attendance, but also consistent with your own beliefs and style of practice—e.g., will you use a colorectal screening handout that recommends a fecal Hemoccult screening test plus a flexible sigmoidoscopy, or one that encourages periodic colonoscopies?

The Recommended Seating Arrangement in the Group Room

In DIGMAs and PSMAs, patients, support persons, the physician, and the behaviorist typically all sit in a circular or elliptical seating arrangement—without any tables or clutter in the middle so that the physician can easily walk over to examine a patient, hand them a prescription, or give them a handout. Ideally, the physician and behaviorist should be sitting next to each other with a small table between them—upon which medical charts, handouts, forms, and any medical equipment that the physician might occasionally want to use in the group (such as a stethoscope, pulse oximeter, frozen nitrogen can, tuning forks for simple hearing tests, filament for diabetic foot exams, device for testing for peripheral neuropathy, etc.) are kept.

It is best for the physician and behaviorist to be seated closest to the door leading from the group room to the exam room, with their backs to the door. In this way, the nurse/MAs (who starts early and typically spends the first part of the DIGMA session in the nearby exam room taking vital signs, updating injections and routine health maintenance, and providing any special duties that the physician might have requested) only needs to walk a short distance to get from the exam room to the group room in order to speak with the physician or place partially completed referral forms on the table. This arrangement also enables the nurse to call patients out of the group room (and then escort them from the group room to the exam room, and back) with a minimal disturbance to the flow of the group. Furthermore, should the nurse or MA need to speak briefly to the physician about a patient they are working with, the physician is located in a convenient seating position within the group room.

The paper forms that could be placed by the nurse upon the table beside the physician might include referral forms, signed confidentiality releases, and a sheet listing any medical concerns that the patients might have disclosed to the nurse(s). In addition, for systems still using paper charts, patients' medical charts could also be placed by the nurse upon the table adjacent to the physician as each patient is returned from the exam room to the group room—along with today's SMA chart note, which is partially completed by the nurse and paper clipped to the front cover (i.e., with the sections for vital signs, injections, performance measures, routine health maintenance, and reasons for today's visit completed by the nurse/MA).

Serve Water, Coffee, and Snacks If Desired, but Make Certain They Are Appropriate

It is a good idea, when it is possible and in the budget, to serve appropriate drinks and snacks as refreshments—such as fruit, yogurt, power bars, decaffeinated coffee, tea, bottled water, etc. Patients appreciate it when even modest snacks and drinks (especially bottled water, coffee, and snack bars) are provided. Be sure to model healthy snacks for the patient populations that will be attending. Be careful not to serve inappropriate refreshments—such as caffeinated coffee for prenatal Physicals SMAs in obstetrics, high caloric snacks at a weight management DIGMA, messy snacks (such as cookies, oranges, or potato chips) in a pediatrics SMA, or candy and soft drinks high in sugar content at an Endocrinology DIGMA for diabetes.

Place drinks and snacks on a table placed in a corner (or to one side) of the group room and make certain that they are readily accessible to all in attendance. It should be pointed out during the behaviorist's introduction that these items are available to all group members and that everyone should feel free to walk over and take some refreshments any time they want to during the session. It is often the case that patients do not get up and go over to get snacks during the SMA session, so that it is a much appreciated gesture when the behaviorist puts several snacks (including bottled water) on a tray and walks it around the group—offering them to one patient and support person after another—a couple of times during the session.

For DIGMAs, a Well-Equipped Exam Room Should Be Located Near the Group Room

For DIGMAs, a private exam room needs to be secured that is located near to the group room. For PSMAs, approximately four exam rooms are typically used;

however, they can be in the provider's own office area. The exam room(s) should be stocked with all necessary equipment and forms for the nurse/MA(s) to take vitals, provide injections, update routine health maintenance, and perform any other special duties requested by the physician just prior to (and during the first part of) the session. It is helpful if the nearby exam room is large enough for both a nurse and MA when both are used in the DIGMA so that, when the MA is finished with vitals and other duties, the patient can then be *handed off* to the nurse—who updates injections, performs any special nursing duties requested by the physician, etc. It is not only more efficient for the nurse and MA to be in the same exam room (assuming that is is large enough for both, and is set up accordingly), it also provides a more enjoyable experience for both—as they are able to talk not only with patients, but also with each other.

The physician can later use the same exam room during DIGMA sessions—i.e., to conduct brief private examinations and discussions as needed, typically toward the end of the session so as to not interrupt the flow of the group. Therefore, the exam room should ideally be fully equipped and have a sink, exam table, chairs, scale, all necessary forms and handouts, a refrigerator (for certain injections)—and any medications, materials, or medical equipment that might be needed. It is advisable for the group room to have a sink as well so that the physician can wash hands after examining a patient. If one is not available, then be sure to use some type of hand sanitizer until one can be installed.

The nurse or medical assistant will use the nearby examination room, typically just prior to and during the first part of each DIGMA session—to take vital signs (and enter them, along with reason for today's visit, into the patients' DIGMA chart notes), conduct special duties (e.g., give injections, examine the feet of diabetic patients, check the peak flow and PO2 levels on asthmatic patients, etc.), update performance measures and routine health maintenance due on each patient, and pull and partially complete referral form for specialists as well as tests and procedures. In a PSMA, these nursing duties would be performed on all patients as they are being individually roomed into one of the exam rooms assigned to the program. Therefore, it is important that a functional computer be located in each exam room (two in case of a larger DIGMA exam room that has been set up with 2 stations for both a nurse and a medical assistant), especially for systems already using electronic medical records.

I have tried virtually every other possible arrangement for taking vital signs—from the nurse/MA/nursing tech. going around the group room and taking vitals while patients are seated during DIGMA sessions to taking patients' vital signs behind a curtain in the corner of the group room. However, no arrangement has worked out as satisfactorily as taking vitals in a separate, nearby exam room—with the door closed, so that privacy can be maintained and talk between the patient and the nurse/MA does not become a source of distraction to the group. After all, we want the DIGMA to be a pleasant experience for all, including the nursing personnel attached to the program. We want nurses to talk to, and laugh with, the patients—and to be able to do so without worrying about being too loud or disruptive to the group process. It is also important to keep in mind that, while patients will talk candidly about virtually anything in the DIGMA group setting (from erectile dysfunction and diarrhea, to menstrual problems and vaginal discharge), few are willing to share their weight and age with others. Therefore, vital signs are best taken in the privacy of a separate exam room located near to the group room.

Step 10: Max-Pack All SMAs to Provide as Much Medical Care as Possible

It is important to the success of a SMA program to *max-pack* all DIGMA and PSMA sessions so that you not only address the medical needs that are bringing the patient in today, but also update their performance measures, routine health maintenance, and injections. The goal is to provide patients with the maximum amount of medical care possible during each and every SMA visit, and consequently to offer them the convenience of a one-stop shopping experience for their healthcare.

Much of this effort can be delegated by the physician to less costly members of the SMA care delivery team, especially to the nurse or medical assistant(s), who then consistently dispatch these duties on all patients once it becomes a part of their protocol—an arragement that is superior in consistency to the often *hit or miss* approach of the individual office visit. This is but one example of how to build maximum quality into your group visit program—which is important because maximum quality, together with optimal group census, is always the goal for every properly designed, supported, and run DIGMA or PSMA that is implemented.. For example, all needed injections can consistently be provided and updated (e.g., flu shots, pneumovax, tetanus, etc.) and all routine health maintenance can be brought current (e.g., referrals for mammograms, colonoscopies, etc.) during each and every session. In addition, prescriptions can be refilled or changed, brief exams (that do not require disrobing) can be conducted

during the group (with private exams provided in the exam room), and referrals to specialists (or for tests and procedures) can be made during group time.

Some systems have also told me about many positive improvements in the consistency with which they are able to update performace measures and routine health maintenance through their relatively new DIGMA and PSMA programs, results they indicate will be published in the not too distant future (also, see Chapter 9, which is the outcomes chapter of this book).

With DIGMAs and PSMAs, Deliver as Much Care as Possible in the Group Room

During each DIGMA and PSMA session, make a point of providing as much medical care and discussion as possible and appropriate in the group setting, where all can listen and learn. For example, in the case of DIGMAs, symptoms can be reviewed, risk assessment and reduction can be conducted, personal and family health histories can be updated, and various questions can be asked and answered in the group setting. History, exam, medical decision-making, and counseling, etc. can all be conducted on patients individually in the DIGMA group setting. The physician can address patients' medical concerns, change and refill prescriptions, discuss treatment options and medication side effects, and provide many types of exams that do not require disrobing in the group setting. Of course, truly private discussions and exams (such as breast and abdominal exams) would be provided in the privacy of the exam room, typically toward the end of the session.

This is one of the great patient education and efficiency benefits of DIGMAs and PSMAs because as much as possible is done in the group room, where all can ask questions, interact, and learn. However, this is often not the case for other group models, such as the CHCC, where the actual delivery of medical care does not efficiently occur in the group setting while the other patients are listening, interacting, and learning.

Finally, a great deal of patient education can be provided (in the context of working with each patient individually) during every DIGMA and PSMA group session. It is not uncommon for patients to bring up medically important issues that have previously gone undisclosed—i.e., because other patients bring them up and discuss them in the group setting. I have quite often found that significant cardiovascular symptoms—which are known to often go underreported or unnoticed in the traditional individual office visit venue of care delivery—are not uncommonly brought up in the DIGMA or PSMA setting for the first time because another patient brings it up first.

Some Minor Procedures Can Also Be Provided During Group Visits

Certain minor procedures (such as trigger point injections, vaccinations, brief hearing tests, nitrogen freezing of skin lesions, etc.) can be provided during most DIGMA and PSMA sessions, sometimes during the group but occasionally (depending upon the physician's preference) in the privacy of the nearby exam room toward the end of the session. Offering simple procedures is another way of enhancing quality and max-packing SMA visits, as it is a convenience to patients and can also reduce patient demand for additional medical services and appointments later on.

During Each Session, Offer Patients Private Time with the Physician as Needed

A characteristic of the DIGMA, CHCC, and PSMA models is that private time with the physician is offered to patients during each and every session—typically for brief private discussions and exams on an as-needed basis toward the end of the session. All patients are told during every DIGMA session that they can speak privately with the physicians toward the end of the session if they so desire (something that is automatically built into the Physicals SMA model, where all patients typically start the session with a private physical examination). Conversely, it is the physician who sometimes asks to meet with the patient in private (again, typically toward the end of the session, so as to not interfere with the flow of the group) for a brief discussion or to conduct a brief private exam—for example, when disrobing is required. In the CHCC model, patients who need to be seen individually are simply scheduled into the individual care segment that follows the group component of the visit as medical care in this model is generally not delivered during the group setting—and is instead delivered to patients individually, generally out of earshot of others.

Although Offered to All, It Is Surprising How Seldom Private Time Is Actually Requested by Patients

What is surprising is how seldom patients actually accept this offer during DIGMAs for private one-on-one time with the physician—i.e., by following through and actually asking to be seen individually by the physician in the privacy of the exam room. In DIGMAs, almost everything occurs in the group room, where efficiency is gained, repetition can be avoided, and all present can simultaneously listen and learn. In a typical well-run primary care DIGMA with 12–15 patients in attendance, physicians contemplating a DIGMA for their practice often fear that all of these patients will want to have private one-on-one time with them. In fact, the opposite is typically true as experience has shown that it is most likely that none of the patients will need to be seen in the privacy of the exam room toward the end of the session. The next most common scenario is that one or two patients will request private time with the physician. It is only on rare occasions that more than 2 of these 12–15 patients will need to be seen privately in a well-run DIGMA session, unless it happens to be something like a physiatry or rheumatology DIGMA in which the physician chooses to provide trigger point injections on some patients toward the end of the session.

Unexpectedly, Patients Often Discuss the Most Personal of Issues in the Group Setting

There are certain occasions where patients might be too embarrassed to bring a particular issue up in the group, and therefore ask to speak to the physician in private. In reality, this happens surprisingly infrequently in a well-run DIGMA as patients are usually remarkably open to discussing even the most personal and private of issues in the group setting, especially when others bring the subject up first. In fact, quite often the opposite is the case. Not uncommonly, patients will say something like the following to the provider: "I didn't feel comfortable bringing this up in our last office visit, doc, but I feel safe with these fine folks here…" and then go on to discuss some of the most personal and private of issues. Patients will often talk about such private issues as erectile dysfunction, vaginal discharge, STDs, depression, incontinence, etc. in the group setting—especially when somebody else brings the topic up.

The fact that even the most intimate and personal of topics are often discussed openly in the group—even by patients who have not previously disclosed these issues to their physician during prior individual office visits—is surprising to many, but just another example of the many ways in which group visits can be counterintuitive. And this typically begins to happen even more often over time—i.e., as the physician and behaviorist gain experience and comfort with the DIGMA or PSMA, and with handling such personal discussions in the group setting.

Occasionally, It Is the Physician Who Asks to See the Patient in Private

Sometimes, it is the physician who wants to speak privately to the patient. This is certainly true when the physician wants to conduct a physical examination that requires disrobing, such as a breast or abdominal exam. Also, physicians would not want to tell a patient in the group setting that their HIV test just came back and that, unfortunately, it was positive. Instead, they would just mention, when working with the patient individually in the group setting, that they would like to talk to them in private for a moment—usually toward the end of the group session.

Just as is the case for individual office visits, physicians continue to use their own best judgment at all times in DIGMAs and Physicals SMAs—including on issues regarding privacy and what to discuss or not discuss in the group setting. Physicians are never asked to go beyond their comfort level—or to depart from their own best judgment, professional ethics, or standards of care—during DIGMA and PSMA sessions. However, I have noticed that—as time goes by and the physician becomes more comfortable with the group visit format—there is frequently a gradual but steady increase both in the amount of medical care delivered and in the amount of sensitive discussion that actually occurs in the group setting.

In the CHCC model, patients who need to be seen individually are simply scheduled into the individual care segment that follows the group component of the visit as medical care in this model is generally not delivered during the group setting—and is instead delivered to patients individually, generally out of earshot of others.

Step 11: Optimize Providers' Mix of Individual and Group Visits

DIGMAs and PSMAs can be used to optimize the mix of appointments offered on the physician's schedule, which is one method that providers can employ to better manage their practice and maximize efficiency, value, and quality in the services they render. DIGMAs and PSMAs are attractive to physicians and administrators alike because, when judiciously used together with individual appointments in a balanced and measured way, they strike an optimal balance between cost, efficiency, and quality care on the one hand—and between the needs of patients, physicians, and healthcare organizations on the other. Efficient, cost-effective DIGMA and PSMA visits provide a nice complement to the judicious use of more costly individual office visits in the physician's schedule.

For example, some specialists and surgeons will want to off-load many lower compensated intake and follow-up visits onto their DIGMAs and PSMAs (with the added benefits of being able to overbook sessions according to the expected number of no-shows and late cancels, and of not having to repeat the same information over and over to different patients individually), and then retool their master schedule to offer more time each week for doing more highly compensated procedures and surgeries.

Similarly, many busy and backlogged primary care providers might want to off-load numerous routine and chronic illness follow-up appointments onto their highly productive and cost-effective DIGMA sessions—and thereby reduce patient demand for precious individual office visit appointments in their schedules. This makes individual appointments more available to those patients truly needing them. In addition, they could then retool their master schedule by reducing the number of individual return visits that they offer each week in order to: (1) make room for administrative, teaching, or research time; (2) open up more individual appointments of the types that are most backlogged; (3) offer more appointments of the type they most enjoy seeing; (4) consolidate several short follow-up visits into a couple of extra physical examination visits offered each week; (5) add additional desktop medicine time; (6) lengthen some of the remaining short individual office visit appointments in their schedule to make them 5 minutes longer; (7) shorten their workweek by an hour or 2 (without any corresponding net decrease in overall productivity for the entire week); or (8) grow their practice by opening up more intake appointments in their master schedule. These are yet other examples of how DIGMAs and PSMAs can be used as excellent practice management tools.

Individual and SMA Visits Each Have Their Advantages and Disadvantages

DIGMAs and PSMAs are meant to complement, not to completely replace, individual office visits, and to provide an additional tool in the physician's black bag for better managing chronic illnesses and a large, busy, and backlogged practice. They are designed to work well in conjunction with the judicious use of individual appointments, as both types of visits have an important role to play in today's rapidly changing and highly competitive healthcare environment. Each has its own advantages and disadvantages, and neither is best for all patients and situations—i.e., neither is a *one size fits all* solution to today's multifarious healthcare challenges. To the contrary, both the individual and the different types of group appointments have something valuable to contribute.

Individual appointments, which are best in many circumstances, provide the traditional venue for medical care and a care setting that patients have become accustomed to and grown to expect. On the other hand, physicians who use DIGMAs and PSMAs effectively can achieve extraordinary access, productivity, economic, and quality of care benefits in their practices. This is because these SMA models are max-packed and excel at containing costs by increasing physician productivity, by leveraging existing resources, by reducing backlogs to follow-up visits and physical exams, and by improving access to care. Properly designed and run DIGMAs and PSMAs can improve service and quality of care, while also making individual appointments more available to those patients who need them most.

DIGMAs for Two-Part Physicals Can Be Used to Improve Access to Physical Exams

When the physician does not run a Physicals SMA but nonetheless needs to improve access to physical examinations, DIGMAs can be (and have been) used for up to 5 *two-part physicals* per session.

What Is a Two-Part Physical?

In two-part physicals, patients are promptly seen for the first part of their physical examination in the physician's DIGMA that week. It is here that much of the discussion transpires that normally occurs in a physical examination between the physician and the patient—e.g., review of systems, history taking, risk assessment and reduction, discussion of treatment options, addressing of medical issues, answering of questions, etc. In addition, vital signs are taken, routine health maintenance is brought current, and lab tests, procedures, and blood screening tests are ordered. Then, a short individual office visit (i.e., rather than a more lengthy physical examination appointment, which might be completely booked months in advance on the physician's schedule) with the physician is scheduled for the patient during the next week or two in order to conduct the private part of the physical examination—i.e., which requires disrobing in the privacy of the exam room.

Two-Part Physicals with DIGMAs Are Less Efficient than Exams in Physicals SMAs

Please note that, when DIGMAs are used in this way, it is very important that the second part of the two-part

physical be scheduled within the next week or two. Do not wait for more than 2 weeks, or else the patient might have many new issues to discuss—and this will make the brief 15- or 20-minute individual office visit too short to complete the private physical examination. The two-part physical is a way of seeing patients promptly for physical examinations when: (1) backlogs to physical exist on the physician's schedule; (2) the physician does run a DIGMA; and (3) when the physician is not running a Physicals SMA (which would otherwise be the preferable option because of its greater efficiency benefits). Two-part physicals can also be used to backfill DIGMA sessions that are not yet full.

However, it is important to note that two-part physicals in the DIGMA model are not nearly as efficient in delivering complete physical examinations as is the Physicals SMA model (see Chapter 5). Whereas physicians can typically only be twice as productive in delivering physical examinations with two-part physicals in DIGMAs, they can often be three or more times as efficient in providing physical exams with the PSMA model.

DIGMAs and PSMAs Are Often a Better Choice than Traditional Office Visits

Anxiety, depression, and significant psychosocial issues are frequently comorbid with having health problems, especially serious chronic conditions. Patients with extensive emotional and psychosocial issues (such as depression, anxiety, loneliness, lack of social support, etc.), who would benefit from the help and support of the behaviorist and other patients, are often ideal candidates for DIGMAs and Physical SMAs. Similarly, patients whose medical condition is affecting their ability to function socially, at work, or at home often benefit from group visits. Likewise, certain types of patients that physicians might find somewhat difficult to treat in traditional individual office visits—such as chronic pain, headache, fibromyalgia, irritable bowel, etc.—often do quite well in a DIGMA. High utilizers and low utilizers alike, along with the *worried well* and patients requiring some additional professional handholding, are often ideal candidates for SMAs (see Table 10.5 for various types of patients who are often best handled through DIGMA and PSMA visits).

Sometimes Individual Office Visits Are Best

Individual office visits are generally best for certain types of patients and situations, such as the following: monolingual

Table 10.5 DIGMAs and PSMAs work exceptionally well for many types of patients

- Patients needing routine follow-up care (DIGMA) or a physical examination (PSMA)
- Physical examinations for established or new patients (PSMAs)
- Relatively stable chronically ill patients
- Most patients telephoning the office for a return visit or physical exam
- Newly diagnosed patients needing information and emotional support
- Patients starting a new medication or treatment who need closer follow-up care
- Medication and laboratory test re-check visits
- The worried well
- Non-compliant patients
- Low and high utilizers alike
- Underserved patients currently "falling between the cracks"
- Homeless, economically disadvantaged, uninsured, or street-involved patients
- Patients with high *no-show* and *late-cancel* rates
- The anxious, depressed, lonely, and psychologically needy
- Difficult, angry, distrustful, demanding, and time-consuming patients
- Patients with extensive informational and psychosocial needs
- Medical patients less able to function at home, at work, or socially
- Patients for whom the physician keeps repeating the same information
- Patients needing a lot of professional handholding
- Patients who feel alone, isolated, or "woe is me"
- Patient telephone calls that can be handled through the DIGMA
- Patients the physician wants to follow more closely
- Patients preferring DIGMAs and PSMAs to individual visits
- Any patients the physician prefers to see in the group visit format

patients who do not speak the language that the DIGMA or PSMA is being conducted in; patients too demented or hearing impaired to benefit (although their support persons and caregivers certainly could); patients with serious acute infectious illnesses that are highly contagious (such as tuberculosis, bird flu, and severe acute respiratory syndrome or SARS, although some healthcare systems do run seasonal cold and flu DIGMAs); rapidly evolving medical conditions requiring emergency care; most complex medical procedures (although some simple procedures such as trigger point injections and nitrogen freezes in dermatology can be conducted in SMAs); palliative care in podiatry (i.e., corns, calluses, and toenails, which are usually better handled through individual office visits); patients the provider prefers to see individually; and patients who are inappropriate for a group visit (such as those unwilling to agree to confidentiality, which seldom if ever happens in practice, or refuse to attend voluntarily).

Step 12: Select Your Initial SMA Providers with Care

For your pilot study (as well as for the *early adopter* physicians that you choose to launch your group visits with soon thereafter), you will want to be especially careful about how you select these providers—as it is in the initial phases of launching DIGMAs and Physicals SMAs that the program is most fragile and vulnerable to failure. Because it is imperative that you select your initial group visit providers with great care, this section is dedicated to examining different possible selection strategies for choosing your initial providers —and to different ways that you can successfully launch your group visit program.

Choose Busy, Backlogged Physicians Respected by Their Peers

Although it is most common to select motivated and interested physicians for the pilot study, it is best if they are well respected by colleagues and have busy, backlogged practices. In addition, there are other physician selection strategies that can be employed for your pilot study, such as selecting physicians having intermediate or even high risk of failure—because these are often the physicians with whom other physicians can identify.

Obviously, before a physician can be selected for the SMA program, they must first be successfully recruited—which requires that their concerns first be addressed and that the many physician benefits that SMAs offer be fully explained (see Chapter 6). This will take some time and the right type of approach, as many physicians feel overwhelmed by the amount of change they have already sustained and are still undergoing.

While It Is Common to Select Motivated Physicians Who Volunteer, There Are Potential Pitfalls

The champion must at all times court, select, and recruit physicians for the group visit program with care—especially in the early stages of developing the DIGMA and Physicals SMA program, as this is when the group visit program is most vulnerable. The normal approach that most medical groups take in establishing their pilot study is the *low-hanging fruit* approach—which typically is to select 1–4 motivated physicians that are willing to step forward and start a SMA for their practice, and then use them as the candidates for their pilot. While this approach can be successfully employed (and is admittedly the simplest and easiest approach to take), it suffers from three potential shortcomings that you must be careful to avoid.

First, if these pilot physicians are seen as being extroverted, gregarious, comfortable in groups, and extremely gifted in their interpersonal skills, it will likely do little to convince other physicians to also try a DIGMA or PSMA for their practices even if they are successful—as others will likely not perceive themselves as possessing these attributes. Simply put, they will not identify with such pilot physicians and will probably hold the view: "Of course it worked for them because they're that type of person, but it won't work for me!"

Second, if the pilot physicians are not highly respected by their peers—but rather are seen as being *kooky, on the fringe*, or *into every new thing that comes along*—then they could actually be a detriment to the overall long-term success of the program. This is because, even if they did prove to be successful with their group visit programs, the success of such providers would be unlikely to motivate their *mainstream* physician colleagues to also try a SMA for their own practices.

Third, if these initial physicians do not have large and busy practices, do not have backlogs or access problems, or do not work full time (or worse yet, only work half-time or less), then they will potentially have fewer patients to recruit into their DIGMAs and PSMAs—and will therefore be at high risk for failure. It is important that all pilot physicians and early adopters have full and busy practices—and preferably be full-time and have seriously backlogged practices. I say this because these busy, backlogged, full-time physicians will have the most patients to recruit into their sessions, and therefore the easiest time in filling their DIGMA and PSMA sessions—and in consistently meeting their census targets, which is the most important key to a successful SMA.

Preferred Strategy for Selecting Physicians for the SMA Pilot Study

My preferred strategy for selecting initial SMA physicians, especially for the pilot study, has been to begin two to four (most commonly three) DIGMAs and/or Physicals SMAs at approximately the same time. Depending on the organization's precise needs, I will often start the pilot by selecting three physicians: one physician from internal medicine; another from family

practice (or a nurse practitioner, osteopath, etc.); and a third provider from one of the medical or surgical subspecialties. The exact mix of primary and specialty care providers would depend both upon which providers are motivated to run a SMA and upon the organization's needs, goals, and resources. It would be best for all three pilot physicians to be well established, busy, full-time providers who are respected by their peers and have both backlogs and access problems to their practices. This will ensure that there will be many patients in their practices to draw from in order to fill all group sessions—so that their SMAs will therefore have a high probability of success.

In my preferred strategy, at least one of the pilot physicians (and often two) should have a high likelihood of success—i.e., be a *low-risk* provider because of the personality, motivation, skill set, and commitment of that physician. Another pilot SMA would typically be selected to have an intermediate likelihood of success—i.e., it would be run by an *intermediate-risk* provider who is somewhat skeptical and possesses a balance between positive and negative attributes.

This is typically a physician who is respected by peers and, while being somewhat hesitant and skeptical, is nonetheless willing to try a DIGMA or Physicals SMA and give it his/her *best shot*. This is the type of physician that other physicians on staff will likely be able to identify with, and possibly even be swayed by, so that they become more willing to also try a SMA for their own practice— that is, in the event that this physician proves to be successful and actually enjoys the SMA. It is, however, very important that all pilot physicians clearly agree to perform the all-important task of inviting all appropriate patients seen during regular individual office visits to have their next follow-up appointment be in the provider's DIGMA (or their next physical examination be in the provider's PSMA)—i.e., so as to ensure consistently full sessions.

When intermediate risk physicians succeed with their DIGMAs and/or Physicals SMAs despite having initial concerns, resistances, and skepticism (especially when they are not seen as being particularly outgoing and comfortable in groups), then their physician colleagues will likely see them as being much like themselves. Therefore, when such intermediate-risk physicians prove to be successful with their group visit programs, especially when they grow to truly enjoy and enthusiastically endorse them, then their reticent physician colleagues are likely to take note and be more willing to also try one for themselves. It is then highly likely that some of these initially reluctant colleagues will gradually be won over and ultimately be willing to also try a SMA for their own practices.

Occasionally Select High-Risk Providers, but Then Do Everything Possible to Ensure Success

The third pilot could also be one of the above two types of providers—i.e., low or intermediate risk. However, on rare occasions, the champion might prefer that the third pilot physician be one that could best be characterized as *high risk*. In the latter case, the physician selected would either have a significant resistance to the SMA program or there would be a perceived mismatch between the program and the physician's personality and practice style. This latter strategy of choosing a high-risk pilot physician, while risky because of the relatively high likelihood of failure, can enable a SMA program to be rapidly advanced throughout a facility with maximum speed if it succeeds. However, while I have done this a couple of times in order to advance a group visit program more rapidly than would otherwise have been possible, I must admit that I more frequently start with all pilot physicians being in the first two categories (i.e., of low or intermediate risk).

Pluses and Minuses to Selecting High-Risk Physicians for the SMA Pilot

The high-risk physician is the one who, while often very busy and respected by colleagues, is frequently seen as the *impossible* physician. This is the type of physician perceived by colleagues as being the least likely to want to run a DIGMA or Physicals SMA for their practice, and highly unlikely to succeed even if they did try to run one. Physician colleagues might hold this view for a variety of reasons, such as this *high-risk* physician's: (1) personality and practice style; (2) sincere lack of interest in starting a SMA, despite possibly having a severe workload and access problems; (3) strong resistance to innovation and change; (4) disinterest in dealing with patients' psychosocial and behavioral health issues; (5) problematic communication style with patients and staff; and (6) colleagues simply not being able, for whatever reason, to envision this particular physician as being able to run a successful group medical appointment for his or her practice.

On rare occasions in the past, I have been privileged to set up DIGMAs with such high-risk physicians—often because I was strongly encouraged to do so by administration due to the heavy workload burden being shouldered by such a physician. While this approach is more difficult at first, when high-risk DIGMAs and PSMAs do in fact succeed, they have often proven in the long run to be the most rewarding SMAs of all. However, it is important to add that when I have employed this high-risk strategy, I personally do everything humanly possible to ensure the success of this high-risk SMA. This is because,

when it does succeed, it is an extremely effective catalyst to the rapid dissemination of the DIGMA and PSMA program throughout the organization.

Obviously, convincing such an unmotivated physician to actually try a SMA can be a difficult, time-consuming, and challenging job for the champion—and will undoubtedly require on-going effort and a *full-court press*. One such physician, who eventually grew to embrace his DIGMA, later said that the only reason he ever started his DIGMA was because "It was just too difficult to say 'No' to Dr. Noffsinger. It seemed like everywhere I went, he was also there preaching the value of group visits and telling me that I should start one for my practice. In the end, I found myself agreeing to do one—not because I wanted to, but just because it was easier than constantly having to say 'No' to him. Now, I'm glad that I did because I have found that there is a lot of benefit to the process."

The caveat here is that every effort must be made to ensure that such a high-risk SMA is in fact successful, because it is at high risk to fail. I would like to add that this approach requires a skilled champion and behaviorist and is best done when there is administrative support, an excellent champion (and program coordinator to assist the champion), and a trained and skilled SMA treatment team available to help this physician.

Can DIGMAs and PSMAs Improve a Physician's Patient Satisfaction Scores?

Past success with physicians perceived by colleagues as *impossible* (or very unlikely to be interested in, or successful with, a DIGMA or Physicals SMA) leads me to the following hypothesis—one that is based upon personal experience, but remains untested to date. It is the author's belief that, when properly run, DIGMAs and PSMAs might someday be tried in an entirely new application: as a benign but effective training tool for improving the low patient satisfaction scores of physicians with poor communication skills. Because a behaviorist is involved in DIGMAs and PSMAs, these two group visit models should be extremely effective and helpful in improving a physician's communication skills—an approach that could be employed without embarrassing the physician or requiring attendance in some sort of remedial training program for improving patient–physician communications.

It seems that this positive result of improved patient satisfaction scores could be achieved effectively with DIGMAs and PSMAs by simply pairing such low-scoring physicians with a behaviorist specifically selected because of his or her exceptional communication skills. Because such a behaviorist could consistently model effective communication techniques throughout the SMA setting and week after week, the communication skills of such low-scoring physicians would likely gradually improve over time—at least this is what I have personally witnessed. This improved ability to communicate occurs almost by osmosis as the physician observes the behaviorist's communication style and means of interacting with patients session after session—and without the concomitant physician embarrassment and resentment that could occur through forced attendance in some sort of remedial training program designed to enhance patient–physician communications. If you consider such an application of SMAs in your healthcare delivery system, I would appreciate hearing from you about your results.

Step 13: Carefully Select and Train the Behaviorist

The role of the behaviorist is critically important in the DIGMA and PSMA models, yet is one that many healthcare organizations pay scant attention to. For this reason, the best available behaviorist—and not the cheapest or most readily available—should be selected based upon skill set, professional experience, scope of practice under licensure, and being well matched to both the physician and the patients. The behaviorist's skills are meant to complement (i.e., not be the same as) those of the physician. The behaviorist and the nurse(s)—both of whom have dramatically expanded roles and responsibilities in the DIGMA and PSMA settings—free the physician up to concentrate on providing those services that the physician alone can provide. The same is true of the documenter.

Healthcare organizations often risk having the wrong behaviorist for the job because they insist on using only readily available or inexpensive personnel in this role, which is a common beginners' mistake. Some systems make an even greater mistake by expecting a provider to run a DIGMA or PSMA alone, i.e., without any behaviorist whatsoever. DIGMAs and PSMAs provide a multidisciplinary team-based approach to care. Consequently, they are not intended to be run by the physician alone. In addition, the behaviorist plays a critically important role in achieving full benefit from DIGMA and PSMA programs. A poor choice as behaviorist (or, worse yet, no behaviorist at all) would greatly reduce both the productivity and the quality of the SMA because the physician could neither delegate nor provide the efficiency and quality benefits that an effective behaviorist can help provide to such a large number of patients in the group setting.

It is true that some nominally increased productivity benefits could still be achieved for physicians willing to deliver care alone in the group setting due to certain efficiency benefits inherent in the group process itself—e.g., the help and support of other patients, a reduced need to repeat information to patients individually, and the ability to overbook sessions according to the expected number of no-shows and late-cancels. Nevertheless, this approach would not begin to match the remarkable efficiency gains that can be achieved by properly run DIGMAs or PSMAs—which represent a major paradigm shift to a multidisciplinary team-based approach to care in which as many physician responsibilities as appropriate and possible are delegated and off-loaded onto less costly personnel with complementary skill sets.

The Behaviorist's Role in a DIGMA or PSMA Is Quite Different from that in a Mental Health Group

The behaviorist's role in a DIGMA or PSMA is dramatically different from both the relatively passive role taken in traditional mental health groups and the more active educator role assumed in cognitive behavioral depression and anxiety programs. First and foremost, the behaviorist's role in a SMA is one of supporting and helping the physician in every possible way—a subordinate role that can be a difficult adjustment for some mental health professionals to make, especially those who are doctoral level and used to being the "doctor" in running their own therapy groups with considerable autonomy. The behaviorist must therefore be selected with great care, as it is known that many mental health professionals are not able to make the transition to primary and specialty care and that the fit here is not always a good one.

Behaviorists Are Often More Directive and Self Disclosing in SMAs

Behaviorists are often more directive and self-disclosing in DIGMAs and PSMAs than in traditional mental health groups. There is no "Uh-huh, uh-huh. And how does that make you feel?" in a DIGMA or Physicals SMA. Here, the behaviorist plays a much more active and structured role by warming the group up, giving the introduction at the beginning of the session, assisting the physician in every possible way, actively managing group dynamic and psychosocial issues, distributing handouts selected by the physician, taking over the group when the physician documents chart notes or steps out of the group room, pacing the group so as to finish on time, and staying after to clear and clean the group room up.

When I have occupied the role of behaviorist, I found that it was often very effective for me to be much more self-disclosing of my own health problems than I ever would have been during a psychotherapy group or behavioral medicine program. Of course this needed to be done with tact, and always with the intent of benefiting the patients rather than myself. Patients generally responded very positively to this, which was important because, unlike the physician, the patients did not know me. Such disclosure tended to help patients more quickly bond with me as they recognized that, while I may not have struggled with the exact same health problems that they have, I nonetheless dealt with enough such health issues that I could understand and appreciate what they are going through. In general, I found that anything that helped to develop a relationship of trust and understanding, and which enabled patients to more quickly bond with me, was helpful.

The Behaviorist Must Be Well Matched to Both the Physician and the Patients

The selection of behaviorist must be a good match to both the physician and the group. A mistake here could be costly as a poor choice could ultimately result in the failure of the group—or it could require the champion to later need to train another behaviorist to replace the original, inappropriate choice once the physician became frustrated enough. The last thing you will want is to have the DIGMA or PSMA unravel because the behaviorist quits or is asked to leave by the physician.

The Behaviorist Has Many Different Responsibilities in a DIGMA or PSMA

DIGMAs and PSMAs are led by the physician with the assistance of a behavioral health professional, such as a health psychologist or social worker experienced in running groups and in working closely with physicians and medically ill patients (as well as their families). The behaviorist has many responsibilities in the DIGMA and PSMA settings, including arriving early and warming the group up by fostering some group interaction; helping patients to focus upon what they want from the physician that day; writing patients' medical concerns down on a whiteboard or flipchart just prior to the session; starting the group on time with an introduction (even if the physician has not yet arrived); identifying and responding to

group dynamic and psychosocial issues; providing behavioral health evaluations and interventions; referring patients to appropriate internal and external resources; handling any psychiatric emergencies that might occur (which rarely happens); helping the physician to deal with patients who are difficult, drug seeking, dissatisfied with medical care, hostile, depressed, distrustful, or anxious; keeping the SMA running smoothly and on time; briefly taking over the group when the physician documents chart notes or steps out of the group room; staying late to address any last-minute questions that patients might have (i.e., that are within the behaviorist's scope of practice); and finally straightening the group room up after the session.

The behaviorist must both establish a supportive collegial relationship with the physician and assist the physician in every way possible. The behaviorist also takes over leading the group (focusing on behavioral health and psychosocial issues of mutual interest to the patients in attendance) when the physician writes the chart note after completing working with each patient in the SMA (Fig. 10.2). In addition, the behaviorist temporarily takes over the group when the physician arrives late, steps out to handle an urgent clinic manner, conducts a brief private medical examination or discussion in the exam room (usually toward the end of the session), or is otherwise temporarily absent. The multiple specific responsibilities of the behaviorist are detailed in Table 10.6. As can be seen, the behaviorist's role in a well-run DIGMA or PSMA differs greatly from the behaviorist's role in a typical mental health group in that it is a more active, structured, and self-disclosing role.

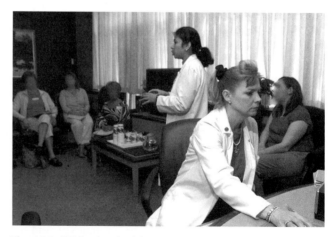

Fig. 10.2 While the physician writes the chart note after working with each patient, the behaviorist temporarily leads the group, focusing on behavioral health and psychosocial issues
(Courtesy of Dr. Holly Thacker, Women's Health Physicals SMA, Cleveland Clinic, Cleveland, OH)

Table 10.6 The behaviorist has many different responsibilities in a DIGMA or PSMA

- The behaviorist's role in a DIGMA or PSMA differs greatly from a typical mental health role in that it is a much more active, structured, and self-disclosing role
- Arrive approximately 15 minutes early to each session
  - Warm group up by fostering some group interaction
  - Write each patient's current medical needs down next to patient's name on a flip chart or whiteboard
- Start on time by giving the "introduction" at the beginning of every DIGMA and PSMA session
  - Numerous different points are covered in the behaviorist's highly structured introduction (see Table 10.7)
  - This saves the physician time and allows the provider to arrive a couple minutes late
- Manage group dynamic, psychosocial, and behavioral health issues—plus foster some group interaction
- Assist physician in dealing with difficult, demanding, hostile, and distrusting patients
- Handle any psychiatric emergencies (which rarely occur)
- Assist in keeping DIGMA running smoothly and on time
- Do everything possible to assist provider
- Temporarily take over running the group while the physician completes each chart note
- Temporarily runs the group alone when the provider steps out of the group room for brief private exams and discussions—or to handle a clinic emergency
- Stays late to clear room and answer any last-minute patient questions
- Straighten the room up afterward and set it up for the next SMA

The Behaviorist's Multiple Responsibilities Enable the Physician to Focus on Providing Personalized Medical Care

This arrangement enables physicians to focus on delivering quality medical care instead of worrying about group dynamic and psychosocial issues that require special expertise. It off-loads many duties from the physician onto the behaviorist and augments the physician's skills in dealing with behavioral health, emotional, and psychosocial issues (such as diagnosing depression or anxiety-related conditions)—issues which often go under-diagnosed and under-treated in primary and specialty care settings. The presence of the behaviorist also relieves many physician anxieties around dealing with patients' psychosocial issues, making embarrassing mistakes in the group setting, or losing control of the group and having it spiral negatively out of control. When physicians enter the DIGMA setting for the first time and see some 15 or 20 sets of eyes staring back at them, this can be an unnerving and disconcerting experience—at least for physicians who do not have a great deal of group experience. Fortunately, these concerns can be ameliorated considerably if the physician has full confidence in the professional skills and abilities of the behaviorist in handling any such problems that might emerge with regard to group dynamic and psychosocial issues.

The Behaviorist Must Use Tact When Addressing Psychosocial Issues in the Group

The behaviorist will sometimes address psychosocial issues in the DIGMA or PSMA and will also recommend internal and external resources such as stop smoking programs, community support groups, cognitive behavioral treatment programs for anxiety and depression, etc. In so doing, the behaviorist must use great tact when addressing depression, anxiety, substance abuse, etc. in the group setting—keeping in mind that this is the physician's practice and these patients have come in for a medical visit (i.e., not for a psychiatric consultation). Never point to a patient and surprise or blindside them by accusingly saying words to the effect that, "You're depressed" or "It sounds as if you're an alcoholic." Nonetheless, by both being extremely tactful and developing a close working relationship with the physician, the behaviorist can develop signals for alerting the physician to patients' emotional and psychosocial issues—and even carefully enter into brief discussions with patients regarding these issues.

However, since there is limited time and this is not the primary purpose of a SMA, the goal is typically not necessarily to treat these conditions in the DIGMA or PSMA group setting (although the physician might choose to start them on a trial of psychotropic medication), but rather to triage them into appropriate internal and external treatment resources. However, when it is the behaviorist that makes such referrals, it is important to resist any temptation to refer patients into one's own practice and treatment programs if there is any chance that this could be perceived by patients as being self-serving. In this way, the behaviorist can tactfully bring psychosocial issues to the attention of patients, alert the physician to them, and even refer the patient when appropriate (but only when this is what the physician wants)—all of which enables the behaviorist to play an important role in addressing the behavioral health and psychosocial issues that drive such a large percentage of all office visits.

Psychologists and Social Workers Are Often Preferred in DIGMAs, but Others Are Sometimes Used

An important part of the behaviorist's job in DIGMA and PSMA settings is managing group dynamics, addressing psychosocial issues, pacing the group, fostering group interaction, and diagnosing depression and anxiety—responsibilities that best fit the scope of practice of experienced and skilled mental health professionals such as psychologists and social workers. However, it is also important to note that many mental health professionals will not transition well into primary or specialty care—or to DIGMAs and PSMAs for that matter. Therefore, it is important to carefully select behaviorists who enjoy working in primary and specialty care, have experience in managing large groups, are empathetic toward medical patients and their families, understand the psychosocial concomitants of illness, and are able to work closely and cooperatively with physicians and other healthcare providers. It is important for mental health behaviorists to have considerable group experience, to enjoy working with medical (and not just mental health) patients, and to understand the differences between the behaviorist role in DIGMAs and PSMAs versus traditional mental health groups.

In fact, it is extremely important that behaviorists thoroughly understand the DIGMA and PSMA models, their role in it, and the importance of staying focused and succinct in their interactions throughout—and to always focus upon leveraging the physician's time. This means that, when temporarily taking over the group while the physician is completing a chart note, to promptly end this discussion and relinquish the floor to the physician as soon as the physician has completed the chart note—i.e., so that the physician can then promptly move on to working with the next patient in the group setting.

Nurses, diabetic nurse educators, nurse practitioners, marriage and family therapists, counselors, Pharm. Ds.., PAs, and others have also sometimes been used successfully as behaviorists. In addition, health educators and nutritionists have also occasionally been used when they are the best resource available because they are familiar with running classes and presenting educational material. However, because they are often more used to giving lectures and running classes, they will likely need some additional training in order to handle some of the behaviorist's responsibilities in the DIGMA setting—such as fostering group interaction, managing group dynamics, addressing psychosocial and behavioral health issues, helping to diagnose depression and anxiety, etc.

While a psychologist or social worker with much experience in conducting groups and working with medical patients is often the preferred choice as behaviorist in a DIGMA, a nurse, nurse practitioner, or diabetic nurse educator is often the preferred choice as behaviorist in a PSMA. However, in order to keep costs down for the SMA program, be certain that if you do use nurse practitioners in this role, their overhead expense to the SMA program is calculated based on their hourly wage—and not upon the revenues that they themselves could have generated during 90 minutes of clinic time if they would have instead been seeing patients individually (which would place an onerous overhead burden upon the SMA program). Be prepared to provide the additional training that might be required in order for this person to effectively and efficiently dispatch the multiple responsibilities that the behaviorist has in the SMA setting.

Points to Cover in the Behaviorist's Introduction

Here, the reader is encouraged to watch the behaviorist training segment of the DVD attached to this book. Because different patients typically attend each DIGMA or PSMA session, several of whom will be attending for the first time, the behaviorist needs to start each and every DIGMA session on time with a brief but thorough introduction that lasts no more than 3–5 minutes. This arrangement also partially covers for the physician, who often enters the group session a few minutes late due to running late in the clinic. The major talking points for the behaviorist's introduction are presented in Table 10.7; however, these points must be covered in the behaviorist's own words and in a manner that feels comfortable to her/him. Personally, when I am a behaviorist, I usually divide the introductions that I give into 4 major segments: 1) the *welcome and WIFFM* (what's in it for me) part; 2) the *what to expect* segment; 3) the *confidentiality* portion; and 4) the *personal comfort* segment.

If the physician also wants the patients to briefly introduce themselves at the beginning of the SMA, then they should each be strictly limited to approximately 30–45 seconds apiece—and be asked to focus upon what health problems they are currently experiencing and specifically what they would like from the doctor today. Usually, I do not recommend that patients introduce themselves at the beginning of the session due to the fact that patients often ramble and do not want to be hurried in their introduction—a process that can therefore take too much time out of the group, and ultimately result in less time for medical care to be delivered (plus fewer patients being seen). Even if the all patients are brief in their personal introductions (which certainly cannot be counted on), this could easily take up as much as ten minutes of the 90-minute group—which represents a major loss of time(which translates into smaller groups and reduced productivity). Instead, what I generally recommend is that the physician (i.e., when this might be helpful to the group,

Table 10.7 Points to be addressed in the behaviorist's introduction

- Welcome all patients in attendance (state it's only for Dr. _____'s patients)
- Behaviorist quickly introduces self, nurse/MA(s), documenter, and any other staff present—and their roles
- Ask that all pagers and cell phones be turned off
- Explain why MD started the DIGMA (in terms of benefits to patients)
  - Too long a wait for patients to be seen
  - Patients feel office visits are too rushed
  - Meet others dealing with similar issues
- Give a brief description of the DIGMA
  - Extended medical appointment
  - Meets weekly for 90 minutes
  - Patients are to attend only as needed, not weekly
  - If patients later choose to *drop-in* to a DIGMA, they should phone the office at least a day in advance to inform staff that they will be coming and to check that the session is going to be held
- Describe a few key intended benefits to patients
  - Prompt access
  - More time with MD
  - Mind–Body care and max-packed visits
  - Closer follow-up care
  - Help and support from other patients
  - Greater patient education
  - Get answers to questions you might not have thought to ask
- Tell patients what to expect during today's session
  - Tell patients that MD will be going around the room and addressing each patients medical needs individually
  - Ask patients to promptly indicate, as soon as the MD focuses upon them, what the 1–3 most important issues are that they want the doctor to address today
  - Encourage patients to actively participate during the session, including sharing any helpful ideas or relevant personal experiences they might have
  - Mention that the nurse/MA will be calling patients out for vital signs, injections, health maintenance updates, and other special duties
  - State that the behaviorist will act as timekeeper to ensure that all can have their needs met and so that the session finishes on time (emphasize that MD has other patients to see in clinic after session ends)
  - State last 5–10 minutes of session will be reserved for brief private exams and discussions (emphasize brief)
  - Tell patients they will be asked to complete a patient satisfaction survey before leaving
- Describe medical services MD will provide
  - Most of the same medical services will be provided as in regular office visits
  - Questions will be answered and medical concerns addressed
  - Prescriptions will be changed or refilled
  - Tests, procedures, and referrals will be ordered and results discussed
  - Many exams will be conducted in group with patients' permission
  - Brief private exams and discussions will be provided by MD as needed toward end of session
- Make clear that private time with the physician will always be made available to any patient requesting it (for brief private discussions or exams requiring disrobing)
- Tell patients that they can still have traditional individual office visits with their doctor as before
- Cover personal comfort issues
  - Location of rest rooms
  - Feel free to stand up, stretch, or move around if uncomfortable
  - Discuss where coffee, soft drinks, and/or snacks are located—and that patients are free to go over and get a snack at any point during the session
- Emphasize the need for confidentiality both inside and outside of the group
  - Discuss limits of confidentiality in group
  - All present must sign a confidentiality release at every DIGMA or PSMA session (check to make certain that all have signed the release and, if not, promptly have them do so)
  - Your medical care will be discussed and delivered in the group setting—and that must be OK with you
  - If any patients are uncomfortable with their medical issues being discussed in front of others, then they will need to reschedule an individual visit instead of attending the group
  - Patients must agree not to reveal other patients' identities outside of group—directly or indirectly
  - Patients must agree to not discuss other people's health problems outside of the session
  - You can leave at any time without any penalty whatsoever should you feel uncomfortable in the group

Table 10.7 (continued)

- Invite patients to return to the DIGMA whenever they have a future medical need. Explain that they can just drop in; however, they need to call a day ahead so that:
    - Charts can be ordered (for systems not yet on EMR)
    - Staff knows they are coming and can prepare for them
    - Patients can check to see if the DIGMA will be meeting that day
    - Staff will call pre-registered patients if the DIGMA is cancelled at the last minute (e.g., if MD is ill)
- For some DIGMAs, ask at the end of the introduction (but only if the physician wants it asked): "Who needs to leave early?"
- Then have the nurse/MA(s) next take those patients next who must leave early, but have not yet had their vitals taken and other nursing duties performed
- Physician then enters group room, briefly says "Hello", welcomes patients, and starts the session—perhaps by calling for a volunteer, preferably someone who needs to leave early and has had vital signs already taken. Or else, the physician might instead start with a patient accompanied by a child, having cold or flu symptoms, or that the physician knows and feels comfortable with

but only with the patient's permission) give a brief, perhaps 10-20 second, introduction on each patient in turn when beginning to work with that patient in the group setting.

Step 14: Select the Best Possible Treatment Team for Each SMA

In addition to the champion and program coordinator in larger systems, every DIGMA and PSMA should have a behaviorist, one or two nursing personnel, a documenter (whenever possible), and a dedicated scheduler attached to the program. For full benefit, select the best personnel for SMA teams and train them well. If it requires spending a few extra dollars to get the right individuals for these jobs, then it is important to spend that money—even if it requires raising the target census level slightly in order to include an additional patient or two during SMA sessions to pay for this additional overhead expense.

Not only must all members of the SMA team be the right people and well trained for their specific responsibilities in the DIGMA or PSMA program, but they must also be provided with sufficient time dedicated to the program each week to appropriately discharge their duties. Because we have just discussed the importance of selecting the best possible behaviorist, and because the roles of the champion and program coordinator have already been discussed earlier in this chapter, let us take a closer look at the other personnel associated with the DIGMA or PSMA: the provider's support staff; the nursing personnel; the documenter and the dedicated scheduler. In addition, let us look at a telephone script and talking points that schedulers can use when scheduling patients into a DIGMA or PSMA.

Consider the Provider's Own Support Staff as Part of the Team

In addition to the SMA team itself, the physician's scheduling and reception staff should also be properly trained

and actively involved in promoting the program to patients—and in scheduling as many appropriate patients as possible into future SMA sessions. Clearly, the provider's entire scheduling staff must be willing to explain the DIGMA and/or PSMA program to all appropriate patients, to invite them to attend, and to promptly pre-schedule any patients who accept this invitation and indicate that they are willing to attend a future SMA session. Simply put, it is the scheduling piece that is the most important component to the success of any well-run DIGMA or PSMA program—i.e., by achieving SMA sessions that are consistently filled to targeted census levels.

Receptionists also need to be trained—i.e., to give invitations to all appropriate patients as they register for regular office visits, to ask patients to read it while waiting in the lobby, to say some well chosen and positive words about the SMA program, and to encourage patients to attend a future DIGMA or PSMA session the next time that they have a medical need to be seen. The reception staff also needs to hand out invitations to all appropriate patients as they register for traditional office visits, and how to be trained in how to register patients into the DIGMA or PSMA—efficiently registering the large number of attendees, distributing the Patient Packets, filling in name tags with a fat felt marker, distributing confidentiality releases and collecting them (after they are signed by both the patient and any support person accompanying him/her), directing patients as to where to go next, etc. It is important for the provider's own scheduling and reception staff to have an opportunity to sit in on a DIGMA or PSMA session (perhaps one or two at a time) so that they can witness first-hand what a warm, pleasant, informative, and helpful service it truly is for patients—and thus be better able to explain and *sell* the program to all suitable patients thereafter. All of these personnel (the SMA team as well as the provider's support staff) play important roles in achieving full benefit from the DIGMA or PSMA and are therefore vital to the overall success of the program.

The Nursing Personnel Are Critically Important to the SMA's Success

The nursing role in a DIGMA or Physicals SMA is typically quite expanded—i.e., beyond typical nursing duties that are conducted during traditional individual office visits in an outpatient ambulatory care setting. The expanded roles of the 1–2 nurses/MAs/nursing techs attached to properly run DIGMAs and PSMAs enable many of the quality, outcome, and productivity goals of the SMA program to be achieved. This includes max-packing visits, providing patients with a comprehensive *one-stop shopping* healthcare experience, taking expanded vital signs, bringing performance measures and routine health maintenance current, updating injections, and performing any *special* nursing duties requested by the physician.

In addition to the myriad of nursing duties conducted during a DIGMA or PSMA, an important nursing function also occurs outside of the SMA session, in between sessions, while the provider's nursing personnel are rooming appropriate patients into exam rooms during regular individual office visits. Here, while rooming patients, the nurse/MA: (1) says a few positive words about the DIGMA or PSMA to inform all suitable patients about the program and encourage them to attend; (2) gives all appropriate patients a program description flier to read while waiting for the doctor to enter the exam room; and (3) invites them to attend the next time they have a medical need and wish to be seen.

For systems still using paper charts, bringing performance measures and health maintenance current involves the nurse/MA(s): (1) searching the medical chart for routine health maintenance due on each patient (colonoscopy, mammogram, PSA, pap smear, etc.); (2) pulling the appropriate referral and/or screening test forms, and then completing the patient information section on each; (3) attaching these partially completed forms onto the front cover of the medical chart, along with the partially completed DIGMA progress note depicting all nursing duties and vitals that have been performed; and then (4) placing the paper medical chart plus forms onto the table located between the physician and behaviorist when escorting the patient back into the group room. For systems using electronic medical records (EMR), the nurse would enter all such information into each patient's EMR chart note for the DIGMA or PSMA.

The nurse/MA might even keep a *crash cart* supplied with all necessary forms, handouts, supplies, and medical equipment for the DIGMA or PSMA—a cart that can then easily be wheeled into the group room at the beginning of each SMA session, and then back again once the session is over. Nursing personnel can also collect signed confidentiality waivers and assist in documenting (by entering vital signs taken, injections provided, and special duties performed; by listing reasons for today's visit as well as allergies to medications; by reviewing personal health history and updating medications, etc.). While some of these SMA nursing duties are normally performed during routine office visits, others are specific to the expanded nursing role in the SMA. The goal of every DIGMA and PSMA is to fully expand these nursing duties to be all that they can be in order to maximally benefit our patients and leverage the physician's time. All of these expanded nursing duties will then greatly assist in enabling the DIGMA or PSMA to achieve its stated goals of enhancing quality, max-packing visits, and optimizing physician productivity.

When Possible, It Is Generally Recommended to Have Two Nurses Rather than One

Having two nursing personnel, such as a medical assistant and a nurse, in DIGMAs and PSMAs is often a good idea (provided that this resource is available) because it allows all nursing responsibilities to be completed in half the time and enables the nurse/MA(s) to divide their expanded duties up between themselves according to experience, skill set, and scope of practice under licensure. In addition, by working with a colleague, the nurse/MA(s) tend to enjoy the SMA experience more and have more fun. However, they must be specifically trained to handle the increased patient volume and expanded responsibilities that occur in this setting. Be careful to select nurse/MA(s) for the SMA who are positive, engaging, motivated, willing to work hard, and welcome the added workload and responsibility that the DIGMA or PSMA involves—preferably those who see it as an opportunity to gain experience, showcase their professional skills, and develop professionally.

Maximizing the Nursing Role Increases the Physician's Productivity

The vast majority of nursing personnel do in fact welcome these added duties, which not only help to maximize the physician's productivity and efficiency but also help to enhance the pleasantness and quality of the SMA experience for nurses and patients alike. This is because the expanded nursing role in the SMA provides an antidote to the boredom that many nurses/MA(s) experience in outpatient ambulatory care settings as a result of repeatedly performing the same limited number of functions—e.g., rooming patients and taking a limited number of vital signs all day long. This expanded nursing role permits an off-loading onto the nurse/MAs of many responsibilities that might otherwise have had to be performed by the physician. Because the physician is thereby freed up to provide only those services which the physician alone can do, more patients are able to be seen—thereby both increasing the SMA's efficiency and enabling the nurse/MA(s) to recognize that they have played an important role in the overall success of the SMA.

Having a Documenter Increases Productivity and Aligns the Physician's Priorities with Administration's

Although optional, it is highly recommended to have a documenter because this will: (1) greatly increase the provider's productivity and efficiency during the DIGMA or PSMA; (2) produce a superior chart note due to its being both comprehensive and contemporaneous; (3) optimize billing because all services provided should all be entered into the chart note in real time; (4) make it easier to recruit physicians into running SMAs (because they will recognize that much of the increased documentation responsibility that comes with seeing so many more patients in the SMA will be done for them during the group time); and (5) align the priorities of the physician with that of administration for full group sessions.

However, it is important to make having a documenter contingent upon meeting pre-established census targets—plus, possibly even seeing an additional patient (or, in a couple of cases, two) in order to cover the additional cost of having a documenter. This also aligns the priorities of the physician with those of administration. I say that priorities would thereby be aligned because, in return for having a documenter, the physician would need to agree to consistently maintain a certain average group size. Otherwise (i.e., without this commitment to maintain group census that comes in return for having a documenter), providers might rationalize that while they could see 13 patients in their DIGMA, they might prefer seeing only eight because it's easier—which, from administration's point of view, could undercut the economic, productivity, and access benefit of the entire SMA program. Because having a documenter available to do most of the charting for them is highly valued by providers (but because this resource is contingent upon maintaining census targets), they frequently become just as interested in consistently achieving target census levels as administration is.

The Dedicated Scheduler Is Critical to Filling All Sessions and Maximizing Economic Gain

The dedicated scheduler, who can be attached to any DIGMA or PSMA for up to 2–4 hours per week (i.e., on weeks when the SMA's census is low and insufficient), plays a critically important role in topping off and filling all sessions so that the profit margin is protected and economic gain is optimized. Dedicated schedulers must be hired based upon their interpersonal, telemarketing, computer, typing, and telephone skills. They should be carefully selected based upon how motivated they are, how pleasant they are with patients, and how persuasive they are in their ability to encourage patients to attend SMA sessions in lieu of individual office visits.

The dedicated scheduler attached to a SMA is typically a motivated scheduler or clerical person specifically trained to telephone and invite patients into future DIGMA and PSMA sessions through a scripted telephone message coupled with talking points—and to answer any patient questions about the program. Having a dedicated scheduler, who is responsible for as many as 15–25 DIGMAs and PSMAs, plays a critical role in ensuring that the desired number of patients attends each SMA session—especially for those sessions that have not been completely filled by the physician and the physician's scheduling staff.

A Sample Script and Talking Points for Schedulers

It is helpful for all schedulers involved with scheduling the physician's patients to be given a sample invitation script (together with some talking points) that they can use when inviting patients into DIGMAs and Physicals SMAs, samples of which are provided on the attached DVD. It is intended that scheduling personnel be able to modify this sample script and put it into their own words, using language that they are content with so that they can be comfortable when using their personalized version of the script.

The Dedicated Scheduler Does Not Take Primary Responsibility for Filling Sessions

No one would expect a physician's individual appointment schedule for the day to be fully booked without patients having first been scheduled by the physician's scheduling staff beforehand. Similarly, the physician and scheduling staff must likewise take primary responsibility for filling group sessions by scheduling enough appropriate patients into the physician's DIGMA or PSMA each week. In addition, for those weeks where the number of patients prescheduled into the DIGMA or PSMA is somewhat less than the targeted census level, the dedicated scheduler needs to spend the time necessary (perhaps 2–6 hours) to telephone enough appropriate patients approved by the physician to *top-off* the group census, keep all sessions filled to capacity, and protect the SMA's profit margin. The dedicated scheduler is only needed in this capacity on those weeks when census for the next session is less than the targeted number of patients, taking into account that sessions need to be overbooked by enough patients to compensate for the expected number of no-shows and late-cancellations (less, of course, the anticipated number of drop-ins).

The Dedicated Scheduler Must Follow-Up with Potentially Interested Patients

The dedicated scheduler must also have the time to follow-up with every telephone contact (especially with patients who agree to attend or for whom telephone messages were left) by sending them a photocopied or computer-generated follow-up letter. This letter needs to include all necessary information about the program, incorporate the physician's signature, and encourage the patient to attend. For those patients that the dedicated scheduler was able to reach and speak with (and who accepted this personal invitation), the time and date of their scheduled SMA visit should also be depicted on the follow-up letter (see example in the Important SMA Department Forms file on the attached DVD).

There is an additional important function that the dedicated scheduler can fulfill just prior to all SMA sessions that will help to optimize census: In addition to activating the normal appointment reminder system for the clinic (automated reminder calls, post cards, etc.), it is also a good idea to have the dedicated scheduler (or a nurse or MA) assigned to the SMA personally call and remind all scheduled patients about their upcoming SMA visit a business day or two beforehand (during which a medication reconciliation can be conducted, HEDIS measures can be updated, and any routine health maintenance or injections due can be determined).

Not Having a Dedicated Scheduler Is a Common Beginner's Mistake

I have found that not having a dedicated scheduler attached to all DIGMAs and PSMAs is a common beginners' mistake that many healthcare systems make. For many, it is an oversight. Some systems do not want to introduce a centralized scheduling function, preferring instead that all scheduling be local and site-based. Other systems simply try to get by without this added expense, small as it might be, and consequently deliberately choose to not have a dedicated scheduler. Still others lose their dedicated scheduler due to competing demands upon this person's time. Although, as a clerical person, the dedicated scheduler represents one of the least expensive personnel resources in the medical center, there are often competing demands throughout the clinic for the scheduler's time. Despite being a comparatively inexpensive resource within the system, the dedicated scheduler can play an important role in leveraging the time of the most expensive resource of all—i.e., the physician's time—by ensuring that all DIGMA and PSMA sessions are filled to capacity.

Despite being comparatively inexpensive, this critically important function nonetheless creates a predictable expense that planners must include in the SMA program's budget. Furthermore, once the service of a dedicated scheduler has been obtained, it is important that the scheduler's time that is attached to the program be given a high priority and protected. Without the dedicated scheduler, DIGMA and PSMA sessions would often be incompletely filled, with the result being a corresponding decrease in the program's productivity and efficiency gains—and thus a reduction in the cost-effectiveness and economic benefit of the program.

Step 15: Custom Design SMAs to Each Provider's Exact Needs

After a physician has been recruited to run a DIGMA or PSMA for his or her practice, the champion and newly recruited physician will need to meet in order to custom designing the DIGMA, CHCC, or PSMA according to the provider's specific needs, goals, practice style, and patient panel constituency. When customizing the design of a SMA for a particular provider's practice (see Table 2.2), it is important that every possible effort be made to design the program in such a way that it is maximally beneficial not only for the provider but also for his or her patients (as well as for the needs of the healthcare organization).

After the physician agrees to run a SMA for his or her practice and the necessary administrative support has been secured, the champion will then need to schedule two or three follow-up meetings with the physician. Whenever possible, these meetings should occur outside of normal working hours so as to minimally impact normal clinic duties. Usually, the first meeting will be between the physician and the champion (and possibly include the program coordinator) in order to more thoroughly familiarize the provider with today's major group visit models and subtypes (as well as their respective strengths and weaknesses) and to determine precisely what the physician's needs and goals are for the program. In addition, the champion and physician will need to determine what SMA model, subtype, and design will best meet these objectives—plus establish all parameters for the group visit program (such as frequency and length of sessions, time of day, day of week, patients to be included, personnel and facilities to be utilized, etc.).

An additional couple of meetings will then need to be held which will variously include the proposed SMA team as well as key personnel from the provider's front and back office staff. During these meetings, the champion, and program coordinator will go over the entire flow of the DIGMA or PSMA and everyone's responsibilities in it. Additional training meetings will need to be scheduled with all of the physician's scheduling and reception staffs (often including half of these staffs at a time so as to not shut down normal clinic operations)—meetings that should also include the office administrator as well as key front and back office staff. The physician would only need to attend some of these meetings and could even come to those for only part of the time. The critical reason for involving the physician at all in these training meetings is for the physician to make it clear to the support staff and SMA team members alike that this SMA is very important to him/her, and it is therefore expected that everyone will do their part in making the program a success. Again, whenever possible, these meetings should be scheduled during lunch or non-clinic hours so as to minimize disruption to the provider and support personnel's schedule during the design and training phases of launching a new DIGMA or Physicals SMA.

Avoid the Common Beginner's Mistake of Limiting the SMA to a Single Condition

During these meetings between the champion and the physician, the appropriate subtype of the DIGMA or PSMA model (heterogeneous, mixed, or homogeneous) needs to be selected to best meet both the provider's and the patients' needs. In addition, the SMA must be designed in such a way as to include the types of patients that the provider most wants to attend each session—but, at the same time, designed in a manner that enables all group sessions to be easily filled. Rather than designing the SMA around conditions that happen to be of particular interest to the provider, be certain to instead design it around where the patient demand is—i.e., so that sessions can be consistently be kept filled.

During these meetings, the champion will often need to strongly encourage the physician to expand the scope of the DIGMA or Physicals SMA to where the patient demand is—i.e., to cover many or even most patients in the physician's practice (or, if the SMA is to be a part of a chronic illness treatment program, most of the patients in the chronic illness population management program). Therefore, be careful to avoid the common beginner's mistake of limiting the SMA to a single condition if the intent is to better manage the physician's practice (for which the heterogeneous subtype is often best), although the homogeneous subtype can often be used with great benefit for chronic disease management programs.

Remember that in order to attend a homogeneous DIGMA session, patients must then not only have that particular condition, but also have a medical need to be seen at that time. In addition, they must know about the SMA program, feel that it holds value for them, and be willing to attend. If the SMA is designed in such a way as to make it unlikely that all sessions will be filled to targeted census levels, then it is at a high risk to fail.

Therefore, if the physician wants to have a DIGMA that is limited to patients with diabetes but has too few of them in the practice to ensure that all future group sessions will be filled (which will certainly be the case when only 10–20% of the physician's entire practice has diabetes), then the champion should propose instead expanding it to be a *Hyperlipidiabesity* DIGMA. The latter DIGMA would cover a much larger group of patients by being open to all of the physician's endocrine syndrome patients (i.e., diabetes, obesity, hypertension, and hyperlipidemia patients). In combination, such a grouping of patients could easily represent perhaps as much as 70% of the physician's entire practice (i.e., rather than the 15% or so that happen to actually have diabetes), thereby making it much easier to consistently fill all group sessions to the SMA's targeted census level—and therefore to have a successful group visit program.

This would make it easy to run an endocrine syndrome group because these patients would identify with one another as well as support and help each other—e.g., by sharing successes, disappointments, encouragement, personal experiences, important disease self-management skills, and helpful tips. In fact, I have run numerous such groups successfully with many different physicians nationally and internationally. Interestingly, for reasons discussed elsewhere in this book, they often evolve into completely heterogeneous DIGMAs within a year's time.

What Should Be Expected from Physicians Running a DIGMA or PSMA?

It is during these early meetings with the physician that the champion personally goes over all of the responsibilities that the physician must assume in order to have a successful DIGMA or Physicals SMA program. The champion usually first points out all of the different types of supports that will be provided to the SMA physician by the champion, program coordinator, behaviorist, nursing personnel, documenter, dedicated scheduler, support staff, etc. These supports are provided during the early planning and design phases of the program, throughout the lengthy process of getting the group visit launched (e.g., see the *pipeline* in the next chapter), and then later on an ongoing basis once the DIGMA or PSMA has been implemented.

Despite all of this support from the multidisciplinary SMA team members that is designed to minimize the physician's time commitment in getting the DIGMA or PSMA launched (and then later is running the group), the champion needs to make absolutely clear that there are certain vitally important duties that the SMA physician must nonetheless personally dispatch in order for the program to succeed. If the provider is not willing to assume these responsibilities, then this is the time to let the champion know they would prefer not to conduct a SMA. Even though every reasonable effort will be made to minimize the physician's time outlay in designing, implementing, and running their DIGMA or Physicals SMA, they will need to personally assume the responsibilities depicted in Table 10.8. The most important of these physician responsibilities is that of personally inviting all appropriate patients seen during regular office visits to

Table 10.8 Responsibilities that all SMA providers must be willing to assume for full success

- Most importantly, to spend 30–60 seconds during every office visit inviting all appropriate patients to have their next visit be in the DIGMA or Physicals SMA. It is absolutely imperative to the success of the program that providers take full responsibility for keeping their SMAs filled to targeted census levels, and that they oversee the performance of their entire support staff in inviting and scheduling patients.
- If you use paper charts but are forgetting to invite all appropriate patients to your SMA, then (first thing in the morning) have your staff paper clip a SMA flier onto the front of each patient's medical chart, which will serve as a reminder when you later see the patient in the exam room.
- If your SMA census is below target, begin submitting your daily schedules to the SMA program coordinator. On them, indicate which patients you invited each day to attend a future SMA and, for patients who accept this offer, when they agreed to attend. This enables SMA staff to check if the patients actually followed through and scheduled the SMA appointment. For those patients who do not, the SMA staff can follow up with a phone call.
- Always remain aware of the census of pre-booked patients for your upcoming DIGMA and PSMA sessions, and promptly let your scheduling staff know whenever your census target is not being met for an upcoming session—encouraging them to get into *high gear* with regards to quickly filling any such sessions (plus, redouble your own efforts in personally inviting patients).
- Agree to let the SMA staff create a roster of your patients with chronic health problems who come regularly for follow-up visits, so they can proactively be offered the SMA for their next visit. If this offer is accepted, then they can be scheduled into the appropriate SMA session—i.e., after their usual follow-up interval.
- Also provide the dedicated scheduler whatever lists of patients they might need so that they can later call and invite sufficient patients into the SMA whenever census is low and needs to be topped off—e.g., patients scheduled more that 2 weeks in advance for an office visit and offering them this week's SMA instead; any diabetic patients who have not been in for 3 or more months, etc.
- Ensure that your behaviorist, nurse/MA(s), documenter, and support staff are all appropriately dispatching their SMA duties, and secure from the champion or program coordinator any additional training they might require.
- Spend a couple minutes each week encouraging your reception staff to keep telling all appropriate patients about your SMA and giving them the invitation letter.
- Take a couple minutes each week to encourage your scheduling staff to keep offering your SMA in a positive manner to all patients requesting an appointment, and then scheduling all appropriate patients who agree to attend into the SMA.
- Be sure to congratulate anyone on your staff or SMA team in a timely manner when they do a good job with regard to inviting patients and filling sessions.
- When things do not go right, which occasionally happens, take corrective action. However, try to avoid getting frustrated and taking it out on your staff (especially your scheduling staff, whose ongoing support is absolutely critical to success) and SMA team, which will only demoralize or anger them—and could even undermine the program.
- Arrange to have all of your key reception and scheduling staff attend one (or at least part of one) of your SMA sessions—perhaps one or two staff members at a time—so they can better inform and tell patients about it.
- Always strive to start and finish your SMA on time; however, recognize that you are likely going to finish late at first (and perhaps even quite late)—at least for the first couple of months, until you gain efficiency and become more comfortable with the new group visit format.
- Learn to delegate fully to your entire SMA team (MA/nurse, behaviorist, and documenter).
- Stay focused and succinct throughout each SMA session. Always strive to start and finish your SMA on time; however, recognize that you are likely going to finish late at first (and perhaps even quite late)—at least for the first couple of months, until you gain efficiency and become more comfortable with the new group visit format.
- Do not cut back on your SMA census targets because you are finishing late—especially during the first couple of months of operations, while you and your SMA team are still learning and trying to get coordinated.
- For the first 2 months of your DIGMA or Physicals SMA, be sure to take a few minutes after each session to debrief with your SMA team and discuss how to make future sessions even better and more efficient—and how to ensure that future sessions will always be filled.

have their next visit be in a DIGMA or PSMA—which requires that the physician take responsibility for ensuring that all sessions are consistently filled to targeted census levels.

To Succeed, Physicians Need to Personally Believe in Their SMA

The bottom line is that, to be successful with their SMA, physicians need to truly believe in their DIGMA or Physicals SMA program. Otherwise, this lack of commitment will somehow get communicated—whether directly or indirectly—to patients and staff. Honestly ask yourself whether you would personally attend a SMA when you need a medical appointment. Do you feel that your DIGMA or Physicals SMA offers patients better care? Do you enjoy running your SMA? Do you believe that you can adequately address most of your patients' medical concerns during your SMA? Personally believing in your SMA program—and being fully committed to making it a success—are absolutely critical to success, and to achieving full benefit from your DIGMA or Physicals SMA.

When Custom Designing SMAs, Also Select the Forms, Handouts, and Marketing Materials

It is here, during the custom-designing phase of conceptualizing your upcoming SMA, when all forms, handouts, and marketing materials need to be selected and configured. The patient packet, educational handouts, promotional materials, and documentation templates to be used in the program constitute major considerations when custom designing a DIGMA or PSMA to the provider's specific needs, goals, practice style, and patient panel constituency. Examples of all of these materials are included on the attached DVD. Other issues that must be addressed when customizing a SMA include identifying the appropriate patient populations for each DIGMA or PSMA (i.e., specifying which patients will and will not be included in each session) and selecting the best available SMA treatment team—behaviorist, nurse/MAs, documenter, and dedicated scheduler. Also, the group and exam rooms need to chosen and reserved, and a realistic start date needs to be determined and agreed upon. Finally, other parameters must also be determined, such as the frequency with which sessions are to be held, the day of the week that the DIGMA will occur, the time of day that works best, and how long sessions are to be.

After These Initial Meetings, the DIGMA Goes into the "Pipeline" for Development

After these initial meetings with the provider and the provider's support staff, the champion and program coordinator place the physician's newly designed DIGMA or Physicals SMA into the *pipeline* that the champion and program coordinator have developed for the program (see Chapter 11, which discusses the pipeline in detail). This process minimizes investment of physician time in the design and planning stages of each new SMA that is to be launched, and simultaneously enables the champion and program coordinator (in larger systems) to systematically and efficiently develop the program until it is launched 8–12 weeks later—i.e., by sequentially attending to all of the numerous detailed steps itemized in the pipeline, and doing so according to the timeline contained therein.

Step 16: Physicians Must Delegate Fully to the Skilled, Trained SMA Team

To maximize quality, outcomes, and physician efficiency, the best available treatment team needs to be assembled for each DIGMA and PSMA that is implemented—behaviorist, nurse/MA(s), documenter, and dedicated scheduler. The entire team needs to be selected by the physician (with the help of the champion and program coordinator), and then appropriately trained by the champion and program coordinator to fully dispatch their respective roles and responsibilities. However, once the best possible SMA team has been assembled, to be optimally efficient it is critically important for the provider to then delegate as much as possible and appropriate to the various team members—which is something that physicians frequently have a difficult time doing.

It Is Only by Delegating Fully to the SMA Team that Physician Productivity Is Optimized

By delegating as much as appropriate and possible to the various members of the SMA team, the physician is able to optimize productivity. The SMA team supports the physician in many ways. The overarching philosophy of this multidisciplinary team-based approach to care is to increase provider efficiency and cost-effectiveness by off-loading onto less expensive, specially trained SMA team members as many provider responsibilities and duties as possible and appropriate. This optimizes efficiency by allowing the physician to do less with each patient—i.e., that which the physician alone can do. However, this "less" is precisely what physicians have gone to medical school to learn to do, what they uniquely can do, and that which they typically most enjoy doing—i.e., to deliver high-quality, high value medical care to each and every patient in attendance.

Because the physician does less with each patient (i.e., only that which the physician alone can do), the physician is therefore able to see many more patients in the DIGMA or PSMA—a process that optimizes efficiency. Table 10.9 shows but a few of the supports that can routinely be provided to the physician by the SMA team.

Table 10.9 DIGMAs and PSMAs provide physicians with many supports

- The champion will help to custom design the DIGMA or Physicals SMA to best meet the physician's particular needs and goals.
- The champion will train the physician on how to successfully refer patients into the SMA (including how to word the referrals) and will provide helpful tips on how to conduct the group successfully, how to document chart notes, and how to solve challenges and problems as they arise.
- The program coordinator will, prior to launching the program, obtain a comprehensive list of all patients (by diagnosis) that can be identified as belonging to the physician's practice—a list that can then be used for mailing announcement letters and for calling patients in order to keep future SMA sessions consistently full.
- The program coordinator will change the provider's master schedule to include the SMA—plus any changes that the provider desires to make as a result of running a SMA.
- The program coordinator will order the posters, fliers, and flier holders for the provider's SMA and will then have them (with the physician's approval) appropriately mounted on the provider's lobby and exam room walls.
- The program coordinator will schedule the group and exam rooms for the physician's SMA program and will also arrange for the coffee, tea, water, and/or snacks that are to be provided during each session.
- Prior to launching the SMA, the program coordinator will provide—for the physician's review and approval—invitations, announcement letters, fliers, forms, chart note template, etc. customized to the physician's needs from templates that have been developed for the SMA program.
- The SMA champion and program coordinator will do everything possible to assist the physician in launching all new DIGMAs and PSMAs within the system, which includes assistance in training all support and SMA team personnel.
- The SMA dedicated scheduler (or else someone from the physician's support staff) will, on an ongoing basis, replenish supplies of the "You Are Invited…" letter being given by receptionists to all of the physician's patients as they register for individual office visits—as well as ensure that flier holders are being kept full in the physician's lobby and exam rooms.
- Nursing personnel will provide a greatly expanded function in the DIGMA or PSMA by taking additional vital signs, updating health maintenance and injections, assisting in the documentation and referral processes, and performing all special nursing duties requested by the physician.
- A behaviorist will be attached to each DIGMA and PSMA to assist the physician in many ways (to arrive early and warm the group up write down patients' health concerns; give the introduction; keep the SMA running smoothly and on time; address group dynamic and psychosocial issues; temporarily take over the group, focusing on behavioral health and psychosocial issues, whenever the physician documents a chart note or provides brief private examinations; stay late to clear and straighten up the group room; etc.
- It is highly recommended that a specifically trained documenter be provided throughout the session, especially in systems using electronic medical records, to assist the physician with most of the documentation responsibilities for the DIGMA or PSMA—generating a superior chart note in real time covering all medical services provided that is both contemporaneous and comprehensive in nature (and one which therefore optimizes billing).
- All of the provider's support staff involved in the program and important to its success (receptionists, schedulers, nurses, medical assistants, office managers, call center personnel, etc.) will receive appropriate training from the champion and program coordinator— both initially and on an ongoing basis.
- The program coordinator will help the physician's nurse/MA design and stock a *crash cart* containing all of the forms, supplies, handouts, equipment, etc. needed for the SMA—a cart that can easily be wheeled in and out of each session.
- The champion and program coordinator will produce a monthly productivity report covering all SMA programs—a report that will provide physicians with ongoing feedback as to how well their SMA is doing (e.g., in achieving the provider's predetermined census targets; patient satisfaction; etc.).
- The dedicated scheduler and program coordinator will generate twice weekly (or weekly) pre-booking census reports so that the provider will know at all times to what degree upcoming SMA sessions are filled.
- The DIGMA champion and program coordinator will meet with the provider and staff as needed to: address any future census problems that might occur; solve system problems as they arise; overcome nonperformance of support staff; train staff regarding how to successfully refer patients; ensure that all members of the support staff and treatment team are dispatching their responsibilities properly; role play difficult situations that might be arising; etc.
- At the physician's request, the dedicated scheduler will help to maintain predetermined census targets by *topping-off* sessions via telephoning patients that the physician has identified as being appropriate (patients on wait-lists; patients already scheduled for future office visits; patients who have failed to return to the office in a timely manner; patients with certain diagnoses or conditions; etc.) and inviting them to attend future DIGMA or PSMA sessions.
- The various members of the SMA team (champion, program coordinator, dedicated scheduler, etc.) will be available to the provider and the provider's staff as needed for assistance and support.

As previously discussed, although some efficiency can be gained in a SMA simply because it occurs in a supportive group setting—where sessions can be over-booked (to compensate for no-shows and late-cancels), repetition can be avoided, patient education can be optimized, and the help and support of others is integrated into each patient's healthcare experience—it is the appropriate delegation of physician duties onto well trained and less costly SMA personnel that is the primary reason for the dramatic productivity gain that DIGMAs and PSMAs offer.

Fully Successful SMAs Require Skilled, Trained, and Well-Functioning Multidisciplinary Teams

Without exception, all staff associated with the SMA must be motivated, competent, well-trained, courteous, and compatible *team players*. Their job is to not only maximize physician productivity, but also foster a pleasant and congenial SMA environment that is satisfying to patients and staff alike. The DIGMA and PSMA models work best with a committed team of trained and capable individuals—each with their own complementary set of skills and responsibilities—and with each having the appropriate amount of dedicated time each week required to fully dispatch their respective duties in the SMA. It is the combined efforts of the champion, program coordinator, and entire SMA team that will be the primary factor in leveraging the physician's time, increasing productivity, and delivering the multiple economic, efficiency, access, satisfaction, and quality of care benefits that a well-run DIGMA or PSMA can provide. All physician responsibilities that can be appropriately off-loaded onto less costly members of the SMA team are to be shifted from the physician to others in order to optimize physician productivity. This not only optimizes efficiency, but also enables everyone to feel that they are valuable and productive members of the SMA team.

Try to engender a positive attitude toward the program among all support staff associated with the SMA. Be certain to confront and promptly resolve any staff negativity toward the program just as soon as it arises. I recommend that all key support personnel attached to the DIGMA or Physicals SMA—especially those who schedule the physician's return appointments and physical examinations (followed by receptionist staff)—sit in on a session or two (one or two staff members per session), or even just a half a session if that is all that is possible. This should occur as soon as possible after the SMA has been launched, so that key support staff (first all scheduling staff, then all receptionists/PSRs, and finally all nursing personnel) can see first-hand what the program is like. By so doing, they will gain a better direct appreciation of: the multiple benefits that a well-run SMA provides; the amount of information and support that it delivers; the warm and pleasant healthcare experience it offers to patients and staff alike; and how satisfied patients are with this new venue of care—even upon experiencing it for the first time. This will enable support staff to better appreciate the multiple benefits that DIGMAs and PSMAs offer to patients—and to better *sell* the program to patients when they subsequently schedule future appointments for their medical care.

Step 17: Develop Policies that Ensure Success, Promptly Solve Any Problems that Arise, and Avoid Common Mistakes

During the design and planning stages, it is wise for the physician and champion to establish in advance the important policy directives for the DIGMA or PSMA—while also incorporating suggestions from the rest of the SMA team (behaviorist, nurse, documenter, support staff, schedulers, and the program coordinator). Many such suggestions regarding developing policies that ensure success, promptly solving any problems that might arise, and avoiding common beginner's mistakes have already been discussed at various points throughout this book.

Twenty-Six Practical Tips for Physicians in Running a DIGMA or PSMA

Since the focus here is upon developing policies that ensure success, promptly solving any problems as they emerge, and avoiding common mistakes, I would like to start this section off by pointing out 24 hard-earned practical tips for physicians to use when setting up and running their DIGMA and/or PSMA program (Table 10.10). Each of these tips has been discussed in detail elsewhere in the book; however, the reader will undoubtedly find it helpful to have all of these practical tips for physicians listed in one place—i.e., where they can all be easily referenced at the same time. In addition to helping you to be successful when you design and launch your own group visit program, these practical tips will also help you to avoid making many problematic beginner's mistakes that could otherwise so easily be made.

Table 10.10 Twenty-Six practical tips for physicians in running a successful DIGMA or Physicals SMA

1. Start by using the established group visit models—do not just "wing it" on your own
2. Select your entire SMA team with great care (see Chapters 2, 3, and 11)
3. Start with a realistic, but slightly high, target census
4. Get the necessary administrative, promotional, and training support before starting
5. Obtain an adequately sized group room with an exam room nearby for DIGMAs, or a smaller group room and 2–5 exam rooms (most commonly 4) for PSMAs
6. Obtain a trained dedicated scheduler to help keep your sessions full
7. Have your entire support staff—especially scheduling, reception, and nursing staff—promote the SMA program effectively to all appropriate patients
8. The physician needs to personally invite all appropriate patients seen individually to have their next visit in the SMA
9. Distribute quality "Patient Packets" to patients when they register for the SMA (and have all patients, as well as their support persons, sign a confidentiality release)
10. Maximally expand the nursing role in every SMA session—and delegate fully to the entire SMA team
11. Similarly maximize the behaviorist's role to make it all that it can be—and then delegate fully
12. Using a documenter can greatly enhance your efficiency—as well as the quality of both your chart note and your DIGMA or PSMA experience
13. Utilize a dedicated scheduler to *top off* SMA sessions whenever census for an upcoming group happens to be low
14. Develop a strategy for the order in which you treat patients in the SMA—especially your more challenging and difficult patients
15. Keep patients engaged by fostering some group interaction and providing abundant patient education throughout
16. Do not spend too much time with the first couple of patients that you treat in the SMA
17. To finish on time, the physician and behaviorist must stay focused and succint, plus pace the group throughout the session
18. Strive to always finish on time with all documentation completed, but expect to finish late at first
19. Whenever appropriate, try to schedule follow-up visits back into a future DIGMA session
20. Do not reduce census targets at first, and later only do so slowly—but only if necessary (instead, try debriefing with your SMA team for 15–20 minutes after sessions for 2 months)
21. The physician must assume primary responsibility for maintaining the SMA's census
22. Have the SMA program coordinator generate a weekly prebooking census report as well as a weekly (or monthly) productivity report so that you can closely monitor census of all of your DIGMA/PSMA sessions
23. Continually improve your SMA over time
24. Consider better managing your practice by eventually offering more than one DIGMA or PSMA per week
25. For large, busy, and backlogged practices, ultimately work toward having a DIGMA or two every day of the week—plus a weekly Physicals SMA
26. Have fun!

With DIGMAs and PSMAs, Deliver as Much Medical Care as Possible in the Group Setting

One such policy is that the physician should attempt to provide as much medical care as possible and appropriate during each and every session, as this is a real convenience to patients—who appreciate the benefits of max-packed visits and this *one-stop shopping* approach to healthcare delivery. Foster some group interaction (but not too much, as it can be time consuming) during the group so as to keep patients attentive and involved. Be certain to deliver as much of this individualized medical care as possible in the group setting—where all can listen and learn, and where repetition can be avoided. It is here, in the group setting, that referrals can be made for tests and procedures, prescriptions can be given and refilled, counseling and brief exams that do not require disrobing can be provided, minor procedures (such as freezing skin tags)

can be delivered, and patients can be referred to specialists, dieticians, smoking cessation programs, etc.

Reduce "No-Shows" by Reminding Patients a Day or Two Prior to Their Upcoming SMA Visit

Another such policy is always achieving the goal of getting the targeted number of patients to attend each and every SMA session—which will optimize the physician's productivity and the quality of the group experience for all. Because consistently full groups are critical to the success of any DIGMA or Physicals SMA program, it is recommended that certain basic policies be put in place to ensure full attendance. For example, all patients pre-registered for the SMA should be given a standard institutional reminder of their upcoming appointment a couple days in advance of the session (automated phone call, post card, etc.). In addition, have a specifically trained nurse or medical assistant make a personal reminder phone call to all patients scheduled for the upcoming SMA session a business day or two before each session—at which time they could also do a medication reconciliation, check whether all previsit labs have been completed, and determine if any injections. Screening tests, or health maintenance needs to be updated during the upcoming SMA visit. This takes a little time on the part of a clerical person; however, it can pay off big in terms of having consistently full groups. These last-minute reminder calls can produce rich dividends in terms of reducing the no-show and late-cancel rates of SMA patients, and therefore in increasing the physician's productivity during sessions.

Whenever Appropriate, Try to Schedule Follow-Up Appointments Back into Future SMA Sessions

Another policy that enhances the likelihood of success is to be certain to encourage all patients in attendance to return to a future DIGMA the next time they have a medical need—or, in the case of a PSMA, the next time they need a physical exam. In other words, make a serious effort to schedule as many appropriate follow-up appointments as possible from the SMA session directly back into future DIGMA sessions (and as many appropriate private physical examinations as possible from the SMA session directly into a future PSMA session). Because patient satisfaction with well-run DIGMAs and PSMAs is so high, patients attending a SMA will almost always like this venue of care once they actually experience it. They will therefore be willing to return, if only they are invited. Hence, it is important to invite all patients in attendance to have their next follow-up visit be a DIGMA visit—i.e., whenever they have a future medical need and want to be seen.

Should the physician happen to forget to invite any particular patient while individually working with each of the patients in the DIGMA or PSMA setting, then the back-up plan could be for the behaviorist to ask: "Is there a follow-up plan, doctor?" This would serve as a reminder to the physician to consider whether a follow-up appointment is needed and, if so, whether or not to invite the patient back into the appropriate future DIGMA session. In addition, patients could also be told in the behaviorist's introduction that they are welcome to return to the DIGMA any time that they have a medical need in the future.

Have Patients Call the Office Before Dropping in

Another policy I recommend is to tell patients that, if they do choose to drop into a DIGMA, to telephone the office a business day or two prior to the session. In the introduction to each SMA session, the behaviorist should point out that—by calling the office a day or two in advance of dropping in—patients will enable staff to monitor group census and, for systems still using paper charts, to order patients' medical charts in time for the session. In addition, telephoning the office also provides patients with an opportunity to confirm that the DIGMA will be meeting that week—as the physician will occasionally cancel due to being ill, on vacation, at an off-site meeting, on sabbatical, etc. Also, by calling the office a day or two in advance and pre-registering for the DIGMA (i.e., rather than just dropping in unannounced), patients are pre-registered for the group and can therefore be notified later in the event that the session needs to be cancelled at the last minute for some reason (such as the physician being ill)—thereby avoiding an unnecessary trip to the clinic.

Consistently Achieving Full Groups Presents an Ongoing Challenge

Always keep in mind that DIGMAs and PSMAs are census driven programs and that it is important to set the necessary policies in place for your SMA so as to ensure that targeted census levels are consistently achieved. While an important goal for every DIGMA and PSMA is to get the pre-determined number of patients to attend each session, there are two reasons that this presents an on-going challenge for these group visit models. First, achieving desired census levels is challenging because different patients typically attend each session—as patients only attend when they actually have a medical need. Second, because patients have a lifetime of expecting individual office visits and they typically know nothing about group visits (which represent a very different paradigm of care delivery), it is difficult to get patients to attend a shared medical appointment for the first time. This is why high-quality promotional materials are required for the SMA program, and why it is so important for the physician and support staff to consistently and effectively promote the DIGMA or PSMA program to all appropriate patients.

In addition, there might be other problems that make it difficult to get the required number of patients consistently scheduled into each and every SMA session. Perhaps the announcements were not mailed out to all of the physician's appropriate patients before the SMA was launched, or the support staff might not be actively recommending the SMA to all suitable patients. Framed posters for the program might not be prominently displayed on the walls in the physician's lobby and exam rooms, or fliers might not be stocked in the dispenser next to them (or the dispensers may not be kept full over time). Most importantly, the physician might not be effectively promoting the SMA by personally inviting all appropriate patients seen during traditional office visits to have their next return visit be in the physician's DIGMA (or their next physical examination in the physician's PSMA). Or else, the physician might not be inviting all appropriate patients when individually treating them during the DIGMA or PSMA session—i.e., to have their next return visit be in a future DIGMA session.

In addition, the receptionist might not be consistently handing out invitations to all of the physician's patients as they register for an office visit, or the nurse/MA might not be handing program description fliers (along with saying a few kind words about the SMA) to all appropriate patients as they are being roomed. Finally, a dedicated scheduler might not have been assigned to the SMA with the responsibility of topping-off sessions to ensure that they are all filled to the desired capacity (in which case, try to get one as soon as possible). Or else, there might be a dedicated scheduler attached to the program, but competing resource demands disallow sufficient time being dedicated to the DIGMA/PSMA to contact enough patients each week so that consistently full sessions can be ensured. When such problems occur, they must be promptly recognized and addressed.

Solve Operational Problems as They Arise

They say that the devil is in the details. With DIGMAs and PSMAs, the success of the entire program lies in paying close attention to all the operational, administrative, and logistical details—and to promptly addressing any operational problems that might arise. Each new SMA that is launched will likely experience some operational problems, especially during the initial design and implementation phases—and most particularly during the first few months of operations.

Operational Problems of All Types Can Arise

Operational problems can arise regarding any aspect of the new SMA program—personnel, facilities, equipment (computers, printers, telephones, medical equipment, etc.), forms and handouts, documentation, scheduling, program promotion, etc. When such operational problems occur, they should promptly be addressed and resolved (preferably by the champion, behaviorist, nurse/MA, or program coordinator)—i.e., rather than by the more costly physician, which helps to leverage the physician's time.

For example, the group room might be too small or it might occasionally be mistakenly scheduled out to others during the timeslot set aside for the DIGMA or PSMA. The group room might need to be set up properly before each session, tables or other clutter will need to be removed from the group room, and additional furnishings and wall hangings might be required in order to create the desired ambiance. The temperature of the group room might not be set at a comfortable level, the required number of chairs might not be consistently available, or the entire issue of snacks might somehow prove to be problematic. The exam room might not be appropriately equipped, the logistics surrounding the Patient Packet might break down, referral forms and handouts might need to be supplied, charts might not be arriving on time (for systems using paper charts), the computer or telephone might not be functional, the printer might not work, or there might not be chalk or colored pens with erasable ink available for writing on the whiteboard or flipchart in the group room. Or else, the physician might be arriving late, the behaviorist and nursing personnel might not be arriving sufficiently early, or the documenter might fail to show up.

The Increased Productivity of the DIGMA or PSMA Can Itself Stress the System

In addition, the major paradigm shift and increased productivity that DIGMAs and PSMAs entail tends to stress the system—and to make unacceptable any inefficiencies that might heretofore have been marginally acceptable when one patient was being seen at a time. For example, a receptionist who has historically been a slow and marginal performer is not likely to suddenly become faster and more efficient when 15 patients (rather than one) are waiting in line to be registered for a DIGMA. Thus, the remarkable efficiency gain of a properly run DIGMA or PSMA can itself stress the system and create certain operational challenges. The *good news* here is that, by promptly solving any such operational problems and inefficiencies as they arise, the whole clinic might thereafter be able to function better throughout the remainder of the workweek. However, the *bad news* here is that, if these operational and administrative problems are not promptly resolved, they can reduce patient and staff satisfaction with the program—and can even end up undercutting the whole SMA program.

Avoid Follow-Up Scheduling Log-Jams After the Session Is Over

In addition, there might be problems scheduling the follow-up appointments of all patients attending the SMA immediately after the DIGMA or PSMA is over. This is especially true if almost all patients end up lining up in front of the scheduler as they simultaneously leave the group room after the session is over. This problem can be greatly ameliorated by having each patient briefly leave the group room immediately after the physician has completed working with them (i.e., to individually schedule their follow-up appointment)—and then return to the group setting after their return appointment has been scheduled. Even though they end up missing a few minutes of the session, this turns out to be a very workable approach to efficiently scheduling follow-up visits. Although temporarily bringing a scheduler into the group room to schedule all the follow-up appointments for patients in attendance might be possible, it would need to be done in such a manner as to not significantly drive up the overhead expense of the SMA program. For systems on EMR, it might also be a viable option to have the documenter in the SMA schedule many follow-up appointments and referrals for attendees during the session—although I do not recommend this approach, as it will likely result in a time consuming distraction that could keep the documenter from getting everything that the physician is doing into the chart note. At Harvard Vanguard Medical Associates/Atrius Health, we use a care coordinator (typically the MA during the last half of the DIGMA or PSMA session, i.e., after all initial MA duties have been completed on all patients) to: call patients out of the group room one by one; promptly schedule all referrals and follow-ups made by the physician; and give all patients an after visit summary (i.e., a copy of those parts of the chart note that the physician wants the patient to have). In the event that no referrals or procedures need to be scheduled, the care coordinator simply takes the AVS to the patient in the group room, as there is no need to call patients out in that case (which could be somewhat disruptive to the flow of the group and would cause the patient to unnecessarily miss part of the group session).

There Can Be Equipment, Medical Chart, and Scheduling Mix-Ups

The physician might want specific medical equipment to be there for his/her DIGMA, or for certain injections requiring refrigeration to be administered—in which case, there needs to be a refrigerator in the group or exam room that can be used for this purpose (plus sufficient injections contained therein for all of the patients attending the SMA that might require them). For systems still using paper charts, the charts might not be arriving at the right place (or at the correct time) for the DIGMA or PSMA session. Also, there might be scheduling mix-ups, or patients might simply be arriving at the wrong place or time. Clearly, all such operational and logical problems would need to be promptly resolved as quickly as possible so as to not interfere with the efficient functioning of the SMA.

The Physician and Entire SMA Team Can Also Have Problems, Especially at the Start

There are many flow problems that the physician and SMA team can face when first launching a DIGMA or PSMA. For example, there might be problems: in getting the confidentiality waivers signed and collected; in having the nurse(s) or behaviorist efficiently dispatch all of their duties in an effective and timely manner; in ensuring that the physician fosters some group interaction and delivers as much medical care as appropriate and possible during the highly productive group setting; in referring patients to specialists, for lab tests, or for procedures; in refilling medications or providing minor procedures toward the end of the session; or in getting patients scheduled into appropriate follow-up appointments during or after the DIGMA or PSMA session. Also, there might be problems with the nurse/MA, behaviorist, documenter, or physician arriving on time or pacing their activities so as to finish on time; and the SMA team itself might have difficulties coalescing into a coordinated and efficient unit. Clearly, all such problems must be promptly addressed as soon as they arise in order for DIGMAs and PSMAs to be as productive, efficient, and enjoyable as possible. By having a debriefing session at the end of all DIGMAs and PSMAs for the first 2 months, all such problems can potentially be expeditiously resolved.

Avoid Making Common Beginners' Mistakes that Can Undermine Your SMA Program

It is very easy to make many common beginners' mistakes when starting a SMA program (Table 10.11). Furthermore, there is much about group visits that is counterintuitive, which can itself lead to many beginners' mistakes. For this reason, I strongly recommend that—before departing from the SMA models as they have been developed and utilized—you first start with the established DIGMA, CHCC, and Physicals SMA models as they are described herein. These models have had a fairly long evolutionary history, have gone through numerous iterations, have been

Table 10.11 Ten common beginner's mistakes

1. Administration demanding that the physician first demonstrate that SMAs work well within the organization—and only then will they support the program
2. Launching SMAs prematurely, before all key supports needed for success are first secured: administrative support; the necessary promotional materials; important patient education materials; the required personnel and facilities; organizational consensus; a billing policy, an easy-to-understand confidentiality release drawn up by system's corporate attorney, etc.
3. Failing to design four major factors into each and every SMA that is launched: (1) optimally build all possible quality in; (2) ensure that targeted census levels are always met; (3) keep overhead costs reasonable; and (4) measure outcomes on an ongoing basis
4. Making the groups too homogeneous, so that too few patients qualify to attend sessions and targeted census levels cannot be consistently achieved; or making it occur on too infrequent a basis, such as every 2 weeks, once a month, or even quarterly
5. Worrying about many small things, but failing to stay focused on the most important key to success—i.e., always having full groups, with a targeted census level selected so as to increase productivity by 200–300% or more. Insufficient census signals a *sick* group; therefore, do not start small with the intention of later working up to larger groups; let your census drop over time; or rationalize small groups because "it's better care," especially after initial success. On the other hand, be certain to use a documenter to gain efficiency (especially in systems having electronic medical records); address the challenge posed by the off-site Call Center in helping to fill sessions; and debrief with your SMA team after sessions for the first couple of months of implementation to increase efficiency and improve the program.
6. Not promoting the SMA effectively to all appropriate patients (e.g., by not prominently displaying the poster on the lobby and exam rooms; not sending out an announcement letter beforehand; not having receptionists hand out invitations; not having the nurse(s) distribute fliers and promote the program when rooming patients; not training the scheduling staff to *sell* the program; not using a dedicated scheduler; not using Patient Packets for the SMA; not informing patients through newsletters as well as the mass media; and most importantly, by the physician not personally inviting all appropriate patients seen during normal office visits)
7. By assembling the cheapest or most available SMA team rather than the best team for you and your practice, one which consists of skilled, trained, and compatible participants (behaviorist; nursing personnel; documenter; dedicated scheduler; your trained support staff; and, in larger systems, a champion and program coordinator)—or, worse yet, trying to do without critically important SMA personnel
8. By the physician not delegating fully to the entire SMA team (in order to optimize efficiency and quality)
9. The physician and behaviorist not starting and finishing on time, and not staying focused and succinct throughout the entire session (e.g., by leaving the group room unnecessarily; losing control of the group; taking too much time with the first couple of patients; not maintaining a workable pace throughout; taking too much time on interesting or problematic patients; using a chair with wheels and rolling over and talking to one patient, but turning one's back to the rest of the group; the behaviorist spending too much time talking; or by not properly managing talkative and dominating patients)
10. Failing to foster enough group interaction, or too much (which can either cause patients to lose interest in what is transpiring in the group or end up slowing the group down to the point where it finishes late, respectively)

fine-tuned over time, and have been demonstrated to work time and time again in actual practice. Only consider departing from these established models later, after you have already had some successes and gained much practical experience with your SMA.

Although there are a myriad of common beginner's mistakes that healthcare organizations and physicians often make when first implementing DIGMA, CHCC, and Physicals SMA programs, they tend to be of two basic types:

1. *Putting too little into the SMA program for it to succeed* (inadequate funding; poor staffing; inadequate training; selecting personnel based upon low cost rather than appropriateness for the job; inadequate group and exam room facilities; inadequate promotion of the program; no posters or fliers; allowing too little time for SMA sessions; not providing all the necessary personnel; not giving the champion, program coordinator, behaviorists, documenters, dedicated schedulers, and support personnel sufficient training and time to adequately dispatch their SMA duties; etc.).
2. *Taking more out of DIGMAs and Physicals SMAs than they were ever intended to give*—i.e., in a futile attempt to extract even more benefit from these efficient programs than they were designed to achieve (requiring too many

patients to attend each SMA; demanding that all patients and providers participate rather than keeping SMAs voluntary for all; etc.).

Both of the above scenarios have the same net result: a program that either fails or is only partially successful. To be fully successful, DIGMAs and PSMAs require that: (1) the necessary budgetary, personnel, promotional, and facilities resources are infused into these programs; and (2) efforts not be made to extract even greater productivity, efficiency, and economic gains than well-run DIGMAs and PSMAs are designed to achieve.

Despite All My SMA Experience, Even I Make Beginners' Mistakes—So Be Careful

Despite my extensive experience with over 20,000 patient visits in the DIGMA and PSMA models (and with over 400 different providers in healthcare systems both nationally and internationally), I made a beginners' mistake in creating the PSMA model in 2001—one that delayed its development by almost a year. This happened because I went with what seemed to me to be intuitively obvious—i.e., having the interactive group segment of the session first (during which all the discussion was to occur), and then following this with the private physical examination segment of the visit (after which patients were free to either leave or return to the small group being led by the behaviorist). I started the early PSMA sessions on time with the behaviorist's introduction—in which I emphasized that all but truly private discussions with the provider were to occur during the initial interactive group segment (and not during the private physical examination that was to follow). In addition, the physician started the session off by repeating this exact same guideline. Unfortunately, by following this intuitively appealing approach of doing the interactive group segment first and the exams last, the result was an unworkable model in which sessions typically finished quite late.

It took many months—and three frustrated physicians who were tired of finishing late—before I reversed *the cart and the horse*. It took over half a year to realize that there was a flaw in the model as initially conceived—and that it could easily be corrected by delivering the private examinations first. This enabled physicians to easily defer most discussions from the inefficient exam room setting to the highly efficient group room setting that followed, where things only needed to be said once to the benefit of all present. The physician could easily accomplish this in the exam room by saying something to the patient like: "Good point! Why don't you bring that up in the group that follows so that everybody can listen and learn?" With my original PSMA model (wherein the exams were performed last), physicians were stuck with inefficiently addressing the additional questions and medical issues that patients always seemed to bring up when they got the physician alone in the exam room—i.e., because the group discussion segment of the visit was already over.

In other words, if the physician detected a problem during the physical examination, then there was no alternative to discussing it with the patient at that time—i.e., in the inefficient exam room (rather than group room) setting. The fact that patients still had additional questions to ask when they got the physician alone in the exam room—which is something that occurred time and again—made it clear that this was an unworkable model in most cases. And this was despite the fact that patients were being told in both the promotional materials and the behaviorist's introduction—as well as by the physician at the start of the SMA—that all discussions, except for truly private matters and that which was necessary in order to conduct the exam, were to occur in the group room during the first part of the visit. Despite these admonitions, patients always seemed to save up a few issues to discuss later when alone with the physician in the exam room—which almost always caused these flawed PSMA sessions to finish late.

Step 18: Start with a Carefully Designed Pilot Study and Evaluate its Success

In order to determine for themselves whether today's major group visit models can work within their system, most healthcare organizations will probably want to first develop a carefully designed pilot study and then evaluate how successful it is when conducted within their own facilities. Certainly, larger group practices and managed-care organizations will probably want to first evaluate the viability of a DIGMA or PSMA program in their organization through a substantial pilot study. Personally, I have found that these SMA models can be designed to work well in any healthcare system. Conversely, I cannot think of a single instance where they did not work, provided that they were appropriately designed, supported, promoted, and run.

First Steps in Starting Your Pilot Study

After securing the necessary administrative support, the champion needs to recruit appropriate physician volunteers for the pilot study by giving presentations to various departments at the targeted facilities. A budget is developed for the pilot program, and the various parameters of the pilot study are carefully defined, e.g., which group visit models to use; which subtypes; what physicians; how many providers; primary or specialty care; which facilities; what behaviorists; which group and exam rooms; what promotional materials to employ; etc. With the help of the pilot physicians and the program coordinator, the champion will need to design and develop all forms to be used in the program—always in template form. Please note that examples of virtually all important DIGMA and PSMA forms that the readers will need in order to start their own group visit program are included in the DVD attached to this book.

Customize Pilot DIGMAs and PSMAs, and Select Both SMA Teams and Outcome Measures

The champion then meets individually with the recruited physicians to custom design their DIGMAs, CHCCs, and PSMAs according to their specific needs, goals, practice styles, and patient panel constituencies. The treatment teams are assigned to the pilot SMAs and then appropriately trained by the champion and program coordinator—i.e., the behaviorist, 1–2 nursing personnel (usually including the physician's own nurse or MA), documenter, and dedicated scheduler.

The pilot study will need to be evaluated according to appropriate criteria of greatest interest to the healthcare organization—e.g., enhanced quality of care, increased provider productivity, improved access, reduced cost of care, improved outcomes, better performance measures, updated injections and routine health maintenance, enhanced patient and physician satisfaction, etc. Clearly, the factors to be assessed will first need to be selected (i.e., factors that are appropriate to the SMA model being selected and of importance to both the pilot physicians and the organization), and then the means of assessing improvements in these areas through the SMA program will need to be determined. In addition, tests, analytic measures, and forms to be used in evaluating the program (such as the patient satisfaction form) will need to be selected, developed, and appropriately utilized.

Select Your Pilot Physicians and Pilot Site(s)

Pilot studies have been conducted with as few as 1 physician and with as many as 12 different providers in primary and specialty care. Usually one or two pilot sites are selected within the organization—based upon administrative priorities, which physicians are willing to participate in the pilot, and where the need is greatest. Only after the pilot study has successfully demonstrated feasibility of the DIGMA, CHCC, and/or Physicals SMA models within their own system will most administrators and executive leaders in integrated healthcare delivery systems want to expand their group visit program to organization-wide implementation.

Evaluate the Pilot's Success Before Expanding the SMA Program Facility and Organization Wide

By having a pilot study, the success of DIGMAs and PSMAs can be evaluated within the organization (according to the potential benefits that are of greatest interest to the organization) before the decision is made to disseminate the program facility- and organization- wide. As is always the case with DIGMAs and PSMAs, each pilot is custom designed to the particular needs, practice style, and patient panel constituency of the individual physician. In addition, the SMA program needs to be fully supported and properly run, and all templates and promotional materials necessary for a successful pilot study must be developed. However, once the pilot has been demonstrated to be successful, the healthcare organization's goal will likely rapidly shift from pilot study to rapid, full-scale, and system-wide deployment of the SMA program throughout both primary and specialty care.

Use Evaluative Measures that Are Appropriate to the SMA Model You Choose

Be certain to use measures for evaluating your SMA program that are appropriate to the particular group visit model that you select so that you do not develop unrealistic and unachievable expectations for the outcomes of your program. For example, whereas one would want CHCCs to reduce use of emergency department, hospital, and nursing home services, one would not expect access to be dramatically improved or physician productivity to be greatly increased—which are strengths of the DIGMA and PSMA models, not CHCCs or Specialty CHCCs. In today's medical environment, operational decisions must increasingly be data driven—with ongoing programs continuously needing to prove their value through appropriate evaluative criteria. It is in this light that I highly recommend appropriate outcome measures be developed for any group visit programs adopted by the organization—evaluative measures that should reflect each model's primary goals in terms of quality, access, service, satisfaction, efficiency, increased capacity, cost savings, and reduced utilization (goals of various group visit models that are often overlapping and synergistic rather than mutually exclusive). However, in the interests of being realistic and keeping costs down, it is important that all such measurements be relatively simple, reliable, readily available, and valid—as well as being aligned to both the organization's priorities and the particular benefits that each group visit model was designed to achieve.

Carefully Evaluate Your Pilot Study, and Then Issue Periodic Reports on the SMA Program Thereafter

The pilot study (as well as all future SMAs) needs to be appropriately evaluated during and after a certain interval of time (often after 6 weeks to one year), and then periodically thereafter—i.e., according to the potential benefits that group visits can offer which are of greatest interest to your healthcare organization. Such benefits can include enhanced care, superior updating of performance measures and health maintenance, increased MD productivity, improved access to care, leveraging of existing staffing, reduced costs, better patient education, improved clinical outcomes, enhanced doctor–patient relationships, reduced utilization, increased patient and physician satisfaction, etc. Forms to be employed in evaluating the pilot, such as the Patient Satisfaction Form, must be selected, developed, and appropriately utilized (see sample patient satisfaction forms on the attached DVD). These forms can be either normed research instruments or specifically developed tools for evaluating the SMA program, although the selection as to which type(s) to use will need to be jointly made by the organization and the SMA champion.

Appropriate outcomes reports must be generated for the pilot study, and the success or failure of the pilot study needs to be fully evaluated by larger organizations—i.e., prior to initially expanding the group visit program from pilot study to facility-wide (and ultimately to organization-wide) implementation. For DIGMA and PSMA programs, periodic reports assessing any increases in physician productivity and access as a result of the SMA program need to be created—reports which should include productivity measures, improvements in backlogs and wait-lists, any decreases in telephone volume or patient complaints, and improvements in patient access to care. Whenever possible, any improvements in injections, health maintenance, performance measures, patient satisfaction, and outcomes should also be included in these reports. Measurements must be taken, data must be collected and analyzed, any cost savings must be evaluated, and appropriate reports need to be periodically generated and distributed.

Step 19: Go from Successful Pilot Study to System-Wide Implementation

Once a pilot study has demonstrated feasibility of the SMA concept within your healthcare organization's own facilities, then the next step will be facility-wide (and ultimately organization-wide) implementation of the SMA program. However, it is important that the expansion of the SMA program be on a voluntary basis—i.e., by securing physician buy-in at the grass roots level rather than dictating participation top-down, and by always making the SMA program voluntary (as well as an extra healthcare choice) to patients. Let us now examine how integrated healthcare delivery systems (group practices, IPAs, PPOs, HMOs, for profits, not for profits, public health facilities, DoD, VA, etc.) can best establish successful primary and specialty care DIGMAs and Physicals SMAs throughout their systems.

The Process of Expanding the SMA Program Organization Wide

Once the pilot study has been demonstrated to be successful and administration has made the decision to advance the SMA program system-wide, the champion moves the

program toward organization-wide dissemination by recruiting more and more interested primary and specialty care providers in the various departments and facilities throughout the entire system on an on-going basis. The goal is for the champion to get physicians throughout the facility (as well as the entire system) to voluntarily launch DIGMAs, CHCCs, and/or PSMAs for their practices. Ultimately, as more and more DIGMAs, CHCCs, and PSMAs are developed, they will be increasingly recognized by patients and staff alike as important elements in how the organization has chosen to deliver mainstream medical care. As more and more DIGMAs and PSMAs are launched throughout the system, behaviorists (typically specifically trained psychologists, licensed clinical social workers, or nurses for DIGMAs, and nurses—but sometimes mental health professionals—in PSMAs), documenters, and dedicated schedulers will need to be hired into the SMA program on an as-needed basis either as employees or on a contractual basis.

If, for some reason, your pilot study should have proven to be unsuccessful, then I would encourage you to carefully examine the underlying reasons for failure and whether errors were made in how the pilot was conducted (e.g., was the design flawed; was the focus upon too narrow of a patient population; were census requirements met; were critical supports not yet in place; were appropriate personnel and facilities secured; was the necessary training provided; were the physician and support staff consistently inviting all appropriate patients to attend; etc.) before abandoning group visits in your organization. Ask whether your pilot was appropriately designed, supported, promoted, and run. Should you find that some oversight or mistake has been made, correct it as soon as possible and then reassess the success of your pilot some time later—i.e., after new data are collected and analyzed. I say this because successful group visit programs have been developed within innumerable healthcare systems (and in primary care and virtually all medical and surgical subspecialties). Therefore, if your SMA program happens to fail for some reason, then there is likely one or more problems contributing to this lack of success which, if only corrected, would greatly enhance the likelihood of success.

Try to Secure Physician Buy-In at the Grass Roots Level, Not Through Administrative Mandates

If the initial DIGMAs, CHCCs, and Physicals SMAs being run within the system are well designed, supported, and run, then it is expected that they will be successful and that a gradual increase in physician buy-in to the SMA program at the grassroots level will gradually begin to occur over time. Furthermore, it is anticipated that this process should steadily increase as more and more successful group visits are eventually implemented throughout the system. This can be expected to occur on several fronts: as a result of positive reports from physician colleagues who are actually running successful group visits; through the champion's efforts in moving the program forward throughout the system; and out of physician self interest due to the multiple patient and physician benefits that properly run group visits can offer (i.e., despite the fact that a major paradigm shift and considerable change is thereby introduced into the system by the SMA program). However, be careful to stick closely (especially at first) with these major SMA models as they have broad applicability, have successfully gone through countless developmental iterations, and can help you to avoid many common beginner's mistakes. Design and run your SMA program appropriately—because it seems that, whereas good news tends to travel painfully slow in an organization, bad news travels extremely fast.

There Will Likely Always Be Some Physician Holdouts to SMAs, Which Is OK

However, it can also be anticipated that there will always be a few physician holdouts remaining—no matter how successful the SMA program might ultimately become—as physician needs and motivations are expected to vary (both between physicians and over time), and differences of opinion are always facts of life that need to be reckoned with. Some physicians will simply not see any need for changing how they do things—and for some, especially those with smaller and unfilled practices which they are not interested in growing, this is probably true. In addition, it is highly probable that there will always be some providers who simply prefer the old way of doing things—i.e., of only providing individual office visits. Perhaps some will always remain convinced that the traditional individual office visit modality in which they have been trained—and may have been practicing for many years—is simply the best method of providing care. Others might feel that they are close to retirement, that there is simply no reason to change at this time, or that they presently have no need for group visits in their practice.

I have always welcomed such dissension, and have even considered it to be a healthy process, because: (1) there is always room for differences of opinion; (2) group visits are meant to be voluntary and not to be imposed upon anyone; (3) this can be a healthy process that

provides an important counterbalance to the SMA program; and (4) experience has demonstrated that over time, even some of the most resistant physicians can eventually be won over to running group visits for their practices—ultimately to the point of actively embracing and recommending them.

The First DIGMAs and PSMAs to Be Launched Are Typically the Most Difficult

No matter what approach the champion adopts for moving the SMA program forward from pilot study to organization-wide implementation, the first set of DIGMAs and PSMAs at each facility will generally be the most difficult and time consuming to establish. In part, this is due to the fact that, at first, patients and providers alike are largely unfamiliar with—and frequently more resistant to—group visits and the voluminous benefits they can offer. Afterward, as experience is gained, protocols are established, patient and physician buy-in progressively increase, forms and promotional materials are developed, training programs for behaviorists and nurses are developed, documenters learn how to best fulfill their function, administrative and operational issues are addressed, and a systematic approach to launching successive SMAs is gradually developed (i.e., a *pipeline*, as described in the next chapter) that subsequent SMAs gradually become easier and easier to launch.

In other words, most of the work for a successful program must be done up-front. During the initial weeks of designing and planning the pilot study—and during the first few weeks of operations for the first SMAs that are run (which is also the time that the most beginner's mistakes can easily be made)—much work needs to be done. For example, in these early months of the SMA program all forms and promotional materials need to be developed in template form, suitable training programs for the SMA team and support staff need to be developed, and the learning curve is greatest with regard to consistently meeting census requirements. There are several reasons, including the following, for this up-front workload bolus that group visit programs entail:

- Administrative support and an adequate budget for the program must first be secured.
- In larger systems, the champion and program coordinator will need to be selected—and then provided with the necessary time and resources.
- The appropriate personnel and facilities required for a successful group visit program need to be obtained from the start.

- All basic policies and procedures must be developed at the beginning of the SMA program, including documentation, billing, and evaluation policies.
- Templates of all forms and promotional materials will need to be created at the outset, which can be a demanding and time-consuming process (examples of all such forms, which are contained in the DVD attached to this book, can be most helpful in this regard).
- Especially in the beginning, the group visit program will need to be aggressively promoted to patients, providers, and support staffs alike in order to familiarize them with SMAs and their many potential benefits—so that acceptance, buy-in, and full groups can all be achieved.
- The amount of change involved (to patients, staff, providers, and the system alike), and therefore the amount of resistance that can be expected to be engendered toward the SMA program, will likely be at its peak at the start of the program—resistance that takes hard work to overcome so that the SMA program can get started.
- The first group visits will likely be the most difficult to launch successfully because, at the inception of the program, providers, champion, program coordinator, and support staffs alike will largely be unfamiliar with SMAs and how to run them. Clearly, learning curves for all concerned will be at their steepest at the beginning of the program; however, things should gradually get easier over time, as interested providers and staff are able to sit in and observe SMAs that have already been established and are being successfully run.
- Because group visits are often counterintuitive and represent a major paradigm shift that introduces a great deal of change, it is likely that many beginner's mistakes will be made when group visits are first being launched and implemented within the system—design flaws that will need to be corrected as soon as they are recognized.
- Effective training programs will need to be developed for all SMA personnel, and this training will need to be embarked upon from the start of the program—i.e., with the first SMA teams selected.
- Initial group visit teams will need to be carefully selected and properly trained. Furthermore, they will need to gain hard-earned practical experience firsthand during their initial SMA sessions—which is particularly important as there will not yet be other successful group visits up and running that they can sit in on and learn from.
- It is likely that many operational, administrative, personnel, training, facilities, IT, and equipment problems will surface during the early stages of the group visit program—all of which will need to be successfully addressed (later on, dealing with such problems will become *second nature*).
- From the beginning, one needs to develop an effective *pipeline* (which is fully discussed in the final chapter of this book) for efficiently launching all subsequent DIGMAs and Physicals SMAs throughout the system—a process that can be very time consuming (especially at first, when the pipeline is initially being developed) and fraught with errors.
- It is in the beginning of the SMA program that one will likely need to design, run, and evaluate a meaningful pilot study—and afterward commence moving the SMA program toward facility- and organization-wide implementation.
- Each DIGMA will become easier to fill over time as evermore patients attend and are willing to return for their follow-up care.

I have found that, if the physician walks into a group room and sees 10–16 patients in attendance for the DIGMA, it will almost certainly be a success—as it will likely be lively, interactive, fast-paced, fun, and economically viable. On the other hand, if only 3–5 patients are present, the DIGMA will almost certainly be a failure (and will likely also be boring)—even if the physician is one of the very best—because more patients could have been seen individually in the clinic during the same amount of time, and without the overhead expense of the SMA program.

Not only are the initial SMAs the most difficult to develop, but it has also been the author's experience that SMAs seldom migrate with any meaningful speed throughout the system to other providers' practices by word-of-mouth recommendations alone. In today's fast-paced healthcare environment, physicians are simply too busy managing their own practices to take much note of their colleagues' successes. It therefore takes a champion (with the help of a program coordinator), at least in larger systems, to advance the SMA program rapidly throughout the system—i.e., by continuously recruiting additional providers and helping them to successfully launch their own group visits.

Develop a Critical Mass of Successful SMAs at Each Facility

Eventually, a critical mass of successful SMAs will ultimately become operational at a given site—thus enabling group visits to become more and more accepted by patients, physicians, and staff alike. As this progressively happens over time, first at a given site and eventually system-wide, SMAs will move gradually into the mainstream of medical care within the organization—i.e., through the efforts of the champion and positive word-of-mouth recommendations from patients as well as physician colleagues already successfully running SMAs for their practices becoming more commonplace. Of course, achieving this result requires that the program be actively promoted by the champion, fully supported by administration, properly run, and appropriated evaluated over time so that its merits can be clearly measured and demonstrated. In addition, it also requires that all SMAs be carefully designed, actively promoted to patients, appropriately housed and staffed, and properly run—and that any system or operational problems be promptly addressed as they arise.

By the time this critical mass of group visits is achieved: SMA teams and support staffs will be familiar with the program and experienced in conducting their responsibilities; promotional materials and templates for the program will be developed; patients will have become increasingly aware and accepting of SMAs; positive comments and recommendations from SMA physicians will be commonplace; and, as a result, other physicians should gradually become more willing to try a DIGMA, CHCC, or Physicals SMA for their own practices. In other words, the whole recruitment and implementation process should gradually become easier overtime, until the supply of providers capable of being persuaded to run a SMA for their practices at that time is ultimately *tapped out* at that facility. Despite this success, it is important to note that ongoing vigilance will nonetheless be required in order to ensure that pre-established census targets for each and every SMA session continue to be met—as having all group sessions consistently full remains an ongoing requirement for success.

Step 20: Determine How Many SMAs You Want to Launch Each Year

It is important, once a successful pilot study has been completed, to determine how rapidly you want to disseminate the SMA program throughout the facility and organization. More specifically, you need to determine how many DIGMAs, CHCCs, and PSMAs you want to develop and launch each year in primary and specialty care (at each facility and throughout the organization). Once you have established your target for the number of new SMAs that you want to launch each year, you must then consistently meet this target each and every year. Having such a launch rate target not only optimizes the speed with which SMAs can be implemented throughout the system, but also allows the champion, administration,

and program coordinator to plan their SMA program's budget (e.g., the rate at which behaviorists, documenters, nursing personnel, and dedicated schedulers will need to be hired or secured). In order to determine this annual launch rate, you will need to first examine how long it will realistically take you to develop and launch a single DIGMA or Physicals SMA in your system.

Meeting this target regarding how many DIGMAs and PSMAs to launch each year will require that the champion recruits providers to run SMAs in their practices on an ongoing basis. To accomplish this, the champion will need to give departmental and grand rounds presentations in both primary care and the various medical and surgical subspecialties on an ongoing basis—and to meet individually with interested providers throughout the organization. Working closely with administration to select the most important sites and best possible physician candidates, the champion preferentially selects busy providers with heavy workloads and severe access problems; however, they must be providers who are highly respected by their peers.

What Is a Realistic Timetable for Launching a Single DIGMA or PSMA in Your System?

Healthcare organizations interested in developing a SMA program and implementing it system-wide as rapidly as possible often ask, once the pilot has been demonstrated to be successful, how quickly can the champion be expected to move DIGMAs and PSMAs forward throughout the organization. The first step in answering this question lies in understanding how long it typically takes to develop and launch a single DIGMA or PSMA—i.e., once experience and comfort has been gained with these new group visit models and the *pipeline* for launching them has been developed (as discussed in Chapter 11).

Through extensive experience in acting as champion, the amount of time that it typically takes (i.e., to go from recruiting a provider and early discussions, through the design and training phases, through the entire pipeline, and ultimately to the start of the first SMA session) averages approximately 8–12 weeks once experience is gained and the *bugs* are worked out of the system.

The Champion Can Help Launch the DIGMA or PSMA by Temporarily Acting as Behaviorist

Once the DIGMA or Physicals SMA is launched, the champion (especially if the champion is an experienced psychologist or social worker) can then assist the physician as needed during the first 1–2 months of operations in two ways. First of all, the champion can possibly act as the behaviorist in the SMA for the first session or two, while the behaviorist-in-training watches and learns. Although optional, this process can be very helpful in setting the SMA up properly from the outset, in keeping the physician relaxed during the first couple of sessions, and in avoiding many common beginners' mistakes. After the first session or two, the champion is then able to switch roles and observe the behaviorist replacement in action—who then acts as the behaviorist from that point forward.

The Champion Can Also Debrief After Sessions with the Physician and SMA Team for the First 2 Months

The second way that the champion can assist the physician during the initial launch of the SMA is by debriefing afterwards (perhaps 2 or 3 times) on an as-needed basis with the physician, behaviorist-in-training, nurse/MA(s), and documenter for approximately 10–20 minutes—i.e., after sessions during the first month or two of operations for each new DIGMA or PSMA that is launched. As a SMA champion, I usually try to attend at least 3 different SMA sessions and debriefings for each new DIGMA and PSMA that is launched–typically the first 2 and then another a couple of weeks later. The focus of these debriefings should be upon how to make the next sessions even better and more efficient. This is important because it allows the program to be improved and *fine-tuned* during the first couple of months of operations, and soon enables the DIGMA or PSMA to end on time with full groups—and to do so even if the first couple of sessions happen to finish quite late.

The Champion and Program Coordinator Help in Many Ways During the First 2 Months of Running Each New SMA

During this first month or two of operations, the champion and program coordinator: address all system and operational problems as they arise; constantly monitor group size (to ensure that pre-established census targets are consistently being met); provide additional training to the SMA team and support staff as needed; and do everything possible to assist the physician and keep the physician comfortable and relaxed in the group setting. This

can be very helpful because physicians frequently have many initial misgivings about launching a group visit in their practice. They worry about saying something stupid in front of 15 patients at once, or about not knowing the answer to a question that might be asked. They worry about making mistakes and embarrassing themselves and fear that the group might spiral negatively out of control. Because of these many physician misgivings, the champion and program coordinator can be most reassuring and helpful in getting a new SMA properly launched and operational.

While the strategy being discussed here represents my own preferred way of doing things as SMA champion, it should be noted that there is wide variability as to how involved different champions will want to be with the launching of each new DIGMA or PSMA in their system—and with regard to the timeframes involved as well as the time commitment they are willing to make to the process.

After 2 Months, the Group Visits Should Be Operating Smoothly Enough for the Champion to Disengage and Start the Next Cohort of SMAs

After approximately 1 or 2 months (i.e., once the behaviorist is trained, any operational problems are resolved, the SMA is running smoothly, census targets are being fairly consistently met, the physician is comfortable with the program, the SMA is starting and ending on time with all documenting done, and debriefing after sessions is no longer necessary), the champion then exits from this initial SMA—which is usually part of the start-up cohort of SMAs—to develop and launch the next cohort of DIGMAs and PSMAs with other providers in the organization (more on this later in this section). It is important to note, however, that neither the champion nor the program coordinator ever fully disengages from any DIGMA or PSMA which has been launched, as they will remain ever vigilant over time to ensure that pre-established census targets are consistently being met—and to take prompt corrective action should census ever begin to drop or operational problems emerge that go unresolved.

The Total Time It Takes to Completely Establish a Successful New SMA Is Therefore Approximately 2–3 Months, Plus 1–2 Months of Follow-Up Attention

As can be seen from the previous discussion, the time that it takes (from start to finish) to launch a single DIGMA or PSMA in primary or specialty care is approximately

2–3 months: from the time a motivated physician is first recruited; through the SMA's design, development, and training stages; and through the time that it takes for the DIGMA or PSMA to actually be launched. Then, it typically takes an additional 1–2 months of the champion and program coordinator's time for: the *bugs* to get worked out; any mistakes to be corrected; the behaviorist to become fully trained; the program to become properly established and run; and the SMA to consistently finish on time with full groups and all chart notes completed. Only then can the champion exit the initially established cohort of DIGMAs and PSMAs to launch yet other cohorts of SMAs with still other providers in primary and specialty care.

However, it is important to note that there can be overlap, as the recruitment and training of the next cohort of providers can be occurring concurrently with the debriefing sessions held with the first cohort during the 1–2 months of follow-up that the champion and program coordinator provide. In addition, the various SMAs in a cohort do not all have to be launched at the same time; instead, they can be implemented on a staggered basis. I have even run such cohorts back-to-back with little or no time between them, so that the end result is an almost continuous launching of DIGMAs and PSMAs—i.e., one after another.

How Rapidly Can You Disseminate Your SMA Program Throughout the Organization?

Integrated healthcare delivery systems will undoubtedly want to estimate how many group visits they can realistically expect to be able to launch in any given year.

Working at an aggressive but realistic pace, a skilled and experienced half- to full-time champion with a program coordinator should be able to establish between 18 and 36 primary and specialty care DIGMAs and PSMAs per year within the organization–i.e., working at maximum speed and a very aggressive pace. For example, while working half-time as Director of Clinical Access Improvement at the Palo Alto Medical Foundation (PAMF), I founded and headed their SMA Department. In this capacity, I worked half-time as champion and was charged with the responsibility of launching 18 DIGMAs and PSMAs per year in primary and specialty care throughout PAMF's various facilities. The remainder of my workweek was spent consulting with healthcare organizations around the country. I launched a similar number of DIGMAs and PSMAs during my first year at Harvard Vanguard Medical Associates/Atrius Health

while working half-time, and expect to launch 30 more next year while working three-fourths time.

By launching programs at this rate, the result was 18, 36, and 54 SMAs launched throughout the PAMF system after 1, 2, and 3 years, respectively. Of course, the net number of functioning SMAs at any given time would then be this number less the number of implemented DIGMAs and PSMAs that had been lost due to a variety of causes—the most important of which was inadequate census, although there were also many other reasons (such as the SMA providers leaving the system, retirements, long absences on year-long sabbaticals, and changing physician and departmental needs).

Under ideal circumstances, large healthcare organizations wanting to aggressively launch SMAs at the fastest possible rate might be able to implement as many as 36 DIGMAs and Physicals SMAs per year. This would only apply to larger systems having a highly skilled and experienced full-time champion who is supported by administration and has an experienced program coordinator providing critically important assistance (plus having adequate SMA personnel and facilities, and sufficient provider and patient buy-in at each facility). If there was a single full-time champion for the entire system, then there could be as many as 36 newly launched SMAs annually in combination across all facilities. On the other hand, if the champion worked less than full time, the pace of rolling out new DIGMAs and PSMAS under ideal circumstances would be proportionately less–such as a half-time provider launching 18 SMAs per year (and most likely, even less).

However, if there was a different SMA site champion trained by the champion at each large facility within the organization having say more than 20 providers (i.e., so as to have one overall champion overseeing the work of all the site champions at the various facilities), then many additional DIGMAs and PSMAs could be launched annually at each facility—i.e., until all providers at each facility interested in launching one or more DIGMAs and/or PSMAs per week have been *tapped out*. Usually, when I am the SMA champion at a larger integrated delivery system, I try to personally launch the first 3-5 DIGMAs and PSMAs at each site before turning things over to the site champion. By doing so, there are then several successful SMAs being run at that site which other interested providers (and SMA team members) can sit in on and learn from. When site champions are utilized, the overall SMA champion can hold monthly meetings (i.e., with all of the SMA site champions present) to exchange helpful tips and discuss problems, difficult situations, progress, and what has been learned at each of the sites.

On the other hand, organizations preferring a slower, more comfortable pace for launching shared medical appointments might instead choose to have the champion launch substantially fewer SMAs annually—i.e., being especially careful to ensure that each DIGMA or PSMA that is launched is done correctly.

How Many DIGMAs and PSMAs Can Be in the "Pipeline" at Once?

Depending upon how well the *pipeline* is set up by the champion and program coordinator (and upon whether they work full time or not, as well as the demands and opportunities of the moment), there could be anywhere from 3 to 12 DIGMAs and/or PSMAs being developed with staggered start dates in the system's *pipeline* at any one time—although I find approximately 6–8 to be the most common number. This number of SMAs simultaneously in the pipeline at any given time depends strongly upon the champion's skillfulness, the helpfulness of the program coordinator, and the champion's mandate from administration regarding the number of SMAs that are to be launched annually. It also depends upon the number of physicians willing to participate that happen to be recruited during any particular timeframe.

Although the number of programs in the pipeline at any one time will vary widely, the most aggressive number for a full-time champion appears to involve launching approximately 1½ to 3 DIGMAs or PSMAs per month—at least in systems where the champion's mandate is to launch 18–36 new primary and specialty care SMAs per year. For pipelines that are 10–12 weeks long, this generally translates to an average of between 4 and 9 DIGMAs and/or PSMAs being in the pipeline at any given time. As previously discussed, most systems and SMA champions will prefer a more relaxed rollout pace than this—often involving substantially smaller numbers than those being discussed here. Be certain to read the final chapter of this book with all due diligence in order to ensure that you set up your *pipeline* as correctly as possible.

Launching SMAs at This Aggressive Pace Requires Experience—and that All Necessary Resources Be in Place

Naturally, this aggressive of a launch rate can only be achieved after considerable experience has been gained, promotional materials and all templates for the SMA program have been developed, ongoing physician and staff buy-in are achieved, the necessary scheduling of patients is occurring, and all necessary operational and administrative supports for the program are in place. In addition, as will be discussed later in this book, a comprehensive SMA *pipeline* will need to be developed for the program by the champion and program coordinator—i.e., a detailed, replicable, and step-by-step guide for efficiently and systematically launching all future DIGMAs and Physicals SMAs within the system.

In addition, rolling out DIGMAs and PSMAs at the aggressive pace of 18 or more per year in larger systems requires that the following resources also be in place: the best possible champion and program coordinator (with adequate time dedicated to the program); appropriate behaviorists (approximately one half-time behaviorist for every 9–10 weekly DIGMAs and PSMAs implemented); dedicated scheduling personnel (approximately one dedicated scheduler for every 15–25 DIGMAs and PSMAs implemented to ensure that full group sessions are consistently achieved and that the profit margin for the SMA program is thereby protected); one or two nursing personnel per DIGMA and PSMA (RN or LVN nurses, medical assistants, nursing techs, etc.); a documenter (whenever possible, especially for PSMAs and systems using electronic medical records); high quality promotional materials; and the necessary group and exam room facilities. All of these supports and resources must be budgeted for and made available as needed to the SMA program on an ongoing basis.

Three Different Approaches to Full-Scale Implementation in Large Systems with Multiple Sites

Depending on the size of the managed-care organization and the number of separate facilities they have (as well as the number of providers at each site), there are at least three different ways in which the champion might approach full-scale SMA implementation.

First, There Is the "One Facility at a Time" Approach

In this approach, the champion focuses upon one facility at a time—and eventually sets up as many SMAs as possible at that facility. This process of launching SMAs at that facility would continue until all physicians that can be recruited at that time to start DIGMAs or Physicals SMAs (i.e., for their own practices or for various chronic illness population management programs at that facility) are in fact running SMAs. At that point, the champion can then shift focus from that facility to starting SMAs in the next highest priority facility within the system—and then, after that, the next highest priority facility, etc.—until all facilities have been covered. This process should ideally occur in some sort of logical sequence, preferably by starting with high-priority sites having motivated providers, heavy workloads, serious backlogs, and severe access problems. Naturally, the champion and program coordinator will need to generate periodic reports on an ongoing basis that will continuously evaluate all established SMAs at each facility.

Consider Training a SMA Site Champion at Each Site Before Moving on to the Next Facility

In addition, the champion might want to select and train a SMA site champion at that facility before moving on to the next site—i.e., so that the site champion can continue to encourage providers to run SMAs (or more SMAs) in their practices. It is possible that, over time, certain newly hired physicians as well as some highly resistant physicians at that site might ultimately be willing to run a SMA for their practice through the ongoing efforts of the SMA site champion.

The First Facilities to Launch SMAs Will Likely Be the Most Difficult

For many of the same reasons that the first few SMAs launched at any given facility are likely to be the most challenging, time consuming, and difficult to establish, the first facilities within a multisite organization to launch a DIGMA and PSMA program and move it toward full-scale implementation will likely involve the most difficulty, the most effort, and the most physician and staff resistance. As experience is gained in this new paradigm of care—and as positive word-of-mouth reports about the program's success start to occur and become more commonplace from patients, staff, and colleagues alike—implementation at each successive site is expected to become progressively easier over time (except for any sites that might remain particularly resistant and hostile toward group visits). Positive reports from patients and physician colleagues, accumulating experience gained at the various facilities already running SMAs, and the champion's continuing efforts to promote the program to patients and staff alike should eventually all converge to successfully spread the SMA program throughout the entire system. However, the word of caution here is that the forward momentum of the SMA program could become bogged down and stalled if the champion and program coordinator's attention needs to constantly be turned backward to dealing with previously established SMAs that are continuously failing to meet census targets.

Subsequent Facilities Should Become Progressively Easier Over Time

Therefore, one can reasonably anticipate that future SMA launches at successive sites should gradually, but progressively, become easier and easier over time—i.e., provided that the initial launches at previous sites have gone well and are successful. In other words, full implementation at the first facility is expected to be the most difficult, with implementation at each successive site becoming progressively easier—until marketing efforts for the program by the champion and positive reports from colleagues and patients alike combine to reach a *critical mass* that helps to spread group visits throughout the entire integrated healthcare delivery system. Of course, this will only occur if positive reports and recommendations begin to surface throughout the organization; therefore, be careful to solve any census problems that might occur in the SMA program just as promptly as possible so that negative reports do not begin to circulate.

If You Cannot Fill Weekly DIGMAs or PSMAs, It Is Unlikely that Reducing Frequency Will Help

As an aside, it is worth noting that it seldom works to have DIGMAs held every other week if full groups cannot be achieved weekly. Most DIGMAs and Physicals SMAs are designed to meet weekly—or even more often, such as two or three times weekly (and, in some cases, even daily). I have found it very difficult to launch successful DIGMAs and PSMAs designed to meet every other week when the reason for meeting bi-weekly is that weekly groups failed to consistently meet census requirements. Experience has demonstrated that, when the provider has problems meeting census requirements for weekly SMAs, the strategy of holding it bi-weekly or monthly rather than weekly in order to better meet census targets seldom works. Although it is not impossible for this strategy to work, the simple fact is that when providers have difficulty filling a weekly DIGMA or PSMA, it is highly unlikely that these same difficulties will not just carry over to the bi-weekly SMA—so that census requirements continue to not be met even if the frequency of SMA sessions is dramatically reduced.

Instead, try other options that are available to you for increasing group census, such as: opening up the DIGMA or PSMA to a larger group of patients by opting for a more heterogeneous SMA design; redoubling personal invitations by the physician and staff during regular individual office visits to help keep all SMA sessions filled; and/or making better use of the dedicated scheduler, the physician's scheduling staff, and promotional materials.

Second, the Champion Can Choose the "Multiple Facilities at a Time" Approach

In this approach, the champion concurrently starts DIGMAs and PSMAs at multiple facilities within the system, and then moves back and forth between sites on a staggered basis (as well as between departments within each site) according to the level of need and physician interest. Although it involves some inefficiency due to travel time, this is the approach that I used in heading the Shared Medical Appointment Department at the Palo Alto Medical Foundation, which is an integrated healthcare delivery system in California that is largely fee-for-service (but partially capitated) in nature and involves a large main campus and several smaller satellite clinics. I am also currently utilizing this *multiple facilities at a time* approach at the various medical centers of Harvard Vanguard Medical Associates/ Atrius Health throughout eastern Massachusetts.

Third, There Is the "Champion of Champions" Approach for Large Systems with Multiple Sites

For larger systems with multiple large facilities, executive leadership might choose to proceed with yet another method for rapidly disseminating a SMA program throughout the organization—one which might best be called a *champion of champions* approach. This third approach to widespread implementation could possibly be used in the largest integrated delivery systems— especially those that have multiple large facilities with perhaps at least 20 or more providers at each site. This approach offers the advantages both of rapid dissemination of the SMA program and of enabling the maximum number of SMAs to be simultaneously launched at various facilities throughout the organization.

In this *champion of champions* approach, most site champions could be psychologists, social workers, nurses, or highly motivated and skilled site administrators. Here, as briefly discussed above, the overall champion responsible for the entire SMA program could select and train a different site champion at each of the major sites within the organization. It is preferable that all such site champions at the various facilities be interested in working closely with physicians and medical patients (and not just with mental health patients), be experienced in running large groups and in working closely with physicians, be able to address the extensive psychosocial needs of medical patients and their families, and be very knowledgeable of the various SMA models (including their respective strengths, weaknesses, flow patterns, and how to set them up). In addition, it is important to the success of the SMA program that both the overall champion and

the various site champions have adequate time available on their schedules to dedicate to the SMA program and fully dispatch their respective duties. It would also be possible to use other disciplines than psychologists and social workers as SMA site champions, such as nurse practitioners, diabetic nurse educators, nurses, or highly motivated administrators, etc. However, experienced mental health professionals are often better choices as site champions because of their skill set, scope of practice under licensure, ability to temporarily act as behaviorist in newly launched DIGMAs and PSMAs and often the amount of time that can potentially be made available to them for discharging their responsibilities in this role of site champion. Together with the "Multiple Facilities at a Time" approach, I am also currently employing this "champion of champions" approach at Harvard Vanguard Medical Associates/Atrius Health.

Some Systems Might Want a Physician Champion Overseeing the Program and Reporting to Executive Leadership

It is worth noting that some larger multifacility organizations might also want to have a physician champion with broad oversight responsibilities for the entire SMA program who can act as a liaison with the organization's high-level executive leadership—a physician with the less time-consuming duty of broad oversight responsibility only for the entire SMA program. It is important to note that, in order to be able to report to executive leadership, this physician champion would have only the broadest oversight responsibility for the program—and would not be responsible for the day-to-day operations or administration of the SMA program at various facilities throughout the system. The physician champion in this arrangement would therefore not have the more time-consuming duties of the behavioral health champion, who is recruiting providers, custom designing their DIGMA and PSMA programs, rapidly expanding the program throughout the organization, handling day-to-day administrative and management duties, and dealing with operational challenges to the SMA program at each facility. These duties would continue to fall on the shoulders of the *champion of champions* (plus the program coordinator) in this design.

The SMA Champion Identifies, Selects, and Trains the Best Site Champion at Each Facility

Here, the overall SMA champion would sequentially select, train, and assist a site champion at each major facility within the organization. In general, the champion would personally launch the first 2–7 or so DIGMAs and PSMAs sequentially at each satellite facility within the system in an effort to get the SMA program off the ground correctly at each site. These initial, correctly launched DIGMAs and PSMAs would then become the several *A-teams* established at each site—i.e., which the site champion could then use as training vehicles for all subsequent SMAs to be launched at that site . This would be accomplished by having subsequently interested providers and SMA team members sit in on these established and correctly run DIGMAs and PSMAs for a session or two in order to learn how it is done and to talk with the various A-team providers and SMA team members regarding what to do and how to do it.

After the site champions in training at the various major facilities that the champion has already launched several successful SMAs in have been identified and fully trained (i.e., for continuing to move the SMA program forward at their respective facilities), the overall SMA champion would then move on to launch additional DIGMAs and PSMAs at yet other satellite facilities within the organization. However, the SMA champion would still continue to oversee the work of each of the previously established site champions at their respective facilities on an ongoing basis—providing important advice, training, and assistance to the site champions at these various facilities as needed. Periodic meetings (perhaps held monthly) would then be held on an ongoing basis that include the overall champion and all of the site champions in order to share ideas, solve problems, help one another, share successes, and coordinate efforts.

The Champion and Site Champion Can Sometimes Act as Behaviorist for the First Couple of Sessions

In addition, the organization might want the SMA program's overall champion (or the site champion at that facility) to temporarily act as the behaviorist in 1 or 2 carefully selected DIGMAs or PSMAs at each of the system's various sites—i.e., while the behaviorist replacement is able to observe and learn, so that there are 1 or 2 well-trained behaviorists in the *A-teams* established at each site for demonstration and training purposes. This can continue until the replacement behaviorist and site champion selected at each facility are thoroughly trained and comfortable with their new roles. In this manner, other interested providers at each facility could subsequently simply sit in on one or two of the *A-team's* DIGMA or PSMA sessions in order to see how they are run, how well they are received by patients, and make a more informed determination as to whether or not they

want to run a SMA in their own practice. Of course, once the site champion at any particular facility is fully trained, the overall champion for the program could then leave that site, step out from these *A-team* training DIGMAs and PSMAs, and let the site champion and specially trained behaviorists at that facility fully take over their new roles and responsibilities.

At Larger Facilities, the Site Champions Will Also Need a Site Program Coordinator to Leverage Their Time

Obviously, to do all of the above at larger facilities, the site champion might also need to have a site program coordinator in order to fully leverage the site champion's time—but only if it is anticipated that a large number of SMAs will be launched at that site. In smaller sites, the overall champion's program coordinator might be able to fulfill that function. Once providers already running DIGMAs and PSMAs at a given facility are comfortable with running their SMAs (and the system problems and operational *bugs* have been worked out), the site champion at that facility can then move on to the next cohort of recruited providers that show interest in implementing DIGMAs or PSMAs in their practices (or in a chronic illness treatment program to which they are attached) at that site. This process would proceed at each major facility within the organization in turn until all physicians at each site who can be recruited into running a SMA have been reached.

These Approaches to Rapidly Deploying SMAs Throughout the Organization Keep the Champion from Becoming Bogged Down

As can be seen, whereas the overall champion for the SMA program would quickly become overwhelmed with the extensive responsibilities of running and expanding the group visit program alone in larger healthcare systems (i.e., regardless of whether the *one facility at a time* approach or the *multiple facilities at a time* approach was used), using the *champion of champions* approach—and selecting and training a capable site champion at each facility—makes the champion's job doable. It does this by breaking the champion's duties down by facility into *bite-sized* chunks that are manageable because they can eventually be delegated to, and handled by, the SMA site champions at the various facilities. Furthermore, the *champion of champions* approach also permits the maximum number of DIGMAs and PSMAs to be rapidly launched at various sites throughout the entire system—and at the fastest possible rate.

The SMA Champion Needs to Think Out the Overall Implementation Plan from the Beginning

A SMA champion should therefore carefully consider from the outset what their implementation plan for organization-wide deployment is to be. The implementation plan needs to be developed before actually launching the DIGMA and PSMA program—with a major focus being upon how the champion intends to accomplish rapid organization-wide expansion of the SMA program without getting *bogged down* in the details (i.e., so that the champion is not limited to launching just 20 or 30 SMAs, and then being maxed out). This can be particularly problematic for a physician SMA champion who has her/his own practice and therefore limited time to devote to the SMA program. Instead, the SMA champion needs to develop a system for organization-wide implementation to efficiently launch hundreds or possibly even thousands of DIGMAs and PSMAs over time throughout the entire system—an approach that will likely require not only the best possible program coordinator, but also capable and well trained site champions for the SMA program at each of the integrated healthcare delivery system's major satellite facilities.

Reference

1. Howard B. Minnesota medicine. Minnesota Medical Association, (Minneapolis) 2002, Vol. 85.

Chapter 11
A 10-Week Pipeline for Launching New DIGMAs and PSMAs

It is here, in Chapter 11, that we pull together all of the information and knowledge that we have gained throughout this entire book to create the all-important "pipeline" consisting of all the key steps that are so critical to the successful launching and running of all DIGMAs and PSMAs (many of which apply equally to CHCCs) implemented within the system. The *pipeline* presented here is simply an implementation tool for the champion and program coordinator to use for efficiently launching numerous DIGMAs and PSMAs throughout the entire system as easily and rapidly as possible, and without having to *reinvent the wheel* time and time again. It is important to note that the pipeline that we discuss in this chapter is not to be viewed as static; in fact, you will undoubtedly find it to be constantly evolving and improving over time in your system through continuous process improvement. It is something that the SMA champion and program coordinator will always be updating, streamlining, and modifying as experience is gained and operational issues are addressed. Therefore, the pipeline is best viewed as a work that will always be in progress.

Ultimately unique to each integrated healthcare delivery system, the pipeline is designed to systematize the entire implementation process in an easily replicated manner—and to thereby save time and money in the launching of all new group visits within the system. This is because it enables less-expensive personnel (especially the program coordinator and champion, rather than the physicians launching SMAs for their practices) to do much of the time-consuming work involved with rolling out every new group visit within the system—i.e., developing forms and promotional materials out of templates already developed for the SMA program, identifying and obtaining the appropriate SMA team members, securing the necessary group and exam rooms, training the provider's support staff, etc.

Table 11.1 presents the 10-week pipeline that is proposed here, which you will see is nothing other than an organized series of steps to be taken—in a particular order and time frame—with each and every new DIGMA and PSMA that is launched within the system. There is also an example of a pipeline included in the DVD attached to this book. As can be seen, the pipeline depicted in Table 11.1 is broken down into several distinct time frames: (1) steps to be taken prior to entering the pipeline; (2) steps to be taken during weeks 1 and 2 after entering the pipeline; (3) steps to be taken during weeks 3–5 after entering the pipeline; (4) steps to be taken during weeks 6–8 after entering the pipeline; (5) steps to be taken during weeks 9 and 10 after entering the pipeline; (6) steps to be taken after launching your new DIGMA and PSMA program; and (7) steps to be taken for continuously evaluating your SMA program on an ongoing basis over time.

Although a few of these steps in the pipeline might involve the champion and physician, most will not—because the program coordinator, dedicated scheduler, and behaviorist (often the senior or lead behaviorist for the SMA program rather than the behaviorist attached to the new SMA) can take care of the majority of the steps in the pipeline. The champion is, however, directly involved at several critical points in this pipeline—i.e., those which require the champion's involvement. The same is true of the physician, some of whose time is nonetheless required even though the SMA champion and program coordinator will do everything possible to minimize the physician's *front-end* time commitment to launching his or her new DIGMA or PSMA. This enables the program coordinator (in some cases, with the help of the dedicated scheduler and lead behaviorist) to leverage the time of the physician and champion. This process reflects one of the important underlying tenets of group visits, which is to always delegate tasks, whenever appropriate and possible, to highly skilled and trained—but less expensive—personnel.

E.B. Noffsinger, *Running Group Visits in Your Practice*, DOI 10.1007/b106441_11,
© Springer Science+Business Media, LLC 2009

Table 11.1 Steps of the Pipeline

A. Steps to be taken with each new DIGMA and PSMA prior to entering the pipeline

1. Complete the 20 key steps to a successful SMA outlined in the previous chapter
2. The champion recruits providers on an ongoing basis
3. The champion meets with physician during off-hours to explain SMA program
4. Champion custom designs SMA (model, subtype, time, day, goals, SMA team members, facilities, census levels, etc.) and develops promotional materials
5. The champion explains what the physician's responsibilities will be for the SMA (and physician selects snacks, promotional materials, handouts, chart note template, etc.)
6. The provider is taught how to refer patients into the SMA
7. The provider begins to mark and invite appropriate patients on the daily schedule
8. The physician establishes lists of patients to be invited to the SMA
9. SMA champion and program coordinator meet with the provider and staff to finalize the custom design of the group visit (to educate everyone about the SMA, their duties, and the need for specific training), which triggers entry into pipeline

B. Weeks 1 and 2 after entering the pipeline

1. All major details of the provider's SMA are established, including the start date
2. DIGMA or PSMA is placed on the schedules of provider and entire SMA team (physician starts inviting patients)
3. Arrange clinic coverage in advance to avoid emergency interruptions during SMA
4. Reserve the group and exam rooms
5. Determine the provider's actual pre-SMA productivity during normal clinic hours
6. Obtain a list of all patients on the provider's panel by diagnosis
7. Continue training provider on how to best word personal invitation to patients
8. Order and mount framed posters onto the provider's lobby and exam room walls (see examples in attached DVD)
9. Order holders for program description fliers and mount them on wall by poster
10. Get two 4×6 foot white boards installed into group room, one with grid lines
11. Select and fully equip a nearby exam room (for DIGMAs and CHCCs)

C. Weeks 3, 4, and 5 after entering the pipeline

1. Establish duties of all support personnel (schedulers, receptionists, nurses, etc.) and provide the necessary training
2. Train all support personnel on how to most effectively invite and schedule patients
3. Staff must continuously schedule patients into SMA—not just into first session
4. Schedulers start making *cold calls* and scheduling patients into initial SMA sessions
5. Provider needs to approve all SMA documents and to select the handouts to be used
6. Discuss billing and documentation protocols with provider, and develop chart note template
7. Set up training sessions for SMA behaviorist and nurse/MA(s) regarding their expanded duties
8. Order required supplies, such as name tags and broad felt markers with dark ink
9. Set up IT infrastructure for computers in group and exam rooms

D. Weeks 6, 7, and 8 after entering the pipeline

1. Print the appropriate number of copies of all forms to be used in the SMA
   a. Program description flier (see examples on attached DVD)
      i. Give provider temporary fliers immediately (approximately 300 copies)
      ii. Initially order or print a relatively small number of final fliers
      iii. A bulk order for the finalized flier is placed later
      iv. Fill flier holders in provider's lobby and exam rooms
      v. Select a staff person to keep flier holders full
      vi. Train MA to promote SMA and give flier to all appropriate patients as they are roomed
   b. Announcement letter (see examples on attached DVD)
      i. Order or print enough copies to mail to all appropriate patients
      ii. Order any inserts to be included in this mailing
      iii. Establish the mailing date(s) for the announcement (perhaps 50 per week)
      iv. Send announcement to all appropriate patients
   c. Invitation letter (see examples on attached DVD)
      i. Make approximately 300 copies to start with
      ii. Receptionists begin giving the invitation letters to all appropriate patients during regular office visits
      iii. One receptionist is assigned to notify the program coordinator when invitations are running low
2. Install two functional computers (a desktop for documenter and a laptop for physician), a printer, and a phone in the group room
3. Develop provider's chart note template for the SMA (an EMR chart note template is often developed for SMA Department for primary care and each medical and surgical subspecialty)

Table 11.1 (continued)

    a. Be sure the provider and documenter are well trained in using this template for:
       i. Paper chart notes, or
       ii. EMR chart notes
       iii. A documenter can optimize charting and billing
    b. Ensure the provider's chart note template is acceptable to documentation as well as billing and compliance leadership
    c. Have documenter examine ~30 of providers current chart notes and then shadow provider 1–2 days (drafting individual chart notes for provider to review)
4. Start monitoring the census of the new provider's SMA on a weekly or twice-weekly basis
    a. Weekly or twice-weekly pre-booking census reports generated by the program coordinator enable the champion to run the SMA program
    b. As needed, coach and train the physician and staff to better refer patients
    c. If upcoming sessions are still not filling, then meet again with the physician and all scheduling staff to continue training
    d. Persist with training until the first session is full and initial sessions are filling well—otherwise, postpone the start date
    e. Consider using a dedicated scheduler to *top off* sessions and ensure full groups
5. Solve any systems problems as they arise
6. If water, coffee, tea, and healthy snacks are to be provided, then schedule them on an ongoing basis
7. The champion should reassure the provider and staff during this period, addressing any concerns and anxieties
8. Develop the outcome measures and methodologies that will be used to evaluate the SMA program, and issue periodic reports
    a. Measure the unique strengths of the group visit model you are using
    b. Also measure the multiple common benefits offered by group visits in general
    c. What tests, measurements, and methodologies will be used—and how will the data be analyzed?
    d. Will you want to access, productivity, measure improvements in quality, clinical outcomes, productivity, access, cost savings, practice or chronic disease management, etc.?
    e. It is generally easier to measure outcomes, cost savings, etc. with CHCCs than DIGMAs and PSMAs—especially the heterogeneous model
    f. Be practical, measure what is easiest and most important, and try to issue monthly, quarterly, and/or annual reports

E. Weeks 9 and 10 after entering the pipeline
1. Hold final training for all support personnel as needed (receptionists, nursing personnel, and all scheduling personnel including the call center)—review census and everybody's roles and responsibilities
2. Check daily to see how many patients are scheduled for the first four SMA sessions
3. If the census is low, alert the provider and schedulers (plus have the dedicated scheduler call patients)—but postpone the SMA if sessions are not filling properly
4. Assemble *Patient Packets* for all patients attending DIGMAs and PSMAs
5. Address any unresolved issues as they arise prior to the launch
6. Just before the launch, conduct a complete *walk-through* and *mock DIGMA* or *PSMA session* with staff acting as patients—a practice *dry run* to detect and correct any existing defects
    a) The patient flow *walk-through*
    b) The *walk-through* process for DIGMAs
    c) *Walk the visit through* from start to finish
    d) Run the *mock* DIGMA or PSMA
    e) Try to detect and solve any problems in the *mock SMA* as soon as possible
    f) The *mock DIGMA* process
    g) Champion points out common beginners' mistakes that physicians and behaviorists often make
    h) Aligning the motivations of patients and physicians to finish on time
    i) Some of the most common beginners' mistakes that physicians make
    j) Some of the most common beginners' mistakes that behaviorists make
    k) Launch DIGMA or PSMA

F. Steps to be taken after launching your new DIGMA or PSMA
1. Are you successfully finishing on time with all chart notes completed?
2. Be flexible and slowly make changes to the SMA as needed—but do not reduce census targets at first
3. Have all staff involved with the SMA sit in on a session or two on a rotating basis—starting with schedulers (and then the receptionists)
4. Always have all attendees sign the confidentiality waiver
5. Whenever possible, schedule appropriate return visits back into a future SMA session
6. Give after visit summary—including copy of provider's treatment recommendation to patients
7. Personally compliment schedulers, receptionists, and nursing staff whenever SMAs are filled
8. Ensure that all SMA materials are replenished as needed
9. Provider, behaviorist, nurse/MA, documenter, and sometimes champion and/or program coordinator debrief after sessions for first 2 months to evaluate and improve program
10. Monitor census for upcoming sessions on an ongoing basis
11. Have billing and compliance monitor all bills for the SMA program during the first 2 months, and periodically thereafter

Table 11.1 (continued)

G. Continuously evaluate the SMA program

1. Measure patient satisfaction after SMA sessions
2. Evaluate the pilot study and determine whether to expand SMA program organization-wide
3. If the program is to be expanded organization-wide, then determine the number of new SMAs to be launched per year
4. Consistently strive to meet this number of new SMAs launched per year
5. Repeat the entire *pipeline* process for all newly recruited providers
6. Generate weekly (or preferably bi-weekly) pre-registration census reports for all SMAs
7. Activate a plan for promptly filling sessions when census is low
8. Terminate any SMAs that consistently fail to meet minimum census requirements
9. Have champion and program coordinator sit in on ~3 of the initial SMA sessions, plus participate in debriefings afterward
10. Periodically assess physician professional satisfaction with SMA program
11. Produce a monthly productivity report covering the entire SMA program and circulate it to both executive leadership and all SMA providers to give ongoing feedback on program

Steps to be Taken with Each New SMA Prior to Entering the Pipeline

First complete all of the 20 major steps described in Chapter 10, each of which is necessary for developing a successful DIGMA or PSMA program (see Table 10.1). I use the form entitled Description of New DIGMA, for custom designing new DIGMAs. On the other hand, for custom designing new PSMAs, I use both this form and the additional form entitled Description of New SMAs (see DVD). Prior to launching each and every new DIGMA and Physicals SMA in the system, the following steps need to be taken by the SMA champion and program coordinator in order to recruit providers and custom design the SMA program to the physician's particular needs and practice (after which the new DIGMA or PSMA enters the pipeline):

- Champion selects a program coordinator and develops all form and promotional materials for the SMA program (in template form whenever possible
- Champion needs to give presentations at departmental meetings so as to recruit interested primary and specialty care physicians on an ongoing basis
- Champion meets with interested providers (typically outside of clinic hours) to explain DIGMAs and PSMAs and the multifarious benefits they offer
- Champion sits down with each recruited provider to custom design their DIGMA, CHCC, or PSMA—with all due consideration being given to the provider's goals; the preferred SMA model and subtype; the time and day of the week that the SMA will be offered; the facilities and SMA team members to be used; the minimum, target, and maximum census levels for the SMA; whether snacks be served and, if so which ones, etc.
- Champion explains physician's responsibilities when running a DIGMA or PSMA—especially how to refer and schedule patients into the SMA so as to consistently fill sessions
- Physician begins to invite all appropriate patients seen during individual office visits
- Physician establishes lists of patients that can appropriately be invited to the SMA (for later use by scheduling staff and dedicated schedulers)
- Physician works with champion and program coordinator to customize the promotional materials, Patient Packets, educational handouts, chart note template, etc. from existing SMA Department templates

After all of the above have been completed, the SMA champion and program coordinator meet with the provider, the various SMA team members, and key support staff members to finalize the custom design of the provider's group visit program (and to educate all about the flow of the SMA, everyone's responsibilities and duties in it, and the need for specific training)—which triggers entry into pipeline.

Weeks 1 and 2 After Entering the Pipeline

We turn next to all of the steps that occur during the first 2 weeks after the provider's DIGMA or PSMA enters the pipeline.

All Major Details of the Provider's SMA Are Established, Including the Start Date

At this previously discussed meeting that signals entry into the pipeline (which is scheduled with the physician, champion, program coordinator, SMA team, and the physician's own nurse MA and support staff), all of the important details regarding the provider's upcoming

DIGMA or PSMA need to be discussed, resolved, and approved by the physician (some of which may already have been determined during earlier meetings between the physician and champion)—including the following:

i. Champion to start meeting off by giving a brief explanation of the basics about group visits, the many benefits they can offer, and the fact that this is a team-based approach to care in which all must play their part—as each person's contributions are important.

ii. Which subtype of the model (i.e., homogeneous, mixed, or heterogeneous) is to be used and precisely what types of patients are (and are not) to be included in the various SMA sessions.

iii. The physician's reasons, goals, and objectives for running the SMA must be clearly stated to enlist the help of the support staff.

iv. The minimum, target, and maximum census levels for the program need to be determined—and the important, ongoing role that everyone needs to play in consistently achieving full groups is emphasized. Remember to overbook sessions by the expected number of no-shows and late-cancels to make the SMA immune to these challenges.

v. The frequency, length, time of day, and the day of the week that the DIGMA or PSMA is to be held need to be determined.

vi. The group and exam rooms to be utilized are selected.

vii. Will snacks be served and, if so, what snacks and who will be responsible for obtaining them?

viii. If a PSMA is being implemented, how will patients be scheduled and how far in advance is the Patient Packet to be sent? In addition, all details surrounding the Patient Packet need to be determined: what patients should attend; when should they be scheduled; what materials will be enclosed in the Patient Packet; who will assemble and mail them; who will receive the completed health history forms; what follow-up system will be put in place to ensure that patients return their completed health history forms to the office (and that someone enters this information into the PSMA chart note) plus complete their blood urine screening tests prior to the session;

ix. Consensus needs to be achieved regarding the start date for the DIGMA or PSMA.

x. The specific roles and responsibilities of the support staff (receptionists, schedulers, office manager, etc.) and the expanded duties of the SMA team (behaviorist, nurse/MA, documenter, and dedicated scheduler) need to be discussed and explained—and any necessary future training sessions need to be scheduled at this time, training that will be lead by the champion and/or program coordinator. If any members of the SMA team are as yet unidentified, then suitable candidates should be discussed (and hopefully selected) at this time.

xi. The importance of all staff promoting the program and inviting patients is emphasized, and various patient invitation materials (including a preliminary invitation letter and telephone scripts) can be distributed. (Samples of the invitation letter and telephone script are included in the Important SMA Department Forms section of the attached DVD.)

xii. Any anticipated system, facilities, IT, equipment, or personnel problems that are expected to occur need to be discussed and resolved.

xiii. The provider is asked to select (or create) any handouts that are to be used in the SMA and to develop a chart note template for the program.

xiv. The time line for launching the SMA is laid out and discussed in this interactive meeting—i.e., in which all staff are encouraged to speak and openly discuss any concerns they may have (all of which need to be addressed by the champion, physician, and program coordinator).

xv. Any details regarding the provider's DIGMA or PSMA that are not fully resolved during this meeting will need to be addressed by the champion, program coordinator, and physician just as quickly as is realistically possible afterward.

The DIGMA or PSMA Is Placed on the Schedules of the Entire SMA Team (Physician Starts Inviting Patients)

A new template of the physician's master schedule, which includes all changes necessary to accommodate the DIGMA or PSMA, needs to be created by the program coordinator and then given to the physician for approval. Once the template is approved by the provider, the provider's master schedule is submitted to scheduling management by the program coordinator so that it can be approved and updated (and once it is approved, the physician starts inviting all appropriate patients seen during normal office visits to upcoming SMA session). In a similar manner, the program coordinator needs to place the DIGMA or PSMA on the master schedules of the behaviorist, nurse/MA(s), and documenter (if one is to be employed)—beginning with the projected start date and continuing thereafter on an ongoing basis.

The nurse/MA(s) master schedules are somewhat different from the master schedules of the rest of the SMA team because they usually arrive 15–30 minutes early to begin their expanded SMA nursing duties on the patients who arrive early. They continue this process even after the session has started, until all vital signs, routine health maintenance, injections, and special nursing duties have been completed on all patients—at which time the nurse/MA(s) are then free to return to normal clinic duties. However, some providers prefer to have a nurse, especially if it is the provider's own nurse, join the group at that time in order to help out in any way that they can—such as acting as a *go-for* or demonstrating certain types of musculoskeletal exercises.

If two nursing personnel are used (which is something that I generally recommend, especially if this resource is available to the provider, as nurses and medical assistants tend to like having the companionship of a colleague), then their SMA duties can be divided between them by interest, skill level, and scope of practice under licensure—and all SMA nursing duties can thereby be finished in approximately half the time. After completing these duties, the MA can recheck any high blood pressures and then become the care coordinator (i.e., scheduling all referrals and follow-ups recommended by the physician, and then giving the patient an "after visit summary" of her/his chart note).

A full 2 hours should be blocked off the master schedule of the physician, behaviorist, and documenter during the first 2 months of the DIGMA or PSMA—not only because these initial sessions will likely finish late, but also because this will allow 15–20 minutes for the treatment team to debrief after sessions for the first couple of months. It is helpful for the champion and the program coordinator to also be scheduled to attend approximately three of the initial SMA sessions, and to debrief occasionally with the physician and SMA team during the first couple of months of implementation.

After the first 2 months, the master schedules of the physician and documenter should only allow 90 min for sessions; however, the behaviorist will continues to need 2 hours for the SMA on an ongoing basis. This is because the behaviorist needs to arrive approximately 15 minutes early to greet patients, warm the group up, and write their health concerns down on a whiteboard—and then to stay approximately 15 minutes after sessions to address any last-minute non-medical questions patients might have (e.g., "Where do I go for the smoking cessation class, depression program, and colonoscopy that the doctor recommended?"). Then, the behaviorist tactfully clears the room and quickly straightens the group room up for the next SMA to be held therein. Also, the nursing personnel might require less time (especially when two nurses are used), although they will need to enter 15–30 minutes prior

to the start of the DIGMA session (or even as much as 45 minutes in the case of a PSMA) in order to begin dispatching nursing duties as quickly as possible on early arrivers. Two nursing personnel (usually one at the RN or an LVN level, and the other at an MA or nursing tech level) should be able to complete their expanded nursing duties on all patients within 30–45 minutes, whereas a single nurse or medical assistant might require as much as 60–90 minutes in order to finish all nursing duties. The important point to notice here is that the master schedules of all nursing personnel associated with DIGMAs and PSMAs need to be offset from that of other SMA participants because the nurse(s) and/or MA(s) enter the session early and then usually complete their nursing duties during the first half of the DIGMA or PSMA. The exceptions here are the MA who becomes a *care coordinator* approximately half way into the SMA session and the doctor's own nurse (who might join the SMA group during the latter part of the session in order to help the physician).

Arrange in Advance for Clinic Coverage During SMA Sessions

It is a very good idea to arrange well in advance for clinic coverage during the time that the provider will be running the DIGMA or PSMA so as to avoid unnecessary interruptions while the session is being run. Although there is the possibility of an emergency interruption that will, on rare occasion, need to be handled by the physician during a SMA session, our goal here is to keep all such interruptions to an absolute minimum. To do otherwise would be to: (1) undercut the SMA program's remarkable efficiency and productivity gains; (2) frustrate both patients and the SMA team, who would now be left for a period of time without the physician; and (3) decrease the high level of physician professional satisfaction with the program (as physicians really appreciate being able to focus upon their patients and having this time away from normal clinic distractions and interruptions). Along a similar line, the entire SMA team will need to understand that they will also be responsible for arranging for cross-coverage whenever they are unable to attend the DIGMA or PSMA due to leave, meetings, or vacation. However, when it comes to last minute cancellations such as those due to sudden illness, this is something that the program coordinator can help in arranging once contacted by the sick SMA employee (i.e., behaviorist, documenter, or nurse) as backup behaviorists, nurses, and documenters need to be trained and available at each facility when this happens.

Reserve the Group and Exam Rooms

The group and exam rooms must be reserved on an ongoing basis. Ensure that the group room is of adequate size (i.e., capable of seating 15–25 attendees in the case of a DIGMA or 10–15 for a PSMA) and has good ventilation. Ensure that the group room is pleasantly decorated and has an appealing ambiance, that it contains enough comfortable chairs, and that it is fittingly equipped with a telephone, two computers (one for the documenter and another for the physician), and a printer. I also find it helpful to have large wall clocks on at least two (if not, three or four) of the walls in the group room so that physician, behaviorist, and patients alike will all remain cognizant of the time. Also, I like to have two 4×6 foot erasable white boards located at convenient locations on the walls of the group room—one with grid lines and the other without. Then, the behaviorist can use the blank one when writing down patients' health concerns before the start of the group, and the nurse/MA can write down lab results and vital signs on the one with grid lines (with patients names beinh in rows and lab results in columns). Be certain to locate these erasable whiteboards in positions where the behaviorist and nurse have ready access to them, and where the physician and documenter can clearly see them.

For a DIGMA, you will also need a nearby exam room that is properly equipped. PSMAs do not require as large a group room as a DIGMA because fewer patients are in attendance (plus spouses are sometimes not invited, especially in primary care PSMAs that are for males or females of a certain age group only). On the other hand, PSMAs typically necessitate two to five fully equipped exam rooms (and most commonly four); however, unlike DIGMAs, these do not need to be near to the group room and can even be in the physician's own office area—although nearer is better.

Determine the Provider's Actual Pre-SMA Productivity During Normal Clinic Hours

In order to establish the minimum and target census levels for the SMA, the provider's actual pre-SMA productivity data need to be determined (covering the previous 2–6 months, if possible) for the types of individual appointments and patients that the DIGMA or PSMA will replace (see Chapter 10). This will allow the provider's pre-SMA productivity to be determined for the types of appointments that will ultimately be seen in the DIGMA or PSMA—so that the physician's current level of clinic productivity for the same types of patient visits as will be seen in the SMA

can be precisely ascertained. It is this actual pre-SMA productivity for return or follow-up appointments that the DIGMA will most often try to triple, and the actual pre-SMA productivity for private physical examinations that the PSMA will typically try to at least triple.

Notice that we need to determine the average number of patients *actually seen* during 90 minutes of clinic time rather than the number of patients who might have been *scheduled* during that amount of clinic time, as the latter number will always be somewhat higher. This is due to the fact that no-shows, late-cancels, open slots, and some possible downtime on the physician's schedule often combine to reduce the physician's actual productivity substantially below the number of patients that could theoretically be scheduled. Determining this lower number (i.e., actual productivity) enables the percentage increase in the physician's productivity that is gained through the DIGMA or PSMA to be accurately evaluated—with the goal being to triple provider productivity whenever appropriate and possible.

Whenever Appropriate, Try to Increase Productivity by 300%

As previously discussed in detail in Chapter 10, the longer the underlying individual appointment that the DIGMA or PSMA is replacing, the easier it is to leverage a physician's time by 300%. For example, experience has shown that primary and specialty care physicians having 15-minute appointments could schedule up to six patients in 90 minutes of clinic time; however, they typically only see between 3.9 and 4.7 patients on average during that amount of time. Serendipitously, tripling the productivity of such providers results in a range of between 11.7 (i.e., $3 \times 3.9 = 11.7$) and 14.1 ($3 \times 4.7 = 14.1$) patients, which is well within the ideal range of 10–16 patients for a DIGMA—and a perfect target census level to strive for. Similarly, physicians with 20-minute office visits could schedule up to 4.5 patients in 90 minutes, but experience has shown that they typically tend to only see approximately 3.0–4.0 patients.

On the other hand, physicians with 30-minute appointments could schedule up to three patients, but typically only see approximately 1.9–2.6 patients in 90 minutes of clinic time. However, in this latter example of 30-minute office visits, I would nonetheless generally recommend a minimum DIGMA group census of 10 patients in most cases—i.e., even though tripling provider productivity in this case would result in an ideal group size range of between 5.7 and 7.8 patients. I say this because such a low DIGMA census (i.e., of between 5.7 and 7.8 patients) can make for a boring and nonproductive group, whereas

10–16 patients generally makes for a more lively, interactive, interesting, and fun group.

Providers often believe that they see more patients than they actually do and therefore are surprised to see their true clinic productivity numbers being as low as they are. In any case, the true number of patients actually seen by the provider on average during 90 minutes of clinic time (i.e., spent on the types of patients and appointments that will be included in the 90-minute DIGMA or PSMA, and in the same proportion) will first need to be accurately determined for any particular provider before the *minimum* and *target* census levels can be accurately established for their DIGMA or PSMA—with target census levels most commonly being set so as to triple provider productivity over individual office visits.

Obtain a List of All Patients on the Provider's Panel by Diagnosis

A list of all patients who can be identified as being on the provider's patient panel (for example, all of the patients assigned to that provider or all of the patients seen by that provider during the past 2 years) needs to be obtained by the program coordinator—i.e., with the provider's consent, assuming that such a list is available. If possible, this list should be broken down by diagnosis and should also include each patient's medical record number, address, phone number, and date of last visit. Such a list can later be most helpful in ensuring that all SMA sessions are filled to the desired census levels—as such a list can be used by the dedicated scheduler for telephoning and inviting these patients (so as to *top off* the census of any upcoming sessions that might still be below targeted census requirements), but only for those patients and conditions approved by the provider for the SMA.

The program coordinator and dedicated scheduler should, at all times, keep *close tabs* on the number of patient's scheduled for the next four SMA sessions. For DIGMAs, what I like to see is that: (1) this week's session is completely full (and even overbooked by one or two patients in order to compensate for the anticipated number of no-shows and late cancellations, but less the anticipated number of drop-ins); (2) next week's session is $^3/_4$ full; (3) the following week's session is half full; and (4) the week after that is already ¼ filled. For PSMAs, I like to see all sessions completely filled (including any overbooking that has been decided upon) approximately 2–3 weeks in advance of the actual PSMA session. This allows enough time for the Patient Packet (which contains the health history form and lab tests to be completed prior to the session) to be sent to the scheduled patients far enough in advance of the session

for them to complete the detailed health history form as well as all lab tests in a timely manner so that they can then be returned to the office on time (i.e., at least a couple of days prior to the session) and duly entered into each patient's upcoming PSMA chart note.

If these census requirements are not being met for all sessions during the upcoming 3–4 weeks, then the physician, scheduling staff, and dedicated scheduler need to *go into high gear* to ensure that all inadequately filled sessions are promptly filled to targeted census levels (plus an additional patient or two in order to overbook sessions to compensate for the expected number of no-shows and late-cancels, less any anticipated drop-ins). If this happens too often, then the program coordinator and champion will need to provide additional training to the provider as well as the provider's scheduling, reception, and nursing staffs on how to effectively invite and schedule patients into their DIGMA or PSMA. It is imperative that the provider and support staff always take primary responsibility for filling all SMA sessions—and that they not expect this responsibility be assumed by the dedicated scheduler, whose job is to simply *top off* those occasional SMA sessions that are not yet quite full.

Continue Training the Provider on How to Best Word the Personal Invitation to Patients

Because this is the single most important duty of physicians in making their DIGMA or PSMA a success (and because this responsibility is ongoing and will last as long as the SMA is run), it is impossible to overstress to the provider how important personally inviting and referring all appropriate patients into the SMA on an ongoing basis is to the success of the program. From early on, the champion should model to the provider how to effectively invite patients into the SMA—and then, especially during initial meetings with the physician, also role play with the physician several different possible scenarios with patients. A sample script for physicians to use when personally inviting patients to attend their SMA can be found in the previous chapter of this book—i.e., in the section entitled "One Physician's Strategy for Successfully promoting—and filling—all DIGMA Sessions," which appears in "Step 8: Promote the Program Effectively to Patients."

Physicians are not used to taking a personal responsibility in filling their normal clinic schedule. Therefore, they can quickly forget to keep consistently inviting all appropriate patients into their SMA—a failure that could quickly undermine the success of their group visit program. The champion should discuss this all-important concern openly with the provider to see if they can jointly come up with some helpful tips in this regard—such as some type of ongoing reminder for the provider to invite all appropriate patients. For example, in systems still using paper charts, a volunteer or motivated member of the physician's staff could come in each morning to paper clip a copy of the SMA program description flier onto the front cover of the medical charts for all patients appropriate to the SMA who will be seen that day. This will later serve as a reminder for the physician to invite all appropriate patients to the DIGMA or PSMA when the physician eventually meets with them in the exam room later on that day.

All providers interested in running a SMA for their practice must agree to personally invite all appropriate patients seen during normal office visits in a positive manner and to actively involve their entire support staff in the referral and scheduling process. This is extremely important as (1) the most common reason for a DIGMA or PSMA to fail is inadequate census, and (2) nothing is more important in getting a patient to attend a SMA than a personal invitation from their own physician. In addition, the entire support staff (especially the scheduling, reception, and nursing staffs) can also play an important role in filling groups and making the SMA a success; however, they will not be able to adequately compensate for the physician who does not invite all appropriate patients seen during normal office visits. Although the SMA staff (champion, program coordinator, and dedicated scheduler) will do everything possible to minimize each new SMA physician's time outlay in starting and running their SMA, some time and energy will nonetheless be required on the physician's part—i.e., in designing the SMA program, developing promotional materials, selecting handouts, attending training sessions, etc. Plus, the physician must make an ongoing commitment to inviting all appropriate patients seen during normal clinic hours to have their next visit be in their DIGMA or PSMA.

patients to get up and go over to read it—Fig. 11.1 (C); see examples provided on the DVD. Actually, it is meant to generate enough interest in the program so that patients go over to read it, and then take a program description flier from the adjacent flier dispenser—and then read it while waiting in the lobby or exam room. The patient could also read the invitation given to them by the receptionist as they registered for their office visit.

While most systems will want to frame the poster and mount it in a prominent location on the physician's lobby and exam room walls (one that is both highly visible and readily accessible to patients), some organizations prefer to either have them on an easel in these areas or be self-standing by means of an attached cardboard stand on the back of the poster. The poster is often generic (i.e., without the physician's name or unique details about any particular physician's SMA program printed on it), so that the same poster can be used over and over for all DIGMA and PSMA programs—unless different photos are used in the generic poster for adult, pediatric, and obsterics–gynecology patients.

However, if it is a computerized template, then all relevant information about any given provider's SMA can be entered into the template with relative ease—and could therefore also be included on the final wall posters that are printed for that provider. However, in this case a new poster will then need to be printed and displayed whenever any significant change occurs in the physician's SMA—which can be both expensive and time consuming. As soon as copies of the posters are produced and delivered, the program coordinator needs to have them mounted and framed—and then make the appropriate arrangements for having them mounted on the provider's lobby and exam room walls (preferably, in prominent and accessible locations that provide maximum visual exposure to patients).

Order and Mount Framed Posters onto the Provider's Lobby and Exam Room Walls

Copies of the poster that has been developed for the system's DIGMA and PSMA program are ordered for the provider's lobby (approximately 30 by 36 inches) and exam room walls (approximately 20 by 24 inches). Although the same poster is used on both the lobby and the exam room walls, their sizes differ—with the smaller sized poster going onto the exam room walls. Recall that the poster is meant to create a trademark look for the SMA program throughout the system (it can even contain the corporate colors) and that its job is designed to act like a *worker bee* selling the program when no staff is present and encouraging

Order Holders for Program Description Fliers and Mount Them Next to the Poster

The program coordinator needs to order the required number of attractive flier holders for the provider's lobby and exam room walls—dispensers capable of holding at least 100 (and preferably 200) copies of the provider's program description flier. Personally, because they were solid, looked nice, and cost about the same, I preferred to have my flier holders custom made by a local craftsman out of thick, clear plastic with rounded edges—holders that were specifically designed for the fliers that I was actually using—rather than ordering standard holders out of a catalog (which are often thin, flimsy, and not necessarily a good fit to the fliers themselves).

Fig. 11.1 (A–C) depict a graphically coordinated announcement letter (A), invitation letter (B), and wall poster (C)—all of which combine to create a trademark look for the SMA program that is designed to sell the program to patients—even when no staff is present. (Courtesy of Mercy Health Partners, Cincinnati, OH.)

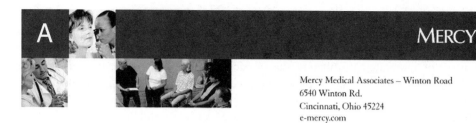

MERCY

Mercy Medical Associates – Winton Road
6540 Winton Rd.
Cincinnati, Ohio 45224
e-mercy.com

Dear Patient,

I would like to introduce a new program at Mercy Medical Associates – Winton Road, designed specifically for patients like you with chronic conditions.

The **Drop-in Shared Medical Appointment Program** provides the opportunity for you to spend up to 90 minutes with me and a small group of other patients with chronic conditions to discuss medical concerns. We also review your recent test results.

The goal of our Shared Medical Appointment program is to provide you with the following:
- timely, high quality medical care
- important medical information
- more time to discuss your concerns
- the opportunity to bring a support person (family member, caregiver, friend, etc.)
- the support of other patients who are dealing with similar issues. You may learn answers to important questions that you might not have thought to ask during previous appointments

I am excited about this new program because a number of patients stated that they preferred these kinds of visits. And there is, in fact, evidence that these types of appointments result in better outcomes.

This program is entirely optional. While many patients prefer group visits, some still choose to have occasional individual office visits — and that is fine!

If you would like to schedule a Shared Medical Appointment or have any questions about our program, please contact one of my staff members at xxx-xxx-xxxx . Information about the program is also available on our website at **www.e-mercy.com**.

Shared Medical Appointments

Because the fliers are meant to form part of an eye-appealing wall display that is graphically coordinated with the poster, this holder should support both sides of the fliers from the front—i.e., high enough up so that the fliers do not droop over, sag, or hang down.

As soon as they are delivered, the program coordinator arranges for these holders to be mounted on the provider's lobby and exam room walls next to the framed wall posters (arrangements that are often made through the organization's facilities department)—i.e., in such a manner that they form a prominent, accessible, and professional appearing display. For those systems choosing to have free-standing posters that are either easel or self-mounted (usually because they lack adequate wall space or because they ban promotional materials from being mounted on the walls of their facilities), the flier holder is typically mounted on the poster itself rather than on the physician's lobby and exam room walls. Such free-standing posters are problematic, however, because they usually are only capable of holding a relatively small number of program description fliers—which often also need to be tri-folded in order to fit into a relatively small

Fig. 11.1 (A–C) (continued)

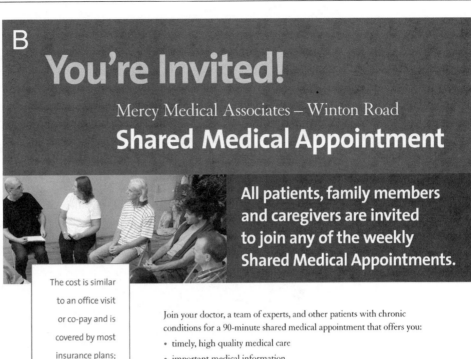

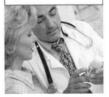

flier holder mounted onto the poster, which represents an additional printing expense.

Weeks 3, 4, and 5 After Entering the Pipeline

During the 3rd, 4th, and 5th weeks after the DIGMA or PSMA enters the pipeline, there are many steps that need to be conducted by the champion and program coordinator—especially by the latter.

Establish the Duties of All Support Personnel (Schedulers, Receptionists, Nurses, etc.) and Provide the Necessary Training

The program coordinator schedules a meeting with the provider (and the provider's office manager, administrator, or operations leader), the champion, and the supervisors of receptionists, schedulers, and nurses in the provider's workplace. The goal of this meeting is to not only secure administrative buy-in, but also establish responsibilities, develop the workflow, and form clear

Fig. 11.1 (A–C) (continued)

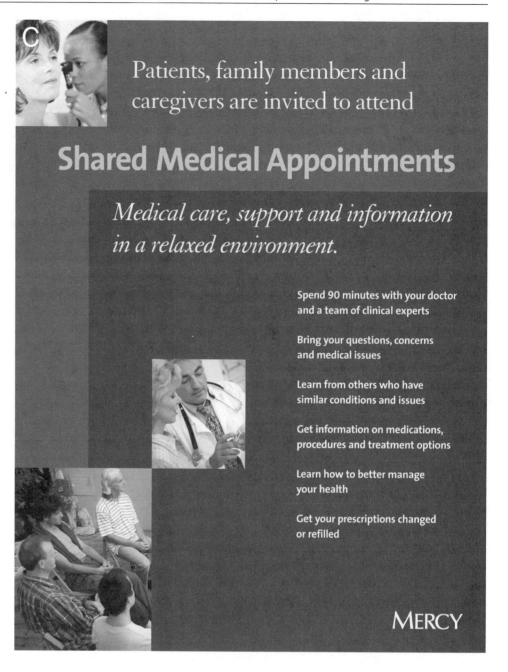

lines of accountability for all support personnel who will be associated with the provider's SMA. During this meeting, the champion also discusses the DIGMA or PSMA program with all of these key administrative personnel and supervisors to ensure that they fully understand: (1) the potential benefits of the program; (2) the physician's desire to see that it succeeds; and (3) that it is very important for all of them to be supportive of the SMA. Questions are to be answered and any resistances addressed. The issue of setting up the IT infrastructure for the computers in group and exam rooms will need to be discussed and resolved. All participants are then asked to sign off on a *statement of work*, which clearly delineates

each person's duties and responsibilities—and establishes accountability (See example in the Important SMA Department Forms section of the attached DVD).

Train All Support Personnel on How to Most Effectively Schedule Patients

The program coordinator needs to subsequently schedule separate training sessions with the physician's receptionists, schedulers, and nurses—all of whom will need to be trained regarding their roles in referring patients (i.e., on how to most effectively invite and schedule patients into the SMA). Often, these training sessions (which are typically run by the program coordinator, sometimes with the assistance of the dedicated scheduler or champion) will need to be done with only half of the schedulers, receptionists, or call center personnel at a time, so that the clinic is still able to function—although this then results in twice as many training sessions. Receptionists must understand that they will be expected, on an ongoing basis, to give an invitation letter to every appropriate patient of the doctors who registers for a traditional individual office visit—along with saying a few kind words about the program (which can be rehearsed and role-played in the training session).

Likewise, the physician's nursing medical assistant staff needs to be responsible for assisting in filling all SMA sessions on an ongoing basis. They should enthusiastically promote the SMA program to all appropriate patients when rooming them during regular office visits—and then give them a program description flier to read while waiting for the physician to enter the exam room. The precise wording of how they recommend the program to patients can be role-played and rehearsed during this training session.

The training meeting(s) with the physician's scheduling staff should include not only on-site scheduling staff, but also any off-site scheduling staff and call center personnel as well (especially any *SMA scheduling angels* selected from the call center, to whom all incoming calls for future appointments with the SMA physician will be directed so that the SMA program can be explained, promoted, and offered to all patients calling in for an appointment)—at least when this is possible. Such meetings can also include the dedicated scheduler attached to the SMA program, who can assist the program coordinator in leading these training sessions for the physician's various scheduling personnel. Sample scheduling scripts as well as talking points can be provided during this training session—a sample of which is included in the DVD attached to this book.

The off-site call center can be particularly problematic for the SMA program because their staff hardly knows anything at all about either the physician or the SMA program—and has minimal, if any, commitment to the program. Furthermore, call center staff is often evaluated based on exactly the opposite criteria from what we would ideally like to have used for the SMA program—i.e., length of telephone queue, average length of call, etc. What we would instead like to see is for the call center personnel to take the extra minute or two necessary to: (1) explain the SMA program to patients in positive terms; (2) answer any patient questions about the program; and (3) schedule appropriate patients into an upcoming SMA session whenever possible. In other words, we would like call center schedulers to take the

extra time necessary to search the computer for next available individual and group appointments, to promote the DIGMA or PSMA program to patients, and to offer patients their choice of either the next available 15–20 minute individual appointment (which might be weeks or months away) or the next available 90-minute group session (which will probably be available that week)—plus add a few positive words about the advantages that the SMA offers to patients. By doing so, the call center can be converted from a potential problem to being a valuable resource in consistently achieving full DIGMA and PSMA sessions.

For this reason, it is advisable to include key call center leadership in the earliest possible meetings when implementing a DIGMA or PSMA program in order to secure buy-in, accountability, and clear lines of responsibility within the call center (i.e., for larger systems having a call center). If possible, try to route all appointment scheduling calls for providers offering DIGMAs and PSMAs through a small number of senior call center personnel having an interest in the SMA program—who could be called *SMA scheduling angels*. They should be selected from the call center's best and most experienced scheduling personnel, especially those showing interest and enthusiasm for the SMA program—and they can then be given the same intense and personalized training as on-site scheduling staff are given.

Designating SMA scheduling angels is helpful because it is easier to train and monitor the efforts of a relatively small number of (i.e., rather than all) call center employees, and then to establish clear lines of responsibility and accountability. This is also true when it comes to arranging for call center personnel—one or two at a time—to actually sit in a DIGMA or PSMA session once it is launched (i.e., so that they can observe its benefits firsthand and later be able to describe and sell the program to patients when they call to schedule an appointment). Here, while it might not be realistic to have all call center personnel sit in a DIGMA or PSMA session, it is usually possible to have a couple of *scheduling angels* selected from the call center attend a session.

Obviously, to be fully effective in referring patients to the SMA, the support staff will need to truly believe in the program—otherwise their body language and tone of voice will reveal their less than enthusiastic endorsement of the program. That is why ample time should be allowed for questions and answers (as well as for addressing any resistances, complaints, or concerns that might exist regarding the SMA program) in these training sessions. In addition, all key support staff should be invited to sit in on one or two SMA sessions just as soon as it is launched and running smoothly—perhaps one or two at a time (typically starting with the most critical scheduling staff, and then including the key reception and nursing staff), so that they can witness firsthand what a wonderful, warm, and caring experience it is for patients.

Staff Needs to Schedule Patients into the SMA on an Ongoing Basis, and Not for Just the First Session

All training sessions with staff that schedules patients into SMAs must emphasize that their scheduling responsibilities will be ongoing. This is because it is not uncommon for scheduling staff to initially get enthused about the DIGMA or PSMA program and to fill the first couple of sessions, but then to gradually lose interest, forget, or turn to competing priorities. When this happens, the inevitable result is that census in subsequent group sessions ultimately begins to decline and dwindle. And once this process of declining census starts, it creates a situation that can deteriorate rapidly—so that future sessions are even less filled by the physician and support staff (and often dramatically less filled).

Be certain to address this challenge and reverse this dangerous trend before insufficient census becomes problematic, which could rapidly result in the SMA's failure. Whenever DIGMA or PSMA sessions start to go unfilled by the physician and support staff, immediate corrective action needs to be taken by the champion and program coordinator—and prompt, appropriate feedback needs to be given to all involved (along with some additional training on scheduling patients into SMAs, if necessary). Again, this is because the physician and support staff—not the dedicated scheduler—must at all times take primary responsibility for filling all SMA sessions.

Start Making "Cold Calls" and Scheduling Patients into the Initial SMA Sessions

It is time to start scheduling patients into the initial DIGMA or PSMA sessions—i.e., just as soon as the start date is established, the provider makes clear which patients are and are not to attend, the computer code for the group visit is entered into the provider's master schedule profile, and all scheduling staff are trained on how to best refer patients. Most patients for the initial group visit sessions will need to be referred by the physician and the physician's support staff according to the protocols developed during the training sessions discussed previously. However, if the provider would like some assistance in this process, the dedicated scheduler could also begin to make some *cold calls* on the physician's behalf to patients on the list(s) provided and approved by the physician.

In larger systems, the program coordinator and champion can also work with the provider to help develop the necessary lists of patients for the dedicated scheduler to call. Although they can still be helpful, cold calls are generally not nearly as successful at recruiting patients into SMAs as personal invitations from the physician and support staff (plus, they often have a higher no-show rate). I say this because it is not uncommon for as many as 10 times as many invitations needing to be made by dedicated schedulers (as compared to personal invitations from the patient's own physician) in order to get a patient to accept, and because the entire process is inefficient anyway because patients are seldom home during working hours (so that *cold call* messages must be left and return calls made). For example, if physicians are 85% successful in inviting patients to attend SMAs, nurses and medical assistants who know the patients might be 40% successful, receptionists knowing the patients might be 20%, and the dedicated scheduler only 5–10% successful through cold calls—as, unlike nurses and receptionists, the patients do not know the dedicated scheduler. This is why it is so important for the physician to assume primary responsibility for filling all SMA sessions.

The dedicated scheduler must be certain to follow up this telephone call with a warm computer-generated or photocopied follow-up letter on the physician's letterhead—a letter initially drafted in template form by the champion and subsequently reviewed, modified, and approved by the physician (see example of a follow-up letter in the Important SMA Department Forms section of the DVD). This letter follows up on the dedicated scheduler's phone call, and it invites/welcomes the patient into the next appropriate DIGMA or PSMA session. This letter can be sent by the dedicated scheduler to all patients contacted by phone—i.e., those who were reached and spoken with as well as those for whom a message was left on their answering machine.

This letter can be personalized by having the patient's name inserted at several points in the text and by including the physician's computer-generated signature at the bottom (plus a small photo of the physician with a pleasant smile, if so desired). Or else, it could simply be photocopied from a signed original that has been approved by the provider. It also contains all necessary details about the SMA program, including when and where it is held, the amount of the co-payment, and how to register. When it is computer-generated (although it can also be simply photocopied, which would result in a less personalized follow-up letter), the letter and accompanying envelope can be efficiently produced with minimum cost. This is done by having the dedicated scheduler simply input a small amount of personalized patient data into the appropriate software field of the computer and then print out an address label.

This combination of a brief initial phone call by the dedicated scheduler and a personalized follow-up letter enhances the likelihood of patients accepting a DIGMA or PSMA appointment in lieu of an individual visit, especially if they have already been personally invited to attend by their physician. When patients do in fact accept this invitation and schedule a IGMA or PSMA appointment, a reminder call a couple of days before the SMA appointment can also help to increase the likelihood of patient follow-through (i.e, by not failing to keep the appointment).

The Provider Needs to Approve All SMA Documents and to Select the Handouts

The program coordinator needs to enter all of the specific details regarding the provider's DIGMA or PSMA into the existing templates previously developed for the SMA program—i.e., wall poster, flier, announcement, invitation, cover letter, follow-up letter, chart note, etc. (see samples of all these materials on the attached DVD). The program coordinator then gives these initial drafts of all forms to the provider as soon as possible to review, make any desired changes or modifications, and then approve. The provider also selects any handouts that he/she wants to use in the SMA—and can personally develop any other handouts that the provider might wish to use which are not readily available. In addition, the provider selects the contents of the Patient Packet for the PSMA or DIGMA (i.e., if one is going to be given to patients at the beginning of DIGMA sessions, which I recommend because it is greatly appreciated by patients and enhances the perceived quality of the visit).

While optional for DIGMAs, a Patient Packet is always used in PSMAs—in which it is typically sent to patients 2 or 3 weeks before their PSMA session. The Patient Packet for PSMAs typically contains a *cover letter* from the physician explaining the program and its many benefits; any *handouts* that the physician wants to have included (on *hot topics*, routine health maintenance guidelines, health education and disease self-management materials, etc.); a *detailed health history form* (addressing current health concerns, recent health changes, family and personal health histories, current medications, allergies to medications, etc.) to be completed and returned to the office at least a couple days prior to the visit; and an *order form for lab tests* (such as routine blood and urine screening tests) that need to be completed prior to the visit.

The health history form enclosed in the Patient Packet is usually the same extensive health history questionnaire as is already being used for individual physical examination appointments, but it is typically even more detailed and comprehensive. Ultimately, as soon as firewall issues are worked out for this process, the entire Patient Packet could be sent to patients—and then the completed health history questionnaire could be returned to the office—electronically. For systems on EMR, the results of the completed lab tests could similarly be returned to the office electronically. Except for the detailed health history form and pre-visit lab order form, the Patient Packet used in DIGMAs typically contains many of the same educational and PR materials as the Patient Packet used in PSMAs (plus a name tag, blank sheet of paper for notes, and confidentiality agreement form—which are normally given to PSMA patients separately as they register for the visit).

Discuss Billing and Documentation Protocols with the Physician, and Develop the Chart Note Template

It is important for the program coordinator to set up another meeting that includes the physician, champion, program coordinator, SMA documenter, and the organization's billing and compliance officer as well as chart note documentation leadership. The purpose of this meeting is to: (1) explain to the provider the billing philosophy and procedures that the organization has developed for billing DIGMA and PSMA group visits; (2) get the provider to develop a highly efficient chart note template for documenting patient visits in the SMA (perhaps by working from their own chart note template for individual visits, or from chart note templates previously developed for the SMA program by other physicians in the same medical subspecialty who are already running DIGMAs and PSMAs for their practices); and (3) enlist the help of the key billing and compliance as well as documentation officers within the organization in order to optimize charting and billing for the provider's SMA.

I have found that including the organization' documentation as well as billing and compliance leadership can be extremely helpful in: (1) *fine-tuning* the chart note template to be used; optimizing the types of medical care that will be delivered in the DIGMA or PSMA; determining the various details of the documentation process; and optimizing billing for the provider's SMA. Once the physician discusses how she/he intends to document the chart note and bill for visits, these organizational leaders can make important positive suggestions and recommendations regarding the SMA chart note and bill—and they can even point out that by including just one or two additional steps that the physician might have forgotten, they might be able to bill at a higher level. I have found this input from the organization's documentation as well as billing and compliance officers to be extremely valuable in helping to optimize the SMA program's billing and charting processes, and in offering providers important and helpful suggestions as to how to conduct, bill, and chart their group visit sessions.

Set Up Training Sessions for the SMA Behaviorist and Nurse/MA(s) Regarding Their Expanded Duties

In addition, the program coordinator should set up separate training sessions—run by the champion, program coordinator, and senior (or lead) behaviorist, if one has been selected—to train the behaviorist and nursing personnel regarding their expanded duties in the provider's upcoming DIGMA or PSMA. Because these expanded behaviorist and nursing duties have been thoroughly discussed earlier in this book, they are not repeated here. However, during this training session, the nurse/MA(s) will also be trained in how to complete their portion of SMA chart note with regards to what they have done (reason for visit, vital signs, flu shot, pneumovax, tetanus, diabetic foot check, diabetic blood glucose level, PO2, peak flow, etc.)—as well as anything else that the provider wants them to provide and document. Of course, the behaviorist and nursing personnel will also need to be fully trained (in this and any additional subsequent meetings that might be needed) for all of their expanded responsibilities in the provider's SMA.

Finally, the behaviorist needs to leave the training session with a clear understanding that the behaviorist's role in the DIGMA or PSMA will be very different from (and much more active and self-disclosing than) their role in traditional mental health groups. They must recognize that even though they might have previously run several mental health or behavioral medicine groups in the past, what they will be doing in the SMA will be quite different. The "Oh yeah, I know how to run groups!" mentality has no place here. In addition, the behaviorist also needs to recognize that his/her primary job in the SMA is to assist the physician in every possible way—and to pace the group so that it runs smoothly and finishes on time. This can be a difficult adjustment for some psychologists and social workers who are used to leading their own groups, and are not used to playing a subordinate or supportive role.

Behaviorists must leave this meeting with the clear recognition that their role in a DIGMA or PSMA is not to bring their own agenda into the group room (especially when it could slow down the pace of the group)—e.g., to train patients in meditation techniques, cognitive behavioral therapy techniques, relaxation techniques. Although such agendas undoubtedly have their place elsewhere, they are not generally appropriate for a DIGMA or PSMA—where the focus from start to finish is upon the provider efficiently delivering high-quality, high-value medical care to all patients in attendance. Instead, the behaviorist must leave with a clear understanding of how to: (1) warm the group up and write down patients' medical issues prior to the session; (2) give the introduction; (3) pace the group to keep it running smoothly and on time; (4) address challenging group dynamic situations that can occur in SMAs; (5) deal with psychosocial issues and any psychiatric emergencies; (6) take over the group temporarily whenever the physician documents a chart note or steps out for a brief private exam or discussion; (7) tactfully handle any last minute patient logistical issues that might arise after the group is over; and then (8) politely clear the group room and quickly straighten it up for the next group. The behaviorist must also understand the dramatically different role that the behaviorist has during the first half of a PSMA, where they are essentially alone with the small, rotating group of unroomed patients while the physician is in the exam rooms conducting private physical examinations thoroughly but rapidly (with a minimum amount of talk and discussion, except for that of a truly private nature or which needs to be discussed in order to conduct the exam).

Generally speaking, the behaviorist's interventions will need to be made briefly (i.e., in 30–90 second sound bytes, so as to not slow the group down)—e.g., while the physician is documenting a chart note or briefly absent from the group room. Furthermore, when the behaviorist does address a patient's psychosocial issues during the SMA session and gently brings them to the attention of the provider, it is usually done for one of three reasons: (1) as a very brief intervention or recommendation during group time; (2) to tactfully bring the patient's emotional or psychological issue to the attention of the physician, who can then decide upon a treatment option such as starting the patient on a psychotropic medication; or (3) to promptly refer patients into appropriate internal or external treatment programs for these issues (i.e., if this is supported by the physician). The goal here is to triage patients into the appropriate treatment venue for such time-consuming emotional and psychosocial issues, but only with the physician's approval.

The goal is certainly not for the behaviorist to take an extended amount of time attempting to solve such problems in the SMA setting—which, after all, is meant to be a shared medical appointment with their own physician focusing upon the delivery of actual medical care to each and every patient in attendance. In other words, the behaviorist must remain cognizant of the fact that, unlike what happens in the psychiatry department, these patients are in general coming in for *body* (not *mind*) issues and care. Therefore, any effort to bring psychosocial and emotional issues to the attention of the physician and patient must be done with extreme tact. On the other hand, because these *mind* issues so often go under-diagnosed and under-treated in the primary care setting (and are often the primary drivers of medical visits, rather than true medical need), one of the important advantages of DIGMAs and PSMAs over individual appointments is this critically important role of recognizing and diagnosing emotional and psychosocial problems that the behaviorist can play.

Unless this is the first SMA being launched in the system, the behaviorist and nurse/MA(s) should be encouraged to attend a couple of other providers' DIGMAs or PSMAs for a session or two (and to do this prior to the start date of the upcoming DIGMA or PSMA of the provider that they will be working with)—to observe how they are doing things and to learn from them. They should also be encouraged to read the relevant literature—including this book as well as any helpful articles published on group visits. If this is the first DIGMA or PSMA in the system, then the nurse/MA(s) and behaviorist—as well as the physician—might want to attend a well-run SMA in a different healthcare organization (or attend training programs at the *Noffsinger Institute for Group Visits*, which is currently (as of May, 2009) in the planning stages at Harvard Vanguard Medical Associates/Atrius Health in Boston, MA).

Order the Necessary Supplies for the Provider's SMA

Finally, the program coordinator should order all the equipment (including any needed medical equipment) and supplies (name tags, felt markers, flip chart, whiteboard, etc.) that will be needed for the provider's SMA. This could include such items as thick felt markers having dark ink and a broad tip (for writing patients' first names in large print on the name tags), erasable markers for the whiteboard, any needed anatomical charts or models, a monofilament for testing for peripheral neuropathy, a frozen nitrogen canister, clocks for the group room walls, etc. More costly durable medical equipment,

such as pulse oximeters and blood glucose meters with test strips, will likely need to come from the physician's own office area.

Weeks 6, 7, and 8 After Entering the Pipeline

Here, we are just past the halfway point in the 10-week pipeline for efficiently developing and launching high-quality DIGMAs and PSMAs throughout the entire healthcare system. As will be seen, this is generally a very active time for the entire SMA department, but most especially for the program coordinator.

Print the Appropriate Number of Copies of All Forms to Be Used in the SMA

Once the provider reviews the initial drafts of all forms and promotional materials to be used in the SMA (which are usually generated from templates already developed for the SMA Depatment)—and then makes any desired changes, approves the updated forms, and returns them to the program coordinator—the appropriate number of copies need to be made or ordered of the final draft of each form. In addition to marketing materials (posters, fliers, invitations, announcements, etc.), this should also include all forms needed in the DIGMA or PSMA—for example, any handouts, health history questionnaires, Patient Packets, or patient satisfaction forms that will be used on an ongoing basis in the SMA program.

Program Description Flier

Every DIGMA and PSMA needs a program description flier containing all necessary details about the program, which has been extensively discussed elsewhere in this book (see samples on the DVD attached to this book).

Give Provider Temporary Fliers Immediately:

The provider can be given 300 or so copies of a temporary flier, so that the provider and staff can immediately begin inviting patients to attend the upcoming DIGMA or PSMA sessions.

Initially Order a Relatively Small Number of Final Fliers:

A small number of the final version of the flier (which must have a high-quality and professional appearance, yet be affordable) is sometimes ordered by the program coordinator at this time. Approximately 300–500 copies are typically procured at this early point—a relatively small number as changes are often made during the first few weeks of actually running a DIGMA or PSMA, changes which can affect the flier and make its original version obsolete.

A Bulk Order for the Finalized Flier Is Placed Later:

Later on, after the program has been running successfully for a couple of months (i.e., after any needed changes have already been made to the SMA and reflected in the flier, and after the DIGMA or PSMA has pretty much achieved its final form), the finalized flier can then be ordered in bulk—perhaps one or two thousand copies.

Fill Flier Holders in the Provider's Lobby and Exam Rooms:

Once the printed fliers are received, the program coordinator ensures that the flier holders in the provider's lobby and exam rooms to capacity—holders that are designed to hold at least 100 copies of the flier.

Select a Staff Person to Keep Flier Holders Full:

A motivated person from the provider's office staff (typically a receptionist, the office manager, a nurse or medical assistant, etc.) must be given primary responsibility for replenishing the fliers in the flier holders that are in the lobby and exam rooms when supplies start to become depleted. In addition, this person must notify the program coordinator when the stock of program description fliers for this provider is running low—so that additional printed fliers can be ordered in a timely manner before the existing supply is completely depleted.

Announcement Letter

It is an excellent idea, just prior to the start of a new SMA, to mail an announcement letter out to all patients on the provider's panel who will qualify to attend the new DIGMA or PSMA the next time that they have a medical need. These announcements can be sent either in a single mailing or, if a large number of patients are involved, by sending them out in batches of 50–100. As extensively discussed elsewhere in this book, this announcement letter will not, by itself, bring patients into the SMA in droves; however, it does serve an important function by making patients aware of this new program (see sample announcement letter in (Fig. 11.1 (A) and DVD).

Order Enough Copies to Mail to All Appropriate Patients:

Make or order the required number of copies of the announcement letter to mail to all appropriate patients on the provider's panel, typically just prior to launching the new DIGMA or PSMA program. These announcement letters are designed to: (1) announce the new SMA to all appropriate patients; (2) describe the program and inform patients of its many benefits; (3) invite patients to attend whenever they have a medical need in the future; and (4) invite patients to attend one of the first sessions. Although the announcement letter, by itself, does not convince many patients to attend a SMA, it does inform patients about the physician's new SMA program—and typically does result in a few direct patient self-referrals.

However, the main benefit of the announcement is that it makes it easier for the physician and staff to refer patients when they later come in for a regular office visit. When the physician then gives patients a personal invitation to attend the DIGMA for their next follow-up visit (or the PSMA for their next private physical examination), patients seem to be a little more willing to accept this invitation as a result of having previously been informed about the SMA through the announcement. It is not uncommon for patients to say something like the following to the physician who has invited them to attend the SMA: "Oh yeah, I remember that you sent me a letter about it earlier. I read it. It sounded intriguing, although I didn't follow up on it. Sure, I'll give it a try. Thanks for thinking about me."

Order Any Inserts to Be Included in This Mailing:

Also order enough copies of any handouts or inserts that the provider might want to include in this announcement letter mailing. See the Fliers folder on the DVD attached to this book for an example of a particularly nice insert that we used at the Palo Alto Medical Foundation (PAMF). It was small and convenient for patients, contained all important details about the program, and was inexpensive to produce since three such inserts fit onto a single printed sheet of heavy paper stock. Many patients told us they would keep it in a prominent location in their houses, with some even using a magnet to keep it on the door of their refrigerator.

Establish the Mailing Date(s) for the Announcement:

Establish the mailing date (or dates) for the announcements. Announcement letters are frequently mailed on a weekly basis in groups of perhaps 50–100 at a time—beginning 2 weeks prior to the first DIGMA or PSMA session, and then continuing in the weeks that follow until they have been sent to all appropriate patients on the physician's panel. This spreads out any patient self-referrals that might be generated by the announcement letter equally over the first few SMA sessions. Alternatively, the announcements could also be mailed either all at once (particularly if there is just a couple hundred of them to be mailed out to patients) or perhaps on a monthly basis for the first few months of the SMA.

Send Announcement to All Appropriate Patients:

Order the envelopes and stamps for mailing the announcement letters. Create the address labels and address the envelopes—stuffing them with the folded announcement letter plus any inserts selected by the provider. Then send this announcement (on the date or dates previously decided upon) to the appropriate patients in the provider's practice. Most of this work can be done by the program coordinator and dedicated scheduler; however, it can also be done by a volunteer or a motivated member of the physician's clerical support staff (which is nice, if there is staff buy-in, because it gets them more invested in the process). For systems that have gone entirely electronic, sending the invitation out electronically will clearly increase efficiency and reduce cost.

Invitation Letter

The invitation letter, which is designed to be given out to all appropriate patients by the receptionist (along with some kind and positive words about the DIGMA or PSMA program) whenever they register for a regular office visit, has been extensively discussed elsewhere in this book (see Chapter 10 and samples on the DVD attached to this book).

Make Approximately 300 Copies to Start with:

The program coordinator photocopies or orders an initial run of approximately 300 copies of the invitation letter for the physician's DIGMA or PSMA—see Fig. 11.1 (B)—which is to be given by the receptionist (along with some kind words about the program) to all appropriate patients whenever they register for a regular office visit. Do not order too many at first, as changes are often made during the first few sessions of a DIGMA or PSMA. Because these invitations do not need to be professionally printed, they are often reproduced on the physician's office copier—often on the preprinted stationary of the SMA Department, which is typically ordered in bulk and printed in just one or two colors (but designed so as to tie into the general look of the SMA program as depicted on the wall poster).

Receptionists Begin Giving the Invitation Letters to All Appropriate Patients During Regular Office Visits:

The program coordinator delivers the 300 or so initial copies of the "You Are Invited…" letter to the receptionists in the provider's front office and reviews the training they received with regards to giving the invitation out to all appropriate patients as they register for a normal office visit—along with how to best say a few positive words about the DIGMA or PSMA. From this point forward, the invitation letter is to be given by receptionists to all appropriate patients being seen for individual office visits as they register for their appointments. This process of the receptionist handing out invitations to all appropriate patients when they register for regular office visits typically occurs during the first year or two subsequent to the launch of the new DIGMA or PSMA, with some providers choosing to make it an ongoing process into the foreseeable future. However, do not keep giving the invitation letter repeatedly to the same patients after office visit.

For example, the receptionist might say: "Hello Mrs. Smith. I see that you are here to see Dr. Jones today. Dr. Jones has just started a new program for some of his/her established patients, a program that he/she is very excited about. Dr. Jones has asked that I give you this invitation to read in the lobby while you are waiting to be seen. The invitation explains the program in detail, and invites you to attend the next time that you have a medical need. Many of Dr. Jones' patients have already told me that they went and really liked it, and that they found it to be very helpful. Actually, I sat in on a session myself and found it to be extremely informative and enjoyable."

One Receptionist Is Assigned to Notify the Program Coordinator when Invitations Are Running Low:

Some one person in the provider's front office (typically a receptionist, but occasionally the office manager) needs to be clearly identified and assigned primary responsibility for ensuring that the reception desk never runs out of these invitations. This person is to inform the SMA program coordinator whenever more invitation letters need to be ordered—usually a week or two before the supply is depleted. In this way, the supply of invitation letters is replenished as needed in a timely manner, and always remains available to receptionists for distributing to patients. When the invitation is simply printed in black ink on white paper (i.e., rather than on the SMA Department Letterhead), these additional copies that need to be printed when the supply of invitation letters is depleted can be made by the physician's own office staff—although the program coordinator will need to check from time to time to ensure that this is happening, and that the supply of invitations never runs out.

Install Two Functional Computers (Desktop for Documenter and Laptop for Physician), a Printer, and a Phone in the Group Room

If not already in the group room, the program coordinator will need to order two appropriate computers (typically a desktop for the documenter and a laptop for the physician), a printer, and a telephone at this point in time—and then have them installed in the group room, plus possibly a computer in each exam room as well. The program coodinator will then need to arrange for the appropriate IT infrastructure for these computers to be set up and installed. Once they are installed and operational, the program coordinator needs to ensure that they are properly set up and completely functional—so that the documenter and provider can access medical records, make referrals, and order any prescriptions, tests, and procedures that might be indicated (as well as print out copies of materials, such as after visit summaries, for patients as desired) during group sessions.

As a consultant for healthcare systems around the nation (and more recently, internationally), it never ceases to amaze me how often computers fail and computer systems crash during the first couple of sessions that a new DIGMA or PSMA is being launched—much to the chagrin of the frustrated provider and staff. Avoid such last minute computer glitches by ensuring that everything is in good working order beforehand, and that the provider and documenter are able to sign on and access patients' chart notes—and then double check this the day before (and even triple check it before the start time on the day of the first SMA session).

In addition to installing the functional computers, be sure to set up whatever type of computer desk configuration is most comfortable and convenient for the documenter and physician when using the computer in the group room. Try to install the printer in a position that is convenient for the physician, documenter, and behaviorist to get at during SMA sessions. In addition, install a telephone in the group room if one is not already there—one that is easily accessible to the provider, as it can also be helpful during the SMA.

Develop the Provider's Chart Note Template for the SMA

It is important at this time for the physician to put any last minute finishing touches upon the chart note template that will be used in the DIGMA or PSMA. An EMR chart note template is typically developed for the SMA Department by the first provider to run a DIGMA or PSMA in each medical subspecialty. Although this original draft of the chart note template would probably be developed in rough form from the existing SMA template of another provider within the same medical subspecialty who has already run a DIGMA or PSMA, this chart note template needs to be *fine-tuned* to the specific needs of the new SMA provider and put into final form. Often, physicians will prefer to continue using their own EMR chart note template for individual office visits, perhaps with some minor changes specific to the DIGMA or PSMA setting.

Be Sure the Provider and Documenter Are Well Trained in the Use of the Chart Note Template

At this point, the champion and program coordinator need to make certain that an appropriate chart note template is fully developed by the provider. Once several operational SMAs exist in primary care and the various medical subspecialties throughout the organization, then the templates used by many other providers within the system will be available to the new provider—i.e., to help in designing the new chart note template for his or her own DIGMA or PSMA. Most systems are now either on electronic medical records or going toward EMR, so that their chart note templates will obviously be in electronic form. In systems that are still using paper charts, this template needs to be largely preprinted and in check-off form in order to optimize charting efficiency. See the DVD attached to this book for examples of a paper chart note templates.

Paper Chart Notes:

Often, providers who still use paper charts will try to keep their SMA chart note template to a single page in length (or even less). Frequently, providers will have a separate section at the top of their chart note template for the SMA nurses/MA(s) to complete—i.e., for all duties performed during their portion of the visit, as well as the patient's reason for today's visit. In addition, providers often have the confidentiality release that patients and their support persons sign printed onto the backside of the paper sheet containing the chart note template. This is convenient because it condenses two sheets of paper into one and because it makes clear that the patient's signature on the release applies to this particular chart note and SMA session.

On each patient's chart note, the nursing personnel can enter vital signs, reason for visit, injections given, special duties performed, performance measures updated, routine health maintenance that needs to be ordered, etc. When finished with each patient, they can attach that patient's paper chart note (with the nursing section of the chart note completed) to the front cover of the paper medical chart, and then return the medical chart to the group room when escorting the patient back from the exam room—typically placing it onto the stack of medical charts on the small table next to the physician. For this reason, it is often recommended that the physician and adjacent behaviorist sit with their backs closest to the door in the group room that leads to the nearby exam room, as it entails a smaller and less distracting walk for the nurse to make when placing paper charts onto the small table between them (or when there is a need for the nurse/MA to say something to the physician). Physicians in systems still using paper charts might want to see the sample chart note template included in the DVD attached to this book.

EMR Chart Notes:

For systems using electronic medical records (EMR), the provider needs to develop an efficient chart note template—one which makes full use of SmartPhrases, SmartText, key-stroke shortcuts, and prepackaged downloadable material that can be efficiently dropped into patients' chart notes. As has been previously discussed, it is wise (especially when using EMR) to employ a documenter in the DIGMA or PSMA. The documenter can then create a comprehensive, contemporaneous chart note on each patient in attendance—i.e., as the care is sequentially being delivered to one patient at a time in the DIGMA or PSMA setting. Also, because charting is all that documenters do in the SMA setting, they soon become quite expert in the process and capable of generating superior chart notes.

However, prior to the actual launch of the DIGMA or PSMA, the documenter will need to be trained as to how to draft chart notes as the physician wants them—i.e. using the physician's own chart note template. This needs to be done prior to the first session as the documenter needs to know what she/he is doing by that time, and is not just trying to learn in the group setting—which will certainly frustrate the physician and cause the SMA to finish late. I recommend having the documenter review perhaps 20–40 of the physician's actual chart notes beforehand to get a clear idea of the physician's documentation style, and then shadow the physician for a day or two. When shadowing the physician during regular office visits, the documenter actually does the chart notes for the physician, using the physician's own template—i.e. for documenters who are licensed to be in exam rooms with disrobed patients (unless, of course, this *shadowing* only occurs for patients who are not undressed and agree to it). This enables the physician to review the chart notes so generated, to give prompt feedback, and to thereby train the documenter as to precisely what the physician wants before the first DIGMA or PSMA session is held.

A Documenter Can Optimize Charting and Billing:

The comprehensive, contemporaneous chart note that is efficiently drafted by the documenter on each patient in attendance can be most helpful in simultaneously optimizing the physician's productivity, the quality of the chart note, and billing. However, the documenter (as well as the provider) must be well trained in utilizing efficient EMR documentation techniques, in navigating through the EMR system, and in using the template that has been developed for the provider's group visit. The documenter is typically trained initially by the provider and program coordinator prior to the first session. Then, additional training from the physician occurs on an ongoing basis in the SMA setting as the physician reviews and modifies each chart note created by the documenter immediately after working with each patient in turn in the group setting—thus providing prompt and immediate feedback to the documenter.

Ensure the Chart Note Template Is Acceptable to Documentation as Well as Billing and Compliance Leadership

It is imperative that the chart notes documented in the DIGMA and PSMA settings be as quick and efficient as possible; however, it is equally important that they also be accurate and complete from the documentation and billing perspectives. Ensure that the chart note template created for each new SMA is acceptable to documentation as well as billing and compliance leadership within the organization—as they can be most helpful in reviewing, modifying, and optimizing the proposed chart note template.

Start Monitoring the Census of the New Provider's SMA on a Weekly Basis

At this point, the program coordinator needs to start monitoring the provider's pre-booking census for all upcoming sessions on a weekly (or, better yet, twice-weekly) basis. When I headed the SMA Department at the Palo Alto Medical Foundation (PAMF), I had my program coordinator (with the help of the dedicated scheduler) produce a twice-weekly report indicating how many patients were pre-registered into each SMA session for the next 2 months for all of the physicians running DIGMAs or PSMAs in their practices. At HVMA/AH, I have my program coordinator generate a weekly report on Monday mornings depicting the census for each and every DIGMA and PSMA in the system covering the next four SMA sessions. These reports are divided by facility, by department within each facility, and alphabetically by individual providers within each department at every facility.

In addition to showing how many patients were in fact prescheduled for each upcoming DIGMA and PSMA session, this weekly (or twice weekly) pre-registration census report also depicted the minimum, target, and maximum census targets for each and every SMA within the system. It could also document the amount that sessions should be overbooked by in order to compensate for the expected number of no-shows and late-cancels (less, of course, the anticipated number of drop-ins in the case of DIGMAs), as well as the average group census for each provider during the past month, past quarter, past year, etc. I typically show the bar graphs in these reports as the percent increase over individual office visits in each provider's productivity that has been accomplished by the DIGMA or PSMA—i.e., for the same types of patients and appointments being seen in the DIGMA or PSMA versus traditional individual office visits (with the most common target being a 300% increase in productivity). The number of patients scheduled into all upcoming SMA sessions during the next month or two should also be included, as well as past performance to date.

Weekly Pre-booking Census Reports Enable the Champion to Run the SMA Program

As the SMA champion, I find these weekly census reports generated by the program coordinator to be the most valuable tool at my disposal for running the SMA program. These reports allow me to: (1) continuously monitor the pre-registration census for all upcoming sessions during the next month or two for all DIGMAs and PSMAs being run in the system (broken out by facility, department within that facility, and alphabetically by provider within each department); (2) determine where to have the dedicated scheduler focus his or her efforts in *topping-off* groups each day; (3) determine which SMA providers and staffs need additional counseling and training regarding how to effectively refer appropriate patients into their SMAs so as to keep their sessions consistently full; (4) assess which SMAs are at greatest risk for failure, so that prompt action can be taken to address this problem; and (5) ultimately determine which SMAs are not economically viable and should therefore be considered for a probationary period (and if poor census persists, ultimately for termination).

As Needed, Coach and Train the Physician and Staff to Better Refer Patients

By starting to monitor the new provider's SMA census every week at this point (i.e., a few weeks before the DIGMA or PSMA is to be launched), you will be able to determine whether the provider and staff need additional coaching and training on referring patients into their SMA weeks before the actual launch date. It therefore provides a *cushion* by allowing some time to take corrective action swiftly in the event that sessions are not filling as rapidly as they should. Consider encouraging patients to arrive 15 minutes early so that the nursing personnel can start with early arrivers—although, in some cases this will not be necessary (i.e. if sufficient patients naturally come to the appointment early).

If Upcoming Sessions Are Still Not Filling, Then Meet Again with the Physician and Staff to Continue Training

If the initial sessions do not start filling a few weeks prior to the start date, and if the initial sessions are not yet close to full, then promptly set up another training meeting with the physician and support staff—i.e., to continue the training on how to effectively refer patients into the SMA. With the provider's permission, the champion and program coordinator can provide an additional helpful service by shadowing the physician and staff for a day or two to watch exactly how they are inviting patients in actual practice—to see what they are doing right, and precisely what they might be doing wrong. This allows the physician and support staff to be given immediate, personalized feedback on how to more effectively invite patients into the DIGMA or PSMA. Also, praise or offer some form of incentive (such as small rewards) to staff for special efforts in successfully recruiting patients into the SMA. It's amazing how effective a pizza, an inexpensive personal item, a certificate for a gourmet cup of coffee, or a personal "thank you" from the physician can be in motivating the physician's schedulers and entire support staff to promote the program.

Persist with Training Until the First Session Is Full and Initial Sessions Are Filling—Otherwise, Postpone the Start Date

Because full sessions are the secret to success with DIGMAs and PSMAs, persist with training the physician and support staff until all initial sessions are filling substantially—and the first session is completely full (plus an extra patient or two to compensate for the anticipated number of no-shows and late-cancels, less drop-ins in the case of DIGMAs). Otherwise, if all of these efforts fail, then the start date will need to be postponed (or else the SMA will need to be redesigned so as to be more heterogeneous in nature, thus enabling a larger number of patients qualify to attend) until full initial sessions can be scheduled with confidence.

Solve Any Systems Problems as They Arise

Because DIGMAs and PSMAs leverage existing resources, dramatically increase physician productivity, and involve multiple patients going through the system at once, they tend to exacerbate any pre-existing system problems. DIGMAs and PSMAs can increase productivity to such a degree that they end up stressing the system—i.e., with the result being that problems begin arising in areas that might heretofore have been marginally functional when one patient was being seen at a time. For example, a receptionist who is slow when one patient is being registered at a time does not suddenly become fast when 15 patients are waiting in line. Additional help, extra training, or a change in personnel may be necessary.

Also, because DIGMAs and PSMAs represent a highly efficient team-based approach to care involving

much change and both group and exam rooms, they can introduce many administrative, equipment, and operational problems that the system does not normally have to deal with. Because they represent such a major paradigm shift, there can be all types of personnel, facilities, promotional, and equipment issues arising from SMAs that the system does not normally have to deal with. For example, is the group room ventilation adequate for large groups and, if not, will adjusting the thermostat or introducing a fan be of help? Are paper charts arriving on time, are there competing organizational demands upon either the SMA personnel or the group and exam rooms, and are the group and exam rooms properly equipped for these large groups? If any such operational problems do in fact arise, then they will need to be promptly addressed by the champion and program coordinator.

For example, consider the variety of operational and logistical problems that can arise around personnel, facilities, census, and patient flow issues within the DIGMA or PSMA setting: have sessions been properly overbooked so that target census is consistently achieved; are patients arriving to register at the right place and time; is the registration process going well; are patients arriving in the group room without getting lost; is the group room properly decorated and set up with enough comfortable chairs in a circular arrangement; are the group and exam rooms properly equipped; are the group and exam rooms available as scheduled (or are they sometimes occupied by others during the group time); are the nursing duties being dispatched in a timely manner; is the behaviorist arriving a few minutes early and starting the group on time; are the physician and documenter arriving on time; is the group running smoothly and on time; are the computer(s) and printer working; is the documentation process going well; are snacks arriving as they are supposed to; are there functional toilet facilities in the area; does the physician leave on time; are patients able to efficiently schedule follow-up appointments during or after group; does the behaviorist stay late to straighten up the group room; etc.? If the myriad potential operational and logistical problems that can arise in DIGMAs and PSMAs are not promptly addressed, they will frustrate patients and staff alike—and could eventually undercut how efficient and enjoyable the group visit program is as well.

If Water, Coffee, Tea, and Healthy Snacks Are to Be Provided, Then Schedule Them on an Ongoing Basis

Because properly run group visits are efficient and cost effective, it is wise to reinvest some of the program's potential savings back into the SMA in the form of snacks—especially healthy snacks that are not too messy—as they are much appreciated by patients and lend themselves nicely to the high-quality image that you want SMAs to have. For one thing, 90 minutes is a fairly long time and patients can get hungry and thirsty—especially when SMAs are held at certain times of the day. Furthermore, having appropriate snacks available can be medically important (or just a wise idea) in some cases—such as diabetes DIGMAs, prenatal PSMAs, pediatric group visits after school, oncology SMAs, etc. In addition, patients truly appreciate the thought when it comes to snacks—and particularly seem to enjoy coffee, water, power bars, and apples or grapes. Although patients would also like cookies, muffins, doughnuts, soft drinks, ice cream, and cake, I generally recommend against them so as to model healthier eating habits. Even when they do not take any, patients still comment on how much they appreciate the fact that snacks are provided.

However if the decision is made to provide snacks at the SMA, then they will need to arrive on time and be provided on an ongoing basis. First, decide which snacks the provider wants to serve (coffee, tea, water, apples, grapes, orange wedges, cheese sticks, power bars, etc.). Try to model healthy eating habits and to avoid unhealthy or messy snacks such as cookies, cupcakes, doughnuts, whole oranges, and ice cream—except under special circumstances. It is also beneficial if the snacks are not particularly perishable, as they can then be brought into the SMA in weeks to come. For this reason, consider snacks such as bottled water, cheese sticks, power bars, etc. because they can be purchased in bulk at a discount store and then kept from one session to the next—at least until they are either consumed or their expiration date occurs.

If you choose to serve snacks, then you will need to develop a budget for them. It is usually the program coordinator who will arrange for snacks to be provided on an ongoing basis; however, it could also be a motivated member of the physician's staff. Determine if they will be catered, brought in by nutritional services, purchased at a discount store by a staff member using the SMA budget, etc. The important point here is that if snacks are to be provided (which is, generally speaking, a good idea), then they need to be within budget and arranged for from the beginning of the new DIGMA or PSMA program—and then, from that point onward (which requires that clear lines of responsibility and accountability for bringing snacks on an ongoing basis be established).

The Champion Should Reassure the Provider and Staff During This Period, Addressing Any Concerns or Anxieties

It is during this intermediate period of planning (i.e. when the prospect of the upcoming SMA looms real, but before the first SMA session is actually run), that provider and staff worries and anxieties can be at their peak—especially just before the first session. Because this is to be expected, it is imperative that the champion, program coordinator, and entire SMA team be sensitive to these anxieties—and that they try to be as reassuring and comforting as possible to the physician and support staff throughout this difficult period.

There will be all types of worries, most of which will ultimately prove to be anxiety based and unimportant in the long run—i.e., due to the SMA being something new and quite different from what the physician and staff are used to. It seems like the unknown is always most scary for us. However, as soon as experience is gained in running the SMA, most of these worries will quickly resolve and vanish. Therefore, most physician worries (e.g., about saying something stupid in front of 15 patients at once; of all patients in the group demanding one-on-one time with the physician at the end of the group; about group visits not working for their practice or personality; of losing control of the group and having it spiral out of control; of not being able to deliver adequate medical care or to complete chart notes on all patients in the allotted time; of catastrophic results from the physician being asked questions in group that he/she does not know the answer to; etc.) typically disappear quite rapidly after only the first couple of sessions have been held.

Physicians will rapidly find that if they do say something they consider to be stupid in front of others in the group, all they have to do is say something lighthearted and humorous like: "Oops, that didn't come out right. Let me try that again." If anything, they will seem more human to their patients—who will typically like them even more as a result. Once they have run one or two successful SMA sessions, physicians will quickly find that most patients will be satisfied with the medical care they receive in the group—and will therefore not generally request private one-on-one time toward the end of the group, unless the physician somehow encourages it. Similarly, physicians will soon find that group visits do in fact work quite well for them and for their practice, just as they have in the practices of hundreds before them—and that the behaviorist' complementary skill set in managing group dynamics and psychosocial issues will be most helpful in preventing the group from spiraling negatively out of control.

Interestingly, although physicians and support staffs appear to worry about everything else, they seldom if ever worry about the one thing they should worry about most—which is how to keep all SMA sessions consistently full. This is because when SMAs do in fact fail, it is almost always for just one reason—insufficient patient attendance. Therefore, this issue of consistently full groups needs to be taken seriously by physician and support staff alike if the SMA program is to succeed in the long run.

Develop the Outcome Measures and Methodologies that Will Be Used to Evaluate the SMA Program on an Ongoing Basis and to Issue Periodic Reports

It is at this point that the outcome measures that will be used to evaluate the SMA program need to be determined, and precisely what types of periodic reports will be issued on the program. Will you want to measure improvements in quality, productivity, access, efficiency, clinical outcomes, practice management, chronic disease management, the bottom line, etc.? This issue of which measures to use in evaluating the SMA should be addressed at this early point—and should include input from the provider, champion, program coordinator, administration, and possibly even the research arm of the organization (assuming that there is one).

Measure the Unique Strengths of the Group Visit Model You Are Using

Group practices and managed care organizations will undoubtedly want to measure the specific strengths of the group visit model that they have selected to use in their SMA program. In the case of *DIGMAs*, increased physician productivity along with the related issues of increased RVUs, enhanced revenues, improved access to care, reduced backlogs, decreased patient telephone volume, fewer work-ins, and improvements in practice and chronic illness management will need to be measured—i.e., along with reported improvements in the patient–physician relationships, clinical outcomes, reduced costs, and increased patient and provider satisfaction. For *CHCCs*, which do not increase productivity or improve access, reductions in the costs of hospital, emergency department, and nursing home care for the

same group of 15–20 high utilizing, multi-morbid geriatric patients being followed over time should be measured. For *PSMAs*, increased productivity in delivering private physical examinations in primary and specialty care, decreased wait lists and backlogs for physicals, and cost savings in delivering physical exams will need to be measured—along with patient and provider professional satisfaction.

Also Measure the Multiple Common Benefits Offered by Group Visits in General

In addition, systems might want to measure improvements in any of the many benefits that today's various group visit models are known to share in common. These shared benefits of all of today's major group visit models (when they are properly run and supported) include potential improvements in quality, outcomes, compliance, patient education, psychosocial issues, self-efficacy, disease self-management, follow-up care, routine health maintenance, injection rates, performance measures, emotional support, cost containment, the patient–physician relationship, patient and provider satisfaction, etc.

What Tests, Measurements, and Methodologies Will Be Used and How Will the Data Be Analyzed?

In terms of data and analysis, precisely what and how things are to be measured needs to be determined—along with which scales, tests, inventories, questionnaires, measures, tools, and protocols are to be used. For example, most systems want to measure patient and provider satisfaction with the SMA program compared to individual appointments—preferably for the same providers during the same period of time. Therefore, they will need to select the patient satisfaction form that they will use, along with the methodology to be employed—e.g. complete the patient satisfaction form after the group and anonymously drop it into a box outside of group room; mail forms to the homes of patients after their visit; test all patients (or just a random sample); will support persons be included; etc. The un-normed sample patient satisfaction forms included in the DVD attached to this book might prove helpful to some organizations, although they might prefer to use normed patient satisfaction forms such as the ones developed by the American Medical Group Association (AMGA) or Press Ganey. However, keep in mind that while unnormed patient satisfaction forms can have high face validity and be specifically designed around group visits, normed patient satisfaction surveys have the advantages of being tested, reliable, normed, and scientifically valid. Unfortunately, normed patient satisfaction questionnaires often contain many items that are not at all relevant to group visits, although they might also include one or two items that could be relevant to both individual and group visits, such as questions like "Overall, how would you rate the quality of care that you received during today's visit."

Will You Want to Measure Outcomes, Productivity, Access, Cost Savings, Quality Improvements, or Enhanced Practice Management?

Then there are the important issues relating to measures of improved quality, clinical outcomes, better access, improved productivity, enhanced practice and chronic illness management, and cost savings—which can also be evaluated, but mostly through use of formal research studies or internal data gathered both within the organization and through the SMA program. For example, we could look at HbA1c control amongst diabetics, improved consistency in screening measures, and percentage of updated injections and health maintenance for patients with diabetes who attended group visits versus a matched control group of diabetic patients who received traditional individual care alone. We could also look at overall costs of caring for diabetic patients attending SMAs compared to the control group—and even examine potential differences in hospital, emergency department, and nursing home utilization and costs. We could measure improvements in access and physician productivity, as well as the strengthening of the bottom line that could potentially come from the group visit program. In addition, we could similarly evaluate the relative efficacy of the homogeneous, heterogeneous, and mixed subtypes of the DIGMA and PSMA models with regards to quality and cost savings.

It Is Generally Easier to Measure Outcomes, Cost Savings, etc. with CHCCs than DIGMAs and PSMAs

Generally speaking, many of these measures (such as outcomes and cost savings) will be easiest to determine for CHCCs because the same 15–20 patients are followed over time—and it is relatively easy to contrast outcomes and cost savings for the experimental group versus a matched control group. DIGMAs and PSMAs will generally take larger, longer, and more costly studies in order to accurately determine these measures—because most, if not all, patients in

the physician's practice (or in the chronic illness population management program) can be impacted by the DIGMA and PSMA program—and because different patients typically attend each session, as they only come in when they have an actual medical need (and then, they might come in with a *laundry list* of health concerns).

However, among the various subtypes of the DIGMA and PSMA models, such studies will be easier for the homogeneous model (which is disease or condition specific) than for the mixed model—which focuses upon four large, but relatively different, groupings or clusters of conditions. Furthermore, studies on both the homogeneous and mixed subtypes will be easier than studies on the heterogeneous subtype of the DIGMA and PSMA models—i.e., due to the fact that many different diseases and conditions are included. For example, in a heterogeneous primary care DIGMA, the patient who comes in today with a URI might not return for 2 years, and then they might return for wrist pain or a skin lesion. So the decision as to what to measure, and how to measure it, is clearly not always an easy one with the heterogeneous subtype. Despite this research challenge, the heterogeneous DIGMA provides physicians with a remarkable practice management (and chronic disease management) tool that can dramatically improve productivity, access, and the bottom line—all of which would be considerably easier to measure with the heterogeneous DIGMA than clinical outcomes.

Be Practical, Measure What Is Easiest and Most Important, and Try to Issue Quarterly or Annual Reports

The possibilities regarding what to measure, what data to collect, what analyses to perform, and what reports to produce regarding the SMA program are almost limitless. Therefore, it is important to be practical by assessing those variables that are both relatively easy to measure and of greatest importance to the organization, provider, and SMA program. Consider what types of data are available or easily obtainable within the system, what types of resources can realistically be utilized for evaluating the program, and how the entire process of evaluation can be streamlined to save time and money. Certainly you will want to address your goals in running the SMA program and how to best measure these goals—e.g., improvements in quality, patient satisfaction, clinical outcomes, productivity, access, cost savings. This emphasis upon being practical and realistic will greatly reduce the types of measures and methodologies that need to be employed to evaluate your SMA program on an ongoing basis. Also, it is advantageous to systematize the entire evaluative process so that periodic reports can be efficiently generated which evaluate the overall progress and success of the SMA program. It is certainly helpful to the organization's executive leadership to have quarterly and annual reports compiled by the champion and program coordinator to evaluate the SMA program on an ongoing basis.

Weeks 9 and 10 After Entering the Pipeline

Here, we are near the end of all the steps contained in the pipeline, and just 2 weeks away from actually launching the DIGMA or PSMA that we have been working so diligently at getting successfully launched. Nonetheless, there are still many last-minutes steps to be taken during these final 2 weeks.

Hold Final Training Sessions for All Support Personnel as Needed—Review Census and Everybody's Roles and Responsibilities

During these last 2 weeks prior to launch, the program coordinator and champion again review census for the upcoming SMA sessions and organize and lead any necessary final training sessions with all support persons involved with the provider's DIGMA or PSMA (receptionists, nursing personnel, and all on- and off-site scheduling personnel, including the call center)—some of whom will need to be trained in shifts so that the clinic's normal daily functioning can continue unhindered.

The degree to which this individualized, final training is necessary will be partially determined by reviewing the census data covering the first few upcoming DIGMA or PSMA sessions. If the first couple of SMA sessions are not yet close to full (as we are now just 2 weeks prior to the start date), then the program coordinator should alert the provider and scheduling staff immediately. In addition, the program coordinator (and possibly the champion) should personally go to the physician's office area and check to make sure that: (1) receptionists are giving out the invitation letter (plus recommending the program) to all appropriate patients as they are registering for their normal office visits with the SMA provider; (2) the nurse/MA is giving all appropriate patients a copy of the SMA flier as they are rooming these patients (plus strong encouragement to attend a session); (3) the provider is personally inviting all patients appropriate for the SMA in an effective and positively worded

manner (this is the most important step of all); and (4) patients who accept this offer are promptly being booked into the appropriate upcoming SMA session.

In addition, the program coordinator should check that the announcements are being mailed on schedule, that the SMA posters are mounted in highly visible locations on the physician's lobby and exam room walls, and that the adjacent program description flier holders are being kept full at all times. The program coordinator should also check on all of the physician's on- and off-site scheduling staff, including any call center personnel involved with scheduling the provider's patients—to ensure that, whenever possible, they are properly referring all appropriate patients calling for an appointment into the SMA. It is also a good idea to similarly hold a final *brush-up* training review at this time on an *as needed* basis for all scheduling and call center staff (making a particular effort to concentrate this training upon the physician's primary scheduling staff as well as the call center's *SMA scheduling angels*)—usually in small groups, but occasionally individually. Meeting with these schedulers individually or in small groups in their regular office environment offers the advantage of enabling the program coordinator and/or champion to observe their work first hand, and to make corrective suggestions accordingly.

Finally, this training should cover other important issues as well as effectively referring all appropriate patients. All of the provider's support staff will have been trained previously in their new roles and responsibilities. They may still have some worries or resistances with regard to these responsibilities which can be addressed now, and there may even be some things about their new SMA duties that the support staff may have forgotten since their last training. There will likely be many last-minute questions and concerns, which should be addressed by the program coordinator, dedicated scheduler, and champion at this time.

Check Daily to See How Many Patients Are Scheduled for the First four SMA Sessions

During weeks 9 and 10 of the pipeline, which represent the final 2 weeks prior to the actual launch, the champion and program coordinator should be checking every day to see how many patients are prescheduled into each of the first four sessions of the provider's new DIGMA or PSMA. If the first session is not yet close to full (and if the following three sessions are not approximately 3/4th, 1/2, and 1/4th full, respectively), then they will need to take the prompt and effective action (or else postpone the launch date until full sessions are assured).

In helping over 400 providers nationally and internationally launch their new DIGMA and PSMA group visit programs, it has been my experience that when census is low at this point, there is a tendency for provider and staff to make excuses—i.e., rather than taking prompt, effective action to solve this patient referral problem. I tend to hear comments like: "My patients are different;" "Our patients aren't interested in a group visit;" "We've called 50 patients, but only 2 have told us that they would come;" "We're waiting for many return phone calls;" "It's OK, we'd rather start off with a small group." The list goes on and on.

When I hear these comments and rationalizations, and then actually investigate what is happening in depth (including personally talking to, and even shadowing, key personnel regarding the manner in which they are referring patients), what I almost always find is that the problem is not with the patients. I do not find that these patients are somehow fundamentally different than other patients around the nation and world in that they really do not want a group visit. Instead, what I typically find is that that the problem lies with the physician and staff—as they are still inexperienced in this new process of referring patients (and might still have some personal reservations about the new SMA program). They could be simply forgetting to invite all appropriate patients, might be nervous themselves about making the referral, may feel inadequate and not up to the task, might not feel comfortable in recommending the program, or might be making some fundamental mistakes in how they are wording invitations and referring patients—all of which could be undercutting their success in referring patients into the SMA.

The worst scenario of all is when the physician or some of the support staff do not really believe in the program and its many patient benefits—in fact, they may hold a deep-seated idea that they would not want to attend a group visit themselves and that others would not want to either (or they might even believe that the whole thing is a dumb idea). When even one person associated with the new SMA holds intense negative feelings or strong reservations about the program, it is amazing how quickly that negativity can begin to affect others. When this happens, it needs to be promptly addressed *before the well gets poisoned*. This is an excellent example of the old adage that "One rotten apple can spoil the bushel."

When we are personally not sold on the program and hold such negative beliefs, it inevitably shows in our demeanor and body language—so that our referrals and recommendations do not ring true to our patients, who then tend to disregard our invitation and decline to attend the SMA. To be enthusiastic in our endorsement of the SMA, and to be fully effective in referring patients into it, we need to truly believe in the program ourselves. One such example of this is the physician who recently told me: "You know, when I invite a patient and they decline to attend the DIGMA, I actually feel bad for them because I know what they are missing." When the physician and staff truly believe in their program (as was the case for this physician), it typically carries over into enthusiastic patient invitations and consequently, full group sessions.

In each of these cases, the program coordinator and champion need to meet with the affected staff members (and sometimes even the provider) to address all of these issues—confronting any resistances, answering any questions, addressing any concerns, and providing whatever additional training might be helpful. In addition, it is important to get any staff member who does not fundamentally believe in the program to actually sit in on a session or two just as soon as the SMA is up and running (or to sit in on another SMA that is already being successfully conducted elsewhere in the system) to personally experience what a warm, pleasant, and educational experience it can be for patients. If this does not work and this person remains a constant source of negativity toward the SMA program, then the physician or administration may soon need to step in to address this problem.

If the Census Is Low, Alert the Provider and Schedulers (Plus Have the Dedicated Scheduler Call Patients Approved by the Provider), but Postpone the SMA if Sessions Are Not Filling Properly

In the event that the census for the first four SMA sessions remains low during these last 2 weeks prior to the launch, then the champion and/or program coordinator should contact the provider and scheduling staff—on a daily basis, if necessary—to keep them appraised of the situation, and the urgent need to rectify it by promptly referring more patients into these initial SMA sessions. The program coordinator needs to enlist their help and support in this regard post-haste—i.e., by encouraging the physician and staff to redouble their referral efforts immediately.

The program coordinator can also offer to have the dedicated scheduler help in this process by calling and inviting patients from the list of approved patients previously provided by the physician. The program coordinator could even offer to have the dedicated scheduler train the physician's scheduling staff by showing them (on a personal one-on-one basis, if necessary) how she/he makes *cold calls* to patients, recommends the SMA, and encourages them to attend.

However, the bottom line remains that if sessions are not being filled by the provider and staff at a rate that the champion and program coordinator are comfortable with, then the launch of the new SMA will need to be postponed accordingly (or else redesigned so as to be more inclusive of patients)—until sessions are being appropriately filled. I have generally found it to be a big mistake to prematurely launch a DIGMA or PSMA before it has clearly been demonstrated that upcoming sessions can be consistently kept full by the physician and support staff. It should also be made clear to all that the dedicated scheduler's job is to *top off* SMA sessions that have already been largely filled by the provider and staff; however, it is not to take primary responsibility for filling the group sessions (which must always remain the physician and support staff's responsibility).

Assemble the "Patient Packets" for All Patients Attending the DIGMA or PSMA

With only 2 weeks to go prior to launching the provider's new DIGMA or PSMA, this is the time to assemble enough Patient Packets to be used in the program for the first couple of sessions—and, in the case of PSMAs, it is important that they be sent to preregistered patients at least 2–3 weeks prior to the session. Patient Packets not only play an important role in the success of a DIGMA or PSMA program but also add to the patients' perception of the quality of that program by giving them important health-related materials to take home with them and read later. While, unlike the case for PSMAs, a Patient Packet is not mandatory for a DIGMA, it does provide a nice touch regarding the quality of the program and how hard the staff has worked to make patients' SMA experience a positive one—i.e., one that patients truly appreciate. This additional patient education is just one other way that DIGMAs and PSMAs strive to enhance quality, max-pack visits, and make them an *one-stop healthcare shopping experience* for patients.

The Patient Packets are typically given to patients when they come in and register for the DIGMA. It contains a variety of enclosures that have been personally selected by the provider, which are presented in a nice folder (see Fig. 2.4 and examples of Patient Packets on the DVD). I generally use a folder that looks expensive but is actually quite cheap. Often in the organization's colors, the folder can also have the organization's logo (and/or the name of the SMA and the doctor printed on it)—creating the impression that these are important, high-quality materials that are to be taken seriously. The folder is usually constructed from heavy, glossy paper that is folded in half, and then bent up on the bottom of both sides on the interior—so that enclosures can be placed inside of the flaps on both sides when it is opened. I usually place materials that the patient will need during the session inside the left flap (name tag, confidentiality release, blank sheet of paper saying "Notes" on top, program description flier, patient satisfaction questionnaire, etc.). On the other hand, I try to place most of the take-home materials, such as PR materials on the organization, list of internal and external resources, educational handouts selected by the physician, etc., inside of the right inside flap.

Clearly, the program coordinator will need to promptly purchase (from the SMA budget) the folders that will contain all of these enclosures that have been selected and approved by the physician. However, somebody still needs to make copies of all the enclosures and then actually assemble the Patient Packets. This person is usually a motivated clerical person on the physician's support staff; however, it could also be someone else, such as the provider's office manager, a medical assistant, or even a volunteer. Furthermore, this needs to be an ongoing responsibility for that staff person—i.e., because enough Patient Packets need to be assembled for each DIGMA or PSMA session, so that every patient gets one during each session. Usually it is the receptionist who: gives the Patient Packet to patients when they register for the DIGMA; collects the signed confidentiality release; and writes the patient's first or last name legibly (depending upon the physician's preference, although I strongly recommend first names only as they are less disclosing of identity) on the name tag in large, bold letters using a fat felt marker with dark ink—so that names can easily be read by the physician from across the group room. While these name tags help patients to get to know each other, they also keep the physician from being embarrassed by not knowing patients' names.

Address Any Unresolved Issues as They Arise Prior to the Launch

There will undoubtedly still be many last minute issues, problems, and concerns that come to the attention of the SMA champion and program coordinator during the last 2 weeks prior to the launch. It is important to address any such unresolved issues as soon as they arise, certainly prior to the launch of the DIGMA or PSMA. For example: computers might not work properly; the provider might not be able to sign on; there might be some scheduling problems; group room furnishings might still need to be installed; someone might need to be found to set the chairs up in a circular or elliptical seating arrangement before sessions; glitches might exist around snacks; or equipment might need to be ordered for the exam room(s), announcement letters might not be going out as planned, Patient Packets may not have been assembled, or getting paper medical charts to the group room might prove problematic (for systems still using paper). When any such problems occur, it is important that they be promptly addressed and completely remedied, preferably prior to that launch of the first SMA session.

Just Before the Launch, Conduct a Complete "Walk-Through" and "Mock" DIGMA or PSMA, with Staff Acting as Patients—a Practice "Dry Run" to Detect Defects

From a couple of days to a week prior to the launch, the champion and program coordinator need to schedule and conduct a complete *walk through* for the SMA—plus a *mock* DIGMA or PSMA with staff acting as patients although some systems choose to do both the walk through and the mock all at once. These are meant to be practice *dry runs* to detect any remaining defects prior to the first SMA session—sort of a *shakedown* cruise, if you will. The *walk-through* involves walking through the entire sequence of steps that patients will soon be going through for the DIGMA or PSMA. This includes: entering the building; finding the right place to register (do directional signs need to be utilized?); actually registering (are the receptionists or PSRs able to handle the anticipated volume of patients efficiently, or is additional help needed?); receiving the Patient Packet (in the case of DIGMAs) and signing the confidentiality release (together with any accompanying support person); getting a name tag and putting it on (be certain it is placed in a highly visible location on the clothing that the patient will be wearing in the group room, and not on a coat or sweater that will be removed); getting to the group room (will patients be escorted or directed to the group room?); being roomed into the exam room (will the MA or nurse be doing this?); going out to the Care Coordinator once the physician has finished working with a patient and completed their chart note; scheduling follow-up appointments, preferably back into the DIGMA whenever appropriate

(how will this scheduling be handled?), and being able to find one's way out of the building after the group session is over.

If they are needed, determine who will be responsible for putting the directional signs up for SMA sessions that direct patients where to go in order to register, to find the group and exam rooms, to schedule any follow-up appointments, and then to exit the building. The same person should be responsible for putting these signs up before all SMA sessions on an ongoing basis, and then for taking them down immediately after sessions.

The walk-through and mock SMA could either be scheduled together (usually a couple of days prior to the first session) or at separate times—in which case, the walk-through would typically occur first (perhaps a week or two prior to the launch date), whereas the mock DIGMA or PSMA would usually occur 1–7 days before the launch. When combined, the walk through and mock SMA are typically scheduled for 2–2½ hours (30–60 minutes for the walk through and 90 minutes for the mock DIGMA or PSMA plus debriefing that follows). The purpose of conducting a complete *walk-through* and *mock* DIGMA or PSMA (i.e., a *dry run* of the SMA, with the provider, SMA team, and all involved support staff being included, plus additional staff acting as patients) just prior to the launch is to detect and correct any defects during the practice session. The intent here is to discover any problems that exist in this benign setting, so that they can be corrected before the first session is actually held. Despite everyone's best efforts, expect that some confusion and mistakes will nonetheless occur at the beginning of every new DIGMA or PSMA—which is something that we are trying to minimize by detecting and correcting them beforehand, prior to the actual launch, through the *walk-through* and *mock DIGMA or PSMA*.

The mock DIGMA or PSMA needs to include the provider, behaviorist, nurse/MA, documenter, receptionists, and key operations and administrative personnel in the provider's workplace. Here—with the physician, behaviorist, documenter, and nursing personnel acting out their actual roles (and with staff role-playing patients)—one is trying to create as realistic of a SMA session as possible, one that mimics what will ultimately be the live SMA as closely as possible. The intent is to not only provide practice for all involved before the actual go-live SMA event occurs, but also detect (and solve) any real-life problems that might emerge beforehand—i.e., in this relatively benign and innocuous environment.

Although they can be stressful (in fact, many providers later say that the mock SMA was harder for them than the actual first session), it usually quickly becomes an enjoyable experience for all participants—and one that includes considerable laughter. Whenever possible, it is also helpful to include as pretend patients in the mock SMA all scheduling personnel who will be involved with scheduling patients into the SMA on an ongoing basis—and to also have them sit in on a SMA session once it is launched and running smoothly, so that they can both appreciate the benefits that it provides and later be able to *sell* it to patients.

The Patient Flow of the Walk-Through

The intent of the *walk-through* is for everyone involved to imagine themselves as being patients, and to walk through all of the steps that patients will take during the actual SMA—i.e., to go through the entire process, from start to finish (from a patient's point of view), in an effort to detect and solve any problems or weak points before the real group visit occurs in a day or two.

It is important to note that the walk-through process would be somewhat different for PSMAs than for DIGMAs. This is because in the PSMA, patients would first receive private physical examinations during the first half of the session (i.e., while the unroomed patients are in the group room with the behaviorist, who would be warming the group up, writing down the issues that patients want addressed during today's visit, discussing patient handouts, etc.). In general, the early arriving patients would register, sign the confidentiality release, receive a name tag, and be roomed into the exam rooms (typically, but not always, four) first. Once the physical examination has been completed, the patient dresses and is escorted back to the group room—and another patient is escorted back from the group room to be roomed in the exam room first for their physical. In the PSMA, once these private physical examinations are completed on all patients in attendance, all patients would be in the group room and basically a small DIGMA would be held during the second half of the session. On the other hand, for DIGMAs, the walk-through process would be as follows.

The Walk-Through Process for DIGMAs from Start to Finish

For DIGMAs, this simulated patient flow would include entering through the front door and finding one's way to the registration desk (do direction signs need to be put up?); then registering, receiving the Patient Packet, signing the confidentiality waiver, putting the name tag on, and being seated in the lobby; and finally being escorted from the lobby to the group room. Also, determine how patients will go from the receptionist to the group room (i.e., whether they will be escorted, or be directed by signs), and whether they will wait in the lobby area for a while after registering but before going to the group room. Be watchful here to determine whether or not the receptionists can handle the expected number of SMA patients (although patients often do arrive in somewhat of a staggered manner, rather than all at once), or will extra help need to be assigned to the reception desk for 20 minutes or so just prior to each SMA session?

Once in the group room, patients would be called out by the nurse/MA(s) to the nearby exam room for vital signs and other nursing duties, and then returned to the group room for the DIGMA. Ensure that the exam room is sufficiently close to the group room for the patients that will be attending (especially if they are anticipated to have mobility problems) and that the exam room is properly equipped. In addition, review the process by which patients will schedule their follow-up visits during the SMA (for example, will a care coordinator be used)—which should be scheduled back into the SMA whenever possible and appropriate.

In particular, will follow up visits be scheduled during or after group—i.e., individually during the group session (i.e., by having patients temporarily step out to schedule their return appointment prior to returning to the group room, perhaps with the care coordinator, who not only schedules any referrals and follow-ups, but also gives them an after-visit summary of the most important parts of the SMA chart note for them to keep) or *en masse* after the group is over (which could overwhelm the scheduling desk)? Or else, will a scheduler be brought in toward the end of the session to schedule follow-ups? Will the documenter actually schedule the returns per the physician's recommendations, or will patients' names be written down on a sheet of paper (or checked off on the attendance roster), along with the date that they are to return, by the physician or behaviorist and later given to a scheduler to actually schedule all follow-up appointments after the DIGMA is over? Finally, make sure that patients know how to get from the group room to the building's exit once the group is over. At Harvard Vanguard Medical Associates/Atrius Health, all of these scheduling functions are handled by the *Care Coordinator*—who also provides each patient with an *after visit summary* of their DIGMA/PSMA visit. See the example of a "walk-through" checklist that is included in the forms section of the DVD attached to this book.

Mock DIGMA or PSMA

The purpose here is to conduct a complete mock DIGMA or PSMA from start to finish—again, making it as realistic as possible, but using staff as patients. In other words, in addition to holding the walk-through that previews the entire patient flow process (i.e., prior to, during, and after the SMA session), it is important to also review the entire flow of the SMA program itself—from start to finish—through a *mock* DIGMA or PSMA. Try to make the mock SMA as realistic as possible by using the same number of patients (acted out by staff) as are actually pre-registered for the SMA and utilizing the same group and exam rooms as will be used for the actual SMA. Have the provider and SMA team members act as themselves—but have staff act as patients, i.e., bringing in an assortment of medical issues that could be either scripted or real. Pay particularly close attention to the entire documentation process during the mock DIGMA, as experience has shown that computer and documentation problems often occur during the initial sessions of a new DIGMA or PSMA.

As was the case for the walk-through, the purpose of the *mock SMA* is to anticipate, detect, and promptly solve any problems that might occur before the program actually starts. Throughout the mock DIGMA, the champion and program coordinator can be interjecting helpful suggestions and tips-and pointing out common pitfalls to be avoided. Be sure to review all of the following during the mock DIGMA:

- When will confidentiality releases be signed and how will they be collected before group?
- Who will fill out the name tags and make sure that the patient puts it on in a highly visible place (e.g. not on a coat that is later taken off)?
- Are the computer and printer completely functional, and are the provider and documenter able to sign-on?
- Are the computers also functional in the exam rooms and can the MA/nurse(s) log on?
- What vital signs, injections, routine health maintenance, and *special duties* are the nurse/MA(s) to provide?
- What documentation, if any, will the MA/nurse(s) provide?
- Where will the behaviorist write down patients' medical issues (flipchart, erasable whiteboard, etc.)?
- What will the precise content of the behaviorist's introduction be, and will patients be told that they can leave early (this needs to be rehearsed in advance and kept to no more than 3–5 minutes in length)?
- By what time must the provider enter the group room and how will he/she start the SMA?

- What types of patients will the physician address first in the group setting (e.g. those who need to leave early; patients who have brought children; patients with colds, flues, or headaches)?
- How much medical care will the provider deliver to each patient in the group setting?
- Will the provider examine each patient in the group room and do something *hands-on* (and, if so, precisely what)?
- How will the provider and behaviorist foster group interaction (and how much)?
- Is the provider making efficient use of both the documenter and the behaviorist?
- Is there good coordination between the provider and behaviorist when a chart note is being documented?
- Are the provider and behaviorist pacing the group so as to finish on time—and, if not, why not?
- Precisely how will follow-up appointments be scheduled during the SMA (e.g. will there be a Care Coordinator and will patients receive an after visit summary)?
- When will the provider see patients needing brief private exams or discussions?
- How and when will the provider exit from the group once the session is over?
- Will patients be asked to complete any forms before or after the session (e.g. patient satisfaction form, quality of life or functional status measures. Or perhaps brief tests for depression, exercise, diet, self-efficacy, or coping skills)?
- How long the behaviorist will stay after group, and how will the group room be cleared and straightened up?
- Will there be a team debriefing afterward (and if so, when, where, and who will attend), and for how long after the launch of the SMA will they be held?

The Mock DIGMA Process

This realistic role play should last as long as the DIGMA, typically 90 minutes, and cover the entire flow of the group as it normally occurs—including the entire sequence of responsibilities of all members of the SMA team. The mock DIGMA starts with patients being called out of the group room, one at a time prior to the session, for their vital signs, injections, and special nursing duties—with the nurse/MA drafting their section of the mock chart note on each patient, and returning patients (and any paper medical charts) to the group room afterward. After all nursing duties are completed on all patients, the SMA nurse/MA(s) could return to normal clinic duties—although one can become the Care Coordinator during the last half of the DIGMA session to schedule all recommended appointments and give patients an after visit summary). However, for the purposes of the mock DIGMA, it is recommended that they be encouraged to stay and join the group as patients or observers. In the real-life DIGMA to follow in a day or two, the nursing personnel will arrive 15–30 minutes early to start their nursing functions on each patient, and then continue with each patient in turn until all are finished—pausing in their process of calling patients out of the group room one at a time only when the behaviorist is giving the introduction, so that all are able to hear the introduction.

The behaviorist arrives early to warm the group up and write down each patient's health concerns on a whiteboard or flip chart, and then starts the group on time with the introduction—which should be role-played in its entirety to ensure that it is comprehensive, yet take no more than 3–5 minutes. The physician then arrives and starts by sequentially delivering medical care to one patient at a time in the group setting (starting with whichever patients the physician wants to begin with, which are often patients saying that they need to leave early or those with cold and flu symptoms), while others are able to listen, interact, and learn—and then reviewing each patient's chart note until all patients are finished (hopefully on time, which probably will not happen at first). Once the provider has finished working with a particular patient in the group setting and completed the chart note on that patient, the Care Coordinator can then call the patient out of the exam room to schedule all appointments and referrals (and to give the patient an after visit summary).

A special focus of the mock DIGMA must be made on the documenter (if one is used) and the entire process of how the chart note is to be efficiently, yet comprehensively, drafted on each patient—i.e., in a timely manner during the group session, using the physician's own chart note template. Also, if a documenter is employed, the physician will need to rehearse, review, and modify the documenter's chart note immediately after working with each patient individually in the group setting—i.e., while the behaviorist temporarily takes over the group, focusing on some behavioral health or psychosocial issue(s). If the physician is not using a documenter, and is instead personally documenting the chart note (regardless of whether this is done with paper, dictation, or EMR), the teamwork between the behaviorist and the physician needs to be thoroughly rehearsed in this mock DIGMA—so that they are reasonably coordinated by the time that the first session is held.

Throughout this process, staff participating in the mock DIGMA or PSMA can be encouraged to act like various patients they actually see in the clinic—or else to discuss any past or present personal health problem that they might feel more comfortable in role-playing. It is important for the provider and behaviorist to develop a sense of timing throughout this mock SMA, so that they begin to develop a cadence and rhythm that enables them to pace themselves and finish on time. They also need to work out the signals which the behaviorist will be using to keep the group moving along smoothly and on time—i.e., in the event that the physician becomes too loquacious, or bogged down, with certain patients in the group.

This is a good time for one or two staff acting as mock patients to act out certain difficult situations that can happen in the group—such as a patient who is overly talkative and dominating, a patient who is reluctant to speak, or two patients who keep starting distracting side-conversations. They can even assume the role of a difficult patient that is currently being seen in the clinic. As soon as the mock SMA is finished, the physician would then role play by pretending to leave the group room—i.e., while the behaviorist lingers to address any last-minute patient questions and issues, to clear the room of patients, and to quickly straighten up the group room. Also role play how patients will schedule their follow-up appointments either during or after the SMA. Be certain to have the provider, SMA team members, involved support staff, program coordinator, and champion debrief thoroughly after the mock SMA.

Usually, there is quite a sense of relief and accomplishment by the time that the mock DIGMA is over, with staff often now feeling energized and more confident—as the mock is not only a rehearsal but often also an enjoyable and successful experience. Because staff and colleagues are there, some physicians later say that the mock DIGMA was harder for them to do than the actual first session—so that their sense of relief afterward is almost palpable. At this point, it is not uncommon for there to be a lot of laughter, a sense of excitement, and some real enthusiasm shared by provider, SMA team, and support staff.

Champion Points Out Common Beginners' Mistakes That Physicians and Behaviorists Often Make

Throughout the mock DIGMA or PSMA, the champion needs to point out common beginners' mistakes that physicians and behaviorists often make so that they can be avoided during the actual SMA session that will soon follow. Remember that group visits represent a major paradigm shift from the traditional office visits that physicians are used to, the result being that they can easily make common beginners' mistakes that interfere with the flow of the group and slow it down. Often, these mistakes are a result of bringing elements of the individual office visit into the group room, where they are frequently counterproductive. Therefore, it is helpful for the champion to point out—as they occur in the mock SMA—some of the most common beginners' mistakes that physicians make when first starting their SMA, most of which end up slowing the group down so that it is difficult to finish on time (and, if left unchecked, can even end up undercutting the entire program). Many common beginners' mistakes are discussed in detail elsewhere in this book (e.g. see Chapter 10).

Aligning the Motivations of Patients and Physicians to Finish on Time

As with individual office visits, finishing on time in a DIGMA or PSMA can also be a problem because, whereas the physician might be motivated to end on time, patients might have the opposite motivation—i.e., by wanting to have more time with their physician. Physicians are often surprised by this because they sometimes almost feel guilty for expecting patients to stay for a 90-minute group visit session—i.e., until they think about the fact that the *cycle time* (i.e., from the minute that the patient enters the doors of the clinic until when they leave) with a short individual office visit is often 90 minutes or more. However, in a DIGMA, the patient is spending the entire 90 minutes with the physician—i.e., rather than being the patient waiting in the lobby, exam room, etc. and just having 7 or 10 minutes with the physician, as is often the case for a short office visit.

What is the solution to this dilemma? One physician had an interesting approach to ensuring that his DIGMA always finished on time. He would simply enter and start the group off by saying something of great interest to the group, such as, "I just read the most interesting article on a promising new treatment for diabetes. I'll tell you what, if we get finished a few minutes early today, I'll tell you about it." This motivates patients to join with the physician in getting the group finished on time, rather than trying to extract even more time from the physician. The champion could remind new SMA providers of this strategy during the mock DIGMA or PSMA—one that can enhance patient education and help them to finish their DIGMA or PSMA on time.

Some of the Most Common Beginners' Mistakes That Physicians Make

The following are some of the most common beginners' mistakes that physicians make when first starting a DIGMA or PSMA program:

- Not staying focused on the medical needs of one patient at a time throughout the DIGMA session (and instead jumping around like a *pinball* from one patient to another, going to the next patient without ever first finishing with the initial patient and completing that patient's chart note), so that documentation is not completed and the group ends up being scattered, fragmented, and disorganized.

- Taking too long on the first couple of patients, so that an unsustainable pace is set from the outset—with the ultimate result being that the group ends up finishing late.

- Sitting on a chair with wheels, and then wheeling over and talking quietly to patients one-on-one, rather than speaking to them clearly from across the room so that all can listen and learn. This results in other patients in the group, who cannot hear what the physician is saying, starting distracting side-conversations with the person next to them—so that the physician quickly loses control of the group. This is an example of carrying forward into the SMA what one normally does during traditional office visits, which often is done to the detriment of the group.

- Slowing the group down—and making it less interesting and beneficial to others—by unnecessarily taking many or even all patients outside of the group room for private one-on-one time during the session for matters that could be handled just as well in the group setting (i.e., where others could listen, interact, and learn). Generally speaking, physicians become increasingly comfortable with delivering evermore care in the DIGMA and PSMA group settings as time passes and experience is gained.

- At most, one or two patients will typically need to be seen by the physician outside of the group room for a brief exam or discussion in the privacy of the exam room. When this does occur, another common beginner's mistake is for the physician to immediately take that patient out of the group room when working with them—i.e., right in the middle of the session. This interrupts the flow of the group and also takes the behaviorist by surprise—thereby leaving the behaviorist with little or no time to prepare what to say when temporarily taking over the group while the physician steps out with the patient. As a result, it is usually best for the physician to wait until towards the end of the session to conduct these 1–2 brief private exams and discussions. There are two exceptions to this: *first*, the patient who needs to leave early but requires a brief private exam or discussion, whom the physician will most likely need to take to the exam room immediately since this patient cannot stay until the end of the session; and *second*, the patient who arrived with the misunderstanding that this was to be an individual office visit rather than a group visit—which is something that should be avoided at all costs, as this does anger and frustrate patients. In the latter case, the physician could offer the patient the choice either of being seen immediately in the privacy of the exam room or of staying for the group and giving it a try since they are there anyway—an option which many such patients do in fact choose.

- Not fostering some group interaction, so as to keep all patients involved and attentive—or fostering too much interaction, as this takes too much time and slows the group down. I am fond of saying that group interaction is like using spice in cooking—a little bit is great, but too much spoils the dish (which, in the case of group visits, means that the group ends up finishing late because too much interaction is very time consuming).
- Not delegating as much as possible and appropriate to other members of the SMA team—the ultimate result of which will be that the physician ends up personally doing more than needs to be done with each patient, and therefore being less efficient and productive. The inevitable result here is that the physician will either finish late or ultimately end up seeing fewer patients during SMA sessions.
- Another common beginners' mistake is taking too much time with patients who happen to have conditions of particular interest to the physician. This makes it important for the behaviorist and physician to work out a signal beforehand by which the behaviorist can interrupt to help keep the group moving along in a timely manner whenever the physician begins to ramble, or gets into a level of detail that is more suitable for a medical grand rounds presentation than for a group visit. This signal can be something as simple as the behaviorist pointing to his/her wristwatch, or saying something like: "So what's the follow-up plan, doctor?" or "That's a very important point, Dr. Jones. But I see that we still have quite a few patients to go. How about moving along now, and then coming back to this very important issue if we have some extra time toward the end of the group?" Other behaviorists simply say: "And what's the follow-up plan, doctor?"
- The physician and behaviorist not pacing themselves throughout the SMA session so as to finish on time—i.e., by the physician not staying focused and succinct, by trying to do too much with certain patients, by not completing the chart note after working with each patient, by giving too much time to dominating or controlling patients, etc. The same net result will occur if the behaviorist takes too much time during interventions and discussions.

Some of the Most Common Beginners' Mistakes That Behaviorists Make

Similar to physicians, behaviorists can also make a host of beginner's mistakes—again, mistakes that all too often end up taking too much time, with the net result being that the group finishes late (or that, ultimately, fewer patients can be seen per session). The following are examples of beginners' mistakes that behaviorists often make:

- Believing that they know how to run groups (i.e., without any special learning or training in the DIGMA/PSMA models, simply because they have run many groups in the past) and not taking the time to fully understand, at both theoretical and operational levels, the details of the behaviorist's role in the DIGMA or PSMA model that they will be participating in—i.e., rather than just gaining a superficial or casual understanding. This is because the behaviorist's role in a SMA is very different from a traditional mental health role and because it is a much more active, directive, and self-disclosing role than they are likely used to.
- Not arriving 10–15 minutes early to welcome patients, warm the group up, and write patients' issues for the day down on a flip chart or whiteboard
- Starting the introduction late (or taking too long with the introduction), so that the group ends up starting and finishing late
- Failing to pace and adequately manage the group, so that the session finishes late
- Fostering too much group interaction
- Refusing to promptly wrap up their discussions around behavioral health and psychosocial issues and move onto the next patient just as soon as the physician has completed reviewing and modifying the previous patient's chart note
- Taking too long in their interventions around psychosocial issues (by and large, the purpose here is to promptly but tactfully bring such issues to the physician's attention so that medications can be started or the physician can refer the patient to the appropriate depression, anxiety, substance abuse, weight loss, or smoking cessation program—not for the behaviorist to attempt to treat these issues in the SMA)
- Failing to see their role as one of assisting the physician in every possible way in the delivery of high-quality medical care to his/her patients—i.e., and not as one of bringing their own agenda into the SMA (e.g., meditation training, relaxation training, depression treatment)
- Appearing in any way self-serving rather than patient centered, such as referring patients into the behaviorist's own private practice

- Feeling intimidated and afraid of actively pacing the group to keep it moving smoothly and on time, even if that might mean tactfully interrupting or cutting the physician off at times. This is especially common with recently licensed and inexperienced behaviorists, as well as those who might be very introverted and shy. I have yet to find the physician who says "Don't interrupt me, I would rather finish late."

The behaviorist needs to understand that not only is his/her role a much more active and directive one in a DIGMA or PSMA, but also that time-consuming, open-ended interventions are usually counterproductive. In other words, there is little room for interventions like "Uh huh, and how does that make you feel?" From start to finish, the focus of a properly conducted DIGMA or PSMA is upon the efficient delivery of high-quality, high-value medical care sequentially delivered to one patient at a time in the supportive group setting while other patients are able to listen, interact, and learn. One must always keep in mind that the DIGMA and PSMA models are actually run like a series of individual office visits with observers in which some group interaction is fostered.

Especially at first, the behaviorist might feel intimidated and hesitate to tactfully interject—i.e., even when it is called for, such as in an effort to keep things moving when the physician is rambling and talking too much. However, almost all physicians prefer to have the behaviorist help them to stay on track and finish on time—even if it means occasionally being interrupted during the session. Like the physician, the behaviorist needs to learn to be clear and focused in his/her interventions, and to speak largely in succinct sound bytes.

Steps to Be Taken After Launching Your New DIGMA or PSMA

Once the DIGMA or PSMA has been successfully launched, there are still several additional steps that are required for the long-term success of the newly implemented program.

After the First SMA Session Has Been Held

Congratulations! It took courage and a lot of effort, but you did it. After completing all the preparations that the 10-week pipeline entailed, your first DIGMA or PSMA session has finally been held. Despite all the worries and anxieties that doing something new and different can

engender, you nonetheless had the courage and intestinal fortitude to make it happen. Now try to improve and refine your SMA during the coming months—and learn to enjoy it and have some fun! However, always try to run your SMA in a way that is maximally beneficial to your patients, yourself, and your practice.

During the next few sessions, be observant, learn from your mistakes, and make any changes necessary to accomplish your goals. Although you probably finished late, felt nervous and pressured, and had many worries and concerns during your first session, the most difficult session is now over. From now on, you can expect your SMA to quickly become easier and more comfortable for you to run as your patients, staff, SMA team, and yourself become more familiar and experienced with it (Fig. 11.2). Now you can see why everybody is not doing group visits already—i.e., because the hardest part, by far, is just getting started properly (and thereafter in maintaining census targets on an ongoing basis).

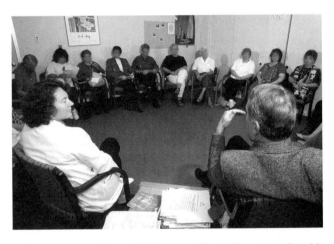

Fig. 11.2 You and your SMA team will quickly get comfortable with this new modality of delivering care and adapt seamlessly to working together to gain full efficiency throughout the session. (Courtesy of American Medical Group Association and Dr. Lynn Dowdell, the Kaiser Permanente Medical Center, San Jose, CA.)

What will surprise you now is how rapidly you and your team will be able to get comfortable with this new modality of delivering care. It is highly likely that, from this point forward, you and your SMA team will quickly become adjusted to one another, adapt to seamlessly coordinating your efforts, and learn to gain full efficiency throughout the session. By following the pointers presented in this book (and by debriefing with your SMA team after sessions for the first 2 months, focusing upon how to make future sessions even better and more productive), you will likely find that within a couple of months you will have made amazing progress with your new DIGMA or PSMA. Furthermore, within 6–12 months, you and your SMA team will likely begin to feel like *old pros* in running it. It's surprising that after going to medical school for so many years to learn how to conduct a traditional individual office visit well, within just a few months you can become very proficient and expert at delivering medical care in a venue that is as different as a group visit.

Try to Finish on Time with Full Groups and All Chart Notes Completed

During these initial SMA sessions, pay special attention to: (1) having full groups; (2) getting finished on time; and (3) completing all chart notes during the session. However, do not be discouraged if you finish late, even very late, during these initial sessions—as you and your team are still learning and unsure of yourselves, and are still not yet fully coordinated and seamless in your work together. Be certain to carefully evaluate how well you are doing with efficiently completing all chart notes during your initial SMA sessions. If you are not yet using a documenter, seriously consider whether having one could be of value to you in increasing your enjoyment and efficiency within the SMA—as the answer here will almost certainly be a resounding "Yes." Having now actually completed your first DIGMA or PSMA session, you can see more clearly than ever why I so strongly recommend having a documenter to make your SMA experience more efficient and enjoyable—to you and your patients alike.

Regardless of whether you use a documenter or choose to do your chart notes yourself immediately after working with each patient, be certain to focus upon enhancing the teamwork you establish with your behaviorist around the charting process. The goal here is to learn to: (1) seamlessly transition from the group to reviewing the chart note while the behaviorist temporarily takes over running the group; (2) complete reviewing and modifying the chart note within a minute or two; and finally (3) go back to the group again, and to the next patient, in a highly efficient manner. It is important that this documentation review and modification process not take more than a minute or two (maximum) on each patient—although, if you do your own charting, you might find yourself doing much of the documenting while actually talking with each patient (just as you most likely normally do when seeing patients individually during regular office visits). The problem with this is that by doing some documentation while speaking with each person in turn, you will also likely get the same complaint as with traditional

individual office visits—i.e., "The doctor looked at the computer the whole time, and never looked at me." Continued practice and efficient teamwork with the behaviorist (and the documenter, when one is used) are the two keys to success when it comes to completing all chart notes during group time.

As experience is gained, the ultimate goal is to eventually learn to pace the group so that it actually finishes a few minutes early. This ensures that there will still be a little time left toward the end of the session in which the physician can conduct brief private exams and discussions as needed. However, when the DIGMA is properly run, there are usually only one or two such private encounters needing to be done toward the end of the group—and most commonly none. If there are one or two patients that need to be seen privately by the physician toward the end of the session, then the behaviorist can temporarily take over leading the group of patients remaining in the group room while the physician is conducting any needed brief private examinations or discussions in the nearby exam room. Again, the behaviorist focuses on behavioral health and psychosocial issues (or nursing issues if the behaviorist is a nurse) of importance to the patients in attendance, and continues to do so until either the physician returns or the group ends.

During upcoming SMA sessions, as additional experience is gained and as you debrief with your team after sessions to discuss how to make future sessions even better and more efficient, you should come closer and closer to finishing on time with full groups—i.e., even if you finished quite late during your first couple of sessions. You will likely be surprised at just how quickly you and your SMA team can become proficient at running your DIGMA or PSMA in a timely manner as a result of having such debriefings after sessions for the first couple of months of operations. Physicians often report becoming comfortable with their SMA in just a couple months, and frequently report feeling like *old pros* in just 6–12 months.

Be Flexible and Slowly Make Changes to the SMA as Needed, but Do Not Reduce Census Targets at First

Be flexible and willing to slowly make any necessary changes in your DIGMA or PSMA that can enhance the success of your group visit, but do not reduce census targets at first. Keep in mind that much about shared medical appointments is counterintuitive and that it is often wise (at least initially) to stay close to the established models to avoid the trap of making common beginners' mistake—i.e., do not just try to *wing it* on your own, especially at first before you know what you are doing. Nonetheless, once you have completed a few SMA sessions, you will likely spot a couple of things that need to be changed. When this does happen, try to be flexible, thoughtful, and deliberate about the changes you do make—and try to make them one at a time, so that you can quickly reverse course if your changes do not work. However, do not rush into reducing your predetermined census levels for your SMA.

Sometimes circumstances (such as the lack of available resources) dictate that you depart from certain aspects of DIGMAs, CHCCs, and PSMAs as they are normally constructed and conducted. When this occurs, it is often worth trying to do the best that you can with the resources at your disposal rather than just giving up entirely on the idea of group visits. Even if what you come up with is less than ideal, it could very well end up being perfectly functional and acceptable—and certainly much better than the alternative of not running a SMA at all for your practice. As I am fond of saying, "A *good enough* SMA is usually better than no SMA at all."

For example, if traditional mental health personnel are not available to you to use as a behaviorist, then consider using a gregarious, interpersonally skilled nurse, nurse practitioner, diabetic nurse educator, medical resident, pharmacist, or fellow with whom you are comfortable working. However, if you do so, be certain that they obtain some training in managing large groups, fostering group interaction, addressing group dynamic and psychosocial issues, etc.

If your census steadily increases over time (e.g., to the point where 14, 15, or 16 patients are attending your DIGMA regularly), then consider starting a second DIGMA in your practice—perhaps having your DIGMAs on Mondays and Thursdays, or on Tuesdays and Fridays. If these sessions also reach the maximum recommended census of 16 patients, then try adding even more DIGMAs to your weekly schedule (plus consider adding a weekly PSMA for your private physical examinations). Keep in mind that some physicians with large practices and demanding workloads have actually run daily DIGMAs to better manage their busy, backlogged practices. There will come a time in the not too distant future when the first physician will choose to run their practice as primarily DIGMAs and PSMAs and secondarily individual office visits (i.e., rather than the opposite, which is presently the case). Should you be that history making physician, be certain to let me know as soon as possible so that we can get an article published on your remarkable achievement.

If you are having problems filling your group because of the time of day or day of the week that it is being held, then consider making the appropriate changes. If no group room is available, consider using lobby space during off hours—or else, consider using any other space that might be available to you which could be converted to a group room, such as a storage area or staff lounge. Be certain to carry any such changes over into fliers, brochures, forms, master schedules, and all related SMA materials so that your patients always remain fully informed about your program.

Have All Staff Involved with Your SMA Sit in on a Session or Two on a Rotating Basis—Starting with Schedulers

I have found that having all support staff attend one or two sessions (i.e., just as soon as the DIGMA or PSMA program has been launched and is running smoothly) is one of the most effective means of getting staff to understand the multiple benefits of the program. This helps to secure staff buy-in, and can even get initially resistant staff members to enthusiastically embrace the program once they experience what a warm and caring experience it is for patients. Thus, try to have all schedulers, receptionists, nursing and support staff associated with the provider's new SMA attend a session or two (or at least a half of a session, if that is not possible)—one or two staff members at a time, starting with those most critical to the success of the program (such as the physician's primary schedulers). By doing so, they become comfortable and familiar with the DIGMA or PSMA and its many benefits firsthand. Thereafter, they can more easily explain the program and refer patients into it with whole-hearted enthusiasm.

The one possible exception here would be for staff members of the opposite sex sitting in on PSMAs that are only for males or for females; however, this would ultimately need to be the provider's decision. If the wrong decision should happen to be made here, it is easy enough to change course for the next PSMA session. The main point here is that whenever possible and appropriate, it is very helpful to have all support staff directly involved with the SMA program—especially those who are inviting and scheduling patients—sit in on a session to see firsthand what a warm, informative, and caring experience it is for patients. By so doing, they can get any questions they might have answered firsthand, plus thereafter be better able to invite and schedule patients into future SMA sessions.

Continue to Have All Attendees Sign the Confidentiality Waiver

Have all patients and support persons sign the confidentiality agreement/release just prior to, or at the very beginning of, each DIGMA or PSMA session. Be certain to also have any observers accompanying the patient to the SMA also sign the confidentiality agreement—usually the same one as the patient (i.e., signing either just above or just below the patient's signature). Determine whether these confidentiality releases are to be filed as hard copies (and, if so, where and how), or whether they are to be scanned into the patient's EMR chart note. If they are to be scanned into the EMR, determine: (1) what process will be used for doing so; (2) who will be responsible for doing it; and (3) when is this to be done. Also establish whether the hard copies are to be kept and filed, or whether they are to be shredded at some later date. For systems still using paper charts, the confidentiality release can actually be preprinted on the back of the paper chart note template being used for each patient in the SMA session, thus both saving a sheet of paper and guaranteeing that the release ends up in patients' medical charts (and clearly identifies the SMA session to which it applies).

A couple of healthcare organizations are looking into having their patients sign confidentiality agreements periodically (such as every 6 months) rather than during each session—something that I find problematic both because it is often difficult and time consuming to locate the previously signed release and because different support persons (all of whom must also sign) sometimes accompany the patient. In addition, at least one system has developed an oral confidentiality release that they feel is sufficient—in which the behaviorist reads the confidentiality release off during the introduction to each SMA, and patients only need to respond in the affirmative. Being conservative by nature, I am not comfortable with this approach and instead make the general recommendation to have all attendees sign a confidentiality agreement/release just prior to the start of each and every SMA session—and not to change this process until it is clearly demonstrated that it is all right to do so (i.e., that there is adequate precedent for doing otherwise and it is clearly accepted practice to do so).

Whenever Possible, Schedule Appropriate Return Visits into a Future SMA Session

Patients attending DIGMAs and PSMAs almost always like them, and are therefore usually willing to return to the SMA setting in the future. Patient satisfaction scores have typically ranged between 4.4 and 4.7 on a 5-point Likert scale, which is often higher than for individual office visits with the same providers. Therefore, for all appropriate patients attending the SMA who need to schedule a follow-up appointment, it is important that the physician offer to schedule their follow-up appointments back into future DIGMA sessions whenever possible (or their next physical examination into an upcoming PSMA session, which likely means that the provider's PSMA schedule will need to be opened at least a year in advance)—as this will be of great help in filling future sessions to desired capacity. Of course, as always, it is important to give patients the choice of having their next visit either be in the SMA or an individual office visit—so that the SMA program remains voluntary to patients and staff at all times.

Give a Copy of the Provider's Treatment Recommendations to Patients

If the physician so desires, the behaviorist can give each patient a written list of treatment recommendations made by the provider during the DIGMA or PSMA, although this list should first be quickly reviewed and signed by the provider. Or else, especially for systems using EMR, patients could be given a copy of their actual SMA chart note—or else, a printed *after visit summary* (AVS). This is especially helpful if these recommendations are complicated, if the patient is unmotivated or noncompliant, or if the patient might have difficulty remembering them. For systems using paper charts, this can be done by having the behaviorist write any such treatment recommendations down onto a sheet of paper (preferably a two copy form) while the physician is making them, a sheet which would then need to be quickly reviewed and signed by the physician before it is given to the patient—with the other copy, if there is one, being placed into the patient's medical chart. Or else, for systems using EMR, a copy of the patient's computerized chart note for the session (or better yet, an *after visit summary*, or AVS) could be printed out at some point during the session and given to the patient—a printout that would contain the provider's treatment recommendations. At Harvard Vanguard Medical Associates/Atrius Health, we have the MA act as a care coordinator during the last half of the DIGMA or PSMA session, calling patients out of the group room (one at a time) to schedule all follow-up appointments and referrals, and give patients their AVS (i.e., a printout of those parts of the SMA chart note that the physician wants the patient to have). For patients only needing to schedule a follow-up appointment with the provider (but not having to schedule any referrals), the care coordinator does not call them out of the group room—but instead takes the AVS into the group room to them (so as to reduce distractions to the group, and keep the patient from needlessly having to miss part of the group session).

Personally Compliment Schedulers, Receptionists, and Nursing Staff Whenever SMAs Are Filled

From now on, the provider should make a point of personally complimenting schedulers, receptionists, and nursing staff whenever full DIGMA or PSMA sessions are achieved—pointing out how much their help is contributing to the program's success. It is amazing how much this is appreciated by the support staff and how it motivates scheduling staff to continue filling upcoming sessions. In addition, it is a nice (and highly motivating) gesture to occasionally buy a lunch or a gourmet cup of coffee for exceptional staff members who refer and schedule many patients into the SMA. Even though saying "thank you" takes little time and is very much appreciated by support staff, it is something that physicians are not used to and are often reluctant to do. Nevertheless, I would strongly recommend that this be done routinely as it definitely contributes to the overall success of the DIGMA/PSMA program.

One final point, never harshly criticize or embarrass your support staff for putting the wrong patient into a group session—unless you want to suddenly find your staff no longer willing to refer patients and, as a result, to having your group sessions unfilled thereafter. I personally witnessed this happen one time when a physician's primary scheduler and receptionist took the challenge upon themselves of personally filling the physician's upcoming DIGMA session, which was to be held in just 2 days but had only one patient pre-registered. This was a physician who had a hard time promoting his DIGMA to patients and consequently often had sessions that were not completely filled. For 2 days they enthusiastically worked hard to fill the session, which eventually resulted in 15 patients actually attending the DIGMA just 2 days later.

Proud of themselves and expecting some praise for their efforts from the physician, what they got instead was a rather harshly worded public criticism to the effect that he would have preferred to have seen 2 of the 15 patients individually. That was it! They never again scheduled any more DIGMA appointments for him: despite his promises to never to do this again; despite

follow-up meetings together with the champion and program coordinator to resolve this matter; and despite the promise of such rewards as an espresso, pizza, free lunch, etc. Instead, they held the view: "Why should I take the chance of getting chewed out again?" As a result, this physician's DIGMA ultimately failed due to lack of adequate attendance, even though he very much liked it and dearly wanted his DIGMA to succeed.

Ensure that All SMA Materials Are Replenished as Needed

It is important that the duties of replenishing all SMA materials be assigned to specific members of the physician's support staff (especially the invitations that receptionists hand out and the program description fliers in the holders located in the provider's lobby and exam rooms), so that clear lines of responsibility and accountability are established. In addition, ensure that all handouts in the group room are replenished as needed, perhaps by the behaviorist, documenter, or nurse. Some healthcare systems organize all of the educational handouts (perhaps 5–30 copies of each) that the provider is likely to use during the SMA by alphabetizing them in file drawers. One provider used only a single file drawer to house all handouts needed during his first session, yet had expanded this to five drawers by the time I returned a year later! Other providers and systems have all of their handouts in electronic form so that they can simply print them out in the group room on an as needed basis.

Similarly replace and replenish any equipment or materials in the exam and group rooms as needed—such as diabetic test strips and frozen nitrogen canisters. Furthermore, if there is a need for any additional equipment or materials for the SMA in either the group or exam rooms, be sure to order them as soon as possible (e.g., stethoscopes, blood pressure cuffs, monofilaments for diabetic foot exams, pulse oximeter, anatomical models or charts, posters, tissues, flip charts, anatomical models or wall charts, erasable whiteboards felt markers).

Nonetheless, the program coordinator should take ultimate responsibility for overseeing all of these efforts by others to ensure that all equipment and materials used in the DIGMA or PSMA (i.e., in the provider's office area, the group room, and the exam rooms) are in fact replenished on an ongoing basis and in a timely manner. The program coordinator will then need to take prompt corrective action if this is not happening—providing additional training, speaking to the physician's office manager, or even reassigning tasks to more responsible personnel, if necessary.

The SMA Team and Provider Debrief After Sessions for 2 Months to Improve the Program and Its Efficiency

For the first 2 months after launching the DIGMA or PSMA, it is recommended that the provider, behaviorist, nursing personnel, and documenter (occasionally joined by the champion and/or program coordinator) debrief after sessions for 10–20 minutes to discuss how to make future SMA sessions even better and more efficient. This is an excellent way to improve efficiency to the point where the SMA is able to finish on time with full groups, even when initial sessions run quite late—and to do so without reducing predetermined census targets (i.e., the size of the DIGMA or PSMA group).

As has been discussed, the first SMA sessions often finish late and the immediate, almost *knee-jerk* reaction is to assume that the group finished late because it was too large—and then to promptly reduce the targeted census level for all future SMAs by several patients. In the vast majority of cases, this would prove to be a terrible mistake because, by so doing, you would undercut both the economic vitality of the SMA and the lively, interactive quality of full group sessions. This is simply a misinterpretation of the fact that this new paradigm of care delivery is still quite new to all, that everyone is anxious and does not yet know what they are doing, and that the physician and SMA team members are not yet fully coordinated and operating as seamlessly and efficiently as possible.

In the majority of cases, debriefing with the SMA team after sessions (focusing upon various ways to increase efficiency) should prove sufficient to gradually learning to finish sessions on time. Remember that you and your team are still new to this very different paradigm of providing medical care, and that you are very likely not yet functioning together optimally in this new SMA care delivery setting. During these debriefing sessions, ask yourselves such questions as the following:

- Did you spend too much time on one or two patients?
- Did everyone arrive when they were supposed to, and did you start on time?
- Were you too slow at various points in the session?
- Is the provider failing to fully delegate to the SMA team?
- Did you use a documenter and, if not, can you now incorporate one?
- Did the behaviorist fail to help pace the group?
- Did a particularly dominating patient manage to control the group?
- Was too much group interaction fostered?
- Were patients unnecessarily seen privately in the exam room?

- Did the behaviorist take too long in the introduction or during psychosocial interventions?
- Did the behaviorist fail to promptly wrap up the discussion when each patient's chart note was completed—so that the physician could immediately move on to the next patient?
- Were the documenter and provider sufficiently coordinated in efficiently completing each chart note?
- Does the documenter need additional training?
- Were there things that wasted time which could be avoided next time?
- Did the physician and/or behaviorist fail to stay focused and succinct throughout?
- Was time wasted looking for medical equipment, materials, or handouts?
- Was there too much social chit-chat?

In other words, resist the temptation to immediately reduce the size of your group and just accept the fact that, despite your best efforts, you will likely finish late at first because you and your team are still learning. Instead, maintain your census requirements and debrief with your team after sessions for the first couple of months. By doing so, you will probably soon find that you are finishing somewhat earlier during each subsequent session, so that you are able to finish on time with full groups within just a few months.

Only in the unlikely event that you find, despite debriefing with your team, that you are still not finishing on time after a couple of months of operations should you consider reducing the size of your group. However, even then, avoid draconian cuts and only reduce targeted census levels by just one or two patients—and then try to adapt to this new census level by finishing on time within another month or two, while continuing to debrief as a team after sessions. Although it is highly unlikely, you could repeat this process again a couple more months later if sessions still finish too late and the group size continues to seem too large. Once you are able to consistently finish on time, there will no longer be a need for you to formally debrief with your team after sessions—although you might still choose to do so occasionally on an as needed basis.

At that point, reduce time allocated to the 90-minute DIGMA or PSMA on the physician's (and the documenter's) schedule from 2 hours to 90 minutes; however, keep the behaviorist's schedule reserved for 2 hours (plus any travel time) on an ongoing basis as he/she will continue to arrive approximately 15 minutes early and leave about 15 minutes late. However, I do recommend initially holding 2 hours on the schedules of the physician, documenter, and behaviorist alike during the first 2 months of implementation (and possibly even 2 hours and 15 minutes initially on the behaviorist's schedule) to allow some extra time because initial sessions will likely finish late and because there is a need to debrief after sessions for the first 2 months.

Continue to Monitor Census for Upcoming Sessions

Finally, once the SMA is launched, you will need to monitor census for all upcoming sessions during the next month or two on an ongoing basis—preferably while also reviewing census levels during past sessions to date. The best way to do this is through periodic reports generated by the program coordinator (with the help of the champion)—such as weekly or twice weekly pre-booking reports on the number of patients pre-registered into all future sessions for the next 1–2 months, plus monthly, quarterly, and or annual productivity reports on all SMAs that currently exist (by facility, department, and provider).

The weekly or twice weekly pre-booking census reports would be looking at the number of patients pre-registered for each DIGMA and PSMA session during the next month or two, so that prompt corrective action could be taken if any upcoming sessions are found to be under-booked with respect to where they should be at that time. On the other hand, the periodic productivity reports (typically generated monthly, quarterly, and or annually) would be examining how many patients have actually been seen on average during DIGMA and PSMA sessions by each SMA provider—perhaps for each quarter since the inception of the program, so as to reveal any important trends regarding attendance. These reports could also be used to compare the average number of actual attendees to the minimum and target census levels for each SMA program. As previously discussed, these productivity reports could be arranged alphabetically by facilities, by departments within each facility, and by SMA providers within each department at each facility.

Have Billing and Compliance Monitor All Bills for Each SMA During the First 2 Months of Operations, and Periodically Thereafter

It is important to have the system's billing and compliance officer review all bills generated during the first 2 months

of each new DIGMA and PSMA that is launched, and then periodically spot-check bills for the SMA thereafter. The intent here is to ensure that all outgoing SMA bills are in compliance with all the various documentation and billing processes, policies, and regulations that are applicable to the SMA program. This would also include those policies that were originally established by the organization at the inception of the SMA program and perhaps updated thereafter (see Chapter 10 covering 20 essential steps to implementing a successful group visit program—especially step 4, which refers to establishing consensus around a comprehensive billing policy for the group visit program).

It is important to note that whenever outgoing bills are checked by billing and compliance (i.e., for both individual office visits and group visits), a certain percentage of bills will likely be found to not be in compliance—in which case appropriate remedial training might need to be provided to certain providers who are frequently submitting bills that are out of compliance. The entire issue of billing is especially important for the SMA program because there are currently are no billing codes available specific either to group visits in general or to each SMA model in particular (although, at least in the case of DIGMAs and PSMAs, many question the need for them as these SMA models are run like a series of individual office visits with observers)—and billing for group visits is still evolving and not completely settled.

Certainly, shared medical appointments represent a dramatically different modality for delivering medical care—and one that physicians, healthcare organizations, and insurers are still adapting to. However, the last thing one would want to see is any billing and compliance problems arise surrounding group visits—or any abuse regarding how group visits are conducted and billed—which could ultimately prove catastrophic at this early stage in their development. Shared medical appointments can offer so many remarkable benefits to patients, physicians, organizations, insurers, and purchasers alike that it would be nothing less than a terrible mistake to have any billing improprieties occur that would darken their image.

DIGMA and PSMA Programs Need to be Evaluated on an Ongoing Basis

Finally, there is a need to continuously monitor and evaluate all DIGMAs and PSMAs that are launched within the system on a periodic and ongoing basis.

Measure Patient Satisfaction After SMA Sessions

While there are many ways to measure patient satisfaction, the most common is through use of a patient satisfaction questionnaire issued to patients and completed anonymously either at the end of SMA sessions or by mailing it to their homes afterward. You can use either a standardized, normed patient satisfaction questionnaire that has been designed for traditional office visits (and is therefore less useful for group visits) or one that is un-normed but designed to be more specific to group visits—such as those provided in the DVD attached to this book. Obviously, both normed and un-normed patient satisfaction questionnaires each have their own respective advantages and disadvantages—and which one to use is often determined by whether one is more interested in a formal research design or in a more informal monitoring of day-to-day operations within the SMA Department. One can also assess patient satisfaction directly or indirectly through structured interviews with patients, focus groups, observing where patients schedule their next appointments, and through various types of questionnaires.

Evaluate the Pilot Study and Determine Whether or Not to Expand SMAs Organization-Wide

If you start with a pilot study, the organization will first need to evaluate all data regarding the SMA pilot as soon as it has been completed, and then make a determination as to whether or not to expand the program organization-wide to full-scale implementation. If the pilot has been carefully designed, adequately supported, well promoted, and properly run, there is every reason to believe that it will have been successful—especially if teams have been well trained and full groups have been consistently achieved. In larger systems, the champion will need to present the results of the pilot study to the organization's executive leadership, who must then decide whether or not to expand the SMA program throughout the organization. The champion and program coordinator will also need to draft a business plan (to be presented to the organization's leadership team) for expanding the SMA program, one that details the anticipated benefits and cost savings of the program along with the personnel, facilities, and budgetary supports that will be required.

If the Program Is to Be Expanded Organization-Wide, then Determine the Number of New SMAs to be Launched Per Year

If organizational leadership has made the decision to expand the SMA program system-wide, then the next decision that needs to be made is at what rate (and therefore how rapidly) the program is to grow—and at what facilities and with which physicians. In particular, organizational leadership needs to decide how many new DIGMAs and PSMAs it wants to have launched each year by the champion and program coordinator—along with a prioritized sequence regarding which facilities, which departments, and which providers they are to include. As a guideline to this decision-making process, keep in mind that a busy, experienced half-time champion (with the able assistance of a capable and experienced program coordinator) can launch up to 18 SMAs per year in larger systems having some degree of physician buy-in—which is what I was able to do during my 3 years as champion of the SMA program at the Palo Alto Medical Foundation (and am currently doing as SMA champion at Harvard Vanguard Medical Associates/Atrius Health, where I am Vice President of Shared Medical Appointments and Group-Based Disease Management—but prorated to three-quarter's time). On the other hand, an experienced and capable full-time champion could launch up to 36 DIGMAs and PSMAs annually under ideal conditions. Of course, if site champions are trained at the organization's larger facilities, and if their efforts are overseen by the overall SMA champion for the organization, than this rollout process of new SMAs could be correspondingly accelerated. However, few systems are able to manage such an aggressive schedule for launching DIGMAs and PSMAs.

Consistently Strive to Meet This Number of New SMAs Launched Per Year

Once the number of new DIGMAs and PSMAs to be launched annually throughout the system has been determined, the champion and program coordinator need to immediately go into high gear to consistently achieve this number of new group visits each and every year. This is especially true during the first year, which will likely be the most difficult as the departmental infrastructure and operational systems will not yet be firmly in place for systematically achieving this number of new launches annually—plus, physician and patient buy-in will likely be at their lowest at the beginning of the SMA program (i.e., due to a lack of familiarity with SMAs and the many benefits that they can provide).

Later, once the *pipeline* is fully developed and the champion and program coordinator gain experience in systematically and efficiently launching new DIGMAs and PSMAs throughout the system, achieving this targeted number of new SMAs per year should become progressively easier over time. It should also prove easier as more and more physicians *buy in* to the model (i.e., as a result of hearing positive reports from their colleagues already running SMAs in their practices), and as patients and staff become more aware and accepting of group visits. Keep in mind that the overall net number of SMAs that are operational within the organization will not just be based upon the number of new SMAs launched per year—i.e., as they will subsequently be reduced somewhat by such factors as physicians already running SMAs leaving the system and by some SMAs failing due to inadequate census. In addition, the rate at which SMAs will be able to be launched throughout the organization will also be largely determined by how successful the physicians and staffs of previously launched DIGMAs and PSMAs are able to run them properly and keep them filled. As SMA champion, I find myself always needing to keep one eye looking forward toward the upcoming DIGMAs and PSMAs needing to be launched, and the other eye looking backward to tend to the difficulties and problems arising from SMAs already launched. Obviously, the more time and energy the champion needs to dedicate to addressing problems emanating from SMAs already established, the less time and energy that is left to put into new SMAs—and therefore, the lower the rollout rate of new SMAs will likely be in the organization.

Once Developed, Simply Repeat the Entire "Pipeline" Process Over and Over with All Newly Recruited Providers

For every new DIGMA and PSMA that is launched (and therefore for every newly recruited provider in either primary care or the various medical and surgical subspecialties), the champion and program coordinator will go through essentially the exact same sequence of steps contained in the *pipeline* as they did for the pilot study. This is the great efficiency advantage of having a pipeline. Of course, as the pipeline is repeated over and over, it will continuously be modified and enhanced (through continuous process improvement)—and will thereby gradually evolve to be even better as experience is gained and evermore SMAs are launched.

Generate Weekly (or Twice-Weekly) Pre-registration Census Reports for All SMAs

This issue has been repeatedly addressed throughout this book; however, because this is such an important issue, it will be summarized here. For all SMAs that have been launched to date, be certain to monitor the census for upcoming sessions on an ongoing basis. Because DIGMAs and PSMAs are census-driven programs, and because full attendance is the single most critical key to achieving the SMA program's goals, the continuous monitoring of census is exceedingly important to the overall success of the program. My preferred way of doing this is through weekly or twice-weekly reports generated by the program coordinator (with the help of the champion) which include the minimum and target census levels that were pre-established for each DIGMA and PSMA that has been implemented—as these reports permit prompt corrective action to be taken if any upcoming sessions are found to be under-booked relative to where they should be at that point in time. These pre-booking census reports not only make it clear to all SMA providers (and their staffs) how well they are doing with regards to achieving full group sessions each week, but also make it clear to the champion and program coordinator which DIGMAs and PSMAs the dedicated scheduler(s) should concentrate their efforts upon each week.

As champion, I always found it very helpful to have the program coordinator generate a weekly or twice-weekly census report on all SMAs being held within the system—i.e., which showed the number of patients pre-registered for each of the various SMA providers' next four to eight sessions. This report was divided up by facility, by departments within each facility, and then alphabetically by physicians within each department who were running DIGMAs or PSMAs. Because this report automatically went out to all providers as well as to me, it alerted all of us as to any upcoming sessions that had low census. For DIGMAs, I always wanted to see this week's sessions completely full, next week's session 3/4ths full, the following session half full, and four sessions out approximately 1/4th full. With PSMAs, I wanted to see sessions completely full 2–3 weeks in advance so that Patient Packets for the session could be mailed out to all pre-registered patients in a timely manner. This way, patients are able to fill out and return the health history form (and complete the blood and urine screening tests) prior to the session. In addition, this provides sufficient time for the information on the returned health history form (as well as from the completed lab tests) to be entered into patients' SMA chart notes by nursing or support personnel on the provider's staff prior to the DIGMA or PSMA session

Activate a Plan for Promptly Filling Sessions when Census Is Low

At the very beginning of the SMA program, the champion and program coordinator need to develop a plan that can be promptly activated whenever upcoming DIGMA or PSMA sessions are found to be inadequately filled. The physician can be contacted, as well as the physician's office manager and key members of the support staff—such as the physician's nurse, the lead receptionist, and the primary scheduler of the physician's appointments. Ideally, all should immediately do everything possible to actively recruit additional patients until the unfilled upcoming sessions are filled to the desired level—including overbooking sessions by an extra patient or two in order to compensate for any no-shows and late-cancels, less any drop-ins in the case of DIGMAs. Secondarily, the program coordinator can also assign the dedicated scheduler the task of calling lists of patients previously provided and approved by the physician (or, with the physicians approval, of calling patients already scheduled for individual office visits 2–4 weeks and further out, and inviting them to attend this week's 90-minute DIGMA or PSMA instead) in order to backfill and *top-off* sessions to achieve targeted census levels.

Terminate Any SMAs That Consistently Fail to Meet Minimum Census Requirements

It is important for the champion and program coordinator to offer physicians every possible support in making their SMA a success. However, as mentioned in detail earlier in this chapter, it is imperative that the physician and support staff assume primary responsibility for personally inviting patients, scheduling them into future SMA appointments, and filling all upcoming SMA sessions. Although the dedicated scheduler can be of help by *topping-off* upcoming sessions that are close to being full, he/she cannot take primary responsibility for filling sessions that go largely unfilled because doing so is simply too inefficient and time consuming of a process. I say this

because, unlike the physician (who is able to efficiently invite patients to attend the SMA for their next visit and to do so with a high likelihood of success), the dedicated scheduler(s) must make *cold calls* to patients they do not know—and who do not know them.

The net result is inefficiency in this backfilling process (including a lot of telephone messages and back and forth phone calls), as the dedicated scheduler must spend considerable time on the phone in order to get even one patient to attend the SMA. Generally speaking, in inviting patients to attend the SMA, even a good and experienced dedicated scheduler will have only 10–20% of the success rate that the physician will likely have (plus higher no-show rates). Whereas the physician can personally invite patients with great success during regular office visits in just 30–60 seconds, the dedicated scheduler will likely have to make 5–15 *cold calls* (and spend a considerable amount of time on each) in order to get a single patient to attend the SMA.

If a particular DIGMA or PSMA continues to fail to meet targeted census level requirements despite the best efforts of the dedicated scheduler and program coordinator, then it needs to be put onto some form of probationary status for a period of time to see if it can be salvaged by the physician and support team. If the nonproductive SMA is of a mixed or homogeneous DIGMA or PSMA design, then—with the provider's approval—consider converting it into a heterogeneous design (because so many more patients then qualify to attend each session) to see if sessions could be filled that way. If the sessions are still lightly attended past the probationary period, even after everything reasonably possible has been done by the program coordinator and champion to correct this census problem, then the tough decision must be made to terminate the SMA because it is economically unviable.

My experience has been that inadequately filled SMAs should be terminated as soon as is reasonably possible with the support of administration and organizational leadership—a decision that needs to be based upon data regarding the meeting of targeted census requirements. This can be difficult because the affected physician and support staff often enjoy the SMA and want it to continue; however, they are unable (or unwilling) to fill sessions to the point where economic viability can be achieved. Unfortunately, much trying experience has shown that once this problem of consistently low census occurs, it does not simply go away—and it is likely to persist into the foreseeable future.

Generally speaking, experience has shown that if the SMA is going to fail, it is almost always due to insufficient group size—and this census problem typically reveals itself soon after the launch. As one might expect, such nonproductive SMAs create an inordinate and ongoing drain (plus an excessive workload demand) upon the champion, program coordinator, and dedicated scheduler. Experience has shown that the constant pressure of trying to fill sessions week after week for a nonproductive SMA takes as much of the champion, program coordinator, and dedicated scheduler's time and energy as overseeing 10 productive SMAs that generally meet their census requirements. This is why census considerations have been emphasized at length both in this chapter and throughout the book.

It is also worth mentioning here that whenever you read or hear about healthcare systems reporting that their DIGMA or PSMA program has not been cost effective, immediately check the data and see whether or not they followed this warning and maintained the recommended census levels on average during all DIGMA and PSMA sessions—which, in such cases, you will find that they almost certainly have not.

I have spent all types of time, energy, and resources on trying to *bail out* a couple of nonproductive SMAs, only to find that they still ultimately failed later on due to continued low census. Of course, this is not always the case, as there have been occasions where physicians and staffs were eventually able to fill their group sessions in the long run (i.e. even when they were unable to do so initially); however, experience has shown this to be a relatively rare occurrence. Therefore, my recommendation is to do everything possible to try to rectify this problem as soon as possible when it does occur but, if that does not work, to *cut your losses* and terminate the nonproductive SMA sooner rather than later. I say this because all that your hard work will likely accomplish is to postpone the inevitable—unless, of course, the physician and support staff should take this matter seriously and redouble their efforts in filling future SMA sessions.

Periodically Assess Physician Professional Satisfaction with the SMA Program

Since enhanced physician professional satisfaction is one of the primary goals for a DIGMA, CHCC, or PSMA program, it is important to periodically assess physician satisfaction with their SMA program. Although there are many methodologies for measuring provider satisfaction with their SMAs, the most popular approaches that most organizations seem to take is through periodic personal discussions or structured interviews—or else through isochronal issuance of a physician professional satisfaction questionnaire of their own design for all SMA providers to complete and return anonymously.

Regardless of the approach taken in assessing physician professional satisfaction with your SMA program, you will want to ask questions like the following of all providers currently running DIGMAs and PSMAs within the system:

- Has it met your expectations?
- Is it helping you to better manage your practice?
- Is it increasing your productivity as you had hoped?
- Has access to care improved in your practice as a result of the SMA?
- Do you find your SMA to be something new, different, and interesting?
- Do you look forward to your group each week?
- Do you leave the group feeling energized?
- Is it helpful for dealing with your chronically ill patients?
- Is it helpful in dealing with angry, demanding, time-consuming, and psychosocially needy patients?
- Does it help you to reach out to underserved patients?
- Does your SMA allow you to provide closer follow-up care?
- Has it reduced patient phone call volume, complaints about poor access, and double bookings (i.e., forced bookings or *work-ins*)?
- Are you able to finish on time with all charting completed?
- Are you able to provide more patient education and disease self-management skills through the SMA?
- Do you find that group visits provide a nice complement to your individual office visits?
- Does the SMA team provide you with real and meaningful help?
- Is your SMA helping to optimize your schedule?
- Are you able to provide a level of medical care that you are satisfied with?
- Are there some things about your SMA that you are dissatisfied with and, if so, what?
- Are you enjoying your group and having some fun?

The data resulting from such periodic assessments of physician professional satisfaction should be compiled and included in the intervallic reports generated by the program coordinator.

Produce Monthly, Quarterly, or Annual Productivity Reports for the Entire SMA Program

With the assistance of the champion, the program coordinator needs to produce ongoing productivity reports for the entire DIGMA and PSMA program on a regular basis—which I like to see done monthly, or at least quarterly—that are to be circulated to both executive leadership and all SMA providers to give ongoing feedback on the program. Try to make this productivity report on the SMA program as helpful and informative as possible—to the SMA providers, administration, organizational leadership, and the SMA program itself. Of course, you can also develop other types of periodic reports as well that might be helpful in evaluating the SMA program on an ongoing basis. The precise format of this report needs to be determined by the champion and program coordinator, with input from administration and executive leadership. For DIGMAs and PSMAs, this report needs to cover the recent (e.g., last month; last quarter) and long-term productivity (last year; since inception of the SMA; etc.) of each and every SMA in the system—broken down by facility, department within that facility, and physician within each department (typically in alphabetical order).

These reports can also include the number of patients who were scheduled to attend each session, the number who actually attended, the number of no-shows and late-cancels, and the number of drop-ins. These reports should also include each provider's pre-SMA productivity, their current average throughput of patients in their DIGMA/PSMA, and the percent increase in their productivity during the 90 minutes of group time as a result of the SMA (and can include their increased productivity for the entire week as well). These monthly, quarterly, and/or annual productivity reports can not only examine how many patients have actually been seen on average over time by each SMA provider during previous sessions, but also compare the average number of patients seen to the minimum and target census levels that were pre-established for each DIGMA or PSMA.

Operational decisions in today's medical environment must be data driven. Ongoing programs, such as group visit programs, must continuously demonstrate and prove their value to the organization. Therefore, appropriate outcome measures need to be developed—measures that reflect not only the primary goals (such as quality, access, productivity, cost savings, clinical outcomes, or satisfaction goals) of the various group visit models, but also the organization's goals for the SMA program. These goals will not be mutually exclusive for the different SMA models (indeed, they are often overlapping); however, all such measures must be relatively simple, obtainable, valid, reliable, and aligned with both the organization's priorities and the specific benefits that each SMA model was designed to achieve.

Interestingly, no matter whether the DIGMA, CHCC, or PSMA model is initially selected as the starting point for an organization's group visit program, most integrated healthcare delivery systems will eventually want to give thorough consideration to using all three of these SMA models—as well as any other models still to be developed. This is the strategy that will ultimately maximize the economic, quality, access, productivity, and satisfaction benefits of the SMA program for patients, physicians, and the organization alike.

Clearly, you will be looking at return on investment for initiating your SMA program—and this requires that appropriate measurements, analyses, and reports be done. This can take the form of improved quality of medical care, greater patient knowledge and self-efficacy, improved clinical outcomes, increased productivity and efficiencies, improved access and service, reduced utilization and costs, enhanced patient and physician satisfaction, etc.. Rather than whether or not to conduct such ongoing assessments of your SMA program, the question therefore becomes one of how to best measure the success of your SMA program. In addition to the average census and increased productivity (which you will undoubtedly want to monitor for a DIGMA and PSMA program), all types of other data and outcomes measures that might have been gathered regarding the SMA program can also be included in these monthly productivity reports—such as the following:

- Decreased wait lists and backlogs
- Improved access (e.g., wait until 3rd available appointments)
- Increased RVUs
- Cost savings (decreased office visits, ER visits, hospitalizations, nursing home care, referrals to specialists, etc.)
- Enhanced service and quality of care
- Improved compliance and adherence to treatment recommendations
- Improved clinical outcome measures
- Improved health maintenance
- Reduced patient phone call volume and complaints about poor access
- Improved patient–physician relationships
- Patient satisfaction
- Provider satisfaction

Appropriate outcome measures need to be developed that reflect not only the primary goals of the group visit model(s) being utilized, but also both the physician's and the organization's goals for the SMA program. Be sure to measure and evaluate that which is practical, realistically achievable, and of greatest importance to your organization. But whatever you do, be sure that you do not overlook this all-important, ongoing evaluative process. After first deciding what to measure and what the baseline is, then go on to measure any important changes resulting from the SMA program on an ongoing, periodic basis. I say this because ongoing measurements and analyses are key not only to determining the value of the SMA program to your organization, but also to continuous process improvement—i.e., toward always enhancing, improving, and making your group visit program better for patients, physicians, and the organization alike.

Conclusion

The pipeline discussed in this chapter should prove most helpful to all SMA champions, program coordinators, and providers—as well as to all healthcare organizations, large and small, in launching their own successful group visit program. This pipeline should also prove invaluable in helping the reader to avoid making many of the frustrating beginners' mistakes that can so easily occur because of both the magnitude of the paradigm shift involved and the counterintuitive nature of group visits. It took me many years to fully conceptualize, formulate, and optimize the DIGMA and PSMA models. After developing these models, it took more than a decade of actual experience *in the trenches* (i.e., with more than 20 thousand patient visits in DIGMAs and PSMAs) designing, adjusting, *tweaking*, fine-tuning, and actually implementing them with more than 400 providers within numerous medical groups both nationally and internationally.

Although my goal has always been to perfect and optimize these group visit models to better serve our patients, I feel that this entire effort still remains very much *a work in progress*—i.e., rather than a *finished product*. The *pipeline* discussed herein is the end product of more than a decade's experience in launching hundreds of DIGMAs and PSMAs in both primary care and the various medical and surgical subspecialties. It covers what you will need to know in order to have your own successful SMA program. I hope that you find it very helpful, and I wish you well in your new group visit endeavor. The practical knowledge contained herein should help you to not only better manage your practice (along with your geriatric, chronically ill, and psychosocially needy patients) while providing better care, but also have years of professional fun and enjoyment. I wish you well on your new professional adventure.

Now that You Have the Knowledge and Tools, JUST DO IT!

To my readers, I can only say in summary that—through this book—we have been able to take a

remarkable journey together. In the Preface, we looked at my personal, almost catastrophic, health experiences and how they provided the rationale, motivation, and foundation for the development of the DIGMA and PSMA models. To this day, these personal *mind/body* medical experiences—together with the knowledge of not only how they affected me, but how they impacted my family as well—continue to serve as the basis for why I remain so passionate about these shared medical appointment models. I fervently believe that, when done properly, these biopsychosocial SMA models not only provide better care to our patients, but can also go a long way toward solving many of the serious healthcare challenges and crises that face us today.

Having read this book, you now understand what you need to know in order to set up and run a successful group visit program for your practice and organization—and how to avoid the many pitfalls that could occur along the way. You now have a thorough working knowledge of today's three major group visit models, of their respective strengths and weaknesses, and of how they can best work not only together but also with traditional one-on-one office visits. You also know, better than anybody else, what the major problems and challenges are in your practice and organization—and consequently, which group visit model (or models) it would be best for you to start with. In the DVD attached to this book, you also have templates and examples of all the forms and promotional materials that you will need in this endeavor—plus edited versions of grand rounds presentations as well as behaviorist training and mock DIGMA training sessions that I have given.

The decision is now yours to make. Needless to say, my hope is that you will choose to start a successful group visit program for your practice—and then perfect and expand it over time, while taking full advantage of the multiple benefits that it can offer to you, your organization, and your patients. However, that choice is now up to you. My recommendation at this point is **JUST DO IT!** You have studied the entire topic of group visits in depth, and you now have all the tools at your disposal that you need in order to proceed with success. If you do choose to move forward with a group visit program in your practice (and if you apply the knowledge that you have gained through this book so that you design, support, and run your SMA program properly), then I believe that you could very well find yourself embarking upon one of the most exciting adventures of your professional lifetime—and one from which you will probably never look back to the *status quo* of the traditional way of delivering medical care.

Suggested Readings

Atkins TN, Noffsinger EB. Implementing a group medical appointment program: a case study at Sutter Medical Foundation. *Group Practice Journal* 2001;50(3):32–39.

Ayoub WT, Newman ED, Blosky MA, Stewart WF, Wood GC. Improving detection and treatment of osteoporosis: redesigning care using the electronic medical record and shared medical appointments. *Osteoporosis International* 2009;20(1): 37–42.

Barud S, Todd, M, Armor, B, et al. Development and Implementation of Group Medical Visits at a Family Medicine Center. *American Journal of Health-System Pharmacy* 2006;63(15):1448–1452.

Beck A, Scott J, Williams P, et al. A Randomized Trial of Group Outpatient Visits for Chronically Ill Older HMO Members: The Cooperative Health Care Clinic. *Journal of the American Geriatric Society* 1997;45(5):543–549.

Beckley, ET. Research Favors Group Diabetes Intervention. Shared appointments improve access and efficiency. *DOC News* 2004;1(1):7.

Belfiglio, G. Crowd control. Group office visits provide efficiencies, patient support. *Modern Physician* 2001;5(9):34–36.

Bell, H. Group appointments – just what the doctor ordered. *Minnesota Medicine* 2002;85: http://policy.mmaonline.net:8080/publications/MNMed2002/June/Bell2.html

Bower, A. The semiprivate checkup: tired of waiting two hours to see the doctor for 10 minutes? Try making your appointments en masse. *Time Magazine* 2003;162(19):71.

Bronson DL, Maxwell, RA. Shared medical appointments: increasing patient access without increasing physician hours. *Cleveland Clinic Journal of Medicine* 2004;71(5):33–37.

Brunk, D. Group appointments may enhance physician-patient relationships. *Family Practice News* 2000;30(6):79.

Brunk, D. Group medical appointments aid communication. *Internal Medicine News* 2000;33(5):50.

Carlson, B. Getting patients in the door faster can boost satisfaction, outcomes. *Managed Care* 2002;11(3):52, 54.

Carlson, B. Shared appointments improve efficiency in the clinic. *Managed Care* 2003;12(5):46–48.

Christianson JB, Warrick, LH. The business case for Drop-In Group Medical Appointments: a case atudy of Luther Midelfort Mayo System. Field Report. *Institute for Healthcare Improvement* Apr 2003;(611). www.cmwf.org

Clancy DE, Cope DW, Magruder KM, Huang P, Salter KH, Fields AW. Evaluating patients in an uninsured or inadequately insured patient population with uncontrolled type 2 diabetes. *The Diabetes Educator* 2003;29(2):292–302.

Clancy DE, Cope DW, Magruder KM, Huang P, Wolfman TE. Evaluating concordance to American Diabetes Association Standards of care for type 2 diabetes through group visits in an uninsured or inadequately insured patient population. *Diabetes Care* 2003;26:2032–2036.

Clancy DE, Dismuke CE, Magruder KM, Simpson KN, Bradford, D. Do diabetes group visits lead to lower medical care charges? *American Journal of Managed Care* 2008;14:39–44.

Clancy DE, Huang P, Okonofua E, Yeager D, Magruder KM. Group visits: promoting adherence to diabetes guidelines. *Journal of General Internal Medicine* 2007;22(5):620–624.

Coleman EA, Eilertsen TB, Kramer AM, Majid DJ, Beck A, Conner D. Reducing emergency visits in older adults with chronic illness – a randomized, controlled trial of group visits. *Effective Clinical Practice* 2001;4(2):49–57.

Cunningham C, Blazer J. Group visits can save you time, but are they right for you. *ACP Observer* Apr 2004. www.acponline.org/journals/news/apr04.htm

Cynkar A. Group doctoring. For psychologists, opportunities may abound as shared medical appointments gain ground. *Monitor on Psychology* 2007;38(8):28–29.

Davis KS, Magruder KM, Lin Y, Powell CK, Clancy, DE. BRIEF REPORT: trainee provider perceptions of group visits. *Journal of General Internal Medicine* 2006;21(4):357–359.

Davis RJ. More physicians hold group checkups. *The Wall Street Journal* Oct 4, 2002:D4.

Dembner A. Patients, doctors turn to care in groups. *The Boston Globe* 2004;265(174):A1, A9.

Domrzalski D. New exam lets you see your doctor faster (with 14 other people). *New Mexico Business Weekly* Mar 29, 2002. www.bizjournals.com/albuquerque/stories/2002/04/01/story6.html?page=3

Donato S. Docs dig the DIGMA (Drop-In Group Medical Appointment). *Physicians Practice Digest* 2001;11(3):A1–A2, A8.

Dornin R. Doctors find quality time with patients in groups. *CNN.com*. Oct 6, 2000.

Doup L. Time share. A growing trend of shared appointments offer patients more time with the doctor and a chance to discuss their ailment in a group setting. *South Florida Sun-Sentinel* Feb 29, 2004:1D–2D

Dreffer, D. Group visits hit the road. *Family Practice Management* 2004;11(8):39–42.

Fairclough J. (Ed). Eight great reasons to try group medical appointments. *Private Practice Success* Aug 2005:1, 4–5.

Fairclough J. (Ed). More crowd-pleasing reasons to offer group visits. *Private Practice Success* Sep 2005:6–7.

Fletcher SG, Clark SJ, Overstreet DL, Steers WD. An improved approach to follow up care for the urological patient: drop-in group medical appointments. *The Journal of Urology* 2006;176(3):1122–1126.

Goff L. The doctor is ready to see all 15 of you now. *Good House-keeping* Jul 2001:187.

Gordon A. Drop-in visits help to improve service. *The Quality Indicator Physician Resource* Dec 2001:1,14–15.

Gordon A. Drop-in visits improve efficiency. *The Quality Indicator Physician Resource* Oct 2001:3–5.

Green L. Shared appointments allow patients to learn from each other's experiences. *San Jose Mercury News* May 6, 2001;1B, 4B.

Gutman J. (Ed). Group visits can lift revenues, efficiency, quality for docs with many kinds of patients. *Physician Compensation Report* 2004;5(10):1–4.

Harris G. (Ed). Bringing patients together can help them and you. *Physician's Managed Care Report* 1999;7(11):165–166, 171–172.

Harris PL. Group sessions are in at the Palo Alto Medical Foundation. *San Jose and Silicon Valley Business Journal* May 5, 2000:8.

Heimoff S. Waiting room crowded? Put a few people in the examining room at once. *Managed Care* 2000;9(6):34–7.

Houck S, Kilo C, Scott J. Improving patient care: group visits 101. *Family Practice Management* 2003;10(5):66–8.

Hines SE. Group medical visits: a glimpse into the future: *Patient Care* 2003;37:18–40.

Jaber R. Group visits offer practical, effective care. *DOC News* 2007;4(2):3.

Jaber R, Braksmajer A, Trilling JS. Group visits: a qualitative review of current research. *Journal of the American Board of Family Medicine* 2006;19(3):276–290.

Kaidar-Person O, Swartz EW, Lefkowitz M, Conigliaro K, Fritz N, Birne J, Alexander C, Szomstein S, Rosenthal R. Shared medical appointments: new concept for high-volume follow-up for bariatric patients. *Surgery for Obesity and Related Dis*ease 2006; 2(5):509–12.

Kirsh S, Watts S, Pascuzzi K, O'Day ME, Davidson D, Strauss G, Kern EO, Aron DC. Shared medical appointments based on the chronic care model: a quality improvement project to address the challenges of patients with diabetes with high cardiovascular risk. *Quality and Safety in Health Care* 2007;16(5):349–53.

Kowalczyki L. The doctor will see all of you now. Amid physician shortage, shared visits get a tryout. *Boston Sunday Globe* Nov 30, 2008;274(153):A1, A6.

Kuiken S, Seiffert D. Thinking outside the box!! Enhance patient education by using shared medical appointments. *Plastic Surgical Nursing* 2005;25(4):191–195.

Lerner M. You, your doctor and a room full of strangers. *Minneapolis Star Tribune* Nov 26, 2000:A1, A18.

Lessig M, Farrell J, Madhavan E, Famy C, Vath B, Holder T, Borsan S. Cooperative dementia care clinics: a new model for managing cognitively impaired patients. *Journal of the American Geriatric Society* 2006;54(12):1937–1942.

Lippman H. Making group visits work. *Hippocrates* 2000;14(7):33–36.

Martinez B. Now it's mass medicine. *Wall Street Journal* Aug 21, 2000:B1, B4.

Masley S, Sokoloff J, Hawes C. Planning group visits for high-risk patients. *Family Practice Management* 2000;7(6):33–37.

McLeod L. (Ed). Launch your group model the right way. *Private Practice Success* Aug 2004:8.

McLeod L. (Ed). Multitask in the exam room: three shared appointment models help physicians see more patients. *Private Practice Success* Jul 2004:6–8.

Meehan KR, Hill JM, Root L, Kimtis E, Patchett L, Noffsinger EB. Group medical appointments: organization and implementation in the bone marrow transplantation clinic. *Supportive Cancer Therapy* 2006;3(2):84–90.

Miller D, Zantop V, Hammer H, Faust S, Grumbach K. Group medical visits for low-income women with chronic disease: a feasibility study. *Journal of Women's Health* 2004;13(2):217–225.

Morelli J. Ladies and gentlemen, the doctor will see you now – Group Appointments May be the Latest Fad. *Web MD*. Atlanta. Aug 2000 http://atlanta.webmd.com/content/article/1728.59931.

Nelson R. Club medical – the new way to get more quality time with your doc: join a group. *Modern Maturity* 2002;45w(6):17–18.

Noffsinger EB. Answering physician concerns about drop-in group medical appointments. *Group Practice Journal* 1999;48(2):14–21.

Noffsinger EB. Benefits of drop-in group medical appointments (DIGMAs) to physicians and patients. *Group Practice Journal* 1999;48(3):21–28.

Noffsinger EB. Drop-In Group Medical Appointments (DIGMAs): history & development. *Counseling for Health – A Newsletter for the Division 17 Section in Counseling Health Psychology*. Spring 1999;(23):3–6.

Noffsinger EB. Enhance satisfaction with drop-in group visits. *Hippocrates* 2001;15(2):30–36.

Noffsinger EB. Establishing successful primary care and subspecialty Drop-in Group Medical Appointments (DIGMAs) in your group practice. *Group Practice Journal* 1999;48(4):20–28.

Noffsinger EB. Group visits for efficient, high-quality chronic disease management. *Group Practice Journal* 2008;57(2):23–40.

Noffsinger EB. Increasing quality of care and access while reducing costs through Drop-In Group Medical Appointments (DIGMAs). *Group Practice Journal* 1999;48(1):12–18.

Noffsinger EB. Operational challenges to implementing a successful Physicals Shared Medical Appointment Program. Part 1: choosing the right type of shared medical appointment. *Group Practice Journal* 2002;51(2):24–34.

Noffsinger EB. Operational challenges to implementing a successful Physicals Shared Medical Appointment Program. Part 2: maximizing efficiency. *Group Practice Journal* 2002;51(3):32–40.

Noffsinger EB. Operational considerations for a Successful Physicals Shared Medical Appointment Program. Part 3: hints and guidelines. *Group Practice Journal* 2002;51(4):22–26.

Noffsinger EB. Physicals Shared Medical Appointments: a revolutionary access solution. *Group Practice Journal* 2002;51(1):16–26.

Noffsinger EB. Solving departmental access problems with DIGMAs. *Group Practice Journal* 2001;50(10):26–36.

Noffsinger EB. Use of group visits in the treatment of the chronically ill. In: Nuovo, J, editor. *Chronic Disease Management*. New York: Springer, 2007. pp. 32–86.

Noffsinger EB. Will Drop-In Group Medical Appointments (DIGMAs) work in practice? *Permanente Journal* 1999;3(3):58–67.

Noffsinger EB. Working smarter: group visits are proving to be a valuable antidote to harried physicians, would a 200 percent increase in productivity make you feel better? *Physicians Practice* 2002;12(3):18–22.

Noffsinger EB, Atkins TN. A business plan for implementing a group medical appointment program: Lessons from a case study at Sutter Medical Foundation. *Group Practice Journal* 2001;50(5):31–38.

Noffsinger EB, Atkins TN. Assessing a Group Medical Appointment Program: a case study at Sutter Medical Foundation. *Group Practice Journal* 2001;50(4):42–50.

Noffsinger EB, Mason JE Jr., Culberson CG, Abel T, Dowdell LA, Peters W, Bhandari R, Donovan M. Physicians evaluate the impact of Drop-in Group Medical Appointments (DIGMAs) on their practices. *Group Practice Journal* 1999;48(8):22–33.

Noffsinger EB, Scott JC. Practical tips for establishing successful group visit programs. Part 1: leadership skills and guidelines. *Group Practice Journal* 2000;49(6):31–37.

Noffsinger EB, Scott JC. Practical tips for establishing successful group visit programs. Part 2: maintaining desired group census. *Group Practice Journal* 2000;49(7):24–27.

Noffsinger EB, Scott, JC. Preventing potential abuses of group visits. *Group Practice Journal* 2000;49(5):37–46.

Noffsinger EB, Scott JC. Understanding today's group visit models. *Group Practice Journal* 2000;49(2):46–58.

Noffsinger EB, Scott JC. Understanding today's group visit models. *The Permanente Journal* 2000;4(2):99–112.

Norbut M. Group appointments have their benefits. *American Medical News* 2003;46(4):14, 18.

Oehlke KJ, Whitehill DM. Shared medical appointments in a pharmacy-based erectile dysfunction clinic. *American Journal of Health-System Pharmacy* 2006;63(12):1165–1166.

Page L. Group visit format raises efficiency & eyebrows. *Internal Medicine News* Oct 15, 2001:39.

Pennachio DL. Should you offer group visits? *Medical Economics* Aug 8, 2003;80(15):70–85.

Schall M, Duffy T, Krishnamurthy A, Levesque O, Mehta P, Murray M, Parlier R, Petzel R, Sanderson J. Improving patient access to the Veterans Health Administration's Primary Care & Specialty Care Clinics. *Joint Commission Journal on Quality and Safety* Aug 2004;30(8):415–423.

Scott J, Gade G, McKenzie M, Venohr I. Cooperative health care clinics: a group approach to individual care. *Geriatrics* 1998;53(5)68–81.

Scott JC, Conner DA, Venohr I, Gade G, McKenzie M, Kramer AM, Bryant L, Beck A. Effectiveness of a group out-patient visit model for chronically ill older health maintenance organization members: a 2-year randomized trial of the cooperative health care clinic. *Journal of the American Geriatric Society* 2004;52(9):1463–1470.

Scott JC, Robertson BJ. Kaiser Colorado's Cooperative Health Care Clinic: a group approach to patient care. *Managed Care Quarterly* 1996;4(3)41–45.

Severns LJ. The doctor is in for group visits. *San Jose Mercury News* 2000 10:5D, 7D.

Shared medical appointments save money for capitated groups. *Capitation Management Report* 2003;10(2):20–4, 17.

Shared medical appointments: will they work for your practice and your patients? *Practice for Patients* 2007;1(2):1–8.

Shute N. That old-time medicine: innovative doctors are rethinking the office visit to put the care back in healthcare. *U.S. News & World Report* 2002;132(13):54–61.

Simon V. (Ed). Group visits can lift revenues, efficiency, quality for docs with many kinds of patients. *Physician Compensation Report* 2004;5(10):1–4.

Slomski AJ. What a behavioral specialist could add to your practice. *Medical Economics* 2000;77(11):149–171.

Stevens S. (Ed). Group visits offer doctors more time for patient care. *Physicians Financial News* 2001;X1X(1):1,18.

Stokes M. Group medical visits offer physicians and their patients greater satisfaction. *Plastic Surgery News* 2007;18(8):1, 36–37.

Sussman D. Group dynamics - new program streamlines care and accommodates more patients in less time. *Nurse Week* 2000;13(23):12,35.

Thacker HL, Maxwell R, Saporito J, Bronson D. Shared medical appointments: facilitating interdisciplinary care for midlife women. *Journal of Women's Health* 2005;14(9):867–870.

Thompson E. The power of group visits. Improved quality of care, increased productivity entice physicians to see up to 15 patients at a time. *Modern Healthcare* 2000;30(23):54,56,62.

Toth CL. You'd better shop around. Pick the right codes for non-traditional patient encounters. *Physicians Practice Digest* 2001;11(6):59–61.

Toto C. Social medicine – group appointments mean more attention. *Washington Times* 2003 Mar 18:B1, B4.

Vesely R. Alternate avenues to access. To ease the path to doc visits, practices are experimenting with care via the internet and group exams. *Modern Healthcare* Mar 16, 2009:32–33.

Victorian B. Group medical visits seek to relieve physician burden, improve care. *Nephrology Times* 2009;2(1):1, 12–15.

Walker T. Medical visits get group mentality approach – group appointments can increase efficiency and patient and physician satisfaction. *Managed Healthcare* Oct 2000:10,13–15.

Walpert B. Patients tired of waiting? Try these strategies. *ACP-ASIM Observer* Oct 1999. http://www.acpinternist.org/archives/1999/10/waiting.htm.

Wax H. The doctor is in. Shared medical appointments help patients, physicians slow down. *Palo Alto Weekly* 2000 Jun 14:42.

Weinger K. Group medical appointments in diabetes care: is there a future? *Diabetes Spectrum* 2003;16(2):104–107.

Wellington M. Stanford health partners: rationale and early experiences in establishing physician group visits and chronic disease self-management workshops. *Journal of Ambulatory Care Management* 2001;24(3):10.

Wheelock C, Savageau JA, Silk H, Lee S. Improving the health of diabetic patients through resident-initiated group visits. *Family Medicine* 2009 Feb;41(2):116–9.

Wolfson BJ. Group visits just what the doctor ordered. *Orange County Register* Apr 14, 2002;414:1, 20–21.

Wysocki B Jr. Doctor prescribes quality control for medicine's ills. *Wall Street Journal* 2002; CCXXX1X:A1, A5.

Yehle KS, Sands LP, Rhynders PA, Newton GD. The effect of shared medical visits on knowledge and self-care in patients with heart failure: a pilot study. *Heart Lung* 2009 Jan–Feb;38(1):25–33.

Zicconi J. The practice revolution. *Unique Opportunities* 2000;10(3):30.

Index

Printed in the United States of America

Springer